emergency care
third edition

TO THE STUDENT

A self-instructional workbook for this text is available through your college bookstore under the title *Self-Instructional Workbook for EMERGENCY CARE, 3rd Edition,* by J. David Bergeron (title code D-1860-8). *Review Questions for the EMT* (title code D-2557-9), a comprehensive question and answer workbook correlated to this text (with sample examination), is also available. If not in stock, ask the bookstore manager to order a copy for you. If your course is being offered off-campus, ask your instructor where to obtain a copy. The Workbook and Review Questions can help you with course material by acting as a tutorial review and study aid.

Executive Editor: Jim Yvorra
Production Editor/Text Designer: Paula Aldrich
Medical Art Director/Designer: Don Sellers, AMI
Art Assistants: Joe Vitek, Robbie Blair, Leslie McMahon, LaWan Singo
Photography Producer: Pat Hansen
Photographers: George Dodson, Rick Brady

Typeface: Palatino (text), Helvetica (display)
Typesetting: CCC—Tele-Comp, Cockeysville, MD
Lithography: Jim Embrey Lithographics, Inc., Beltsville, MD
Printing: Columbia Planograph, Beltsville, MD

emergency
care
third edition

**Harvey D. Grant
Robert H. Murray, Jr.
J. David Bergeron**

Robert J. Brady Co., Bowie, Maryland 20715
A Prentice-Hall Publishing and Communications Company

NOTICE

It is the intent of the authors and publisher that this textbook be used as part of a formal Emergency Medical Technician course taught by a qualified instructor. The care procedures presented here represent accepted practices in the United States. They are not offered as a standard of care. EMT-level emergency care is to be performed under the authority and guidance of a licensed physician. It is the reader's responsibility to know and follow local care protocols as provided by the medical advisors directing the system to which he belongs. Also, it is the reader's responsibility to stay informed of emergency care procedure changes.

Emergency Care, 3rd edition.

Copyright© 1982 by Robert J. Brady Co.
All rights reserved. No part of this publication may be reproduced or transmitted in any form or by any means, electronic or mechanical, including photocopying and recording, or by any information storage and retrieval system, without permission in writing from the publisher. For information, address the Robert J. Brady Co., Bowie, Maryland 20715.

Library of Congress Cataloging in Publication Data

Grant, Harvey, 1934-
    Emergency care.
    Bibliography: p.
    Includes index.
    1. Emergency medicine. 2. First aid in illness and injury. 3. Rescue work. 4. Emergency medical personnel. I. Murray, Robert, 1934- . II. Bergeron, J. David, 1944-
      III. Title. [DNLM: 1: Emergencies. 2. Emergency medical services. 3. First aid. WX 215 G762e]
RC86.7.G7 1982   616'.025   82-4529
                                       AACR2

ISBN 0-89303-116-X

Prentice-Hall International, Inc., London
Prentice-Hall Canada, Inc., Scarborough, Ontario
Prentice-Hall of Australia, Pty., Ltd., Sydney
Prentice-Hall of India Private Limited, New Delhi
Prentice-Hall of Japan, Inc., Tokyo
Prentice-Hall of Southeast Asia Pte. Ltd., Singapore
Whitehall Books, Limited, Petone, New Zealand

Printed in the United States of America

    84 85 86 87 88 89 90 91 92 10 9 8 7 6 5

contents

18. MOVING AND TRANSFERRING PATIENTS

19. TRANSPORT AND TERMINATION OF ACTIVITIES

20. COMMUNICATIONS AND REPORTS

SCANSHEETS

foreword

The Emergency Medical Technician, as a class, continues to be the fastest growing body of allied health professionals in the nation.

This statement stands in stark contrast to the grim evaluation of the nation's emergency medical services only 16 years ago as provided by the National Academy of Sciences in their historic document, "Accidental Death and Disability: The Neglected Disease of Modern Society."

In the early sixties, the American Academy of Orthopedic Surgeons addressed this crisis by offering training programs for emergency care providers across the country. These efforts were followed by the development of the Highway Safety Act of 1966, which charged the Department of Transportation with establishing the Emergency Medical Standard. The Standard provided the impetus to assist state and local communities in the upgrading of prehospital emergency medical services through the development and publication of a national training program. For the first time, the EMT was recognized as a professional who was a true extension of the hospital emergency department.

Today, all states, including Washington D.C., Puerto Rico, the Virgin Islands, and Guam provide state-level EMS program management, including EMT courses meeting national standards. Recently, the development of First Responder training on a national scale has added yet another link to the EMS delivery chain.

The future of the EMT as a public service provider is bright. Increasing numbers of EMTs are receiving certification as EMT ambulance/advanced (EMT-AA) or EMT-Paramedics. It is anticipated that most of the ambulance services in the nation will be providing advanced life support over the next five years. Other areas of growth for the EMT, EMT-AA and EMT-P include industry, coal mining, hospital emergency departments and coronary care units along with the large international energy industries.

Although a great deal of progress has been made in a relatively short time, the job is not complete. EMT, EMT-AA and EMT-P training programs are not readily available to many EMS providers. In addition, the reduction of EMS funds on a national, State and local level have further challenged the EMT to work to correct these deficiencies and to maintain the hard fought fight for professional status.

The Third Edition of *Emergency Care* by Harvey D. Grant, Robert H. Murray, and J. David Bergeron represents a major re-evaluation of both the role of the EMT and the current medical "state of the art." The authors have addressed all aspects of EMT training as defined by the U.S. Department of Transportation. This text will challenge the EMS provider to promote growth and change in his Emergency Medical Services System.

Cecil Arnold
Highway Safety Management Specialist
Emergency Medical Services Branch
National Highway Traffic Safety Administration
Washington, D.C.

preface

You are about to begin your training to become an emergency medical technician (EMT). EMT courses range from 81 to 130 hours in length, with the typical EMT course being 100 hours long. Regardless of the hours you spend in class, your course is most likely based on guidelines set by the Department of Transportation (DOT). This is not to say that there is one universal EMT course. Using the DOT guidelines as a foundation, physicians and instructors in your local Emergency Medical Services System have designed your course to meet specific needs of your community. The basic training is the same, but there are differences in each state as to what materials are presented.

This textbook takes into account some of the variations in emergency care procedures used in different states. That is why you will find alternative methods cited throughout the text. There are some procedures that vary so much that only the most common methods in use are discussed. For such cases, you will be directed to follow local protocols.

Why is there no one method of providing care for certain illnesses and injuries? First of all, there are cases where more than one procedure works. Your EMS System may have tested only one procedure and decided that it was efficient, easy to learn, and simple to use. A different EMS System may have tested a second method and had the same results. This means that you will be trained to use the methods in which your local EMS System has confidence based upon its own rigorous testing.

Methods change as studies are performed to find ways of improving care. Your EMS System may be conducting research on injuries to the extremities, while another EMS System is concentrating on injuries to the soft tissues of the face. As you can see, your course might contain more new information on the emergency care for a patient with a fractured limb, while a course in another EMS System could contain more on injuries to the eye. With time, each system will present its findings nationally and have its methods evaluated. Since this is an ongoing process, it is doubtful that any two EMS Systems will have the same training program.

One thing is certain; not all the methods you learn in your training will stay the same during your career as an EMT. You must keep up to date with local procedures. Your instructor will tell you how continuing education programs for EMTs are presented in your locality.

Who is the authority for your course? Your instructor. As new information is gained and new procedures are developed, your instructor is kept informed. Even new textbooks may not be 100% up to date; and, as we have explained, no textbook can cover the specific protocols for all 50 states. Should you have any questions about sources saying different things, ask your instructor. If this text takes one approach to an emergency and your instructor takes a different one, follow your instructor. We ask you to do this, not to please your instructor, but because a textbook cannot be easily changed to reflect up-to-the-minute information on all emergency care procedures.

Objectives and Skills

At the start of each chapter or section, you will find a list of objectives. These objectives tell you specifically what you should be able to do by the end of the chapter. The objectives used in this text are called behavioral or performance objectives. They state the things you should be able to do that can be measured by you and others to determine if you are learning the materials.

Each chapter or section also has a list of skills to inform you of what procedures you must be able to do as an EMT. In addition to these lists, there is a complete list of EMT skills in the appendix. Before you can become an EMT, you will have to pass a practical examination. Keep a close check on your ability to perform a given procedure as it is covered in you course. If you find you cannot do one of the skills listed for a chapter, see your instructor for additional help.

Terms

To become an EMT, you will have to be able to read and understand many medical terms. As an EMT, you will have to use these terms when communicating with other professionals in the EMS System. Each chapter has its own list of new terms. In addition, there is a section in the appendix to help you learn medical terminology. A full glossary of terms is provided at the end of the text.

When a medical term is used for the first time, a

pronunciation guide will be given. For example, the medical term for chest is ''thoracic.'' The first time this term is used, you will see the following:

thoracic (tho-RAS-ik)

The capital letters indicate the portion of the word that is to be emphasized. Since you will have to use medical terminology when speaking with other emergency care professionals, you should practice saying these words, and using them in conversations with your fellow students and your instructor.

Scansheets

There are many facts and procedures that are easier to learn if you can see them presented in one place, in a manner that allows for quick study. This is why we have developed scansheets for this textbook. A scansheet is a one- or two-page method of covering a complete procedure of care, or reviewing essential information related to assessment and care. Many of the emergency care procedures covered in this text are presented as scansheets. By looking at the illustrations and reading the text on a scansheet, you will be able to study most, if not all of what you will need to know about the procedure being presented. Since all the information for a topic is shown on one or two pages, you will also be able to use a scansheet to help you with the practical training portions of your course.

Using This Textbook

As you read and study each chapter, you should:

1. Read the list of objectives found at the beginning of the chapter.

2. Be certain you understand all the objectives before reading the chapter.

3. Read through the list of terms to familiarize yourself with the new terminology to be used in the chapter.

4. Read the chapter, keeping the list of objectives in mind. Pay close attention to the illustrations, charts, and lists.

5. Spend extra time on each scansheet. The information covered on a scansheet is very important.

6. Read through the summary at the end of the chapter.

7. After reading the chapter, go back over the list of objectives and see if you can accomplish each one. Use the list of objectives as a self-test.

8. Go back over the sections of the chapter that deal with the objectives you could not meet.

9. Read the list of skills and make certain that you can find all the procedures listed in the chapter or

presented on scansheets that will allow you to practice during the laboratory portions of your course. Know what is required to carry out a procedure before you attend the lab.

How To Study

The responsibility for teaching is the teacher's and the responsibility for learning is that of the student. Since it is your responsibility to learn what your instructor teaches, you will have to study the materials presented in this text and in class. There is too much material presented in a short period of time to allow you to remember all that you hear, see, and read without well-organized periods of study.

Every person is unique. How a person studies is a very personal thing; different methods work for each individual. There are, however, some standard recommendations that you may find helpful:

• Always follow the directions given by your instructor and the objectives in this text. Otherwise, you may spend too much time on minor points and not enough on what is critical for the EMT to know.

• Take notes during your training. You should have lecture, reading, and practical laboratory notes.

• Have your own place to study, removed from other activities.

• Study by yourself until you are able to meet all the chapter objectives.

• After you have studied on your own, talk with fellow students and your instructor about what you have learned. These conversations will help you to retain what you have learned and will give you practice using medical terminology.

• When you do not understand something, ask your instructor. Other students in the course may not understand any more than you do. They also lack the experience your instructor will have.

Improving Future Training

Not all the ideas for better methods of training come from physicians, committees, and instructors. Some of the best ideas come from students who can tell us what areas of study caused them the most trouble. Other good ideas come from practicing EMTs who let us know what problems they face in the field.

Any student, practicing EMT, or instructor who has an idea on how to improve EMT training, this textbook, or the emergency care provided to patients should write to the author in care of the Robert J. Brady Co., Bowie, MD 20715.

acknowledgments

FIRST AND SECOND EDITIONS

Before we thank all those who worked on the Third Edition of the "yellow book," it would be fitting to once again express our appreciation to those individuals who helped with the First and Second Editions of *Emergency Care*.

A number of people gave us some thoughts as to what they would like to see in a textbook for EMTs. Robert E. Motley, EMS Advisor at the U.S. Department of Transportation, was one such person. Bob's death leaves a void in the development of emergency medical services. We will miss his advice and support.

Many ideas were given to us by Carole Founds, RN, and Ben Corbalis, MD, both of the Wilmington Medical Center, Wilmington, Delaware. William Duncan, MD, of the St. Francis Hospital in Wilmington, served as an advisor and the principal reviewer for the First Edition. Our major consultant for the First Edition was J.D. Farrington, MD, who was serving as the Chairman, Subcommittee on Emergency Services—Pre-hospital, Committee on Trauma, American College of Surgeons and a member of the Committee on Emergency Medical Services, National Research Council, National Academy of Sciences. Henry C. Huntley, MD, who was Director, Division of Emergency Health Services, Robert Stewart, then Chief of the Training Branch, and other members of their staff at the U.S. Public Health Service read and commented on the manuscript.

At the Brady Company, the Brady family provided us with confidence and support to transform the original manuscript into the First Edition. Donald E. Sellers, PA, was the Art Director who began the tradition of fine illustrations and design for Emergency Care.

Four dedicated reviewers helped with the Second Edition. They were: Charles Phillips, MD, Marilyn Gifford, MD, Don Sleeper, First Aid Instructor Trainer, and Frank Poliafico, RN. Lt. Dan Irvine of the Glen Echo Fire Department, Maryland, was our technical advisor for photography.

Others who helped with the project included: Gladys Boluda, Bernard Vervin, Fred Palmai, and Worta Stevens; Captain Don Hinrichs; Bob Hague; Carolyn Bennett, RN; Ellen Hinrichs, RN; Florence Gilkey, RN and Donna Chitwood; Joel Saltzmann; Gail Walraven, RN; Lt. Larry Shamer; Charles Nabb; Doug Williams and Captain Stu Newman; Edgar "Puddinhead" Miles; and Rocco Morando.

At the Brady Company, we again had the patience, support, and understanding of the Brady family. Others at the Brady Company deserving of our praise included: Al Belskie, Richard Weimer, Brenda Teague, Marlise Reidenbach, Peggy Smith, Herb Ballinger, Bernard Vervin, Laura Lemmens, Ann Szymkowicz, Barbara Cosgrove, Elaine Stonebreaker, and Wayne Lewis.

Again, a special thanks must go to Donald E. Sellers, PA, AMI, NREMT-A. Don was the medical Art Director and designer for the project, assisted with photography, and provided many comments based upon his paramedic background.

The photography for the project was handled by Rick Brady, Director, and by staff photographer, George Dodson.

We also thank the members of the Glen Echo (Maryland) Fire Department, Maryland Fire and Rescue Institute, Glenn Dale (Maryland) Fire Department, Bowie (Maryland) Fire Department, Orlando (Florida) Fire Department, Killarney (Florida) Fire Department, and Altamont Springs (Florida) Fire Department for helping with equipment needs and assisting with special photography.

We owe much to all these people for the success of the first two editions of Emergency Care.

THIRD EDITION

The Brady Company Executive Producer for the Third Edition was Jim Yvorra. Jim is an EMT, a former Senior Instructor of the Maryland Fire and Rescue Institute, and Assistant Chief at the Berwyn Heights Volunteer Fire Department, Prince Georges County, Maryland. Jim's backgrounds in publishing and emergency services came together to provide us with resource personnel, reviewers, and advisors. He also was a source of advice and provided content review for each chapter. His daily concern, interest, and resourcefulness proved to be the difference in the development of the project.

At the company, Jim found support and assistance from Harry Gaines, President of Brady, and David Culverwell, Vice President and Editor-in-Chief.

The Editor and Text Designer for the Third Edition was Paula Aldrich. She is a high-energy person, skillful and disciplined in the art of turning a manuscript into a textbook. Her long hours of work and her dedication to the project were key factors in the completion of this edition.

The Medical Art Director for the Third Edition was Don Sellers, PA, AMI, NREMT-A, former Deputy Chief of the Glenn Dale Rescue Squad, Prince Georges County, Maryland, and former U.S. Navy Corpsman with combat medical training. There is no doubt that Don is the finest emergency care illustrator, designer, and director in the country. He was a part of all aspects of design, photography, and illustration. In addition to the visuals in the book, his paramedic background allowed him to review the text of the first eight chapters, looking for problem areas experienced by the EMT student.

Pat Hansen was the Producer of Photography, working with George Dodson, Director of Photography, to add the many new photographs to this edition. They make a fine team, dedicated to accuracy and improving the learning experience for users of Brady textbooks.

The Brady Company helped from the beginning by finding us Barry Foy, instructional technologist, of Annapolis, Maryland. He provided us with ideas on instructional format and coordinated questionnaires and pre-rough manuscript reviews. The crucial task of coordinating manuscript reviews was given to Jessie Katz at the Brady Company. She provided us with the information we needed from reviewers, promptly and efficiently.

Many fine reviewers and advisors worked on this edition, including:

Section Advisors and Reviewers

Jesse A. Weigel, MD—Primary and Secondary Survey/Patient Assessment

Medical Director, Emergency Health Services, Pa. Dept. of Health, Harrisburg, PA

Mark A. Shaffer, MD—Basic Life Support

Assistant Professor, Project Medical Director, University of Chicago Dept. of Emergency Medicine, Chicago, IL

Frank T. Barranco, MD, AAOS—Orthopedics

Chief Surgeon, Baltimore Co. Fire Dept., Baltimore, MD

Michael V. Vance, MD—Medical Emergencies

Director, Paramedic Program, St. Luke's Hospital, Phoenix, AZ

Specialty Reviewers

Ron Moore—Rescue

Senior Training Technician, Office of Fire Prevention and Control, State of New York

Charles Wood—Rescue

Senior Instructor, EMS Division, Maryland Fire and Rescue Institute

Jeffrey Mitchell—Crisis Intervention

Senior Instructor, Emergency Health Services Program/MIEMS, University of Maryland Baltimore County

Regine Aronaw, MD—Poisons

Poison Control Center, Children's Hospital of Michigan, Detroit, MI

Sallyann Sohr—SIDS

Executive Director, National Sudden Infant Death Syndrome Foundation, Landover, MD

Charles E. Hutcheson, Jr., DDS, RPh— Dental and Oral Emergencies, Drug Abuse, and Poisons

Richmond, VA

Michael S. Hildebrand—Hazardous Materials

Safety and Fire Protection Associate, American Petroleum Institute, Washington, DC

John Hess—Hazardous Materials

Senior Instructor, Maryland Fire and Rescue Institute, College Park, MD

William H. Montgomery, MD—CPR

Director, Surgical Intensive Care Unit, Chief, Department of Anesthesiology, Straub Clinic and Hospital, Honolulu, HI

Full Manuscript Reviewers

Gloria Balducci and *Robert Wright*

Senior Instructors, Maryland Fire & Rescue Institute, Emergency Care Div., College Park, MD

Nels Sanddal

Past Chairman, National Council of EMS Training Coordinators, Helena, MT

The Prepublication Review Committee

The National Council of State EMS Training Coordinators, Basking Ridge, NJ

Phil G. Petty, EMT

Project Director, EMS Training Programs, Georgia Dept. of Education, Atlanta, GA

Judith A. Reid, BSN, EMT-P

Training Coordinator, Emergency Medical Service, Grady Memorial Hospital, Atlanta, GA

Ilene Foster, RN

Instructor, Maryland Institute for Emergency Medical Services, Westminster, MD

Stephen S. Carter

Director, Emergency Services Div., Indian Development District of Arizona, Inc., Phoenix, AZ

Cyril T.M. Cameron, MD, FRCS, FACS

Chief, Dept. of Emergency Medicine, Samaritan Hospital, Troy, NY

Charles B. Gillespie, MD, FACS

Albany, GA

Daniel H. Becker

Past President, American Ambulance Association, Youngstown, OH

Diane Reid, REMT-P

EMT Coordinator, University of Texas Health Science Center, Dallas, TX

Don Sleeper

First Aid CPR, and Water Safety Instructor/Trainer and Teaching Staff, Prince Georges Community College, Prince Georges County, MD

David E. Best

Director, Apprenticeship Program, International Association of Fire Fighters, Washington, DC

James Page, JD

Executive Director, ACT Foundation, Basking Ridge, NJ

Roger Dean White, MD, FACC

Associate Professor of Anesthesiology, Mayo Medical School, Rochester, MN

Gary Termeer

International Rescue and Emergency Care Association, Worthington, OH

Barbara A. Knezevich, RN, MS, CEN

Director, Professional Services, Emergency Department Nurses Association, Chicago, IL

Alisdair Conn, MD

Director, Field Operations Program, Maryland Institute for Emergency Medical Services, Baltimore, MD

Bruce W. Edwards

Coordinator, Emergency Medical Services, City of Virginia Beach, VA

K. Joanne McGlown, RN

EMS Planning and Management Consultant, Federal Emergency Management Agency, Washington, DC

George L. Johnson

Chief, EMS Certification, State of New York, Dept. of Health, Bureau of Emergency Health Services, Albany, NY

Marvin E. Reed

State EMS Training Coordinator, Springfield, IL

Pamela Bakhaus doCarmo, MS, REMT-A

Associate Professor, Emergency Medical Services Technology, Northern Virginia Community College, Annandale, VA

Daniel A. Garman

Training Director, State of Indiana, Emergency Medical Services Commission, Indianapolis, IN

Mary Beth Michos

Captain, Montgomery County Fire/Rescue Services, Rockville, MD

Frank Poliafico, RN

Emergency and Safety Programs, Inc., Miami, FL

Some of the above reviewers did so much additional work on the manuscript that they must be cited as advisors. These are: Cyril Cameron, MD, Stephen Carter, Gloria Balducci, Nels Sanddal, David Best, Phil Petty, Judith Reid, RN, Ilene Foster, Ron Moore, and John Hess. We appreciate the time, content information, and style comments to the rough drafts.

We also thank John Gould, Associate Director, Office of Community Programs, American Heart Association, Dallas, Texas, for finding reviewers for the CPR material.

A special thanks to Bettie Elliott, EMT-A, and Gilbert Elliott, NREMT-P, two very successful and dedicated Virginia EMT instructors and active members in the Bensley-Bermuda Volunteer Rescue Squad, Chesterfield County, Virginia. These two fine instructors allowed us to interact with their students during the writing of this text, providing additional insight to the problems faced by the EMT student. They also shared their teaching approaches that have helped give them such a high success rate.

We are grateful for the equipment and help provided us by the University of Maryland Department of Environmental Safety, Bowie (Maryland) Volunteer Fire Department, Berwyn Heights (Maryland) Volunteer Fire Department, Glenn Dale (Maryland) Volunteer Fire Department, Riverdale (Maryland) Volunteer Fire Department, and the Allsafe Fire Equipment Company of Hagerstown, Maryland.

To Nels Sanddal, Don Horton, James Hendrickson, Patrick Cole, and Steve LeFever, we remember your recommendations during our conversations at Virginia Beach in 1980.

Finally, a special thanks to Gloria Balducci, Senior Instructor, Maryland Fire and Rescue Institute, for serving as our technical advisor for photography. She spent many hours making certain that procedures were correct before and during photography sessions.

1 the emergency medical technician

OBJECTIVES By the end of this chapter, you should be able to:

1. Define emergency medical services (EMS) systems. (p. 4)
2. Define emergency care. (p. 3)
3. Define Emergency Medical Technician (EMT). (p. 8)
4. List the NINE major duties of an EMT. (p. 8)
5. List the major responsibilities of the EMT. (p. 8)
6. List those activities that fall under the heading of EMT duties. (p. 8)
7. Describe the desirable traits of an EMT. (p. 11)
8. Relate EMT responsibilities to Good Samaritan laws and the Standard of Care. (pp. 12–13)
9. Define informed consent, and distinguish between actual and implied consent. (p. 13)
10. Define duty to act and abandonment. (pp. 12, 14)
11. List SIX emergencies that may require you to file special reports. (p. 14)
12. Describe the procedures that an EMT should follow at the crime scene. (p. 15)
13. Describe the role and actions of an EMT when caring for a deceased person. (p. 15)
14. Describe THREE types of ambulances. (pp. 15 16)
15. Categorize the medical equipment, basic tools, and supplies used by the EMT. (pp. 16–17)

SKILLS As an EMT, you should be able to:

1. Display the desirable traits of an EMT.
2. Provide care as defined by law.

TERMS   you may be using for the first time:

Morbidity—the occurrence of illness.

Emergency Care—the prehospital assessment and treatment of the sick or injured patient. This care is initiated at the emergency scene and is continued through transport and transfer at a medical facility. The physical and emotional needs of the patient are considered during care.

Emergency Medical Services System (EMS System)—the complete chain of human and physical resources that provides patient care in cases of sudden illness and injury.

Emergency Medical Technician (EMT)—a professional-level provider of emergency care. This individual has received formal training and is state certified. An EMT can be a volunteer or a paid career professional.

Abandonment—to leave an injured or ill patient before the responsibility for care is handed over to someone of equal or superior training. Leaving the hospital without giving patient information to the staff may be viewed by some legal experts as a form of abandonment.

Duty to Act—typically a local law that states which agencies have a legal responsibility to provide emergency care. If an EMT is a member of such an agency, he has a legal responsibility to render emergency care.

Good Samaritan Laws—a series of laws, varying in each state, designed to protect health care personnel administering emergency care. These laws require a person to act in good faith, and provide care to the level of his training, to the best of his abilities. In some states, these laws do not apply to the paid EMT.

Standard of Care—the minimum accepted level of emergency care to be provided as set forth by law, administrative orders, and guidelines published by emergency care organizations and societies. Each state has its own defined standard of care.

Informed Consent—agreement by a rational adult patient to accept emergency care, after you state your name, the level of your training, and what you plan to do.

Actual Consent—consent given by the adult patient, usually in oral form, accepting emergency care. This must be informed consent.

Implied Consent—a legal position that assumes an unconscious patient (or one so badly injured or ill that he cannot respond) would consent to receiving emergency care if he could do so. Implied consent applies to children when parents or guardians are not at the scene, the mentally retarded, and the mentally disturbed.

THE EMERGENCY MEDICAL SERVICES SYSTEM

HOW IT BEGAN

Most of the techniques and procedures used in medicine are rather new, with the majority of these methods developed since the 1940s. Each new decade increases our scientific knowledge and techniques. Much of this carries over into the field of medicine. Today's hospitals are staffed by highly trained health care teams who use complex medical procedures, accurate methods of detecting disease, elaborate equipment, and new "wonder" drugs. This is a far cry from the hospital of the last century where most patients who entered expected to die.

Sudden illness or severe injury often can cause irreversible damage to the patient or even death, unless appropriate care is initiated as soon as possible. The concept of providing professional-level care at the scene and en route to the hospital is one of the newest in total patient care. The emergency medical services system (EMS System) now reaches out to the patient, assuming responsibility for care at the emergency scene.

Historians are unable to document specific systems for transporting patients before the 1790s. The need to provide care for battlefield casualities inspired the French to begin the transport of patients so they could be cared for by physicians away from the scene of battle. The concern for suffering soldiers on the battlefield continued into the next century, leading to the formation of what was to become the International Red Cross in 1863. This organization saw that there was a responsibility to provide care for the wounded as soon as possible.

In the United States, emergency care also began during time of war. A dedicated nurse, Clara Barton, started professional-level care for the wounded during the Civil War. She was a prime mover in the United States joining the International Red Cross, working from 1881 until 1905 to have the Congress grant a charter for the American Red Cross. Her efforts, and the work of another nurse, Jane Delano, firmly established the American Red Cross. The major thrust of this organization's efforts to provide initial care for accident victims and those taken suddenly ill developed after World War II.

Ambulance service in this country began in a few major cities at the turn of the century. They were transport systems only, offering little or no emergency care. Smaller cities, towns, and rural areas did not begin to develop ambulance services until after World War II. Where services developed to provide emergency care with transport, the fire service was usually responsible to render care.

The American Heart Association (AHA) began to produce training materials and programs for cardiopulmonary resuscitation and basic life support in 1966. Their efforts were directed at prehospital emergency care. A program for public education in basic life support came from the AHA and the National Academy of Sciences' National Research Council recommendations in 1973. By 1977, the AHA and the American Red Cross had trained over 12 million health care professionals and private citizens in basic life support. Their mission is to train 80 million people, providing the skills that may save as many as 100,000 to 200,000 lives each year.

Also during the mid-1960s, the National Academy of Sciences' National Research Council studied the problem of emergency care. Their intent was to establish standards for prehospital care. Modern emergency medical services began when they issued the following statement:

Employees or volunteer members of public and private organizations having a responsibility for the delivery of health services must be trained in and held accountable for administration of specialized care and delivery of the victims of acute illness or injury to a medical facility. This category of lay persons includes ambulance personnel, rescue squad workers, policemen, firemen, lifeguards, workers in first aid or health facilities of public buildings and industrial plants, attendants at sports events, civil defense workers, paramedic personnel, and employees of public or private health service agencies. Specialized training, retraining and accreditation of such persons necessitate development of training courses, manuals and training aids adequate to provide instruction in all emergency care short of that rendered by physicians or by paramedic personnel under their direct supervision.

Ambulance personnel are responsible for all lay emergency care from the time they first see the victim through transportation and delivery to care of a physician. They must therefore be able not only to appraise the extent of first aid rendered by others, but also to carry out what additional measures will make it safe to move the victim and minimize morbidity and mortality. They must operate the vehicle safely and efficiently; maintain communication between the scene of the emergency, traffic authorities, dispatchers, and emergency departments; render necessary additional care enroute; and transmit records and reports to medical and other authorities. Although the emphasis on certain subjects will vary with the nature of employment of those who are not ambulance personnel but who have a responsibility for delivery of health services, they should be equally trained so that minimum care can be assured, whether they transfer responsibility to the ambulance attendant, or, in his absence, carry out the functions required of him.

Training of Ambulance Personnel and Others Responsible for Emergency Care of the Sick and Injured at the Scene and During Transportation. Division of Medical Services, National Academy of Sciences' National Research Council, March, 1968.

The above may not have much meaning so early in your training. However, once you become an EMT, come back to this quotation. You will note that it is the framework on which your course is based. Also, keep in mind what emergency care must have been like in many areas of the country before direction, standards, and a national commitment were developed. With the preceding statment, the longheld concept of ambulance service as a means merely for transporting the sick and injured passed into oblivion. No longer could people view the ambulance attendant as someone with little more than the physical strength required to lift a victim in and out of the ambulance. Victims now became patients, receiving prehospital emergency care from highly trained professional personnel. Emergency care included treating both the sick and injured at the emergency scene and during transport. The providers of this care had to be trained to consider the physical and emotional needs of the patient. The hospital emergency department was extended, through emergency medical services, to reach the sick and injured at the emergency scene and begin immediate care. The ambulance attendant was replaced by the **Emergency Medical Technician (EMT).**

The National Highway Safety Act of 1966 charged the United States Department of Transportation (DOT) with developing Emergency Medical Services (EMS) standards and assisting the states to upgrade their prehospital emergency care. The DOT created the 81-hour EMT course that is the basis for your training.

In 1970, the National Registry of Emergency Medical Technicians was founded. One of the goals of this organization was to establish professional standards for EMTs and to provide services for local

EMS Systems wishing to upgrade their EMT training programs. Other national organizations were created to consider what could be done to improve prehospital emergency care (see page 17).

The National Health Planning and Resources Development Act of 1974 increased planning activities and services to help the states develop their EMS Systems. Today, each state has its own quality EMS System, offering basic, advanced, and continuing education programs to most providers of prehospital emergency care.

Members of this country's EMS Systems are proud of their history and what they have been able to accomplish in the ongoing effort to improve prehospital emergency care.

EMERGENCY MEDICAL SERVICES SYSTEM

The EMS System is more than EMTs and emergency department personnel. It is a chain of human and physical resources, brought together to provide total patient care. To better understand this chain of resources, let us consider an event in the life of Mr. Tom Henderson. Note how all the links of the chain of resorces joined to carry Tom through an unfortunate experience.

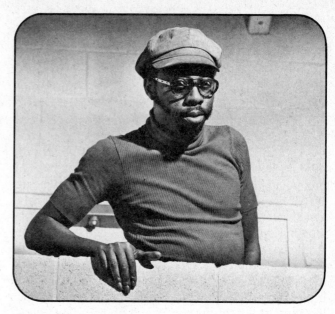

Figure 1-2

11:51 A.M. A workman nearby sees Tom fall. Before going to Tom's assistance, he quickly calls the floor supervisor, who, in turn, notifies the nurse on duty in the plant infirmary. Before she leaves the infirmary, the nurse dials 911 and requests assistance from the local EMS System. (1-2)

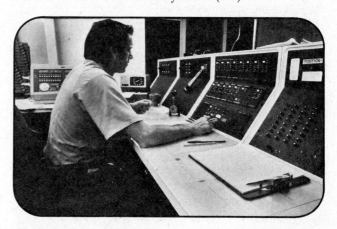

Figure 1-3

11:51 A.M. The regional emergency communications center dispatcher receives the call from the plant nurse. He gathers as much information about the accident as he can, and passes this information on as he alerts the ambulance and rescue squad. (1-3)

11:52 A.M. The workman who witnessed the accident reaches Tom's side. A quick assessment shows him that there are not only serious injuries, but that Tom is having difficulty breathing! He quickly positions himself at Tom's side and opens Tom's airway by using a modified jaw-thrust maneuver that he learned in a plant-sponsored First Responder course. He is careful not to move Tom's head any more than absolutely necessary because of possible spinal injuries. This simple maneuver reduces Tom's problems with breathing. The work-

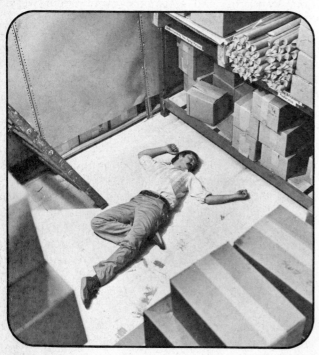

Figure 1-1

Wednesday, June 21, 11:50 A.M. Tom is working on a ladder in the warehouse of the Acme Paper Products Company. While replacing an overhead conduit, he leans too far from his ladder and falls nearly 20 feet to the concrete floor below. He lands on his right leg, and falls backward, striking his head on the concrete. (1-1)

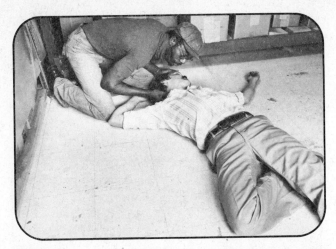

Figure 1-4

man does not move Tom; instead, he closely watches Tom's breathing efforts. He is ready to assist Tom in the event that respirations stop. (1-4)

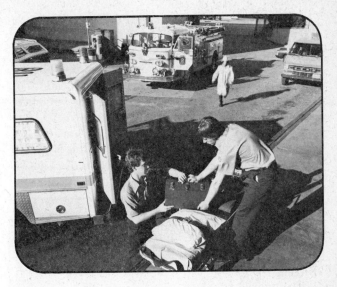

Figure 1-6

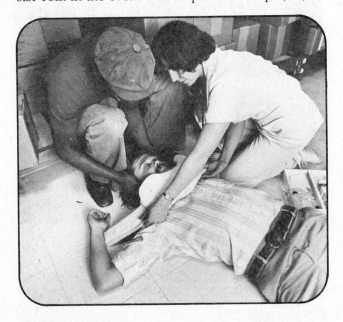

Figure 1-5

11:56 A.M. The plant nurse arrives with a first aid kit and blankets. She too makes a quick assessment and, based on her observation of the mechanism of injury, has the First Responder stabilize Tom's head and neck while she secures an extrication collar around Tom's neck. Knowing that EMTs will soon arrive, she does not move Tom. However, she does begin to treat him for shock. (1-5)

12:01 P.M. The ambulance and rescue unit arrive on the scene. The EMTs and rescue officer enter the building, bringing with them a wheeled stretcher, a long spine board, and a trauma kit. (1-6)

12:03 P.M. The EMTs and the rescue officer reach the site of Tom's accident and squeeze past pallets of stacked cartons in order to reach the patient. A quick primary survey shows that Tom is breathing, he has strong heart action, and that he

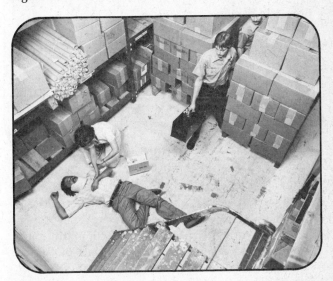

Figure 1-7

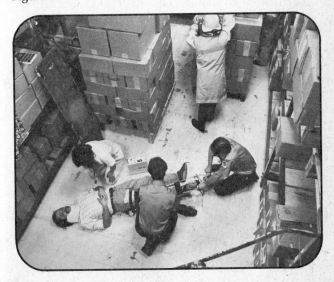

Figure 1-8

has no serious bleeding wounds. They conduct a secondary survey and find that Tom has a possible closed fracture of the right femur (thigh bone). They elect to leave the extrication collar in place and immobilize Tom on a long spine board. Meanwhile, the rescue officer orders his squadmen into the building and directs them to assist with the relocation of those pallets that will block the way of the stretcher. (1-7, 1-8)

12:09 P.M. The EMTs begin to administer oxygen to help prevent shock. Properly splinted, placed on a stretcher, covered, and secured, Tom is wheeled from the accident site. (1-9)

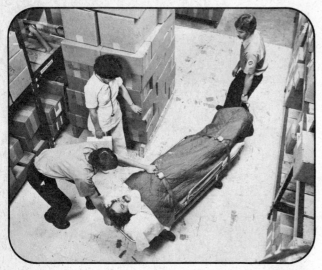

Figure 1-9

12:13 P.M. Tom is loaded into the ambulance and transported to the hospital. He is attended during transport in case additional emergency care is required. During transport, radio communications inform the emergency department staff of the circumstances of Tom's accident, the extent of his injuries, his condition, the care provided, and the estimated time of arrival. The emergency department staff will be alerted if there is any change in Tom's condition during transport. (1-10)

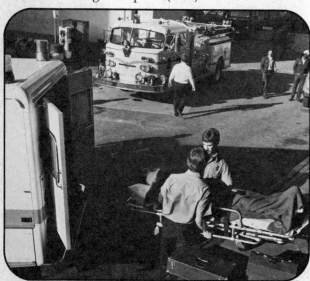

Figure 1-10

12:30 P.M. The ambulance arrives at the medical facility. The EMTs transfer Tom to the emergency department, providing the staff with an oral and written report of the accident, patient assessment, and care rendered. (1-11)

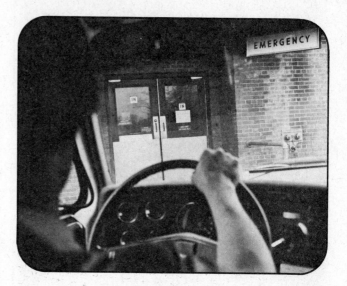

Figure 1-11

Tom's immediate needs are cared for by the emergency department staff. Tests are performed and X-rays are taken. He is then wheeled to an operating room where an orthopedic surgeon cares for Tom's fracture and the damage the sharp bone ends have done to blood vessels and soft tissues around the fracture site. (1-12)

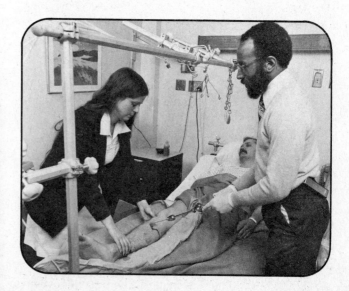

Figure 1-12

Tom is moved to a recovery room and placed in traction. A nurse closely observes him until he is completely recovered from the anesthesia. When appropriate, he will be moved to a room in an area of the hospital where the staff specializes in orthopedic injuries. (1-13)

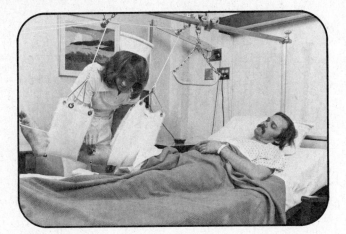

Figure 1-13

Monday, August 14. Tom begins a program of rehabilitation under the supervision of a physical therapist. (1-14)

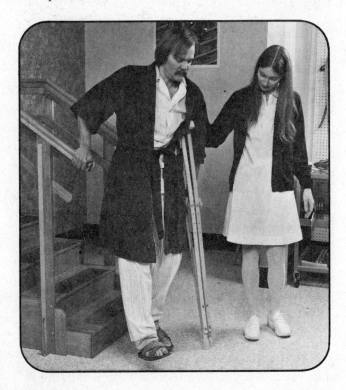

Figure 1-14

Sunday, August 20. Tom has received total patient care while he was in the hospital, and is now ready to be discharged. He will be away from work for some time and he will have to return to the hospital periodically for therapy. But . . .he is alive, and he can walk! (1-15)

Having read of Tom's plight, consider how many different people were involved with his care from accident through recovery. AT ANY POINT, TOM COULD HAVE SUSTAINED IRREVERSIBLE INJURY IF ANY ONE OF THESE PERSONS FAILED TO ACT, OR PROVIDED IMPROPER CARE. The chain of human and physical resources, the EMS System, in Tom's community held together because none of the links failed. Figure 1-16 reviews this chain of resources.

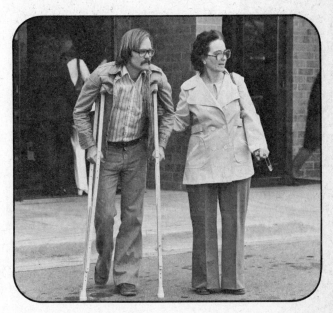

Figure 1-15

Some parts of the EMS System were not visible in the preceding example. An advisory council for EMS decided how the system was to respond and what care procedures were to be used. Public information officers had provided the citizens with the knowledge of what the EMS System is, what it could do, and how to seek assistance. The EMS System trained instructors, who then trained the EMTs who responded to help Tom. Many other people, including those involved with personnel, record keeping, and equipment and supplies were an important part of the EMS System being able to help Tom.

As an EMT, you will be part of the EMS System. More specifically, you will carry out your duties as a part of the prehospital emergency care delivery subsystem. There are three components to this subsystem:

- the EMT
- the ambulance
- the supplies and equipment carried on the ambulance

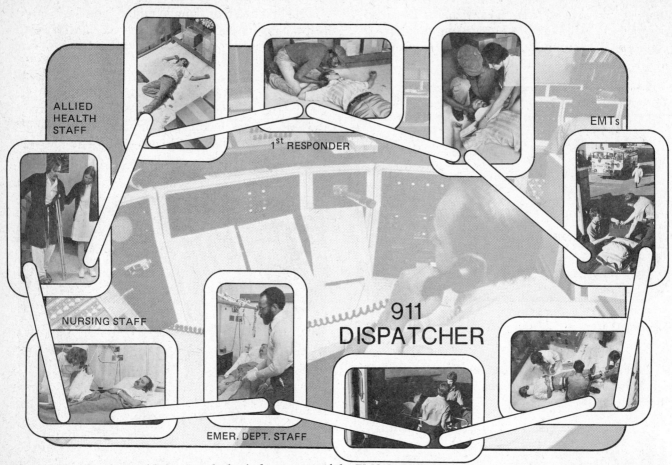

ALLIED
HEALTH
STAFF

1ˢᵗ RESPONDER

EMTs

911
DISPATCHER

NURSING STAFF

EMER. DEPT. STAFF

Figure 1-16: The chain of human and physical resources of the EMS System.

THE EMERGENCY MEDICAL TECHNICIAN

The EMT is a *professional* provider of emergency care. Both the volunteer and paid EMT are considered to be professional members of the EMS System. The term ''professional'' does not imply payment for services. It refers to training, dedication, desire to perform to the best of one's abilities, and the willingness to continue with formal training. Working within the EMS System, the EMT is a team member helping to provide total patient care. Trained and state *certified*, the EMT is capable of providing emergency care at the scene, en route, and, when called upon to do so, at the hospital emergency department. A person who has an accident, or a person who is ill, is called a ''victim.'' Once the EMT begins care, the ''victim'' becomes a ''patient.''

There is more than one level of EMT. In this book, we will use the term to mean the basic level, or EMT-A, unless otherwise stated. The levels of EMTs include:

1. *EMT-A, Emergency Medical Technician-Ambulance*—anyone who has successfully completed a DOT 81-hour course or its equivalent and has been certified as an EMT by a state emergency medical services board.

2. *EMT-I, Emergency Medical Technician-Intermediate* and *A-EMT, Advanced Emergency Medical Technician*—any EMT-A who has passed specific training programs to provide locally determined procedures in intermediate and advanced life support. In some states, this level includes those EMTs who are given the title of Cardiac Technician or Cardiac Rescue Technician.

3. *EMT-P, Emergency Medical Technician-Paramedic*—anyone who has successfully completed paramedic training including or equal to the DOT 15-module program.

The EMT deals with both injury and illness. The care provided can range from basic life support to emotional support. You will have to provide care for cuts, bruises, fractures, burns, and internal injuries. You will be called upon to deal with heart attacks, strokes, respiratory illnesses, seizures, diabetic coma, insulin shock, childbirth, poisoning, drug abuse, and problems due to excessive heat and cold. In addition to these problems, you will have to provide care for patients suffering emotional or psychiatric emergencies. Some problems will be simple, while others will be life-threatening. All will require professional-level emergency care.

THE EMT - NINE MAIN DUTIES

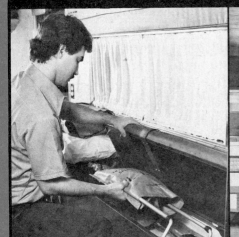
PREPARATION

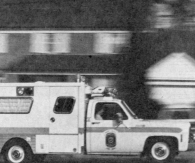
RESPONSE

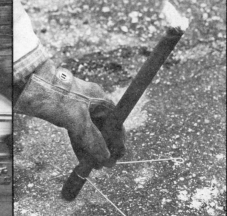
SCENE CONTROL

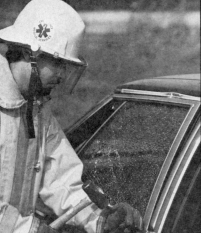
GAINING ACCESS

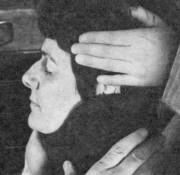
ASSESSMENT AND EMERGENCY CARE

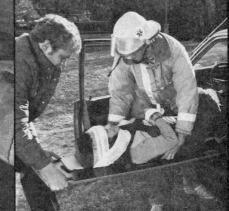
DIS-ENTANGLEMENT

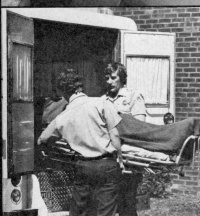
TRANSFER AND TRANSPORT

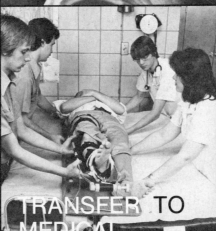
TRANSFER TO MEDICAL FACILITY

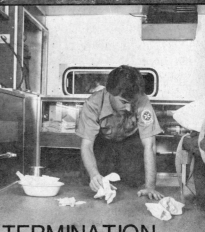
TERMINATION OF ACTIVITIES

SCAN 1-1

Roles and Responsibilities

At an emergency scene, the primary concern is the *patient.* In addition to hands-on care, each aspect of the activities carried out by EMTs is done to assure care, safety, and comfort to the patient.

As an EMT, you will have nine main duties. They are:

1. Be prepared to respond.
2. Respond swiftly but safely to the scene.
3. Make certain that the scene is safe, by either assisting in the control of, or by controlling the activities at the scene.
4. Gain access to patients, using special tools when necessary.
5. Determine what is wrong with the patient and provide appropriate emergency care.
6. Free, lift, and move the patient, when required, and do so without causing additional injury to the patient, or to yourself. These procedures are also called disentanglement, extrication, and transfer.
7. Prepare and properly transfer the patient to the ambulance.
8. Transport the patient safely to the appropriate medical facility, providing en route communications, and handing the patient and patient information over to more highly trained personnel.
9. Return safely from the run, complete records and reports, and prepare for the next response.

Depending on your training and where you will be working as an EMT, you may be called upon to do any or all of the following:

- Function as a driver EMT, who is familiar with driving techniques, traffic regulations, how to select the best route depending on traffic conditions, weather, and other factors, and how to approach, park at, and leave the scene.
- Control an emergency scene in order to protect yourself and the patient, and to prevent additional accidents.
- Assess an emergency scene, knowing when you will need additional assistance from law enforcement, fire services, utility companies, or others that may be needed at the scene.
- Gain access to the patient in situations such as motor vehicle accidents, water and ice accidents, cave-ins, and crime scenes.
- Determine what is wrong with the patient by gathering information from the scene, bystanders, and the patient, and by examining the patient.

- To the best of your ability, provide emergency care at the level of your training.
- Reassure the patient, relatives, and bystanders, providing emotional support as part of your care.
- Free a trapped patient using the techniques and tools of extrication.
- Safely transport a patient to the correct medical facility, monitoring the patient, providing needed emergency care, and communicating with the emergency department staff while en route.
- Transfer the patient, patient information, and personal effects to the emergency department staff, and, on request, assist the emergency department staff.

These are only a few of the many things an EMT must be able to do. Some duties, such as basic life support, are dramatic. Report writing and taking inventory are far less glamorous. All duties are important to providing patient care. You should stop now and turn to Appendix 1. Here you will find a list of all the skills and duties to be performed by an EMT. As you go through your training, check off the items you feel you can accomplish at the professional level of the Emergency Medical Technician.

NOTE: Duties and skills may vary among localities. Within any given area, specific policies determine which member of an EMT team has what duties. Usually, all personnel are equally trained in all duties and responsibilities so that they can function independently or interchangeably.

Background, Training, and Experience

Most areas in the country use a job description for the EMT based on that prepared by the United States Department of Transportation and supported by the National Highway Traffic Safety Administration. In most localities, the minimum levels of education, training, and experience required for the EMT include:

- A high school education or its equivalent
- Age of 18 years or older
- Training to the level recognized as the DOT 81-hour course for EMT-Ambulance personnel
- Practical experience in the care and use of emergency care equipment commonly used by EMTs (suction devices, installed and portable oxygen delivery systems, splints and immobilization equipment, emergency medical kits, obstetric kits, patient transfer devices, and basic rescue tools)
- Practical experience in sanitizing and disin-

fecting procedures for all equipment, including the ambulance

- Knowledge of safety and security procedures to allow for duties to be carried out in hostile environments
- Knowledge of the territory within the EMT's service area
- A driver's license and other professional certificate or license as required by law indicating that the EMT knows the motor vehicle codes and that the EMT-driver can skillfully and safely operate an ambulance
- Ability to use communications equipment
- State certification

EMT Traits

There are certain physical traits and aspects of personality that are desirable for the EMT. Physically, you should be in good health. You have a responsibility to stay in shape so that you can carry out your duties. If you are unable to provide needed care because you cannot bend over or catch your breath, then all your training is worthless.

You should be able to lift and carry up to 100 pounds. Practice with other EMTs is essential so that you can learn how to carry your share of the combined weight of patient, stretcher, linens, and blankets. For such moves, coordination and dexterity are needed, as well as strength. You will have to perform basic rescue procedures, lower stretcher patients from upper levels, and negotiate fire escapes and stairways while carrying patients.

Your eyesight is very important as an EMT. Make certain that you can see distant objects clearly, as well as those close at hand. Both types of vision are needed for patient assessment, driving, and controlling the emergency scene. Should you have any eyesight problems, they must be corrected with prescription glasses or contact lenses.

Be aware of any problems you may have with color vision. Not only is this important to driving, but it could be critical for patient assessment. Colors seen on the patient's skin, lips, nailbeds, ear lobes, and eyelids often provide valuable clues to a patient's condition.

You should be able to give and receive oral and written instructions. Eyesight, hearing, and speech are important to the EMT, thus all problems must be corrected if you are to be an EMT.

Good personality traits are very important to the EMT. You should be:

- Pleasant—inspire confidence and help to calm the sick and injured.
- Cooperative—allow for faster and better care, establish better coordination with other members of the EMS System, and bolster the confidence of patients and bystanders.
- Resourceful—you can adapt a tool or technique to fit an unusual situation.
- A self-starter—you show initiative and accomplish what must be done without having to depend upon someone else starting procedures.
- Emotionally stable—overcome the unpleasant aspects of an emergency to provide needed care and to resolve any uneasy feelings you may have after care has been provided.
- Able to lead—take the steps necessary to control a scene, to organize bystanders to deliver care, and when necessary, to take complete charge of an emergency.
- Proud of a neat and clean appearance—promote confidence in both patients and bystanders and reduce the possibility of contamination.
- Of good moral character with respect for others—that you can be trusted in situations when the patient cannot protect himself or valuables, and so that all information relayed is truthful and accurate.
- In control of personal habits—prevent discomfort to the patient by not smoking when providing care (REMEMBER: smoking may contaminate wounds and is dangerous around oxygen delivery systems), and never consuming alcohol within two hours of duty.
- Controlled in conversation—communicate properly, to inspire confidence, and to avoid inappropriate conversation that may upset or anger the patient or bystanders.
- Able to listen to others—be accurate with interviews and inspire confidence.

All of this helps to developing a CALM, PROFESSIONAL MANNER that will lead to better patient care.

At first some students do not see the importance of the above. They feel that all they need to worry about is how to efficiently provide the correct care procedure. Experience has shown that *all* of the traits listed are needed in the complex world of the emergency scene.

For example, consider leadership ability. Some students believe that *others* will be in charge at the scene. However, YOU may have to take control of an accident scene. YOU may have to initiate rescue efforts. YOU may have to direct the sorting and removal of multiple casualties from the scene. YOU may have to deal with distraught relatives. YOU may have to cope with spectators who are disrupting an otherwise smooth-running operation. YOU may have to make unpleasant decisions. In short, at one time or another, YOU may be in charge and there will be no one else to take over for you. In those instances you must be able to lead calmly, decisively, and firmly if you are to assure cooperation, teamwork, and the best patient care.

Some students believe the EMS System places too much emphasis on a neat clean appearance and good personal grooming. Put yourself in the place of an injured but conscious patient. If one EMT arrives in a clean uniform and another arrives in greasy overalls, which one would you want to help you? You would probably pick the uniformed EMT, if for no other reason than he *looks* the part! The uniform indicates disciplined training, quality, and organization. Be it a full uniform, a jacket, or simply a cap with a badge, a uniform helps to put the patient at ease and to gain the cooperation of bystanders.

Neatness and personal grooming not only inspire confidence, they serve to protect the patient

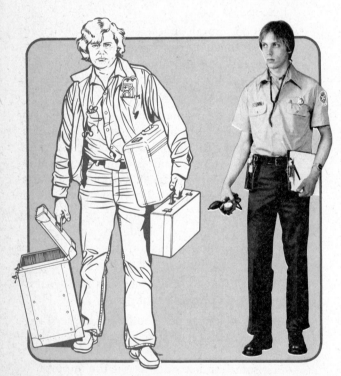

Figure 1-17: A professional appearance inspires confidence.

from contamination that may come from dirty clothing, hands and fingernails, and the unkempt hair of the rescuer.

One of the biggest mistakes made by new EMTs is *inappropriate conversation.* Saying the wrong thing or using the wrong words may upset a patient and worsen his condition. Inappropriate conversation also may upset relatives or bystanders, lessening any chances you may have to gain their confidence and help. Remember, it is not only *what* you say, but *how* you say it. Shouting only leads to confusion. A

harsh voice may make others uncooperative or reluctant to accept your help. The tone of you voice may be the key that allows you to provide proper care.

Imagine how you would feel if you were injured and someone looked at you and yelled, ''Hey Joe, look at the leg on this poor guy here! Ain't that an awful sight!'' You wouldn't do this? Fine, but would you bend over a patient who has just wrecked a new car and has broken his leg and say to him, ''Relax, everything is all right. There's nothing to worry about.''? Saying this would probably produce doubts as to your ability to provide care. Obviously, everything is not all right, or the person would not be lying on the ground in great pain with his leg bent at an odd angle. And as far as worrying is concerned, does your statement mean that the patient should give not a thought to the heap of metal that was once his $20,000 car? The inappropriate statement that you thought showed concern will not gain confidence or cooperation from the patient.

Learning to use appropriate, calm, **neutral** conversation is part of becoming a professional EMT. Conversation can help a patient to relax, if you are calm and honest. Telling the patient that you are trained in emergency care and that you will help him eases fears and inspires confidence. Telling the patient what you are going to do helps him to believe that you are competent.

As you can see, to provide emergency care, you must be able to do more than apply the correct procedure. You must do so as a professional, thus providing TOTAL PATIENT CARE.

THE EMT AND THE LAW

When it comes to the law, a textbook can offer only general guidelines. Each state has its own laws in regard to emergency care provided by the non-physician. We will cover some of the basics, but your instructor will have to provide you with the specifics that apply to your state.

Most individuals involved in providing emergency care are concerned with the legal aspects of care. Often, they are concerned with being sued. No one will tell you to think lightly of this problem. You *can* be sued; however, you will probably be able to defend yourself if you provided proper care to the level of your training, within the laws of your state. *You can be sued and held liable for:*

- *Not* providing care
- Rendering *improper* care when what was needed should have been obvious to a trained EMT
- *Abusing* or mistreating a patient
- Providing care *above* the level of your training
- *Forcing* care upon a competent adult who has refused your care

- *Irresponsible or wreckless driving,* or violating other laws that apply to emergency driving

There are other activities that can lead to a lawsuit. Your instructor can inform you of recent problems in your own state. Keep in mind that the laws have been written so that you can carry out your duties and provide emergency care. If you know the law and act as a professional EMT should, you should have little to worry about in terms of lawsuits. Your concern should not be so great that it prevents you from caring for sick and injured patients.

The Standard of Care

State laws require that a standard of care be provided to patients. This is the *minimum* accepted care based on state laws, administrative orders, and locally accepted guidelines published by emergency care organizations and societies. This standard of care allows you to be judged based on what is expected of someone with your training and experience acting in the same situation. Your course is based on the guidelines originally proposed by the DOT and other authorities who have studied what training, skills, and equipment are required for the EMT to provide the standard of care at the EMT level. You will be trained so you can provide this standard of care. Training and retraining are the best ways to assure that you will be able to provide the standard of care required in your state.

Duty to Act

Laws vary from state to state as to the responsibility an individual has to attempt to help someone in an emergency. As an EMT, more is expected of you than of the general public. In your state you may be required to respond and to provide care. Usually these laws have been written considering the level of your training and your emergency care skills. The safety of the care provider also is considered. Your instructor can inform you of the laws concerning the duty to act that apply to your locality. In most cases, if an agency is given the responsibility to provide care, and you are an EMT in that agency, you have a responsibility to provide care at emergencies, even when off duty.

Consent

Adults, when conscious and mentally competent, have the RIGHT TO REFUSE CARE. Adults who are mentally and physically able to make judgments are assumed to be competent and cannot be forced by an EMT to accept emergency care. Their reasons may be based on religious beliefs or a lack of trust. In some cases, you may find their reasoning to be senseless. For whatever reasons, though, a com-

petent adult can refuse care. You cannot treat such patients, nor can you restrain them. If the patient is fearful or lacks confidence in your abilities, conversation may help you gain trust and approval for care. Do NOT argue with a patient, particularly if his reasons are based on religious belief. To do so will add stress that may intensify the patient's problem.

When a patient refuses your care, you should document this by having him sign a *release form.* In rare cases, a patient may refuse your care and also refuse to sign the form. You will have to rely on eyewitnesses to verify that the patient refused care.

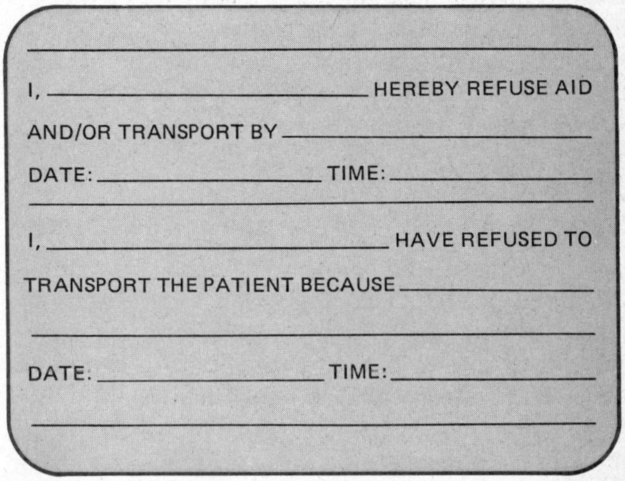

Figure 1-18: A standard consent form.

Parents or legal guardians can refuse to let you treat their child. Once again, if fear or lack of confidence is the apparent reason, try simple conversation. Do not try to make the adult feel guilty of wrong-doing, particularly if religious reasons are the basis of the decision. In some states you must report any case where a parent or legal guardian refuses emergency care for a minor. These states have special laws governing the welfare of children. The information you provide may be passed on to the courts to find out if the child received proper care or is still in need of care.

An adult patient, when conscious and mentally competent, can give you **actual consent** to provide care. Oral consent is considered to be valid; however, a signed consent form provides you with more protection. This consent must be **informed consent** meaning that the patient knows who you are, the level of your training, what is wrong, and what you are going to do.

In cases where the adult is unconscious or for some other reason unable to give you his actual consent, the law assumes that the patient, if able to do so, would want to receive treatment. This is known as **implied consent.** Typically, the law requires that there be an emergency where there is a significant risk of death, deterioration, or of some disability resulting if care is not initiated.

Minor's consent is not viewed as actual consent except in certain situations in certain states (for example, a married minor's consent may be viewed as actual consent in your state). In most cases, a child can refuse care, but if his parent or legal guardian consents to your providing care, then you have received actual consent. The adult can refuse to have you treat his child, but refusal by the child is not a right given to the child (with certain exceptions given in certain states). If the child's parents or legal guardians are not at the scene and they cannot be contacted with the speed needed so that care can be initiated immediately, *implied consent* takes on a special form. The law assumes that the parents or guardians would want care provided for their child. The same holds true for patients who are mentally ill, emotionally disturbed, or mentally retarded.

Immunities

Each state has its own laws in terms of immunity granted to those who provide emergency care. Such laws spell out when you are *immune to liability* in cases where you rendered care or were unable to render care. It is your responsibility to know the laws for your state. Note, too, that there is also governmental immunity provided to some government and military agencies.

Good Samaritan laws have been developed in most states to provide immunity to individuals trying to help people in emergencies. Most of these laws will grant you immunity from liability if you act in good faith to provide care to the level of your training, to the best of your ability. As you might expect, these laws are tied to the standard of care laws. You must familiarize yourself with the laws that govern your state. In some states, the Good Samaritan laws apply only to volunteers. If you are a paid EMT, different laws and regulations may apply.

Some states have specific EMT and paramedic statutes that authorize, regulate, and protect EMTs and paramedics (and the physicians who give instructions to these individuals by radio). To be protected by such laws, you must be recognized as an EMT or paramedic in the state where care has been provided. Some states have specific licensing and certification requirements that must be met, and that obligate the holder to the standard of care recognized in the state.

Take care that you receive your information from your instructor or from a legal authority. If you try researching the law books, you may overlook or misinterpret something of importance. Much of what is written is related to the Medical Practices Act, which requires licensure to practice medicine. Since most states exempt EMTs from the Medical Practices Act for the provisions of emergency care to their level of training, you may find a law that applies to the physician, but not to the EMT.

Abandonment

Once you stop to help someone in a medical emergency or someone who is injured, you have legally initiated care. If you leave this patient before completing care or handing care over to someone with at least your level of training, then you have **abandoned** the patient and may be subject to legal action. This concept exists to ensure that required care is complete and to avoid situations where someone else does not stop to provide care, thinking that you are taking responsibility for the patient and will stay with him.

Some states view as abandonment a situation where you leave a medical facility after bringing in a patient, but you have failed to turn over your information about the patient's problem and the care you provided. There are also states where abandonment may apply if you do not respond to a call or fail to complete a run unless ordered to do so. Abandonment may even apply if equipment failure or your own health prevents you from completing a response and you do not immediately report this failure.

Confidentiality

Many geographical areas have yet to write specific laws about the confidentiality due a patient receiving emergency care from an EMT. However, individuals in emergency care feel very strongly about protecting the patient's right to privacy. You must not care for a patient and then speak to your friends, family, or other members of the public about the details of your care. If you speak of the emergency, you must not relate specifics about what patients may have said, who they were with, any unusual aspects of behavior, or any descriptions of personal appearance. The same holds true if another member of the EMS System provides you with this information.

Responsibility for Possessions

Some care procedures require you to remove articles of the patient's clothing and jewelry. When you do, you are legally responsible for these articles. You must record what articles were removed from the patient and safeguard them until you transfer the patient to the medical facility. At such time, you are to hand the possessions over to the emergency department staff and receive a signed receipt for the articles.

Records and Reporting Requirements

The information you gather when assessing and monitoring a patient is to be written down on a standard form. This form becomes part of the patient's medical records. It is a legal document that must be complete and accurate.

There are situations that may require you to file a special report with the medical facility, the police, or a government agency. This varies from state to state. You may be required to report: child abuse, rape, assault, drug-related injuries, injury received during the commission of a crime, attempted suicide, communicable diseases, and animal bites.

Legal Implications in Special Patient Situations

There are special patients and special care situations where specific laws may apply. Some of these are described below.

Mentally Disturbed Patients Care is usually provided under the laws of implied consent. If the patient is violent and likely to hurt himself or others, then restraint may be necessary. The law does not expect the EMT to risk his own safety to care for any patient. Typically, local laws will not allow an EMT to apply restraints unless ordered to do so by a physician or by the police. In some cases, a court order may be required. The restraints must be applied so as not to harm the patient (police handcuffs may injure a person who is violent. . .wide strips of cloth or leather are usually recommended). Once restraints are in place, they should be kept in place until the patient is handed over to more highly trained personnel at a medical facility. See Chapter 14 for more information concerning these patients.

Female Patients Some localities still have specific rules about the transport of female patients by male EMTs. These areas require another female (usually not a relative of the patient) to be present with the patient during transport. When possible, this other woman should be an EMT. This is strongly advised in cases where the patient is emotionally disturbed, mentally ill, or mentally retarded. Most EMS Systems have the crew radio their time and mileage at the scene and their time and mileage on arrival at the medical facility. This indicates that no delays in transport took place. These special rules are designed to protect you.

Alcohol and Drug Abuse Patients You must, when possible, carry out a complete patient assessment and provide needed care for patients who are under the influence of alcohol or drugs, or who have been injured while under such influence. Since medicine views both alcohol and drug abuse as illnesses and not crimes, you should know if your state requires you to report cases of alcohol and drug abuse to legal authorities. See Chapter 11, Section 2 for more information on the care of these patients.

Attempted Suicide Patients Specific care for such patients is covered in Chapter 14, Section 2. You are not required to endanger yourself to reach and care for patients attempting suicide (unless your duties spell out such responsibility). If you believe an injury or poisoning was due to an attempted sui-

cide, your state may require you to report your suspicions to the emergency department staff or the police.

Felony-Related Cases If you have any reason to believe that the patient is the victim of a crime or was injured while committing a crime, then you must report this suspicion to the police. This holds true for possible cases of assault, rape, or child abuse, gunshot wounds, knife wounds, and any suspicious wound or injury. Your best course of action is to report to the emergency department staff and the police any cases where you feel a possible crime is related to the patient's problem. EMT actions at the crime scene will be covered in Chapter 14.

Animal Bite Patients Such cases usually must be reported to the hospital personnel or to the police. If the animal is dead, you should protect the carcass so that it can be examined by medical authorities. If the animal is at the scene, you should protect yourself first, then the patient and bystanders. Do NOT try to capture the animal unless you are specifically trained to do so.

Disposition of the Deceased In most states, an EMT does not have the authority to pronounce a patient dead. Therefore, if there is any chance of life still existing, you must provide basic life support measures (in cold water drowning, the patient may be resuscitated up to one hour after breathing has stopped). There are cases of obvious death, as when a person is decapitated, his body is severed, or he is virtually cremated. It is recommended and may be legally required that you do not move such bodies so as not to hinder possible police investigations.

In some states, you can phone the coroner or medical examiner and receive permission to declare a patient dead. There are even localities that allow EMTs to independently declare death. You will have to follow local guidelines on this matter.

A major problem now exists because of home care programs for terminally ill patients. The patient may have requested and the doctor may have ordered that no resuscitative measures be taken when the patient's lungs and heart cease to function. Obtaining legal proof of this request and order may prove to be a difficult task. Unless proof can be obtained and relayed to you, resuscitative measures have to be initiated.

EQUIPMENT

It is doubtful that you will have time early in your course to go over all the equipment used by today's EMTs. The information provided in this section is presented to let you look over the equipment you will be using and to cover only what your instructor wishes to introduce at this time. Throughout your course, return to this list to check off the equipment you have learned to use.

The Ambulance

The **ambulance** is a vehicle for emergency care with a driver's compartment and a patient's compartment that can accommodate two EMTs and two litter patients. At least one of these patients must be able to be positioned so that intensive life-support measures can be given during transit. The vehicle must be able to carry, at the same time, equipment and supplies needed to provide optimum EMT-level emergency care at the scene and during transport. Equipment for light rescue procedures is recommended. Two-way radio communication must be provided.

An ambulance must be designed and constructed to provide maximum safety and comfort to patients and EMTs, and to avoid aggravation of the patient's condition and exposure to any factors that may complicate the patient's condition or threaten his survival.

According to federal specifications for emergency care vehicles (KKK-A-1822-A, revised April, 1982), there are three types of ambulances. These are shown and described in Figures 1-19, 20, and 21. The vehicle is identified by "the star of life." The word "AMBULANCE" should appear in mirror image on the front so that the drivers of other vehicles can identify the unit as seen in their rear view mirrors. The vehicle is to have warning lights, including flashing lights (parabolic) in the upper corners of the vehicle body.

More will be said about ambulance driving and vehicle maintenance in Chapter 15.

Equipment and Supplies

Federal specifications must be met when federal funding is used in the purchasing of EMS System supplies. However, many ambulances and supplies are bought without federal funding. For this reason,

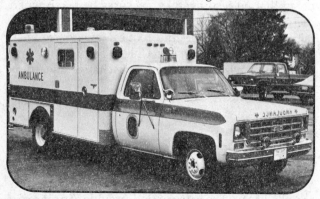

Figure 1-19: A type-I ambulance has a conventional cab and chassis, on which is mounted a modular ambulance body. There is no passageway between the driver's and patient's compartments.

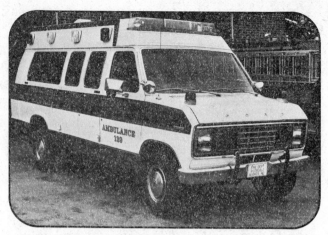

Figure 1-20: A type-II ambulance is commonly called a van-type ambulance. The body and cab form an integral unit, and most models have a raised roof.

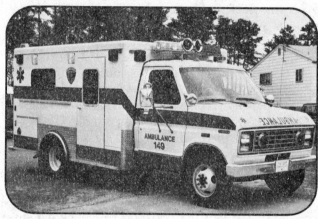

Figure 1-21: A type-III ambulance is commonly called a specialty van ambulance. It has a forward cab and an integral body that is generally larger than that of a type-II ambulance. There is a walk-through compartment.

the lists of equipment and supplies are presented as those items that *should* be carried, not those items that must be carried. A complete list with photographs is provided in Appendix 2. Your instructor will be able to tell you what is considered mandatory for your area.

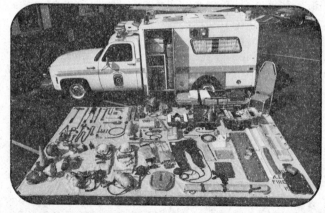

Figure 1-22: The well-equipped ambulance.

The equipment and supplies carried may be categorized as follows:

1. Basic Supplies—those items carried to protect

the patient (linens, pillows, blankets), provide for patient needs (emesis bags, tissues, bedpans, towels), and to monitor the patient (stethoscope, thermometer, and blood pressure measuring devices).

2. Equipment for Patient Transfer—including spine boards, wheeled stretchers, folding stretchers and stair chair, and scoop-style stretchers.

3. Equipment for Ventilation and Resuscitation—including airways, artificial ventilation devices, fixed and portable oxygen delivery systems, fixed and portable suction equipment, spine or CPR boards for chest compression.

4. Supplies for Immobilizing Fractures—including lower extremity traction splints, padded board splints for upper and lower extremities, air inflated splints, and triangular bandages for slings and swathes.

5. Supplies for Wound Care—including sterile gauze pads, sterile universal or multi-trauma dressings, self-adhering roller bandages, sterile nonporous occlusive dressings; along with adhesive tape, safety pins, and bandage shears.

6. Supplies for Childbirth—a sterile childbirth (OB) kit, including all necessary gloves, towels, baby blankets, bags, sanitary napkins, gauze pads, surgical scissors, cord tape or clamps, and rubber bulb syringes.

7. Supplies for Poisonings—including Syrup of Ipecac, activated charcoal, and drinking water.

8. Intermediate-Level Care Supplies—mainly for the treatment of shock, including intravenous agents, sterile IV administration kits, and anti-shock garment sets.

9. Physician and Paramedic Supplies (when carried)—including tracheal intubation kits, pleural decompression kits, drug injection kits, cardioscope and defibrillator, and a surgical kit.

10. Equipment for Gaining Access and Disentanglement—to include hand tools, power tools, and required rope, blocks, wedges, chains, and straps.

11. Equipment for Safegarding Ambulance Personnel—including gloves, safety goggles, helmets, tested lineman's gloves, and raingear.

12. Equipment for Warning and Signaling—to include flares, battery-powered hand lights, and floodlights.

13. Equipment to Extinguish Fire—to include the fire extinguishers required by local orders.

Remember that an EMT must be able to do more than carry out emergency care procedures. Gaining access, disentanglement and extrication, moving patients, and transferring patients are all part of the duties rendered.

NATIONAL ORGANIZATIONS

The National Registry of Emergency Medical Technicians (NREMT) exists to promote the improved delivery of emergency medical services by:

- Assisting in the development and evaluation of educational programs to train Emergency Medical Technicians
- Establishing qualifications for eligibility to apply for registration
- Preparing and conducting examinations designed to ensure the competency of Emergency Medical Technicians
- Establishing a system for biennial registration
- Establishing procedures for revocation of certificates of registration for cause
- Maintaining a directory of registered Emergency Medical Technicians.

Those applicants with the proper training must complete both written and practical examinations to be registered as an EMT-Ambulance, EMT-Intermediate, or EMT-Paramedic. The identification devices for members of the National Registry are shown in Figure 1-23. For more information, write:

The National Registry of Emergency
Medical Technicians
6610 Busch Blvd. P.O. Box 29233
Columbus, OH 43229

The National Association of Emergency Medical Technicians (NAEMT) promotes the professional status of EMTs, encouraging the constant upgrading of skills, abilities, qualifications, and educational requirements of EMTs. The NAEMT provides support for the creation and upgrading of EMS Systems. The association has state chapters open to any nationally or state certified EMT. For more information, write:

The National Association of Emergency
Medical Technicians
P.O. Box 334
Newton Highlands, MA 02161

The American Trauma Society is concerned with many aspects of emergency care, including educating the public as to the care of injured persons prior to the arrival of trained personnel. They are greatly concerned with specialized burn and trauma units for the critically injured. For more information, write:

Amercian Trauma Society
875 N. Michigan Avenue
Chicago, IL 60611

The National Association for Search and Rescue collects data, develops training programs, and participates in public education to help promote the im-

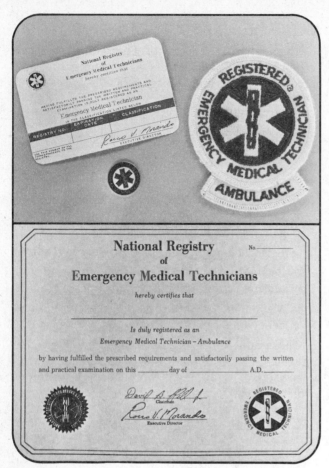

Figure 1-23: Identification devices for members of the National Registry of Emergency Medical Technicians.

plementation of a total, coordinated emergency response, rescue, and recovery system. For more information, write:

National Association for Search and Rescue
P.O. Box 2123
La Jolla, CA 92038

The National Council of State EMS Training Coordinators is involved with the national promotion of EMTs through standarization of courses, certification, reciprocity, and recertification. Concerned with more than training alone, the Council works with all activities required to upgrade the profession and to gain greater public recognition of the EMT and the EMS System. For more information, write:

The National Council of State EMS
  Training Coordinators
P.O. Box 197
Basking Ridge, NJ 07927

SUMMARY

The Emergency Medical Services System is a chain of human and physical resources established to provide complete emergency care. The Emergency Medical Technician is trained and certified to provide professional-level emergency care at the scene and during transport to a medical facility.

The primary concern of the EMT is the patient. To provide proper care, the EMT must carry out nine main duties. These duties include preparation to respond, responding, making certain the scene is safe, gaining access to the patient, finding out what is wrong with the patient and providing emergency care, freeing and moving the patient, transfer to the ambulance, transport and handing over the patient and patient information, and to return and prepare for the next run.

As an EMT, you may be called on to: drive an ambulance, control an accident scene, gain access in special situations, gather patient information, provide emergency care, provide emotional support, perform extrication, transport while monitoring the patient and communicating with the medical facility, transfer the patient over to the medical staff, and many other duties such as report writing and equipment inventory.

EMT-level emergency care deals with both injury and illness, ranging from emotional support to life support. Your duties are performed as part of an emergency care delivery subsystem consisting of EMTs, the ambulance, and equipment and supplies.

As an EMT, you are a professional, required to be pleasant, cooperative, resourceful, emotionally stable, and of good moral character. You must have leadership abilities and be a self-starter. You must be concerned with your personal appearance, your personal habits, and your conversation at the scene. All of these traits allow you to develop the calm professional manner needed to provide proper care.

In most states, specific laws have been written to allow you to provide emergency care. Good Samaritan laws provide most EMTs with immunity from civil liability. You are protected if you act in good faith, providing the EMT standard of care, to your level of training and to the best of your abilities.

Some patients can refuse your care. You must have actual consent from a conscious, clear-thinking adult patient. It must be informed consent, with the patient knowing your level of training and what you are going to do.

In cases when the patient is unable to give consent, you may care for the patient under the law of implied consent.

Implied consent can also apply to children, mentally disturbed, and mentally retarded patients when parents or legal guardians are not present.

When you begin to care for a patient, you have the responsibility to continue care until you are relieved by more highly trained personnel or until you have handed over the patient and patient information to the staff of a medical facility. If you start care and then stop, or if you leave the scene, you can be charged with abandonment.

Patients have a right to privacy. EMTs must respect patient confidentiality.

2 the human body

SKILLS As an EMT, you should be able to:

1. Apply the knowledge gained in this chapter so that you can look at a patient's body and mentally determine the positions of the major organs of the chest and abdomen.
2. Use correct terminology when communicating with other members of the patient care team.

TERMS you may be using for the first time:

Anatomical Position—the standard reference position for the body in the study of anatomy. The body is standing erect, facing the observer. The arms are down at the sides and the palms of the hands face forward.

Anterior—the front of the body or body part.

Posterior—the back of the body or body part.

Superior—toward the head. Often used in reference with inferior.

Inferior—away from the head. Usually compared with another structure which is closer to the head.

Midline—an imaginary line down the center of the body, dividing it into right and left halves.

Medial—toward the vertical midline of the body. Used only in reference to another body part. Thus, you can have a medial side to the arm.

Lateral—to the side, away from the midline of the body. Used only in reference to another body part.

Proximal—close to a point of reference or attachment (e.g., the shoulder or hip joint). Used as a comparison with distal.

Distal—away from a point of reference or attachment (e.g., the shoulder or hip joint). Used as a comparison with proximal.

Abduction—movement away from the midline.

Adduction—movement toward the midline.

Lateral Rotation—to turn the foot or hand outward away from the midline.

Medial Rotation—to turn the foot or hand inward toward the midline.

Flexion—to bend at a joint.

Extension—to straighten a joint.

Erect—the upright position.

Supine—lying on the back.

Prone—lying face down.

Lateral Recumbent—lying on the side.

Thorax (THO-raks)—the chest.

Diaphragm (DI-ah-fram)—the dome-shaped muscle of respiration that separates the chest and abdomen.

Thoracic (tho-RAS-ik) **Cavity**—the anterior body cavity above the diaphragm, containing the heart and the lungs.

Abdominopelvic (AB-dom-i-no-PEL-vik) **Cavity**—the anterior cavity below the diaphragm, made up of the abdominal portion and the pelvic portion. It is often referred to as two separate cavities.

Cranial (KRAY-ne-al) **Cavity**—the area within the braincase of the skull.

Spinal Cavity—the area within the spinal column that contains the spinal cord.

Abdominal Quadrants—the four zones of the abdomen used for quick reference.

Xiphoid (ZI-foyd) **Process**—the lower (inferior) extension of the sternum (breastbone).

Duodenum (du-o-DE-num or du-OD-e-num)—the first portion of the small intestine, beginning with its connection to the inferior portion of the stomach.

OVERVIEW OF THE HUMAN BODY

THE LANGUAGE OF EMERGENCY MEDICAL CARE

To learn the materials presented in your EMT course, you will have to understand what you hear and read. This chapter is an introduction to many of the terms used in your training. You need to be able to define these terms and apply them to your activities as an EMT.

Since you will be communicating with other professionals, you will have to use the vocabulary that is part of your profession. Written and oral reports will require you to use *medical terminology*. In addition, as an EMT, you will have many opportunities to read publications on emergency care and attend continuing education programs taught by physicians and other professionals in the EMS System. You will not be able to develop as a professional EMT unless you understand the terminology that applies to emergency medical care.

Appendix 3 contains a section on the formation of medical terms. You should read through the introduction to this section early in your course to see how medical terms can be divided into parts. Each week, you should go through part of the list provided in this appendix to increase your knowledge of medical terminology.

THE STUDY OF ANATOMY AND PHYSIOLOGY

Two terms appear early and often in an EMT training program. They are anatomy and physiology. **Anatomy** is the study of body structure, while **physiology** is the study of body function. As an EMT, you will have to know the major body structures and systems, and how these parts function. In general you will need a working knowledge of the body in order to do accurate patient assessments and provide efficient care.

It is impossible to learn all of basic anatomy in the standard EMT course. Nursing students average 180 classroom hours of anatomy and physiology study. This is more time than you will have for the entire EMT course. However, you will learn enough to understand EMT activities and care.

This chapter will not attempt to cover *all* the anatomy that is included in your training. Instead, it is meant to serve as a foundation for your studies. At the end of the chapter, additional illustrations are provided as quick references for anatomical landmarks and several of the body systems. In later chapters, we will present entire body systems, important aspects of physiology, and expand on the anatomy here. Throughout the text, anatomy and physiology will be related to patient assessment and specific care procedures.

First, learn to visualize where structures are located as you view a person who is fully clothed. This is the way you will find most patients. Then, start

looking for specific external body landmarks. These will help you locate structures within the body. Keep in mind that the patient's problem may be internal, but all you will be able to see is the external body.

Directional Terms

The following is a set of very basic terms to use when referring to the human body:

Anatomical (AN-a-tom-i-kal) **Position**—Consider the human body, standing erect, facing you. The arms are down at the sides with the palms of the hands facing forward. Unless otherwise indicated, all references to body structures are made when the body is in the anatomical position. This is very important when considering anatomical structures.

Right and **Left**—Always make reference to the patient's right and patient's left.

Anterior and **Posterior**—Anterior means the front of the body and posterior is used to indi-

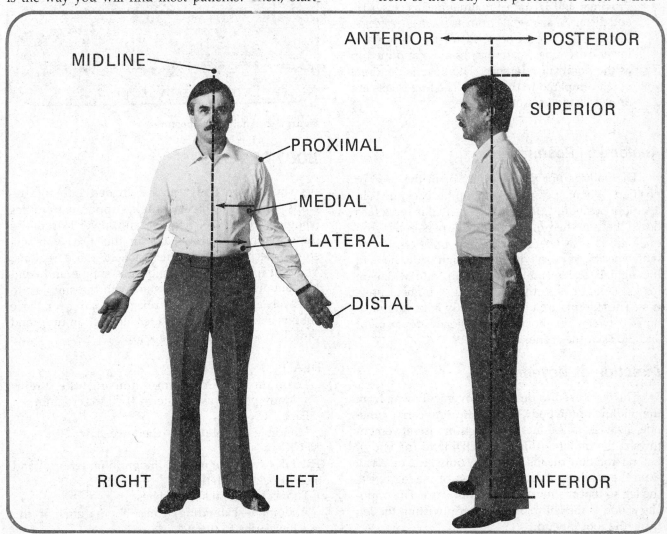

Figure 2-1: Directional terms.

cate the back of the body. For the head, the face and top are considered anterior, while all the remaining structures are posterior. The rest of the body can be divided easily into anterior and posterior by following the seams of your clothing.

Midline—Dividing the body into right and left halves with a vertical line. Anything toward the midline is said to be medial, while anything away from the midline is said to be lateral. Remember the anatomical position, with the thumb on the lateral side of the hand and the little finger on the medial side of the hand.

Superior and Inferior—Superior means toward the top or toward the head, as in the eyes are superior to the nose. Inferior means toward the bottom or toward the feet, as in the mouth is inferior to the nose. (Note: you cannot correctly say something is superior or inferior unless you are comparing at least two structures. The heart is not superior by itself; it is superior to the stomach.)

Proximal and Distal—Proximal means closer to, and distal means away from a *point of reference*. These terms are to be used for the upper and lower extremities, with the shoulder and the hip as the points of reference. The knee is proximal when compared to the ankle. The fingernails are on the distal ends of the fingers.

Anatomical Postures

The body is not always erect, or in the upright position. When a person is lying on his back, he is in a supine position. Conversely, when he is lying face down, he is in the prone position. A person lying on one side is in a lateral recumbent position. To be more specific, if he is lying on his right side, he is in the right lateral recumbent position, and when on his left side, he is in the left lateral recumbent position. These terms are used frequently in communications between the hospital emergency department and EMTs at the scene.

Direction of Movement

The term used to describe movement away from the midline of the body is abduction (to carry someone away is to ABduct). Adduction is movement toward the midline (think of ADDing to the body). Lateral rotation means to rotate outward, or away from the midline. A lateral rotation of the leg twists the leg so that the foot is turned outward. The opposite action is medial rotation, where twisting the leg turns the foot inward.

Flexion is the act of bending at a joint, and extension is the act of straightening. In following sec-

tions on basic life support, you will learn that the airway can become obstructed when the head is flexed forward.

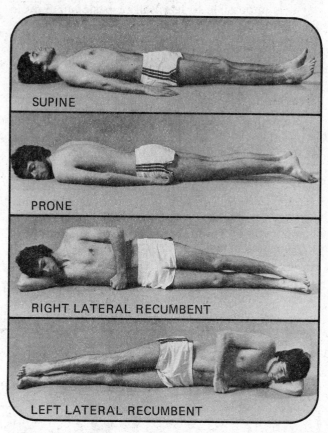

Figure 2-2: Anatomical postures.

BODY REGIONS

The human body can be divided into five regions: the head, neck, trunk, upper extremities (shoulders to tips of fingers), and lower extremities (hips to tips of toes). Later in this text, you will study specific areas within each of these regions. You will find that each region has simple and complex subdivisions. We will start with the simplest to give you an opportunity to begin looking for these subdivisions as you consider illness, injury, and care. For now, you need to know:

HEAD
  Cranium (KRAY-ne-um)—housing the brain. Many people use the term skull for cranium.
  Face
  Mandible (MAN-di-b'l)—the lower jaw
NECK
TRUNK—from the neck to the groin (anteriorly) and the buttocks (posteriorly)
  Thorax (THO-raks)—the chest
  Abdomen—extending from the margins of the lower ribs to the pelvis
  Pelvis—formed and protected by the bones of the pelvic girdle.

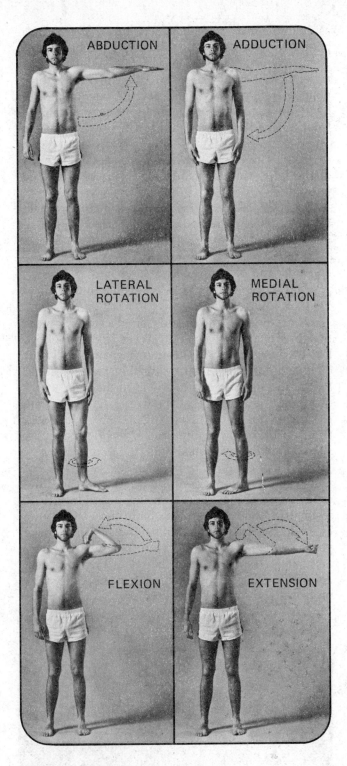

Figure 2-3: Directions of movement.

UPPER EXTREMITIES (as found on each side)
> Shoulder girdle and joint—composed of the scapula (SKAP-u-lah, shoulder blade) posteriorly, the clavicle (KLAV-i-kul, collarbone) anteriorly, and the joint formed by the head of the humerus (HU-mer-us, arm bone) and the scapula.
> Arm—sometimes referred to as the upper arm

Elbow	Hand
Forearm	Fingers
Wrist	

LOWER EXTREMITIES
> Pelvic girdle and joint—composed of the fused bones of the pelvis and lower spine, and the joint made with the femur (FE-mur, thigh bone)
> Thigh—extends from hip to knee
> Knee
> Leg—also called the lower leg or shin and calf
> Ankle
> Foot
> Toes

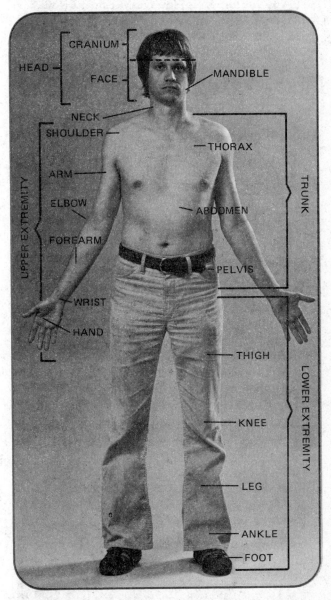

Figure 2-4: Body regions.

BODY CAVITIES

There are four major body cavities, two anterior and two posterior. They can also be called **ventral** (front) and **dorsal** (back) cavities. Housed in these cavities are the vital organs, glands, blood vessels and nerves.

Anterior Cavities

- **Thoracic** (tho-RAS-ik) **Cavity**—this is the entire chest cavity, enclosed by the rib cage, protecting the lungs, heart, great blood vessels, part of the **trachea** (windpipe), and most of the esophagus. The lower border of the thoracic cavity is the **diaphragm,** a dome-shaped muscle used in breathing. The diaphragm separates the thoracic cavity from the lower anterior cavity.

- **Abdominopelvic** (ab-DOM-i-no-PEL-vik) **Cavity**—The anterior body cavity below the diaphragm. There are two portions of the abdominopelvic cavity, abdominal and pelvic. Most people use the terms abdominal cavity and pelvic cavity as if they were two distinct cavities.

    Abdominal Cavity—Extending from the diaphragm to the rim formed by the pelvic bones. The liver, stomach, gallbladder, pancreas, spleen, small intestine, and most of the large intestine are found in this cavity. The abdominal cavity, unlike the other body cavities, is not surrounded by bones. If you consider all the organs in this cavity and the lack of bony protection, it is easy to see why blows to the abdomen can be so severe.

    Pelvic Cavity—Protected by the bones of the pelvic girdle, this cavity houses the urinary bladder, portions of the large intestine, and the internal reproductive organs.

Posterior Cavities

- **Cranial Cavity**—This is the braincase of the skull, housing the brain and its specialized membranes.

- **Spinal Cavity**—This cavity runs through the center of the backbone, protecting the spinal cord and its specialized membranes.

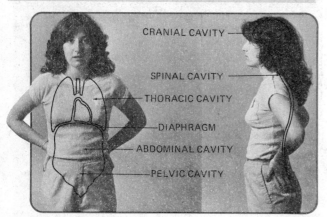

Figure 2-5: Body cavities.

Abdominal Quadrants

The abdomen is a large body region and the abdominal cavity contains many vital organs. In other body regions, bones may be used for reference, such

as counting ribs or feeling a bump or notch on a bone. This is not the case when trying to be specific about references to the areas of the abdomen. The navel or **umbilicus (um-BIL-i-kus)** is the only quick point of reference available for the beginning student. To improve this situation, four quadrants have been assigned to the abdominal wall (see Figure 2-6). These are the:

   Right Upper Quadrant (RUQ)—containing most of the liver, the gallbladder and part of the large intestine.

   Left Upper Quadrant (LUQ)—containing most of the stomach, the spleen, and part of the large intestine.

   Right Lower Quadrant (RLQ)—containing the appendix and part of the large intestine.

   Left Lower Quadrant (LLQ)—containing part of the large intestine.

Some organs and glands are located in more than one quadrant. As you can see from the above list, the large intestine is found, in part, in all four quadrants. The same is true for the small intestine. Part of the stomach can be found in the right upper quadrant. The left lobe of the liver extends into the left upper quadrant. Pelvic organs are included in these quadrants, with the urinary bladder being assigned to both lower quadrants.

The kidneys are a special case. They are not within the abdominal cavity, but located behind the cavity's membrane lining. Consider one kidney to be in the RUQ and the other to be in the LUQ. However, do not let this abdominal classification make you forget that the kidneys are behind the cavity and subject to injury from blows to the mid-back. Any pain or ache in the back may be caused by problems with the kidneys.

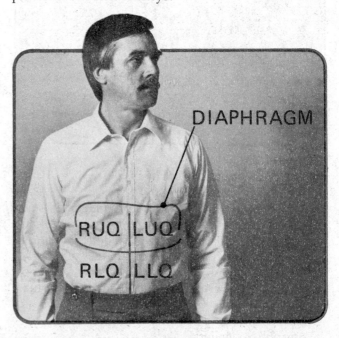

Figure 2-6: Abdominal quadrants.

BODY SYSTEMS

Knowing as much as you can about the body systems and their functions will prove to be of great value when you begin to provide emergency care. Remembering the different body functions can be useful when trying to determine the extent of injury or the nature of a medical emergency. Following is a list of the major body systems and their primary functions:

- *Circulatory System*—moves blood carrying oxygen and foods to the body's cells and removes wastes and carbon dioxide from these cells.

- *Respiratory System*—exchanges air to bring in oxygen and expel carbon dioxide. Oxygen is put into the bloodstream as carbon dioxide is removed to be expelled into the atmosphere.

- *Digestive System*—enables us to eat, digest, and absorb foods and provides for the removal of wastes.

- *Urinary System*—removes chemical wastes from the blood and helps balance water and salt levels of the blood.

- *Reproductive System*—the structures of the body involved with sexual reproduction. Sometimes classified with the urinary system as the genito-urinary (jen-E-to-U-re-NER-e) system.

- *Nervous System*—controls movement, interprets sensations, regulates body activities, and generates memory and thought.

- *Special Senses*—various organs that link with the nervous system to provide sight, hearing, taste, smell and the sensations of pain, cold, heat and tactile (touch) responses.

- *Endocrine* (EN-do-krin) *System*—produces the chemicals called hormones that help regulate most body activities and functions.

- *Musculoskeletal System*—bones provide protection and support, and skeletal muscles act with the bones to permit body movement.

- *Integumentary* (in-TEG-u-MEN-ta-re) *System*—the skin and its accessories (hair, oil glands, sweat glands, and nails).

- *Reticuloendothelial* (re-TIK-u-lo-EN-do-THE-li-al) *System*—a network of specialized cells found throughout the body's connective tissues. These cells function mainly to kill microorganisms (germs).

RELATING STRUCTURES TO THE BODY

In this section we will use a series of illustrations to show what you, as an EMT, should know about the general anatomy of the human body. Your problem is a complex one that requires much thought and practice before you are comfortable with the new knowledge gained in your training. Basically, you will be asked to consider your own body and the bodies of others, to visualize where structures are located within the body. As stated earlier, your job is to know where these structures are, in general, as you view the external body. On many of these illustrations, you will see a broken line representing the diaphragm. Being able to visualize the position of the diaphragm will greatly help you understand how the various organs and glands fit into the body.

Begin with Figure 2-7. Here we see the position of the *heart* in the thoracic cavity. As a quick point of reference, use your fingers to find a small hard spot just below your sternum (breastbone). This is the **xiphoid** (ZI-foyd) **process,** a major body landmark. You can find a point directly over the heart by measuring two finger-widths up from this point. Look at yourself in a mirror and find this point. Each time you look in the mirror during your training, try to visualize where your heart is located.

Figure 2-8 shows you the position of the *lungs* in the chest cavity. Notice that the lungs do not extend downward to the end of the rib cage. You have seen the anterior position of the diaphragm. This is the inferior border of the anterior lungs (note the use of the directional terms). By studying the illustration

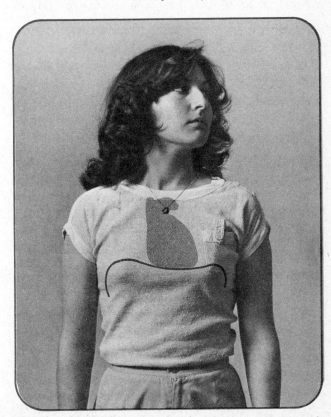

Figure 2-7: Position of the heart.

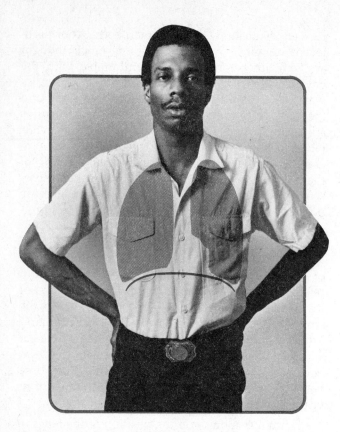

Figure 2-8: Position of the lungs.

in Figure 2-8, you will know the size, shape, and position of the lungs.

The two illustrations in Figure 2-9 show the positioning of the *stomach, liver,* and the first portion of

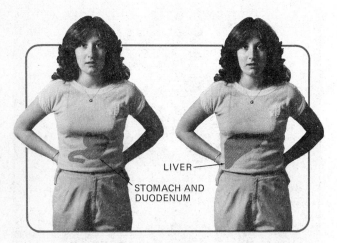

LIVER

STOMACH AND DUODENUM

Figure 2-9: Position of the stomach, duodenum, and liver.

the small intestine (called the **duodenum,** du-o-DEnum). Note how the lower ribs partially protect the stomach and liver. The point at which the esophagus enters the stomach, immediately after passing through the diaphragm, is at the level of the xiphoid process.

The duodenum is important in emergency medical care because it is held in a more rigid position than the rest of the small intestine. Forceful blows to

the abdomen, often received in motor vehicle accidents, may damage the duodenum without causing any significant damage to the rest of the intestine.

Before moving to the next illustration, you can add the positions of three other structures based on what you have already learned. Think of the *gallbladder* as being behind the liver, the *pancreas* as being behind the lower part of the stomach, and the *spleen* being behind the left side of the stomach. These descriptions are very general, but they will do for this stage of your training.

Figure 2-10 shows, on the left, the space occupied by the *small intestine.* As you can see, most of the abdominal cavity is filled with this structure. On

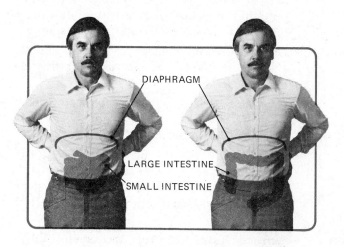

DIAPHRAGM

LARGE INTESTINE

SMALL INTESTINE

Figure 2-10: Position of the small and large intestines.

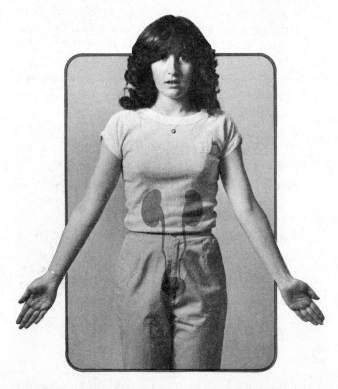

Figure 2-11: The urinary system.

MAJOR BODY ORGANS

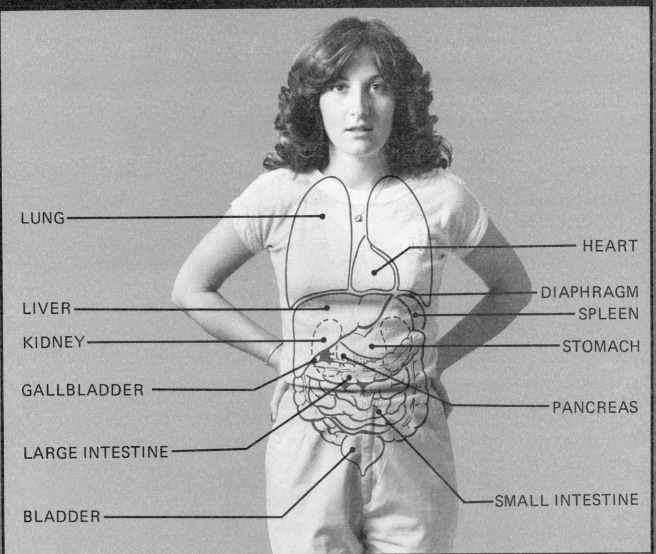

LUNG

LIVER

KIDNEY

GALLBLADDER

LARGE INTESTINE

BLADDER

HEART

DIAPHRAGM

SPLEEN

STOMACH

PANCREAS

SMALL INTESTINE

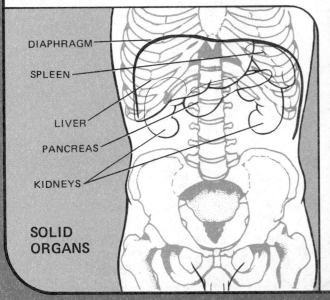

DIAPHRAGM

SPLEEN

LIVER

PANCREAS

KIDNEYS

SOLID ORGANS

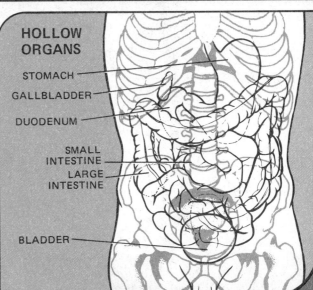

HOLLOW ORGANS

STOMACH

GALLBLADDER

DUODENUM

SMALL INTESTINE

LARGE INTESTINE

BLADDER

SCAN 2-1

the right you can see the space occupied by the *large intestine*. Do not try to memorize its shape, but do note how it passes through each of the four abdominal quadrants.

The *kidneys* and the *urinary bladder* are shown in Figure 2-11. Remember, the kidneys are behind the abdominal cavity and the bladder is in the pelvic cavity. Can you see why a lap seatbelt worn too tightly may cause a ruptured bladder during an auto accident?

You have spent a good deal of your time and effort on the illustrations dealing with the anterior cavities and their structures. Scansheet 2-1 sums up this material with an internal view of the hollow and solid organs. This is added here to review all that you have covered. Try to relate the position of those organs to the body's exterior.

SUMMARY

All references made to body structures consider the body to be in the anatomical position. Always use patient right and patient left. Remember that medial is toward the midline, while lateral is away from the midline.

1. ANTERIOR = front
2. POSTERIOR = back

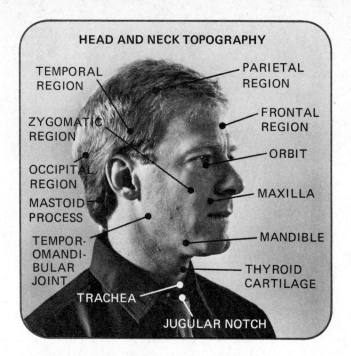

Figure 2-12: The head and neck.

3. SUPERIOR = top
4. INFERIOR = bottom
5. PROXIMAL = closest to the point of origin
6. DISTAL = farthest away from the origin

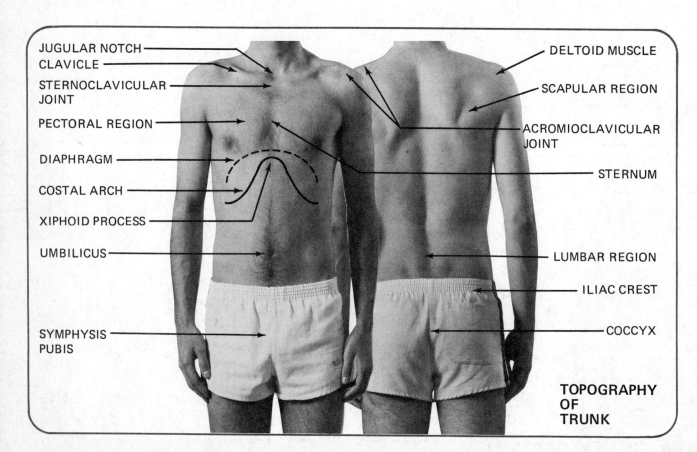

Figure 2-13: The chest, abdomen, and back.

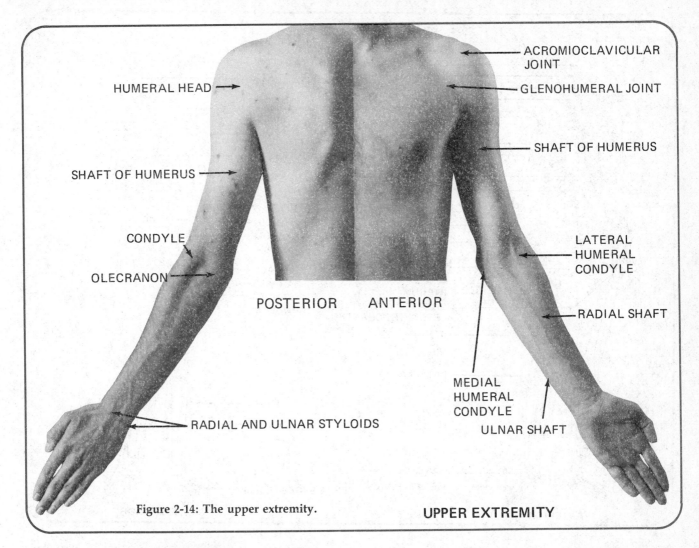

HUMERAL HEAD →

ACROMIOCLAVICULAR JOINT

GLENOHUMERAL JOINT

SHAFT OF HUMERUS

SHAFT OF HUMERUS →

CONDYLE

OLECRANON →

LATERAL HUMERAL CONDYLE

RADIAL SHAFT

POSTERIOR   ANTERIOR

MEDIAL HUMERAL CONDYLE

RADIAL AND ULNAR STYLOIDS

ULNAR SHAFT

Figure 2-14: The upper extremity.

UPPER EXTREMITY

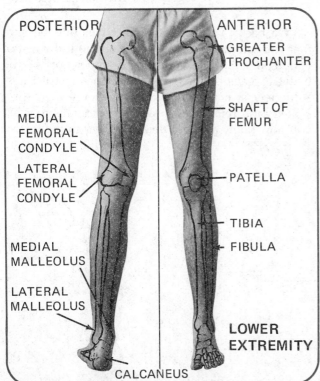

POSTERIOR   ANTERIOR

GREATER TROCHANTER

MEDIAL FEMORAL CONDYLE

LATERAL FEMORAL CONDYLE

SHAFT OF FEMUR

PATELLA

TIBIA

FIBULA

MEDIAL MALLEOLUS

LATERAL MALLEOLUS

LOWER EXTREMITY

CALCANEUS

Figure 2-15: The lower extremity.

There are two anterior body cavities: thoracic and abdominopelvic (abdominal and pelvic). The posterior body cavities are the cranial and the spinal.

Divide the abdomen into abdominal quadrants, right and left upper (RUQ, LUQ), and right and left lower (RLQ, LLQ).

Before returning to the list of objectives for Chapter 2, use your own body as a reference and:

1. Use the terms anterior, posterior, medial, and lateral.

2. Use the terms superior, inferior, proximal, and distal.

3. Outline your own major body cavities. Trace the anterior position of your diaphragm. Can you name the organs found in each cavity?

4. Point to each of your abdominal quadrants. Can you name the organs found in each quadrant?

5. Look in a mirror. Where are your heart, lungs, xiphoid process, liver, stomach, gallbladder, spleen, pancreas, small intestine, and large intestine? Can you locate your kidneys and your urinary bladder?

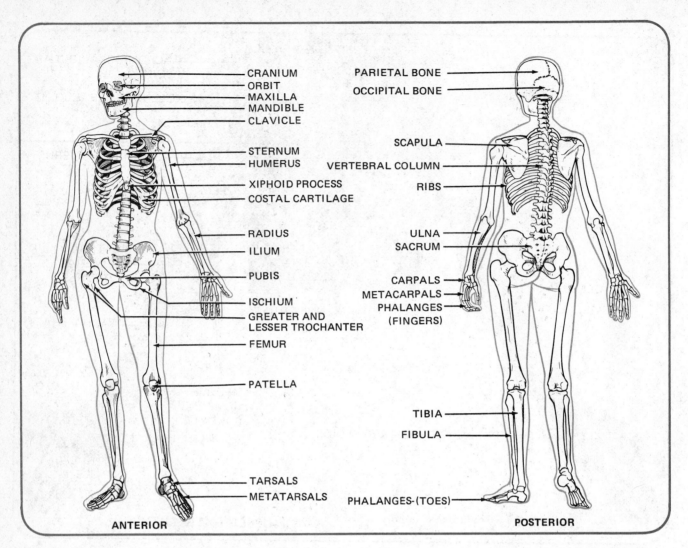

CRANIUM
ORBIT
MAXILLA
MANDIBLE
CLAVICLE

STERNUM
HUMERUS

XIPHOID PROCESS
COSTAL CARTILAGE

RADIUS
ILIUM

PUBIS

ISCHIUM
GREATER AND
LESSER TROCHANTER
FEMUR

PATELLA

TARSALS
METATARSALS

ANTERIOR

PARIETAL BONE
OCCIPITAL BONE

SCAPULA
VERTEBRAL COLUMN
RIBS

ULNA
SACRUM

CARPALS
METACARPALS
PHALANGES
(FINGERS)

TIBIA

FIBULA

PHALANGES-(TOES)

POSTERIOR

Figure 2-16: The skeletal system.

Go back to the chapter objectives and be sure that you can meet every one. Throughout the rest of your course, practice locating the position of the body's organs, glands, and other major structures. Add new structures to your list as they are presented, and remember to add more details to what you now know as these details appear in the text.

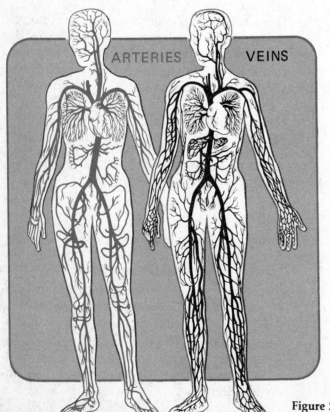

ARTERIES   VEINS

Figure 2-17: The circulatory system.

3 patient assessment

OBJECTIVES By the end of this chapter, you should be able to:

1. List the THREE major concerns you have as an EMT gathering information. (p. 32)

2. List at least FIVE problems at the emergency scene that can complicate the information gathering process. (p. 33)

3. State how you should identify yourself upon arrival at the emergency scene. (p. 33)

4. List SEVEN quick sources of patient information. (p.34)

5. Define mechanism of injury and relate types of accidents to types of injuries. (pp. 34–35)

6. Define primary survey, stating its purpose and indicating when it is done during the patient assessment. (pp. 36–39)

7. Describe how to determine patient responsiveness and indicate how you can tell if a patient is alert and oriented. (pp. 36, 43–44)

8. Describe how to assure an open airway and check a patient for adequate breathing. (pp. 36–37)

9. Describe how to detect a carotid pulse. (p. 37)

10. Define secondary survey, stating its purpose and when it is done during the patient assessment. (p. 39)

11. List the equipment an EMT should have for the secondary survey. (p. 40)

12. Define subjective interview and objective examination. (pp. 39–40)

13. Define symptom, sign, and vital sign. (p. 43)

14. List the major facts that should be sought during your interviews of patients and bystanders. (pp. 41–43)

15. Describe all the procedures used by an EMT in the gathering of vital signs. (pp. 43–49)

16. List, in the correct order, the steps of the head-to-toe survey. (pp. 49–59)

17. State the NINE examination rules you must consider when conducting the patient assessment. (pp. 44, 49, 51, 59)

SKILLS As an EMT, you must be able to:

1. Assure an open airway.

2. Take a carotid pulse, radial pulse, and pedal pulse, and determine rate, rhythm, and character of the radial pulse.

3. Determine respiratory rate and character.

4. Measure blood pressure by auscultation and palpation.

5. Determine relative skin temperature.

6. Gather information and conduct a primary survey and a secondary survey at the emergency scene.

7. Record and communicate the information gained from the patient assessment.

NOTE: In this chapter you will learn about patient assessment, including the physical examination of patients. We have presented the assessment in detail. Read through the chapter once, then use the SCANSHEETS and the SUMMARY to study each aspect of an assessment. Once you can list all the steps, go back and reread the detailed description, adding the additional information presented to your basic list of procedures.

TERMS you may be using for the first time.

Patient Assessment—the systematic gathering of information in order to determine a patient's illness or injury.

Mechanisms of Injury—what caused the injury, allowing you to relate types of accidents to certain types of injuries.

Primary Survey—a patient assessment process carried out to detect life-threatening problems. Basic life support is provided as needed during the primary survey.

Airway—the pathway from nose and mouth that carries air to the exchange levels of the lungs.

Carotid (kah-ROT-id) **Pulse**—the pulse that can be felt on each side of the patient's neck.

Secondary Survey—the procedure of the subjective interview, the taking of vital signs, and the head-to-toe survey of the patient.

Subjective Interview—using the patient and bystanders as sources of information by having them answer specific questions.

Objective Examination—a hands-on survey of the patient when you determine vital signs and do a head-to-toe survey.

Sphygmomanometer (SFIG-mo-mah-NOM-e-ter)—the cuff and gauge used in blood pressure determination.

Sign—what you see, hear, feel, and smell in relation to a patient's problem.

Vital Sign—pulse rate, rhythm, and character, respiratory rate and character, blood pressure, and temperature. Some approaches consider level of consciousness and pupils of the eyes to be part of the vital signs.

Symptom—what the patient tells you about his problem.

Radial Pulse—the wrist pulse.

Systolic (sis-TOL-ik) **Blood Pressure**—the pressure created in arteries when the lower left chamber of the heart contracts and forces blood out into circulation.

Diastolic (di-as-TOL-ik) **Blood Pressure**—the pressure in the arteries when the lower left chamber of the heart is refilling.

Auscultation (os-skul-TAY-shun)—the procedure using a blood pressure cuff and a stethoscope to determine blood pressure. This method requires you to listen for certain sounds in order to read systolic and diastolic blood pressure.

Palpate, Palpation—to feel, as to palpate the radial pulse. Also, to use the blood pressure cuff and the feeling of the radial pulse to determine approximate patient systolic blood pressure

Brachial (BRAY-key-al) **Artery**—the major artery supplying blood in the upper arm.

Cerebrospinal (ser-e-bro-SPI-nal) **Fluid**—the watery fluid that surrounds and protects the brain and spinal cord.

Stoma (STO-mah)—a permanent surgical opening made in the neck. A ''neck breather'' patient breathes through this opening.

Tracheostomy (TRA-ke-OS-to-me)—a surgical opening made through the anterior neck, entering into the windpipe (trachea).

Cervical (SER-ve-kal)—in reference to that portion of the spine which passes through the neck.

Clavicle (KLAV-i-kal)—collarbone.

Sternum (STER-num)—breastbone.

Pedal (PEED-al) **Pulse**—a foot pulse. There are two types, the dorsal pedis and the posterior tibial.

OBTAINING INFORMATION

Patient assessment is the gathering of the information needed to help determine what is wrong with the patient. During this process, your first concern is to detect and correct any life-threatening problems. Always keep this is mind. It is foolish to be gathering information from bystanders when the patient is in cardiac arrest (his heart has stopped beating). You would be a poor EMT if you checked a patient's pulse once and assumed it would not change. A patient assessment is a systematic procedure, but it is not always done step-by-step. A patient's condition may change, requiring you to stop

in the middle of an assessment and repeat a procedure you completed only seconds after you arrived. No matter where you are in the information gathering process, you must remember:

- Your First Concern is to identify and correct life-threatening problems.
- Your Second Concern is to identify any other injuries or medical problems and to provide basic EMT-level care to meet the needs of the patient.
- Your Third Concern is to keep the patient stable and continue monitoring the patient in case conditions worsen or improve.

PROBLEMS WITH ASSESSMENT

As an EMT, you may face all the problems that interfere with patient assessment in the hospital emergency department. In addition, you will have to overcome other problems that may be found at the emergency scene. Problems with assessment can include:

- Dangerous scenes (fires, collapsing buildings, etc.)
- Harsh environments (including unfavorable weather conditions)
- Uncooperative bystanders and motorists
- Uncooperative patients
- Special patients (children, elderly, blind, deaf, chronically ill, handicapped, and those affected by drugs, including alcohol)
- More than one patient
- Severe injuries (especially spinal injuries)
- Patients with more than one serious injury (multi-trauma)
- Grotesque injuries that tax your emotional stability

Each of these problems will be considered at various points throughout this text. Many are covered in Chapters 14 and 15. For now, we will *assume* that there are no problems at the scene of an accident or medical emergency. We will not worry about traffic, crowd control, fire, toxic gases, or possible falling objects. We will mention some special problems, such as spinal injury, but we will delay indepth studies of these problems until later.

ARRIVAL AT THE SCENE

Again, let us assume that the only problems at the scene will be injuries or medical emergencies. If you receive your calls from an efficient dispatching center, you may learn something of a person's illness or injury before leaving quarters. Even though this information can later prove to be erroneous, you can at least be thinking of what equipment you will have to remove from the ambulance and what special procedures may be required immediately upon arrival.

When you arrive at the scene, stay alert and begin to gather information. Do not allow the dispatcher's report or information given to you by untrained bystanders to be the basis of a quick conclusion. You will have to consider many factors before you will know what is wrong with a patient and what course of action you will take in order to provide emergency care.

Upon arrival you must:

1. State your name (and rank or classification, and the organization you represent).
2. Identify yourself as a trained Emergency Medical Technician (not everyone knows what "EMT" means).
3. Ask the patient if you may help.

While doing the above, remember to be looking for any obvious life-threatening problems.

Identifying yourself is very important, even if you believe the patient is unconscious. If you are in uniform, most patients and bystanders will respond to the uniform and let you take charge. When out of uniform, identifying yourself may be the only way you will be allowed to provide care. State your name and the name of your organization, and then the following: "I am an Emergency Medical Technician. I have been trained to provide emergency care." Even if you believe the patient to be unconscious, your next statement should be, "May I help you?" Keep in mind that some patients who appear to be unconscious may respond to your voice. Many patients maintain a functional sense of hearing, even when near death.

Surprisingly, some patients will say no to your offer of help. Usually, their fear is so great that they are confused. Simple conversation works best in gaining confidence. Even if the patient says no to your offer of help, continue to talk to him quietly, offering reassurance. In the vast majority of cases, the patient will allow you to help.

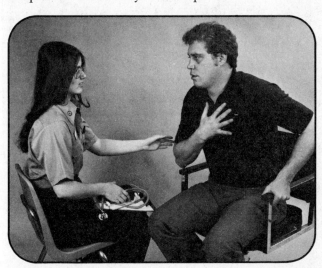

Figure 3-1: Proper identification is needed to enable you to provide patient care.

QUICK SOURCES OF INFORMATION

In a few seconds, you can gain valuable information as to what may be wrong with a patient. Now is not the time to ask a lot of questions, or to look over the entire scene trying to detect all possible causes of injury. You should not delay detection of life-threatening problems. Clues to the patient's problem will come from:

THE SCENE—Is it safe? Does the patient have to be moved? Are conditions harsh?

THE PATIENT—Is he alert, trying to tell you something or pointing to a part of his body?

BYSTANDERS—Are they trying to tell you something? Listen, they might be saying, "He's had a bad heart for years," "He was having chest pains before he fell," "He fell off that ladder."

MECHANISMS OF INJURY—Has something fallen on the patient? Is this a burn injury? Has the patient been thrown against the steering column?

DEFORMITIES OR INJURIES—Does the patient's body appear to be lying in a strange position? Is there blood around the patient? Are there burns, crushed limbs, or any obvious wounds?

SIGNS—What do you quickly see, hear, or smell when approaching the patient? Is there blood around the patient? Has he vomited? Is the patient having convulsions? Is there obvious pain?

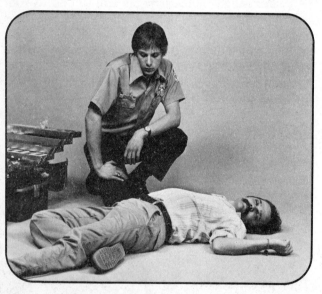

Figure 3-2. Obvious deformities and injuries may tell the extent of a patient's problem.

FIRST RESPONDERS

There will be times when the first person on the scene is someone with formal training in first aid, basic life support, or elementary emergency care. This person may be a police officer, a firefighter, or an industrial health officer. In some cases, this person may have advanced training, such as nursing. These people have traditionally been called first responders.

As an EMT, you will interact with first responders who have had American Red Cross training,

American Heart Association basic life support training, or special industrial first responder training. Today, many police officers, firefighters, and industrial health personnel are trained to Department of Transportation guidelines and are certified First Responders. As a member of the EMS System, you should respect the work done by all of these individuals as they attempt to help the patient and you at the emergency scene.

First responders can provide you with valuable information about the emergency, how the patient was acting when they arrived, what they found to be wrong with the patient, and what care procedures have been started. True, you will still have to do a patient assessment and you must evaluate the care already provided, but you should appreciate what the first responders have done before you arrived. Tactfully assume responsibility for the patient, remembering to thank the first responders and to give them credit for any prompt and efficient care they provided for the patient. Allow first responders to help when you need supervised assistance. When practical, point out any errors made by first responders, but do so tactfully and in private.

MECHANISMS OF INJURY

What caused the injury? If you know this, you can suspect certain types of injuries and be able to decide the possible extent of them.

All injuries can be classified into four broad categories. These are soft tissue injuries, fractures, dislocations, and internal injuries. The accidents that produce these injuries can also be categorized. According to the National Safety Council, people usually are injured in:

- Motor vehicle accidents
- Falls
- Fires and explosions
- Swimming and boating accidents
- Firearms accidents
- Poisonings by solids, liquids, and gases
- Machinery accidents
- Accidents involving electricity

Certain injuries must be considered "common" to each of the above accident situations. Fractured bones are usually associated with falls and motor vehicle accidents; burns are common to fires and explosions; soft tissue injuries can be associated with gunshot wounds, and so on.

Such an approach can be helpful, but do not allow yourself to develop "tunnel vision." Do not become so busy looking at or for one thing that you forget to consider all the major possibilities. A variety of injuries can be produced in any accident situation. For example, a patient who was in a fire may have burns, and he might also have lung damage from smoke and hot gases. Perhaps he fell trying to escape and fractured his leg. Appreciate what an accident can do to the human body, then you will not be easily led into missing an obvious injury, or overlooking hidden injuries.

Table 3.1: Types of Accidents and Their Expected Injuries

TYPES OF ACCIDENTS	THE EXPECTED INJURY (USUALLY OBVIOUS)	OTHER POSSIBLE INJURIES (NOT NECESSARILY OBVIOUS)
MOTOR VEHICLES	1,2,3,4	4
FALLS	2,3	4
FIRES, EXPLOSIONS	1	2,3,4
SWIMMING AND BOATING	4 (DROWNING)	1,2,3
FIREARMS	1	2,4
POISONING BY SOLIDS, LIQUIDS, GASES	4	1
MACHINERY	1,2,3,4	
ELECTRIC SHOCK	4 (CARDIAC ARREST)	1,2,3

1—*Soft Tissue Injuries*   3—*Dislocations*
2—*Fractures*   4—*Internal Injuries*

Knowing mechanisms of injury is very important when dealing with motor vehicle accidents. A collapsed or bent steering column suggests that the

driver has suffered a chest wall injury, possible lung damage, and perhaps damage to the heart. A bent steering wheel tells of the possibility of fractured ribs. A shattered, blood-spattered windshield may point to the likelihood of a forehead or scalp **laceration** (cut), and possibly a severe blow to the head that may have caused brain damage. A lap belt too tightly applied can produce abdominal and pelvic injuries, while an improperly applied shoulder belt may cause fractures to the **clavicle** (collarbone).

REMEMBER: For every obvious injury, there may be a number of hidden ones. Knowing what an accident can do and being able to recognize the mechanisms of injury are important to the patient assessment procedure.

THE FIELD ASSESSMENT

The quick sources of information provide you with a starting point to begin your field assessment of a patient. This assessment must:

- Be appropriate for both medical and trauma emergencies.
- Allow for the quick detection of life-threatening problems.
- Enable you to detect problems that are not immediately life-threatening, but may be if they are allowed to remain uncorrected.
- Be organized to allow for effective communications with the emergency department.
- Include questioning of the conscious patient as well as a hands-on physical examination.
- Take only a few minutes to carefully complete.

Not every person requiring emergency care will have to be surveyed to the depth suggested in this chapter. When a patient's problem is purely medical, and he or she is able to tell you so, there will probably be no need for an in-depth survey. Keep in mind that some medical emergencies may cause a person to fall and injure himself. You must rule out this possibility by questioning the patient. Accident victims, on the other hand, should always be surveyed even when they are conscious and coherent. Of course, if a life-threatening problem is found, it is to be corrected immediately. You should never delay basic life support in order to conduct a complete hands-on examination. Every unconscious patient should be thoroughly examined, regardless of whether the emergency is due to illness or injury.

The field examination consists of the primary survey and the secondary survey.

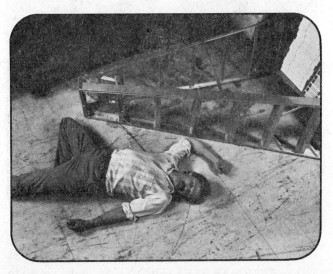

Figure 3-3: Mechanisms of injury provide valuable clues to the nature of a person's injury.

REMEMBER: Learning the steps of the field examination is a simple matter, but you must know more than how to conduct a primary and secondary survey. Unless you understand the significance of the information gathered during a patient assessment, you may not be able to provide the proper care for the patient.

THE PRIMARY SURVEY

The **primary survey** is a process carried out to detect life-threatening problems. As these problems are detected, lifesaving measures are taken. Many conditions can become life-threatening if they remain uncorrected; however, certain problems require immediate attention. An obstructed airway quickly leads to respiratory arrest. Cardiac arrest will occur shortly after respiratory arrest. If a patient's heart is not beating, changes will begin to occur in the brain in four to six minutes. Brain cell death will begin within ten minutes of cardiac arrest. Profuse bleeding is another problem requiring immediate attention. Such bleeding will quickly produce severe shock, leading to death within a few minutes.

The primary survey does not require any special instruments or equipment. You are concerned with the **ABC's of emergency care:**

> **A = AIRWAY:** You must assure an open airway.
> **B = BREATHING:** You must assure adequate breathing.
> **C = CIRCULATION:** You must be sure the heart is beating and that bleeding is not profuse.

Your course and local requirements may state that you should check the patient's pupils and look for medical identification devices during the primary survey. Your instructor is the authority on such matters.

As an EMT, the primary survey procedures you should follow are:

1. Check for RESPONSIVENESS. A conscious patient indicates breathing and circulation. Breathing may not be adequate and you may have to clear the airway, but the patient is breathing. Keep in mind that consciousness may be lost quickly, breathing may change, and circulation may stop. To check for responsiveness, gently tap the patient's shoulders and shout: ''Are you okay? . . . Are you okay? . . . Are you okay?''

2. If the patient is unresponsive, check for BREATHING by assuring an open airway and determining adequate breathing.

OPEN AIRWAY—For cases in which you do not suspect spinal injury, position yourself at the patient's side. Perform a **Head Tilt-Neck Lift** by placing one hand on his forehead and your other hand behind his neck. With your hands so positioned, gently push down on the forehead and lift the neck. This *hyperextends* the neck and places the airway in a favorable position for air flow. Another method, the **Head Tilt-Chin Lift**, may be suggested in your course. If so, see Chapter 4. For patients with possible spinal injury, you should use the **Modified Jaw-Thrust** described in Chapter 4. Most EMS Systems treat all unconscious accident victims as if they have spinal injuries.

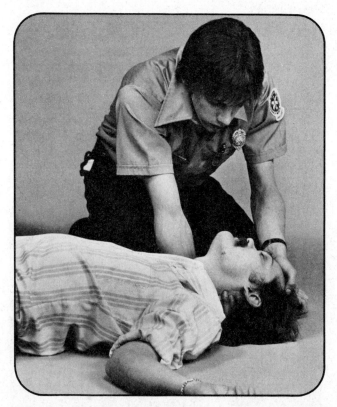

Figure 3-5: Assure an open airway.

ADEQUATE BREATHING—You must check to assure that there is sufficient air exchange. Posi-

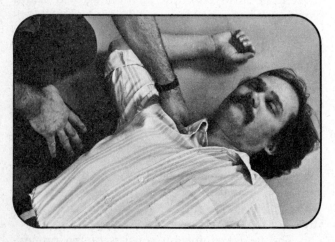

Figure 3-4: Establish responsiveness.

tion the side of your head close to the patient's face, then LOOK, LISTEN, and FEEL.

LOOK for chest movements that are associated with breathing. (NOTE: Males show the most pronounced respiratory movement at the level of the diaphragm. Females show more pronounced movement at the clavicles.)

LISTEN for air moving at the patient's mouth and nose.

FEEL for air being expired through the patient's nose and mouth.

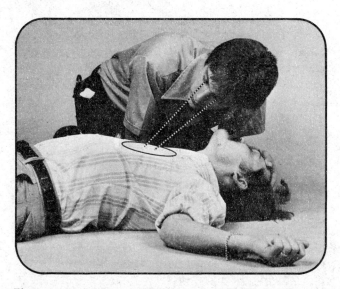

Figure 3-6: LOOK, LISTEN, and FEEL for adequate breathing.

If the patient is not breathing, or if there is an airway obstruction, YOU MUST TAKE IMMEDIATE ACTION. The procedures to follow are covered in Chapter 4. If the patient is breathing adequately through an open airway, continue the primary survey.

You may find it difficult to determine if an unconscious patient in the prone position has an open airway and adequate breathing. Even though you have not surveyed the patient for possible spinal and other serious injuries, you may have to place him in a supine position. If the patient is not breathing, or you cannot tell if he is breathing, use a simple **log-roll maneuver** to move the patient from a prone to a supine position. This can be done by using the four-rescuer log roll described in Chapter 10. If you are working alone, kneel at the patient's side, leaving enough room so that he will not roll onto your lap. Gently straighten his legs and position the arm that is closest to you above his head. Place one of your hands so that it cradles the head and neck from behind. Place your other hand on the patient's distant shoulder. Move the patient as a unit onto his side and then onto his back. You must move his head, neck, and torso as a unit to reduce aggravations to spinal column injuries.

3. Check for CIRCULATION. If the patient has been in respiratory arrest for a few minutes, he may have developed cardiac arrest as well. Also, some patients with very erratic chest movements may not be exchanging air and may have developed cardiac arrest. Determine if there is heart action and blood circulation by palpating (feeling for) a **carotid** (kah-ROT-id) **pulse.** Locate the patient's "Adam's apple" (the most prominent part of the thyroid cartilage) and place the tips of your index and middle fingers directly over the midline of this structure. Slide your fingertips to the side of the patient's neck closest to you. Keep the palm side of your fingertips against the patient's neck.

Do NOT slide your fingertips to the opposite side of the patient's neck. A sudden movement or convulsion by the patient may cause you to inflict further injury. Very little pressure need be applied to the neck to feel the carotid pulse. Do not use your thumb to feel for the carotid pulse. Precise pulse rate is not important.

If there is no carotid pulse, basic life support measures, in the form of **cardiopulmonary resuscitation** (KAR-de-o-PUL-mo-ner-e re-SUS-ci-TA-shun), known as CPR, will have to be initiated. If there is a pulse, but no breathing, continue efforts at artificial ventilation, checking periodically for a carotid pulse. If the patient is breathing and has a carotid pulse, then continue with the primary survey.

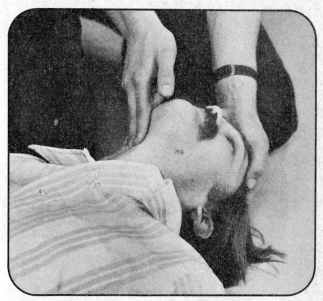

Figure 3-7: A quick check of the carotid pulse confirms circulation.

4. Check for PROFUSE BLEEDING. Only *profuse* bleeding is considered during the primary survey. Look and feel for this bleeding, but do so with extreme care. Keep in mind that the patient may have spinal injuries and other serious injuries requiring him to be kept still.

PRIMARY SURVEY

A ESTABLISH AIRWAY

B LOOK, LISTEN AND FEEL FOR BREATHING

C CIRCULATION
• PULSE
• PROFUSE BLEEDING

SCAN 3-1

Bleeding wounds are not always as severe as they may first appear, so be certain that you are dealing with bleeding that requires immediate action. Look for wounds from which blood is *spurting* or *flowing freely*. Methods to control such bleeding will be covered in Chapter 7.

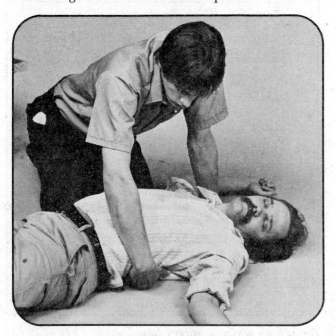

Figure 3-8: Locate and control all profuse bleeding.

There are special cases when you find a patient has been bleeding slowly for a long period of time. Such cases require you to consider any additional bleeding as life-threatening. Taking care not to aggravate spinal and other serious injuries, control bleeding and begin to treat for shock immediately following the primary survey.

In situations where you immediately notice profuse bleeding you may have to begin to control it while, at the same time, you begin to check for respiration. Keep in mind that severe bleeding, with blood spurting from a wound, indicates some heart action (circulation). Remember, even though bleeding is occurring, respiration cannot be ignored.

Upon completing the primary survey, assured that the patient has an open airway, adequate breathing, a carotid pulse, and any profuse bleeding is controlled, you should proceed to the next phase of patient assessment.

THE SECONDARY SURVEY

The objective of the secondary survey is to discover medical and injury-related problems that do not pose an immediate threat to survival, but *may* if allowed to go untreated. There are two parts to the secondary survey, the subjective interview and the objective examination.

The **subjective interview** is not unlike that conducted by a physician prior to a complete physical examination. During the interview, whenever possible, use the patient as a source of information. Relatives and bystanders also may serve as sources of information.

The **objective examination** is a comprehensive hands-on, head-to-toe survey, during which you check the patient's body for less-than-obvious injuries or the effects of illness. The findings from the interview and the examination are combined and related to allow you to make an assessment of your patient's condition and form a plan of emergency care.

You must be realistic when conducting a secondary survey. If you are too systematic, you may find yourself asking the patient a lot of questions while he becomes upset because he simply wants you to look at his leg. In such cases, you may find yourself doing two things at once during the survey. Your activities must fit the situation.

Keep in mind that you will have to reconsider and re-evaluate some of the things you did upon arrival at the scene. Since the primary survey has to begin as soon as possible, you may have missed something, or something may have changed. Before starting the secondary survey, always:

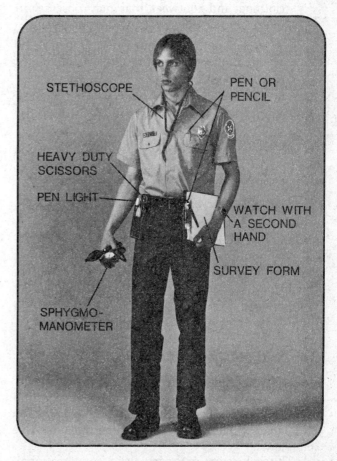

Figure 3-9: A few items are needed for the secondary survey.

- Look over the scene—Is it still safe? Did you overlook a mechanism of injury? Are there any other patients in need of attention?
- Look over your patient—Are there obvious injuries or indications of illness? Is his condition deteriorating? Is the patient wearing a medical identification necklace or bracelet you can read without moving the patient?

Examination Equipment.   Unlike the primary survey, which required no special equipment or instruments, the secondary survey requires some basic items, including:

- A **sphygmomanometer** (SFIG-mo-mah-NOM-e-ter), commonly called a blood pressure cuff—required to measure and monitor blood pressure.
- A stethoscope—used in conjunction with a blood pressure cuff in the determination of blood pressure. A stethoscope can also be used for listening to the sounds of air entering and leaving the lungs.
- A pen light—useful not only in poorly lighted situations, but also for examining the mouth, nose, ears, and pupils.
- Heavy duty bandage scissors—to cut away clothing and footwear that may obscure an injury site, or prevent access to a pulse site.
- A pocket notebook and a pen or pencil—to record the results of the survey and to list actions taken.
- A watch with either a sweep second hand or digital seconds counter—to measure pulse and respiration rates.

Several examination instruments can be carried in a handy belt holster.

The Survey Form.   A standard survey form provides a quick, positive means of recording information obtained during the interview and examination. This form is a legal document and becomes part of the patient's medical records. Findings should be recorded as they are found. The survey procedure can be speeded up if one EMT conducts the survey while another records the findings.

The Subjective Interview

Use your time wisely at the emergency scene. As you become an experienced EMT, you will find that it is possible to begin the physical examination of a patient while you are conducting the subjective interview.

The subjective interview is a conversational, information-gathering effort. When a patient is un-

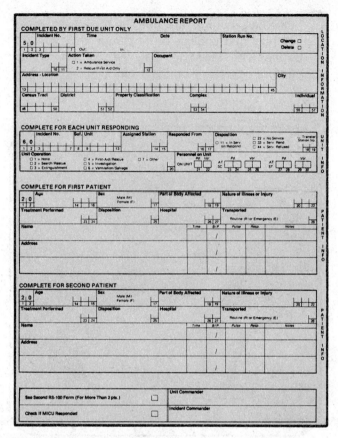

Figure 3-10: A typical survey form.

conscious, you may gain some of this same type of information from bystanders and medical identification devices. However, with the unconscious patient, this information will have to be gained while the physical examination is taking place. With a conscious patient, you should conduct an interview. Not only will you gain needed information, but you will also reduce the patient's fear and promote cooperation.

When conducting a patient interview, you should:

1. *Position yourself close to the patient.* Depending upon the patient's situation, kneel or stand close to him. If possible, position yourself so that the sun or bright lights are not at your back. When practical, allow the patient to see your face.
2. *Identify yourself and reassure your patient.* It is important that the patient know he is in competent hands. Maintain eye contact with the patient and state your name, that you are an Emergency Medical Technician, and the organization you represent.

Speak in your normal voice. If you ask a question, wait for a reply. Remember, at first the patient may not want you to help. Work to gain his confidence through calm conversation. Avoid inappropriate remarks like ''Don't worry,'' and ''Everything is all right.''

Gently touch the patient's shoulder, or rest your hand over his. A simple touch is comforting to most people. Keep in mind that a sign of caring for the sick and injured is to place the back of your hand on a person's forehead. Not only will you help reassure the patient, but you will also gain information about his skin temperature.

3. *Learn your patient's name.* Once you know it, use it in the rest of your conversations. You need the patient's name for completion of your evaluation forms and to give a personal touch that is often very reassuring to the patient.

4. *Learn your patient's age.* This may not be required in your locality, but some areas need this for reports and transmissions to the medical facility. If you cannot judge your patient as to a general age (early adulthood, middle adulthood, late adulthood, etc.), always ask his age.

Children expect to be asked their age. To do so will help keep a "normal" tone to the conversation. You should ask adolescents their age to be certain you are dealing with a minor.

It is a good idea to ask minors how you can contact their parents. Sometimes this question upsets children because it intensifies their fear of being sick or hurt without their parents being there to help. Be prepared to offer comfort and assure the child that someone will contact the parents.

5. *Seek out what is wrong.* This is the patient's primary complaint. Ask your patient where he hurts. Unless the pain of one injury masks that of another, or unless a spinal injury has interrupted nerve pathways, most injured people will be able to tell you of painful areas. A sick person will be able to tell you of pain or discomfort.

When your patient has been injured in an accident, ask him if he has numbness, tingling, burning, or any other unusual sensations in his arms or legs. Such sensations in the extremities suggest damage to the spinal cord and warn you against moving the patient any more than necessary during the remainder of the survey.

As you learn more about specific illnesses and injuries, you will see what additional questions can be asked to develop a list of symptoms.

6. *In cases of injury—ask how it happened.* You are trying to learn the circumstances of the complaint. In an accident, try to determine exactly how the injury was sustained. Knowing how the patient was injured will help direct you to problems that may not be noticeable to you or the patient. Anytime you come upon a patient who is lying down, always find out if he lay down,

was knocked down, fell, or was thrown into that position. Do this even if the patient's primary complaint appears to be medical. The knowledge gained could help direct you to possible spinal injuries and internal bleeding.

In accidents involving two parties, such as automobile accidents, word your questions with great care. If you say, "What happened?", you may find yourself listening to a story of how 'the other person was wrong.' Some bystanders wait for the question to be asked so they can tell their stories. Learn to ask specific questions such as, "Did you hit the dash (windshield, steering wheel)?," and "Were you thrown from the car?" to provide you with better information.

In cases of illness—how long has he felt ill. You will need to know if the problem occurred suddenly, has been developing over the past few days, or has taken some time to develop.

7. *Learn if the problem has happened before or if the patient has ever felt this way before.* You are seeking any previous relevant experience. Injuries and illness alike can sometimes be attributed to a past medical condition. Certain accidents, such as falling from a ladder, may keep happening to a patient, indicating a possible medical problem. If the patient complains of shortness of breath, dizziness or chills, chest pains, or some other medical problem, then you need to know if this is the first time or a recurring problem.

8. *Determine current medical status.* Find out if the patient has been having any medical problems. Has he been feeling ill? Has he been seeing a doctor? If so, then ask the patient for the name of his physician. Keep in mind that you may need to transmit this information to the emergency department staff, so they can contact the doctor and possibly learn what may be critical in helping the patient.

9. *Find out if any medications are being taken.* Again, such information could prove to be critical to the emergency department staff. If you fail to ask and the patient becomes unconscious, this information may take hours, if not days, to determine. Use the word "medication." The word "drugs" implies illicit use. If the patient is on medications that are at the scene, gather all the containers and transport them with the patient.

10. *Ask if the patient has any known allergies.* Any medical problem or injury may prove to be enough for a patient to handle. The health care team needs to know if a patient is allergic to a medication or some other substances or foods so that these things can be kept away from the patient.

You may question the need for the subjective

interview and even argue the merit of asking questions that appear to have no direct bearing on emergency care measures. It takes only a few minutes to conduct the interview, however, and the brief history obtained may gain information that is essential to patient care. This is especially true if the patient loses consciousness before he can be interviewed by the emergency department staff.

Remember, conduct the interview in a calm, professional manner. Avoid inappropriate conversation. A typical interview might be as follows:

EMT: Good morning, I'm Mark Bennett. I'm an Emergency Medical Technician with the Glen Echo Fire Department. May I help you?

PT: Please!

EMT: Sir, would you tell me your name?

PT: I'm Tom Henderson.

EMT: Mr. Henderson, I'd like to ask you a few questions. Would that be all right with you?

PT: Sure. (If the patient says, "Look! I'm in pain!", then skip to his primary complaint.)

EMT: Would you tell me how old you are?

PT: I'm 34.

EMT: Mr. Henderson, can you tell me where you hurt?

PT: My right leg hurts, and I have an awful headache.

EMT: Do you have any numbness, or is there any tingling or burning in your arms or legs?

PT: No.

EMT: Do you remember what happened, Mr. Henderson?

PT: I was up on the ladder working on the light.

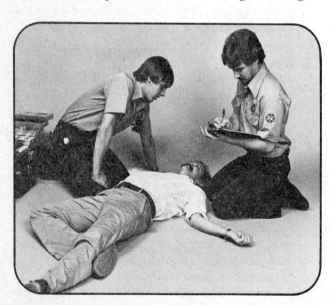

Figure 3-11: A carefully conducted interview can be as important as the physical examination.

I don't remember whether I leaned over too far, or whether I got dizzy and slipped.

EMT: You said you may have had a dizzy spell, Mr. Henderson. Have you ever had a dizzy spell before?

PT: I get light-headed every once in a while, but the spell usually passes quickly.

EMT: Mr. Henderson, are you under a doctor's care at this time?

PT: Yes, Dr. Johnson.

EMT: What is Dr. Johnson treating you for?

PT: High blood pressure.

EMT: Are you taking any medications?

PT: Water pills.

EMT: Are you allergic to anything, Mr. Henderson?

PT: Not that I know of.

The above interview went well and information was gathered by the EMT. However, what if Mr. Henderson were unconscious? In such cases, you will have to depend on first responders, bystanders, medical identification devices, and your own suspicions based upon the mechanism of injury.

When interviewing bystanders, determine if any are relatives or friends of the patient. They usually have more information to provide about past problems. See which of the bystanders saw what happened. When questioning bystanders, you should ask:

1. *The patient's name.* If the patient is obviously a minor, you should ask if the parents are present, or if they have been contacted.

2. *What happened?* You may be told that the patient fell off a ladder, appeared to faint, was hit on the head by a falling object, or any other possible clues.

3. *Did they see anything else?* For example, was the patient clutching his chest or head before he fell?

4. *Did the patient complain of anything before this happened?* You may learn of chest pains, nausea, concern about odors where he was working, or other clues to the problem.

5. *Did the patient have known illnesses or problems?* This may provide you with information about heart problems, alcohol abuse, or other problems that could cause a change in the patient's condition.

6. *Do they know if the patient was taking any medications?* Be sure to use the words "medications" or "medicines." If you say "drugs" or some other term, bystanders may not answer you, thinking that you are asking questions as part of a criminal investigation. In rare cases, you may feel that the bystanders are holding back information because

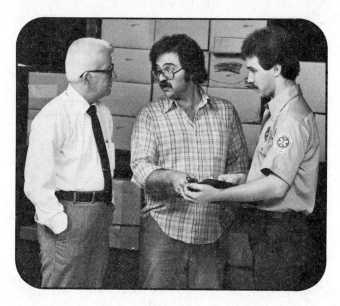

Figure 3-12: Relatives, witnesses, and other bystanders may be able to provide important information.

the patient was abusing drugs. Remind them that you are an EMT and you need all the information they can give you so proper care can begin.

If your patient is the victim of a motor vehicle accident and was taken from the wreckage prior to your arrival, ask if he was the driver or a passenger. You can often associate the mechanism of injury with where a person was sitting in a vehicle. Also ask if the person was alert when he was extricated and if he has lost consciousness, even for a brief moment.

Do NOT ask questions as an isolated part of the secondary survey. You can be active, beginning the examination while you ask questions and listen to bystanders' answers.

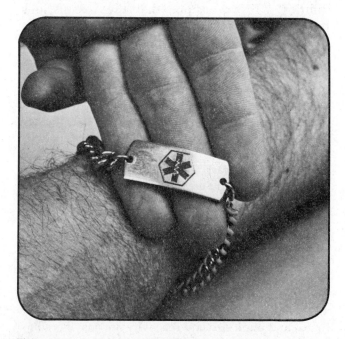

Figure 3-13: A medical identification device.

Medical identification devices can provide needed information. One of the most commonly used medical-alerting devices is the Medic Alert emblem shown in Figure 3-13. Over one million people wear a medical identification device in the form of a necklace, wrist, or ankle bracelet. One side of the device has a star of life emblem. The patient's medical problem is engraved on the reverse side, along with a telephone number to call for additional information. Look for necklaces and bracelets. Never assume you know the form of every medical identification device. Check carefully, without moving the patient or any of his extremities, for any necklace or bracelet. You should alert the emergency department staff (usually by radio transmission) that the patient is wearing a medical identification device. Give the staff the wearer's identification number, the nature of the problem, and the phone number they are to call.

Do not move the patient to reach for his wallet to find a medical alert card. You should not check his wallet unless you are directed to do so on the bracelet or necklace. If there is any chance of spinal injury, you should not move the patient to gain access to his wallet. To do so may cause severe injury to the patient.

The Objective Examination

The objective examination begins the search for very specific signs and symptoms. Before going on, make certain you understand the following terms:

Symptoms—What the patient tells you is wrong. Such things as chest pains, dizziness, and nausea are considered symptoms. Many of these may have been gathered through the interview with the patient. Others can be gained by continuing to ask questions during the examination.

Signs—What you see, hear, feel, and smell when examining the patient. Since you will use these signs to try to determine what is wrong with the patient, they are sometimes called diagnostic signs.

Vital Signs—Pulse, respiration, blood pressure, and skin temperature. Some localities also use pupils, skin color, and level of consciousness.

The objective examination of your patient begins with taking vital signs and continues with a head-to-toe examination. When the patient is alert, be certain to obtain actual consent before starting your examination. Before you obtain vital signs, lean back and TAKE A GOOD LOOK AT YOUR PATIENT. Note whatever you can that is obvious about his condition.

First, determine the patient's **level of consciousness** and orientation. Determining if the patient is conscious or unconscious is no problem; it is the *level* of consciousness that requires special skills.

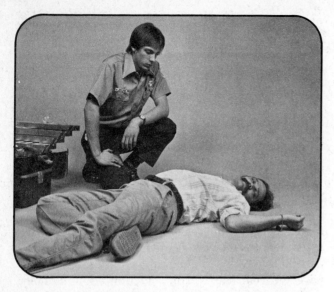

Figure 3-14: Briefly observe the patient before beginning the objective examination.

Table 3.2: Medical Significance of Changes in Skin Color

Skin Color	Possible Cause of Abnormality
Red	High blood pressure, stroke, heart attack, alcohol abuse, sunburn, infectious disease, simple blushing
Cherry red	Carbon monoxide poisoning
White	Shock, heart attack, fright, anemia, simple fainting, emotional distress
Blue	Asphyxia (suffocation), hypoxia (lack of oxygen), heart attack, poisoning
Yellow	Liver disease
Black and blue	Seepage of blood under skin surface

Many terms are used to describe a person's level of consciousness—semiconscious, incoherent, hysterical, stuporous, and so on. Do NOT depend upon these terms to give you a quick classification of the patient. Instead, as you ask questions and ask the patient to do specific things, simply note whether he is alert and oriented to what you are doing. An alert person is aware of what is going on around him. He knows who he is, where he is, the day's date, and he can respond quickly to both vocal and physical stimuli. A confused, disoriented person usually has trouble answering questions and responding to specific instructions. Experience will soon allow you to determine easily a person's level of consciousness.

EXAMINATION RULE #1: If you notice anything unusual about a patient's awareness or behavior, consider that something may be seriously wrong with the patient.

Look for *change* as you continue the survey. Be on the alert for loss of awareness, failing respiration, distress due to pain, new bleeding, and indications of the onset of shock, such as restlessness, anxiety, and profuse sweating. Remember that patient improvement is also a change to be noted.

EXAMINATION RULE #2: Even patients who appear to be stable may worsen rapidly. An EMT must always be aware of changes in a patient's condition. Constant monitoring of patients is an essential part of basic emergency care.

Observe your patient's *skin color and condition.* A great deal of emphasis is often placed on the significance of a sick or injured person's color. Skin color suggests a variety of medical problems.

You need to note any odd colorations of the patient's skin and stay alert for changes. When a person has deeply pigmented or dark skin, it may be necessary to look for color changes in the lips, nailbeds, earlobes, tongue, and whites of the eyes.

EXAMINATION RULE #3: You must watch the patient's skin for color changes.

Quickly look for obvious wound sites, burns, fractures and any obvious deformities, swellings and puffiness, ulcers and blotches on the skin, and any blood-soaked areas.

EXAMINATION RULE #4: You must look over the patient and note ANYTHING that looks wrong.

Spinal injuries can occur during accidents, even in apparently minor accidents. Keep in mind that a patient with a medical emergency may have fallen and hurt his spine. You must conduct the physical examination *without* aggravating spinal injuries.

EXAMINATION RULE #5: Unless you are certain that you are dealing with a patient free from serious spinal injury, *assume* the patient has such injuries. Always assume that the unconscious trauma patient has a spinal injury.

Tell the patient what you are going to do. Let him know if there may be pain or discomfort. Always let the patient know if you must lift, rearrange, or remove any article of his clothing. Do all you can to assure privacy for the patient. Stress the importance of the examination and work to build the patient's confidence. Ask the patient if he understands what you are doing, seeking his response. Try to maintain eye contact whenever possible, and never turn away while you are talking, or while the patient is answering your questions.

EXAMINATION RULE #6: Fully explain what you will be doing during the examination.

Vital Signs. Vital signs are pulse, respiration, blood pressure, and temperature. In basic EMT-level emergency care, relative skin temperature is usually measured. In some localities, level of consciousness (LOC) and pupil size and reactivity are considered to be vital signs.

Your EMS System may have you take vital signs after the physical examination, thus having an assessment protocol of primary survey, secondary survey, and vital signs. In some areas of the country, vital signs are taken for conscious patients after the subjective interview and for unconscious patients after the physical examination. This is done to reduce the risk of aggravating spinal injuries and fractures, and dislocations of the extremities. Most EMS Systems use variations in the approach to patient assessment based upon consciousness or unconsciousness, and trauma or medical emergency.

As an EMT, you should follow a simple procedure in determining vital signs. This procedure allows you to quickly gather the needed measurements in an uninterrupted manner. First, place the stethoscope around your neck. Position yourself at the patient's side and place the blood pressure cuff on his arm. Be certain that there are no suspected or obvious injuries to this arm. There must be no clothing under the cuff. If you can expose the arm sufficiently by rolling the sleeve up, do so, but make sure that this rolled sleeve does not become a constricting band.

Wrap the cuff around the patient's upper arm so that the lower edge of the cuff is about 1 inch above the crease of the elbow. Know the equipment you are using. The center of the cuff bladder must be placed over the brachial (BRAY-key-al) artery. The marker on the cuff (if provided) should indicate where you place the cuff in relation to the artery, but many cuffs do not have markers in the correct location. Tubes entering the bladder are not always in the right location either. The American Heart Association states that the only accurate method is finding

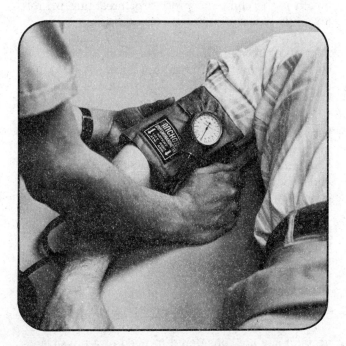

Figure 3-15: Positioning the blood pressure cuff.

the bladder center. If you know your equipment, then you will know if the markers are correct, if you can use the tubes entering the bladder, or if you will have to find the center of the bladder. Always apply the cuff securely, but not overly tight. You are now ready to begin your determination of the patient's vital signs.

Determine Pulse Rate and Character. The pumping action of the heart is normally rhythmic, causing blood to move through the arteries in waves, not smoothly and continuously like water flowing through a pipe. A fingertip held over an artery where it lies close to the body's surface and where it crosses over a bone, can easily feel characteristic "beats" as the surging blood causes the artery to expand. What you feel is called the pulse.

When "taking a patient's pulse," you are concerned with two factors, rate and character. For **pulse rate,** you will have to determine the number of beats per minute. This will allow you to decide if the patient's pulse rate is *normal, rapid,* or *slow.* The rhythm and force of the pulse are considered for **pulse character.** You will have to judge the patient's pulse as *regular* or *irregular* in regard to rhythm, and *full* (strong) or *thready* (weak) in regard to force.

Pulse rate varies among individuals. Factors such as age, sex, physical condition, degree of exercise just completed, medications being taken, blood loss, and stress all have an influence on the rate. The normal rate for an *adult at rest* is between 60 and 80 beats per minute. In an emergency, it is not unusual for this rate to be between 100 and 150 beats per minute. A true emergency, where the patient must see a physician as soon as possible, exists whenever you have an adult patient with a pulse rate above 150 beats per minute. If you take a patient's pulse several times during care at the scene and find him holding a pulse rate above 120 beats or below 50 beats per minute, you must consider this to be a sign that something may be seriously wrong with the patient. Transport as soon as possible.

Any pulse rate above 80 is **rapid,** while a rate below 60 is **slow.** Someone with a normal pulse rate of 85 has a rapid pulse, but this is not considered to be a serious health problem. An athlete may have a pulse rate between 40 and 50 beats per minute. This is a slow pulse rate, but it is certainly not an indication of poor health. As an EMT, you are concerned with the typical adult having pulse rates that stay above 100 and below 60 beats per minute.

The normal pulse rate for children from ages 1–5 years is between 80 and 150 beats per minute. Some newborns may reach as high as 180 beats per minute. Rates above or below this range are considered to be serious, with the patient needing to see a physician as soon as possible. For children from 5-12

Table 3.3: Pulse Variations and Medical Conditions

Pulse	Possible Cause of Abnormality
Rapid, regular and full	May be caused by nothing more than exertion, may also be caused by fright, hypertension (high blood pressure), or first stage of blood loss
Rapid, regular and thready	Reliable sign of shock; often evident in later stage of blood loss
No pulse	Cardiac arrest leading to death

years of age, the rate is usually between 60 and 120 beats per minute. Again, rates above or below this range require immediate medical care rendered by a physician.

Pulse rhythm relates to regularity. A pulse is said to be regular when the intervals between beats are constant. When the intervals are not constant, the pulse is irregular. You should report irregular pulse rate and if you felt what seemed to be a skipping of a beat or beats.

Pulse force refers to the pressure of the pulse wave as it expands the artery. Normally, the pulse should feel as if a strong wave has passed under your fingertips. This is a full pulse. When the pulse feels weak and thin, the patient has a thready pulse.

Many disorders can be related to variations in pulse rate, rhythm, and force.

Pulse rate and character can be determined at a number of points throughout the body. During the secondary survey, a **radial pulse** is measured. This is the wrist pulse, named for the radial artery found in the lateral portion of the forearm (remember the anatomical position). Do NOT attempt to measure a radial pulse if you have to move the patient or an injured limb in order to do so. If you cannot measure one radial pulse, try the other arm. When you cannot measure either radial, use the carotid pulse as described earlier on page 37.

To measure a radial pulse, find the pulse site by placing your first three fingers on the middle of the patient's wrist, just above the crease. Do not use your thumb. It has its own pulse that may cause you to measure your own pulse rate. Slide your fingertips toward the lateral (thumb) side of the patient's wrist, keeping one finger over the crease. Apply moderate pressure to feel the pulse beats. A weak pulse may require applying greater pressure, but take care. If you experience difficulty, try the patient's other arm. Count the pulsations for 15 seconds and multiply by 4 to determine the

beats per minute. While you are counting, judge the rhythm and force. Record the information, e.g., "Pulse 72, regular and full." It is best to wait until you also have determined respiratory rate and character before recording pulse information (see below).

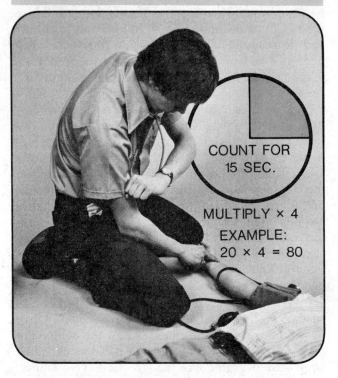

Figure 3-16: Pulse rate and character are vital signs.

Determine Respiratory Rate and Character.
During the secondary survey, you are concerned with the rate and character of breathing. **Respiration** is the act of breathing in and out; therefore, a single breath is the complete process of breathing in, followed by breathing out.

Respiratory rate is the number of breaths a patient takes in one minute. The rate of respiration is classified as normal, rapid, or slow. **Respiratory character** includes rhythm, depth, sounds, and ease of breathing.

The normal respiration rate for an adult at rest is between 12 and 20 breaths per minute. Keep in mind that age, sex, size, physical conditioning, and emotional state can influence breathing rates. Fear and other emotions experienced during an emergency can increase the respiratory rate. However, if you have a patient maintaining a rate above 28 breaths per minute, you must consider this to be a true emergency in need of a physician's care as soon as possible. The same holds true for rates that stay below 10 breaths per minute.

Children breathe more quickly than adults. For children from 1-5, a respiratory rate above 44 breaths per minute is considered serious. Children from 5-12 years of age are considered in need of a physician's

Table 3.4: Variations in Respiration and Medical Conditions

Respirations	Possible Cause of Abnormality
Deep, gasping, labored	Airway obstruction, heart failure, asthma
Rapid, shallow	Shock, cardiac problems
Painful, difficult, labored	Dyspnea (labored or difficult breathing)
Difficulty in breathing while lying down	Heart failure
Stertorous (snoring)	Stroke, fractured skull, drug influence and alcohol intoxication
Gurgling (as though the breaths are passing through water)	Foreign matter in throat, pulmonary edema (accumulation of fluid in lungs)
Crowing (bird-like sounds)	Spasms of the larynx
Temporary cessation of respirations	Hypoxia (lack of oxygen)
No respirations	Respiratory arrest

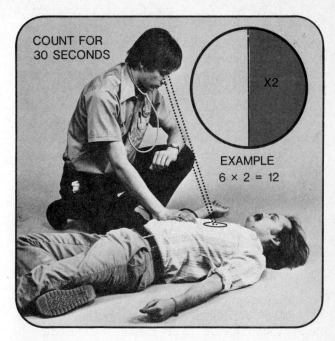

COUNT FOR 30 SECONDS

X2

EXAMPLE
6 × 2 = 12

Figure 3-17: Breathing rate and character are vital signs.

care when their respiratory rate exceeds 36 breaths per minute.

Rhythm refers to the manner in which a person breathes. Breathing is considered *regular* when the interval between breaths is constant, and *irregular* when the interval varies.

Depth relates to the amount of air moved with each breath. Normal breathing is something you will have to judge for yourself by watching many people breathe when at rest. Then you will be able to differentiate between *deep* and *shallow* respirations. While judging depth, also note the ease of respirations. Does the patient exhibit *labored* breathing, *difficult* breathing, or *painful* breathing?

Listen for any sounds of respiration such as *snoring*, *crowing*, and *gurgling*. More will be said about these sounds in Chapter 4.

> As soon as you have determined pulse rate, start counting respirations. Many individuals change their breathing rate if they know someone is watching them breathe. For this reason, do not move your hand from the patient's wrist. After you have counted pulse beats, immediately begin to watch the patient's chest for breathing movements. Count the number of breaths taken by the patient during 30 seconds and multiply by 2 to obtain the breaths per minute. While counting, note rhythm, depth, ease, and sounds of respiration. Record your results. For example, ''Respirations are 16, regular and normal.''

Measure Blood Pressure. Since the blood pressure cuff is already in place, you can begin to measure blood pressure as soon as you determine pulse and respirations. Keep in mind that you have no way of knowing the patient's *normal* blood pressure, unless the patient is alert and knows this information. For this reason, one reading of blood pressure is not very meaningful. You will have to make several readings over a period of time while care is provided at the scene and during transport. Remember that changes in blood pressure are diagnostically significant.

Each time the lower chamber of the left side of the heart contracts, it forces blood out into circulation. The pressure created in the arteries by this blood is called the **systolic** (sis-TOL-ik) blood pressure. When the lower left chamber of the heart is relaxed and refilling, the pressure in the arteries is called the **diastolic** (di-as-TOL-ic) blood pressure. The systolic pressure is reported first, as in 120 over 80.

Just as pulse and respiratory rates vary among individuals, so does blood pressure. There is a generally accepted rule for estimating blood pressure of adults up to the age 40. For an adult male at rest, add his age to 100 to estimate his systolic pressure. For an adult female at rest, add her age to 90 to estimate her systolic pressure. Thus, a 36-year-old man would have an estimated normal systolic blood pressure of 136 millimeters of mercury (mmHg). **Millimeters of mercury** refers to the units of the blood pressure gauge. A 36-year-old woman would have an estimated normal systolic pressure of 126 mmHg. Normal diastolic pressures usually range between 60 and 90 mmHg.

Serious low blood pressure (hypotension) is generally considered to be below 90 mmHg, systolic. High blood pressure (hypertension) exists once the pressure rises above 145/95. Keep in mind that many individuals in emergency situations will show a temporary rise in blood pressure. More than one reading will be necessary to decide if a high or low reading is only temporary. Anytime your patient's blood pressure drops to 90/60 or below, it is almost certain that the patient is going into shock. Report any major changes in blood pressure to emergency department personnel without delay.

In adults, consider *any* systolic reading above 180 and below 90 to be serious. A diastolic reading above 105 or below 60 also must be considered to be serious. For children from 1 to 5, any systolic reading above 120 or below 70 means that the child should be seen by a physician as soon as possible. In this age group, diastolic readings above 75 or below 50 must be considered as indications of serious problems. Children 5 to 12 are classified as needing to see a physician as soon as possible when their systolic pressure is above 150 or below 90. The same is true in cases where the diastolic pressure is above 85 or below 60.

There are three common techniques used to measure blood pressure with a sphygmomanometer: 1) **auscultation** (os-skul-TAY-shun), when a stethoscope is used to listen for characteristic sounds; 2) **palpation,** when the radial pulse is palpated (felt) with the fingertips; and 3) **oscillation**, when movement of the cuff gauge needle or column is noted. Oscillation is rarely used in emergency care.

Determining Blood Pressure by Auscultation. Begin by placing the ends of the stethoscope arms in your ears. With your fingertips, palpate the brachial artery at the crease of the elbow. Position the diaphragm or bell of the stethoscope directly over the brachial pulse site. With the bulb valve closed, inflate the cuff. As you do so, you will be able to hear pulse sounds. Inflate the cuff, watching the gauge. At a certain point, you will no longer hear the brachial pulse. Continue to inflate the cuff until the gauge reads 20 mmHg higher than the point where the pulse sound disappeared.

Slowly release air from the cuff by opening the bulb valve, allowing the pressure to fall smoothly at the rate of 2 to 3 mmHg per second.

Listen for the start of clicking or tapping sounds. When you hear the beginning of these sounds, note the reading on the gauge. This is the systolic pressure. Continue to deflate the cuff, listening for when these distinctive sounds *fade* (not when they disappear). When the sounds turn to dull, muffled thuds, the reading on the gauge is the diastolic pressure. After obtaining the diastolic pressure, let the cuff deflate. If you are not certain of a reading, repeat the procedure. You should use the other arm, or wait one minute before reinflating the cuff. Otherwise, you will tend to obtain an erroneously high reading.

Record the measurements and the time of determination, e.g., ''B.P. is 140/90, fourteen-hundred hours.''

Some people have great difficulty hearing the pulse sounds when they inflate the cuff. If you do, use your fingertips to find the patient's radial pulse at the wrist of the arm to which the cuff has been applied. Make certain that the adjustable valve on the rubber bulb assembly is closed, then inflate the cuff. Note the point at which the radial pulse disappears. Continue inflating the cuff until the needle or column shows 20 mmHg higher than the point of radial pulse cut-off. The rest of the procedure remains the same.

REMEMBER: Blood pressure must be measured while a person is seated or lying down. Do NOT move a patient simply to determine blood pressure. To do so may aggravate existing injuries. Always try to keep the cuff at heart level. If the patient is sitting up, support his arm (e.g. on the arm of a chair) or hold the patient's arm during the entire procedure.

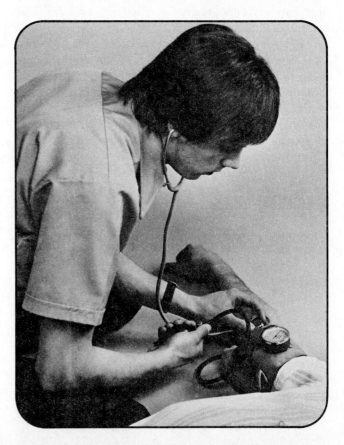

Figure 3-18: Measuring blood pressure by auscultation.

Determining Blood Pressure by Palpation.
This method is not as accurate as the auscultation method, since only an *approximate* systolic pressure can be determined. The technique is used when there is too much noise around a patient to allow the use of the stethoscope, or when the situation involves many patients and too few people to deliver care.

Begin by finding the radial pulse site on the limb to which the blood pressure cuff has been applied. Make certain that the adjustable valve is closed on the bulb, and inflate the cuff to a point where you can no longer feel the radial pulse. Note this point on the gauge and continue to inflate the cuff 20 mmHg beyond this point.

Slowly deflate the cuff, noting the reading at which the radial pulse returns. This reading is the patient's systolic pressure. Record your findings, e.g., ''Blood pressure by palpation, fourteen-hundred hours.''

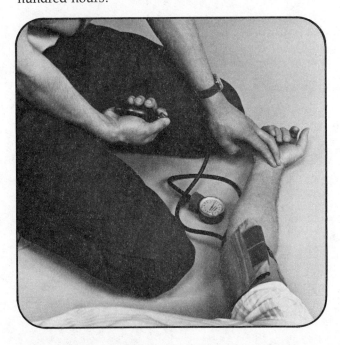

Figure 3-19: Measuring blood pressure by palpation.

Determining Skin Temperature. Some areas have EMTs measure oral, axillary (armpit), or rectal temperatures for a determination of body temperature. However, most area guidelines for basic EMT-level care call for measurement of relative skin temperature. This is not a true vital sign in higher levels of care, but in the field it is useful to find abnormally high and low temperatures.

To determine skin temperature, feel the patient's forehead with the back of your hand. Note if his skin feels *normal, warm, hot, cool,* or *cold.* At the same time, notice if his skin is *dry, moist,* or *clammy.* Look for ''goose pimples'' often associated with chills. Many patient problems are exhibited by changes in skin temperature and condition. As you

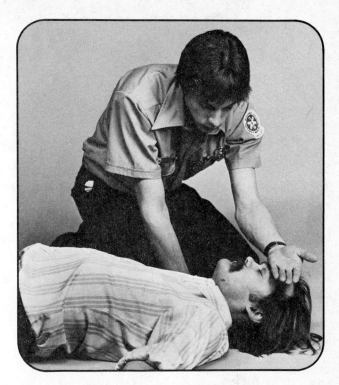

Figure 3-20: Determining relative skin temperature.

continue with the assessment of the patient, be alert for major temperature differences on various parts of the body. For example, you may note that the patient's trunk is warm, but his left arm feels cold. Such a finding can direct you to detecting problems with circulation. A relatively hot area on the abdomen may indicate inflammation or infection within the cavity.

EXAMINATION RULE #7: Take vital signs. The process will take you a little over one minute. The information gained could save a patient's life.

The Head-to-Toe Survey. Immediately after measuring vital signs, you should begin a head-to-toe survey of the patient. Take great care during this procedure. You have yet to determine if there are

Table 3.5: Temperature Variations and Relevant Medical Conditions

Skin Temperature	Possible Cause of Abnormality
Cool, clammy	Usual sign of shock
Cold, moist	Body is losing heat
Cold, dry	Body has been exposed to cold and has lost considerable heat
Hot, dry	Excessive body heat (as in heatstroke and high fever)
''Goose pimples'' accompanied by shivering, chattering teeth, blue lips and pale skin	Chills caused (among other things) by malaria, communicable disease, pneumonia, pain, or fear

VITAL SIGNS

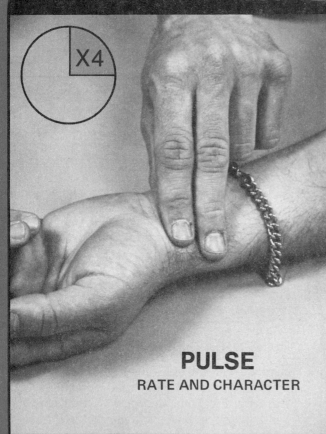

PULSE
RATE AND CHARACTER

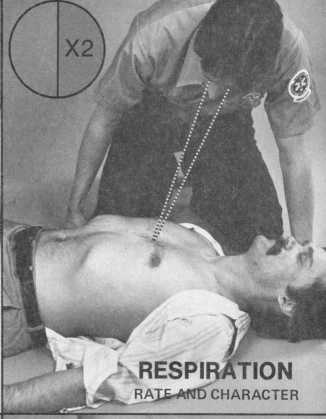

RESPIRATION
RATE AND CHARACTER

TEMPERATURE

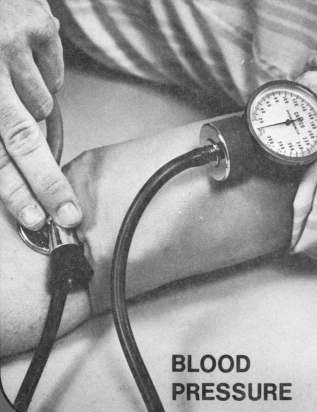

BLOOD PRESSURE

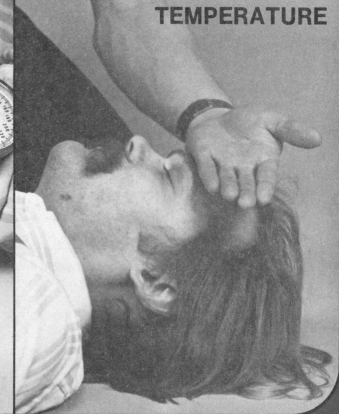

any neck or spinal injuries. You must be very careful not to move the patient until certain findings are reached during the examination.

The head-to-toe procedure may cause the patient some pain and discomfort. Warn the patient of these possibilities. The more systematic you are in your approach, and the better you know how to conduct each aspect of the examination, the less likely you are to cause discomfort. As an EMT, you MUST know the head-to-toe procedures, and be able to perform each move without any hesitation.

Take care not to contaminate wounds and aggravate injuries. If bleeding has obviously stopped, do NOT pull the clothing or skin around the site. Do NOT probe into the site.

Readjust, remove, or cut away only those articles of patient clothing that interfere with your ability to examine the patient. Be certain to tell the patient that you have to rearrange his clothing and explain why this must be done. Do all you can to insure the patient's privacy, even if it means asking bystanders to face away from the patient. Do NOT try to pull clothing off the limbs of a patient. Such procedures could increase bleeding and worsen existing injuries. Some local authorities recommend that a woman EMT be present during the examination of a female patient. However, no one recommends delaying the examination or care of a patient of the opposite sex. As a professional EMT, your intentions should be respected.

During the head-to-toe survey:

- LOOK—for discolorations, deformities, penetrations, wounds, openings in the neck, and any unusual chest movements.
- FEEL—for deformities, tenderness, pulsations, abnormal hardness or softness, and spasms.
- LISTEN—for changes in breathing patterns, unusual breathing sounds, and any grating noises made by the ends of broken bones.
- SMELL—for any unusual odors coming from the patient's body, breath, or clothing.

EXAMINATION RULE #8: Conduct a head-to-toe examination. If ANYTHING looks, feels, sounds, or smells strange to you, assume that there is something seriously wrong with the patient.

There may be some variation in the head-to-toe survey, depending upon local guidelines. Traditionally, examination of the neck is done during Steps 8 and 9 of the survey. We will present the traditional procedure since it is used by most localities. However, many medical authorities now recommend that the neck be examined first in an effort to detect possible spinal injuries. When such injuries are detected, the head and neck can be immobilized to reduce chances of aggravating spinal injury during the rest of the survey.

Begin your head-to-toe survey by once again taking a quick overview of the patient's body. You should then:

1. Inspect the Scalp for Wounds—Extreme care must be exercised so as not to move the patient's head, aggravating possible spinal injuries. Run your fingers gently through the patient's hair, feeling for blood, cuts, swellings or "goose eggs," deformities, and any other indications of injury. If you believe you have found an injury site, do NOT separate strands of hair matted over the site. To do so may re-start bleeding. When the patient is found lying on his back, check the hidden part of his scalp by placing your fingers behind his neck. Slide them upward toward the top of his head. If you have any reason to believe there are spinal or neck injuries, DELAY this procedure until the head and neck are immobilized.

WARNING: Take great care not to drive bone fragments or dirt into any wound.

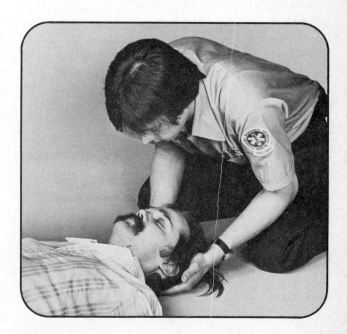

Figure 3-21: Begin the head-to-toe examination by inspecting the scalp.

2. Check the Skull for Deformities and Depressions—While checking the scalp, note any depressions or bony projections that would indicate possible injury to the skull. Check the facial bones for any signs of fractures (obvious breaks in the bones, swellings, heavy discolorations, depressions, or obvious crushing of bones).

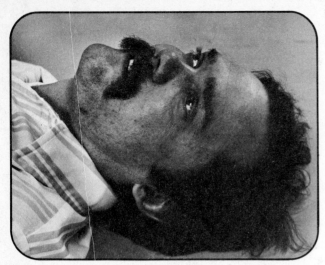

Figure 3-22: After examining the scalp, visually inspect the skull and face.

3. Examine the Patient's Eyes—Begin by looking for cuts, impaled objects, and any signs of burns on the patient's eyelids. Have the patient open his eyes, or, with unresponsive patients, gently open the eyes by sliding back the upper eyelids. Check the globe of each eye for cuts, foreign objects, impaled objects, and burns.

   Next, check the pupils for *size*, *equality*, and *reactivity*. Examine both eyes and note if the pupils are *normal*, *constricted* (small), or *dilated* (large). Are both pupils *equal* in size? Do the pupils *react* to the beam of light from your pen light?

NOTE: Check the unconscious patient for contact lenses. Many areas recommend prompt removal of these lenses to help prevent damage to the patient's eyes. Contact lens removal procedures are described in Chapter 8.

Table 3.6: Medical Significance of Changes in Pupil Size

Pupil Size	Possible Cause of Abnormality
Dilated, unresponsive	Cardiac arrest, influence of drugs such as LSD and amphetamines, unconsciousness from numerous causes
Constricted, unresponsive	Central nervous system disease or disorder, influence of narcotic such as heroin, morphine, or codeine
Unequal	Stroke, head injury
Lackluster, pupils do not appear to focus	Shock, coma

4. Inspect the Inner Surfaces of the Eyelids—Normally these surfaces should be pink. However, with blood loss they become pale. Gently

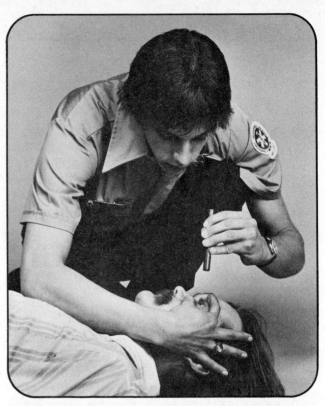

Figure 3-23: Examine the eyelids, eyes, and pupils.

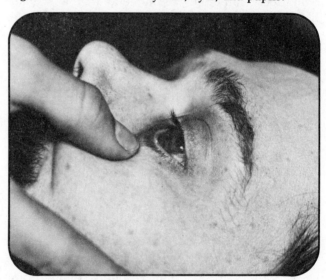

Figure 3-24: Are the inner eyelids pale?

pull down either lower eyelid and check the color of the inner surface.

5. Inspect the Ears and Nose for Blood or Clear Fluids—Observe the ears and nose for blood, clear fluids, or bloody fluids. Blood in the nose may be the result of simple nasal tissue injury (a bloody nose). It could also indicate a skull fracture. Blood in the ears, and clear fluids in the ears or nose are strong indicators of skull fracture. This clear fluid may be **cerebrospinal** (ser-e-bro-SPI-nal) **fluid**, a watery substance that surrounds the brain and the spinal cord.

WARNING: Do NOT rotate the patient's head to inspect the ears.

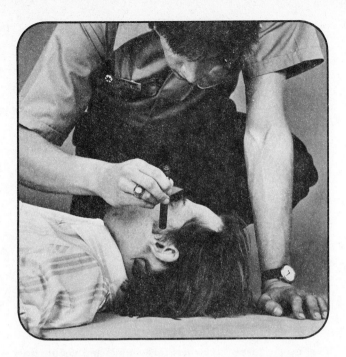

Figure 3-25: Check the ears and nose for blood and clear fluids.

6. Inspect the Mouth—Look for any foreign objects, broken teeth, broken dentures, or vomitus that may be causing airway obstruction. At the same time, look for blood. Take care not to move the patient's head during this inspection.

7. Sniff for Odd Breath Odor—Note any unusual odors such as a fruity smell (diabetic coma), pe-

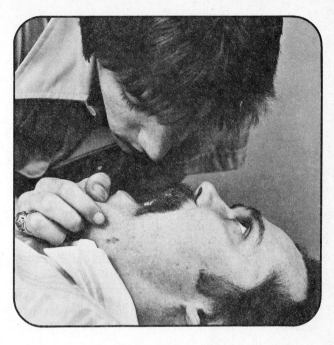

Figure 3-27: Is there any unusual breath odor?

troleum products (ingested poisoning), or alcohol (alcohol intoxication).

NOTE: You will need to expose examination areas. The anterior neck must be exposed so that you can check for surgical openings or a metal tube that indicates the patient is a "neck-breather." The lower chest and abdomen must be exposed to observe chest movements, listen for equal air entry, check

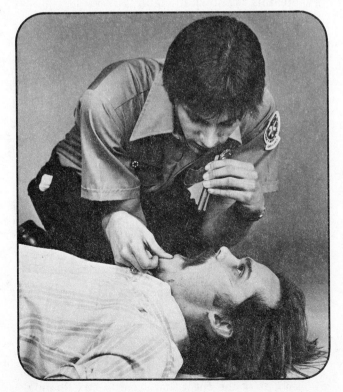

Figure 3-26: Inspect the mouth for obstructions and blood.

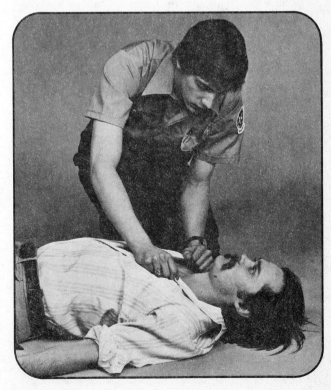

Figure 3-28: Gently check the front of the neck for injuries and surgical openings. Is the patient a neck-breather?

for penetrations, and palpate the abdomen for tenderness. Be certain to protect the patient from the stares of onlookers. Remember, clothing that cannot easily be rearranged should be cut away.

8. Inspect the Anterior Neck for Indications of Injury—Look for cuts, bruises, discolorations, and deformities. Does the larynx (voicebox) or trachea (windpipe) appear to deviate from the midline of the neck? If so, the patient may have an obstructed airway.

   See if the patient has a **stoma** (STO-mah) (permanent surgical opening) in the neck through which he breathes. He may have a **tracheostomy** (TRA-ke-OS-to-me). This is a surgical incision held open by a metal tube or tubes. In either case, the patient will breath through the opening.

   Look for a medical identification necklace. Note the information provided, but do NOT remove the necklace.

9. Check the Cervical Spine for Point Tenderness and Deformity—The portion of the spinal column that runs through the neck is called the **cervical** (SER-ve-cal) **spine**. A painful response to gentle finger pressure is **point tenderness.** You should prepare the patient for possible pain, steady his chin with one hand, then check for midline deformities and point tenderness with your other hand. Slide your fingertips toward the patient's cervical midline, at the point where the head and neck meet. Do this for both sides of the neck.

NOTE: Cervical point tenderness and deformity indicate spinal injury. Most EMS systems recommend stopping the head-to-toe survey at this point if there are signs of spinal injury to provide temporary immobilization for the head and neck. The survey is then continued.

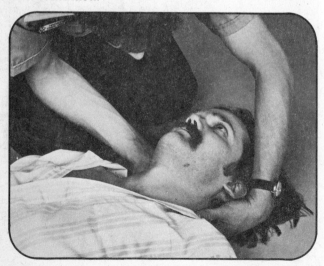

Figure 3-29: Check the back of the neck for point tenderness.

10. Inspect the Chest for Wounds—Look for cuts, bruises, penetrations, and impaled objects. If need be, completely bare the patient's chest.

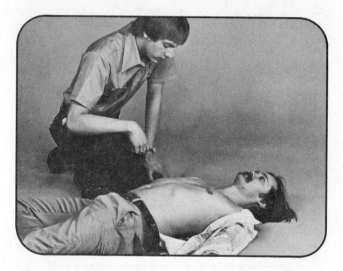

Figure 3-30: Inspect the chest for wounds and visible deformities.

11. Examine the Chest for Fractures—Warn the patient of possible pain and gently feel the clavicles (KLAV-i-kuls) or collarbones. Next, gently feel the sternum (STER-num) or breastbone. Gently apply pressure with your hands to the sides of the rib cage. This process, known as **compression**, usually produces pain in cases of fractured ribs. When applying compression, position your forearms as shown in Figure 3-31.

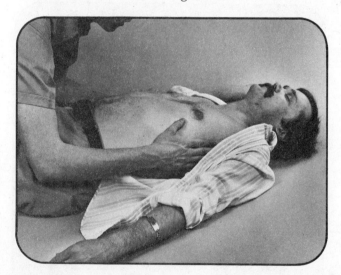

Figure 3-31: Apply compression to the sides of the chest to check for fractures.

12. Check for Equal Expansion of the Chest—While in the same position, look for chest movements and feel for equal expansion. Be on the alert for sections of the chest that seem to be "floating" or moving in opposite directions to the rest of the chest.

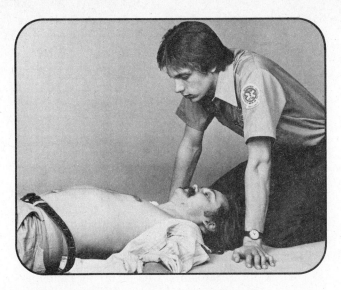

Figure 3-32: Check for equal chest expansion.

13. Listen for Sounds of Equal Air Entry—Use your stethoscope to listen to both sides of the chest. Sounds of air entry usually will be clearly present or absent. Absence of air movement indicates injury or illness to the internal chest or lungs.

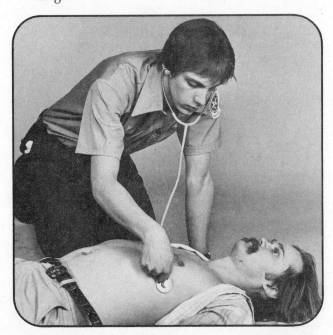

Figure 3-33: Is there equal air entry?

14. Inspect the Abdomen for Wounds—Look for cuts, bruises, penetrations, and impaled objects.

15. Feel the Abdomen for Tenderness—Prepare the patient for possible pain and then *gently* feel his entire abdomen. If the patient tells you he has pain limited to a specific area of the abdomen, palpate this site last. When practical, make sure your hands are warm. Press in on the abdomen with the palm side of your fingers, noting any

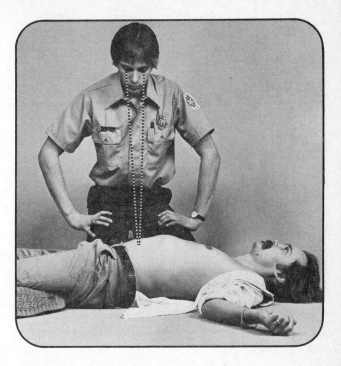

Figure 3-34: Carefully inspect the abdomen for wounds and visible deformities.

painful response. If the pain is confined to one spot, it is said to be **local**. Should it be spread over the entire abdomen, it is classified as **general** or **diffuse**. Relate painful responses to the abdominal quadrants.

While feeling the abdomen for tenderness, note any rigid or distended (swollen) areas. Stay alert for any masses (lumps) that may be felt through the abdominal wall.

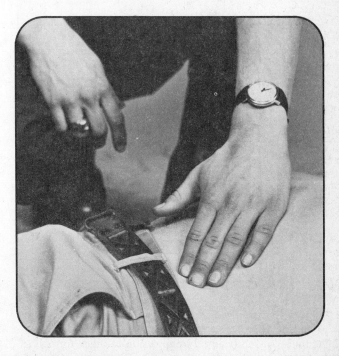

Figure 3-35: Check for abdominal tenderness.

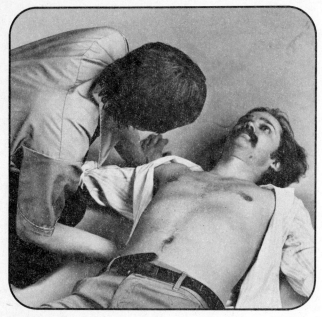

Figure 3-36: Palpate the lower back for point tenderness and deformity.

16. Feel the Lower Back for Point Tenderness and Deformity—Prepare the patient for possible pain and gently slide your hand under the void created by the curve of the spine. Check for both tenderness and deformity. Either suggests possible spinal injury and may require you to immobilize the patient's spine before continuing the survey.

WARNING: Do NOT attempt to inspect the upper

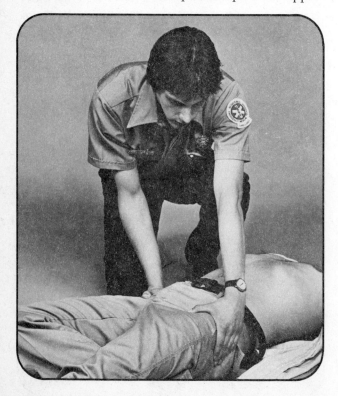

Figure 3-37: Gently apply compression to check for pelvic fractures.

back of the patient at this time. To do so will require you to lift the patient slightly. You have yet to rule out spinal injury and damage to the upper extremities that could be aggravated by such a procedure.

17. Feel the Pelvis for Fractures—Gently slide your hands from the small of the patient's back to the lateral wings of the pelvis. Again, warn the patient of possible pain, then lightly apply compression to the pelvis. Note any painful response and pelvic deformities.

18. Note Any Obvious Injury to the Genital (Groin) Region—Look for bleeding and impaled objects, but do not expose the area unless you are reasonably sure that an injury has been sustained.

    Look for **priapism** (PRI-a-pizm) in male patients. This is a persistent erection of the penis often brought about by spinal injury. If the mechanism of injury, or any signs gathered to this point in the survey, indicate possible spinal injury, and clothing prevents you from being able to see an erect penis, gently brush the genital region, using the back of your hand.

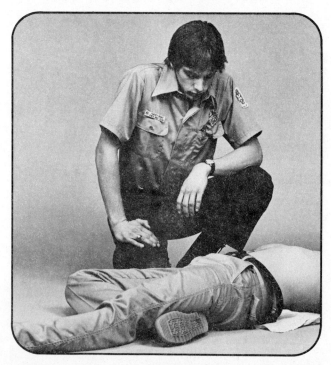

Figure 3-38: Look for obvious injury to the genital region.

NOTE: When examining the lower limbs and feet, it may be necessary to rearrange or cut away clothing. Injury to a lower limb is best observed with little additional aggravation if pants legs are cut away from the site. Cutting is best done along the seams. If there is a painful response to your feeling the patient's foot, or no sign of injury, you need not try to remove shoes. A pulse can be taken without removing low cut shoes. If the patient is wearing gym shoes, high top shoes, or boots it may be necessary to cut away the footwear if unlacing and removal might aggravate an injury. Do NOT attempt to remove ski boots unless you are specifically trained in the procedure.

19. Examine the Lower Limbs and Feet—Inspect each limb from hip to foot, looking for deformities, bleeding, bone protrusions, swellings, and discolorations. Gently palpate any suspected fracture site for point tenderness, warning the patient beforehand.

WARNING: Do NOT move or lift the patient's lower limbs. Do NOT change the position of the limbs or feet from the position they were in at the beginning of the examination.

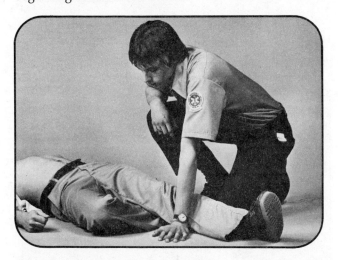

Figure 3-39: Examine the lower limbs and feet, but do NOT lift or move them.

20. Check for a Distal Pulse—You need to know if circulation to both feet is impaired or interrupted. Palpate the distal pulse for each foot either behind the ankle (posterior tibial pulse) or at the juncture of the great and second toes (pedal pulse). Presence of a pulse indicates that circulation is intact. No pulse suggests that a major artery supplying the limb has been pinched or severed, usually by a broken or displaced bone end.

21. Check for Nerve Activity and Possible Paralysis

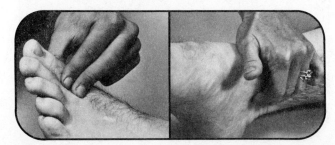

Figure 3-40: The two methods of establishing a distal pulse.

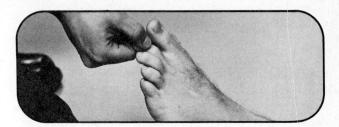

Figure 3-41: Check for sensitivity in the toes of a conscious, responsive patient.

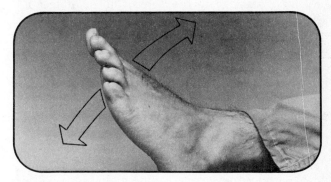

Figure 3-42: Can the patient wave each foot?

to the Lower Extremities—Touch a toe and ask the patient to identify which toe you touched. Do this for each foot. If the patient cannot feel your touch, assume nerve damage in the limb or spinal damage (it is best to assume spinal damage). If sensation appears normal, have the patient wave his feet. Finally, ask the patient to press the sole of his foot gently against the palm of your hand. Do this for each foot. Failure to accomplish any of these tasks indicates the pos-

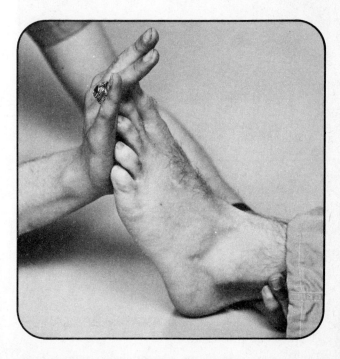

Figure 3-43: Can the patient push his foot against the palm of your hand?

sibility of injury to nerve pathways. At this point, ASSUME SPINAL DAMAGE.

Most EMS guidelines now recommend treating an unconscious patient as if he has spinal injuries. When the patient is unconscious, or unresponsive, then the above tests are of no use. For such patients, you will have to perform different ones. However, these tests are not very reliable in field situations. If you have reason to believe that there is spinal injury, or if damage to the pelvis, limbs, or feet is severe, do not try to cut away or remove the patient's footwear. Instead, ASSUME THERE IS SPINAL DAMAGE and treat accordingly. If you can remove the patient's footwear, grasp the patient's leg at the ankle and scratch the sole of his foot with a broken applicator stick or the cap of a ball point pen. Do NOT use a sharp object, such as a badge pin; the patient, even though unconscious, may show a reflex action by pulling the leg away from the object, or by making a pronounced upward or downward toe movement. Failure to do so MUST be assumed to be the result of spinal injury. Upward movement of the toe may be due to brain injury, while the downward movement is normal.

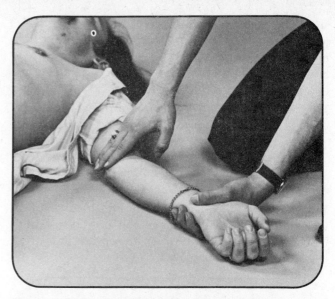

Figure 3-45: Check the arm and hands for injuries.

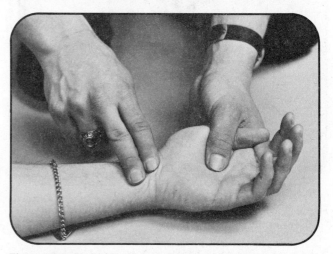

Figure 3-46: Establish a radial pulse for each arm.

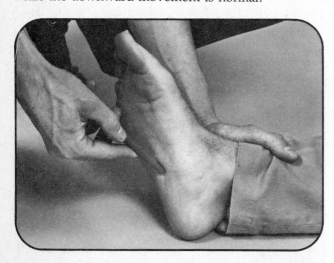

Figure 3-44: If the patient is unconscious, you will have to scratch the sole of each foot to check for nerve function. Keep in mind that this test is not very reliable.

22. Examine the Upper Extremities—Check the patient from clavicles (collarbones) to the fingertips. You should:

- Note any deformities, bleeding, bone protrusions, swellings, or discolorations.
- Check for point tenderness at the site of possible fractures.
- Confirm a radial pulse for each arm. Do not measure pulse rate.
- Have the conscious, responsive patient identify the finger you touch, wave his hand, and

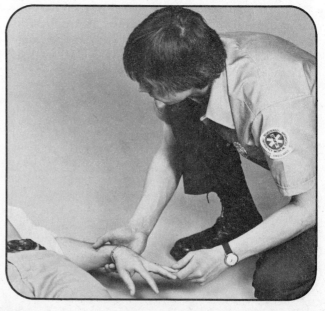

Figure 3-47: Can the patient tell which finger you touched?

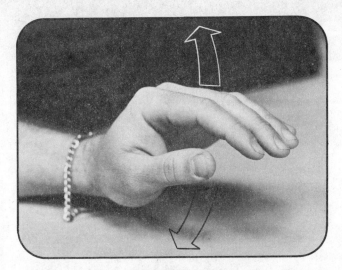

Figure 3-48: Can the patient wave each hand?

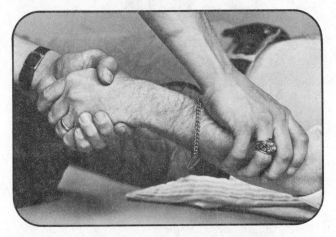

Figure 3-49: Can the patient grasp your hand?

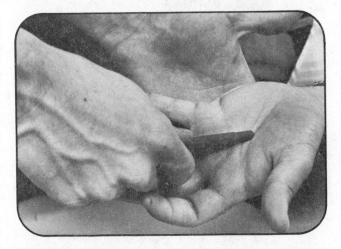

Figure 3-50: To test for nerve function in the unconscious patient, scratch the palms of his hands. This is not a reliable field test.

grasp your hand. Do this for each arm, if the extremity is uninjured.

• Look for a medical identification bracelet.

If the patient is unconscious or unresponsive, grasp his wrist and stroke the palm of his hand with

a broken applicator stick or the cap of a ball point pen. Do this for each hand. The patient may try to pull his hand away from the object used. Do NOT use the point of a badge pin or any other sharp object. If the patient is deeply unconscious, he will not move his hand. This test must be considered to be unreliable under field conditions.

EXAMINATION RULE #9: If a patient fails to respond properly on any test for upper or lower extremity nerve function, you MUST consider this to be a sign of spinal injury.

23. Inspect the Back Surface for Injury—Provided there are no injuries to the skull, neck, spine, or extremities, and you have no evidence of severe injury to the chest or abdomen, gently roll the patient as a unit toward your knees and inspect the back surfaces for bleeding and obvious injuries. Since neck injuries are difficult to detect with some unconscious patients, your local guidelines may state that this procedure should not be done unless you need to control profuse bleeding.

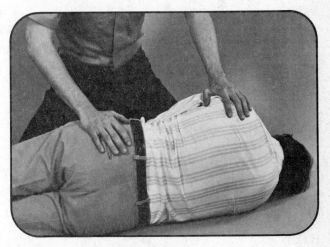

Figure 3-51: Inspect the back surfaces.

The head-to-toe survey appears to be a long process, but as you practice the procedure, you will find that it can be done in a few minutes.

After completing the secondary survey, you will have to consider all the signs you have found and the combinations of these signs that may point the way to specific illness or injury. A *lack* of certain findings also may prove to be important. For example, if the patient has severe obvious injury, but shows no reactions to indicate pain, you will have to consider problems such as spinal injury, brain damage, shock, or drug abuse. Later in this text, we will explain what care you should provide based on your findings during the patient assessment procedures.

Triage, the assessment and grouping of patients when there are a number of patients, is sometimes taught at this point. The section on triage is found in Chapter 14.

SECONDARY SURVEY

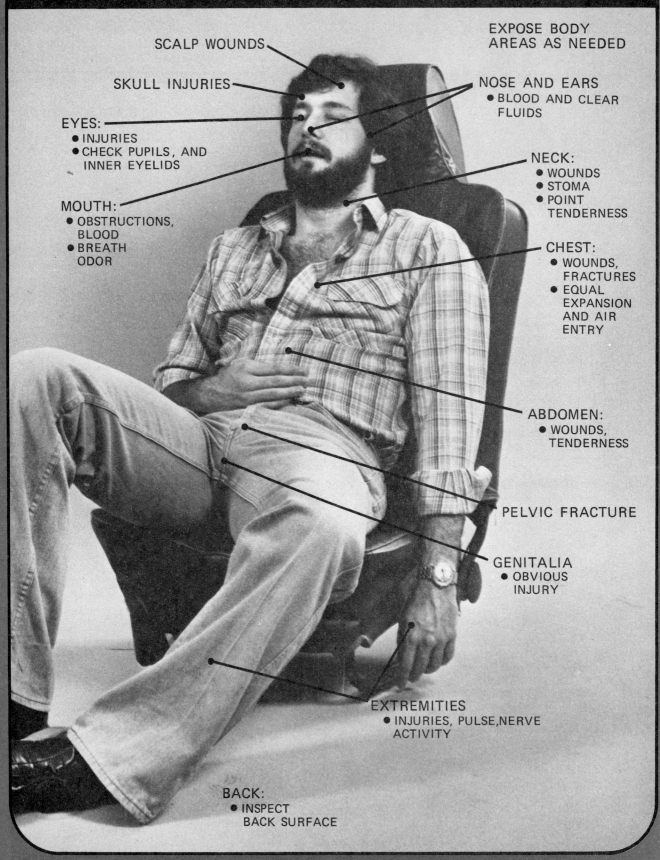

EXPOSE BODY
AREAS AS NEEDED

SCALP WOUNDS

SKULL INJURIES

NOSE AND EARS
- BLOOD AND CLEAR
  FLUIDS

EYES:
- INJURIES
- CHECK PUPILS, AND
  INNER EYELIDS

NECK:
- WOUNDS
- STOMA
- POINT
  TENDERNESS

MOUTH:
- OBSTRUCTIONS,
  BLOOD
- BREATH
  ODOR

CHEST:
- WOUNDS,
  FRACTURES
- EQUAL
  EXPANSION
  AND AIR
  ENTRY

ABDOMEN:
- WOUNDS,
  TENDERNESS

PELVIC FRACTURE

GENITALIA
- OBVIOUS
  INJURY

EXTREMITIES
- INJURIES, PULSE, NERVE
  ACTIVITY

BACK:
- INSPECT
  BACK SURFACE

SCAN 3-3

SUMMARY

Patient assessment is one of the most important things you will learn in your EMT training. Before going back to the chapter objectives, you should review the following:

ARRIVAL—Gain information quickly from the scene, the patient, bystanders, mechanisms of injury, and obvious deformities and signs of injury or illness.

PRIMARY SURVEY—This involves assessment of the airway, breathing, circulation, and profuse bleeding. You must make certain that there is an open airway and adequate breathing. You have to confirm a carotid pulse. You must detect and stop all life-threatening bleeding.

SECONDARY SURVEY—Interview: Look over the scene, look over the patient, and look for medical identification devices. Now, gather information by asking specific questions and listening to the patient's and bystanders' responses. The more organized you are in the interview, the better your chances of gaining needed information.

SECONDARY SURVEY—Vital signs: As part of the examination phase of the secondary survey, you must take vital signs. You have to determine radial pulse rate and character. You must measure respiratory rate and note the character of respirations. You will have to measure blood pressure by auscultation or palpation. You will have to determine relative skin temperature. At this time also note skin color and the general condition of the skin.

SECONDARY SURVEY—Head to Toe Survey:

HEAD—Check scalp for cuts, bruises, swellings, and other signs of injury. Examine the skull for deformities, depressions, and other signs of injury. Include the facial bones. Inspect the eyelids for injury and do the same for the eyes. Determine pupil size, equality, and reactivity. Note any discoloration on the inner eyelid. Look for blood, clear fluids, or bloody fluids in the ears and nose. Examine the mouth for obstructions, bleeding, and any odd odors.

NECK—Check to see if the patient is a neck-breather, examine for neck injury and cervical point tenderness. Look for a medical identification necklace.

CHEST—Examine for injury (cuts, bruise, penetrations, impaled objects, and fractures). Use chest compression as a test for fractures. Check for equal expansion and watch for unusual chest movements. Listen for equal air entry.

ABDOMEN—Examine for injuries (cuts, bruises, penetrations, and impaled objects). Check for local and general pain as you examine the abdomen for tenderness, distension, masses, and rigid areas.

LOWER BACK—Feel for deformity and point tenderness.

PELVIS—Use compression to check for fractures and look for signs of injury.

GENITAL REGION—Note any obvious injury. Look for priapism when assessing male patients.

LOWER EXTREMITIES—Examine for injury (deformities, swellings, discolorations, bone protrusions, and fractures). Run point tenderness tests on suspected fracture sites. Confirm a distal pulse in each limb and check each leg for nerve function.

UPPER EXTREMITIES—Examine for injury (deformities, swellings discolorations, bone protrusions, and fractures). Run point tenderness tests on suspected fracture sites. Confirm a radial pulse for each wrist and check for nerve function. Check for a medical identification bracelet.

BACK SURFACES—Examine for bleeding and obvious injury.

Remember to explain to the patient what you are going to do before you perform the head-to-toe survey. Warn the patient when there is the possibility of pain. Be reassuring at all times.

4 basic life support i: the airway and pulmonary resuscitation

OBJECTIVES By the end of this chapter, you should be able to:

1. State THREE reasons why breathing is essential to life. (pp. 64-5)
2. Define and compare clinical death and biological death. (p. 65)
3. Name and label the major structures of the respiratory system. (pp. 65-6)
4. Name the major muscle used in breathing. (p. 66)
5. Relate in general terms, changes in volume and pressure to the process of breathing. (pp. 66-7)
6. List the FIVE signs of adequate breathing. (p. 67)
7. List the SIX signs of inadequate breathing. (p. 67)
8. List FOUR factors that may cause partial or full airway obstruction. (p. 68)
9. List the THREE major signs of partial airway obstruction. (p. 68)
10. State when you must treat a partial airway obstruction as if it were a full airway obstruction. (p. 68)
11. Describe TWO signs displayed by a conscious patient with a full airway obstruction. (p. 69)
12. Describe, step by step, the head-tilt, neck-lift maneuver; the head-tilt, chin-lift maneuver; and the modified jaw-thrust. (pp. 69-70)
13. Describe, step by step, the procedures used in correcting airway obstructions, including:
    • back blows
    • manual thrusts
    • finger sweeps (pp. 70-5)
14. State the FOUR-step sequence of combined procedures used for correcting an airway obstruction in a conscious patient. (p. 75)
15. List, as NINE steps, the procedures used when a conscious patient with an airway obstruction becomes unconscious. (p. 75)
16. State the SIX-step sequence of combined procedures used for correcting an airway obstruction when the patient is found unconscious. (p. 77)
17. List, step by step, the actions taken when providing mouth-to-mouth ventilation. (pp. 77-8)
18. Compare and contrast mouth-to-nose ventilation and mouth-to-stoma ventilation with the mouth-to-mouth techniques. (pp. 77-81)
19. List, step by step, the actions taken when providing rescue breathing to an infant or a small child. (p. 79)
20. State what the EMT can do to correct problems of gastric distention caused by artificial ventilation. (p. 82)

SKILLS As an EMT, you should be able to:

1. Determine if a patient has an airway obstruction and if there is adequate breathing.
2. Apply the proper techniques in the correct sequence necessary to correct airway obstruction.
3. Properly employ the head-tilt, chin-lift maneuver; the head-tilt, neck-lift maneuver; and the modified jaw-thrust.
4. Determine respiratory arrest.
5. Correctly perform mouth-to-mouth, mouth-to-nose, and mouth-to-stoma ventilations.

6. Correctly perform pulmonary resuscitation techniques on infants and small children.
7. Correct gastric distention brought about by artificial ventilations.

8. Provide airway care and resuscitation for patients with neck and spinal injuries.

TERMS   you may be using for the first time:

Clinical Death—when breathing and heart action stop.
Biological Death—when the brain cells begin to die.
Respiratory Arrest—when a patient stops breathing.

Pleura (PLOOR-ah)—a double-layered membranous sac. The outer layer lines the thoracic cavity. The inner layer clings to the outside of the lungs. Between the two layers lies the pleural space.
Pleural Cavity—the right and left portions of the thoracic cavity, containing the lungs.

Pharynx (FAR-inks)—the throat.
Larynx (LAR-inks)—that portion of the airway connecting the pharynx and the trachea. It contains the voicebox.
Thyroid (THI-roid) **Cartilage**—the Adam's apple.
Trachea (TRAY-ke-ah)—the windpipe.
Bronchus (BRON-kus)—one of the first two large branches that come off the trachea and enter the lungs. There are right and left primary bronchi.

Bronchiole (BRONG-key-ol)—the smaller branches of the airway that connect the bronchi to the airsacs of the lungs. The plural is bronchioles.
Alveoli (al-VE-o-li)—the microscopic airsacs of the lungs where gas exchange with the bloodstream takes place.
Cyanosis (sigh-ah-NO-sis)—when the skin, lips, earlobes, or nailbeds turn blue or gray due to a lack of oxygen in circulation.
Edema (e-DE-mah)—swelling due to excess fluid in the tissues.

Resuscitation (re-SUS-si-TAY-shun)—any efforts used to restore normal lung or lung and heart function.
Pulmonary (PUL-mo-ner-e) **Resuscitation**—providing artificial ventilation (rescue breathing) to the patient in an attempt to restore normal lung function.

Laryngectomee (LAR-in-JEK-to-me)—a "neck breather." A patient who has had surgical cutting into or removal of the larynx.

THE RESPIRATORY SYSTEM

There are several conditions that can cause death quickly, including the cessation of breathing, the absence of breathing and circulation, severe bleeding, and shock. You must be able to detect these problems quickly and take prompt and efficient action.

Keeping a patient alive when he has a life-threatening problem is known as **basic life support.** As an EMT, you must know how to provide basic life support using a minimum of equipment. In some cases, you will have to sustain life with no more than your hands, your breath, a great deal of common sense, and a few basic supplies.

There is more gained by the application of basic life support measures than simply keeping a patient alive. It may help stabilize the patient, or allow him to improve during care and transport.

The Importance of Breathing

The assurance of breathing takes precedence over all other emergency care measures. The reason is simple: if a person cannot breathe, he cannot survive.

The body's cells must be provided with oxygen and have carbon dioxide removed by means of circulating blood. The act of breathing, or **respiration,** is the process that carries oxygen from the atmosphere to the exchange levels of the lungs, where it is diffused into the bloodstream. The process of respiration continues as carbon dioxide is removed from the blood and carried out into the atmosphere.

A series of chemical processes continually converts food into the energy needed for life. These processes are collectively called **metabolism.** Oxygen is required for many of the metabolic processes occurring within the body's cells. An adequate and continuing supply of oxygen is needed to make energy-rich compounds. When these compounds are broken down, the cells again need oxygen for the process. The energy released is used to contract muscles, send nerve impulses, build new tissues, digest foods, and to carry out all life processes.

Carbon dioxide is a waste product released as a result of certain metabolic processes. If allowed to accumulate in the body, carbon dioxide can become a deadly poison. As the concentration of carbon dioxide increases, a person will start panting, trying to rid the body of the carbon dioxide. Soon, brain cells will start to malfunction. The person may start to hallucinate due to the narcotic effects of the excess carbon dioxide. Coma becomes a strong possibility. Unless corrected, body functions, including respiration, will fail, and the person will die.

The process of respiration does more than supply oxygen and remove carbon dioxide. It is difficult for things to stay in balance when there is constant change. Many chemical reactions take place in our bodies, causing such change. Some of these reactions make the blood too acidic, while others make it too basic (alkaline). The respiratory system plays a key role in preventing this. Should breathing become inadequate, the acid-base balance of the blood is upset, causing cells to die. Some of the cells most sensitive to this imbalance are those in the brain. **REMEMBER:** Breathing provides needed oxygen for the cells, removes potentially poisonous carbon dioxide, and helps to maintain the acid-base balance of the blood.

Biological Death

The process of respiration cannot be separated from circulation. It is not enough to receive oxygen at the exchange level of the lungs. This oxygen must be transported by the blood to the cells. Likewise, carbon dioxide must be carried to the lungs for removal from the body. You must always relate breathing to circulation, making sure that both processes are taking place. Chapter 5 will consider heart action and circulation.

As an EMT, you must know the difference between clinical death and biological death.

CLINICAL DEATH—a patient is clinically dead the moment breathing stops and the heart stops beating.
BIOLOGICAL DEATH—if a patient is not breathing and the heart is not circulating oxygenated blood, lethal changes begin to take place in the brain within *four to six minutes.* Biological death occurs with the death of the patient's brain cells. Usually, brain cell death begins *ten minutes* after the heart stops beating. You may be able to reverse clinical death, but biological death is irreversible.

RESPIRATORY SYSTEM ANATOMY

The major structures of the airway include:
- NOSE—the primary pathway for air to enter and leave the system.
- MOUTH—the secondary pathway for air.
- PHARYNX (FAR-inks)—the throat. The common passageway for air and food.
- LARYNX (LAR-inks)—the neck structure that connects the pharynx and the trachea. The voicebox is contained in the larynx. When

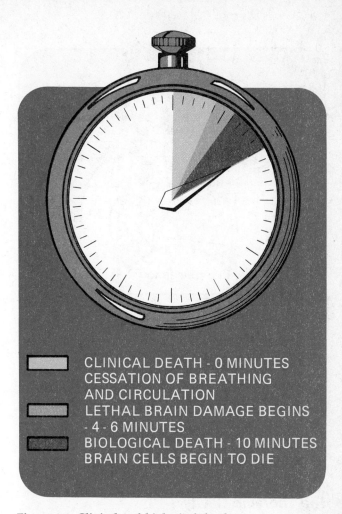

Figure 4-1: Clinical and biological death.

viewed externally, the most prominent feature is the **thyroid** (THI-roid) **cartilage,** or Adam's apple. A trapdoor-like structure, the **epiglottis** (EP-i-GLOT-is), normally prevents food, liquids, and foreign objects from entering the airway as they pass through the pharynx.
- TRACHEA (TRAY-ke-ah)—the windpipe.
- BRONCHIAL TREE—branching from the trachea to the microscopic airsacs of the lungs. The first branches are the right and left primary **bronchi** (BRONG-ki). These branch into secondary bronchi. The smaller branches coming off the secondary bronchi are called the **bronchioles** (BRONG-key-ols).
- LUNGS—the spongy, elastic organs containing **alveoli** (al-VE-o-li), the microscopic airsacs where oxygen and carbon dioxide exchange takes place.

Those structures found superior to the larynx are called the *upper airway.* The *lower airway* is composed of all the structures from the larynx to the alveoli. The structures of the airway do more than provide a passageway for air to and from the lungs. As air passes through the upper airway, it is filtered, adjusted to body temperature, and humidified. Hairs

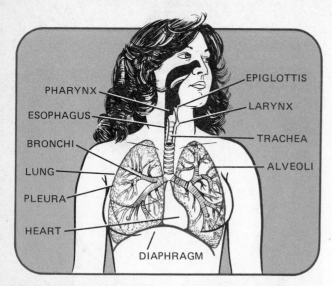

Figure 4-2: The major structures of the airway.

in the nose start the filtration process, trapping large particles. The mucus on the surface of the airway lining picks up most of the smaller particles. The blood vessels in the airway lining can either provide heat to air that is below body temperature, or absorb heat from air that is too warm. The tissues of the lining add water to the air so that it is nearly saturated with moisture. These processes combine to condition the air to reduce lung damage.

The Thoracic Cavity

Most of the trachea and all of the lungs are situated in the thoracic cavity (see Chapter 2). A double-layered membrane sac, the **pleura** (PLOOR-ah), is found inside this cavity. One layer lines the cavity, while the other layer coats the outside of the lungs. The pleural membrane protects the lungs and gives them an attachment with the chest wall.

The portion of the thoracic cavity containing the lungs is called the **pleural portion** of the thoracic cavity.

The thoracic cavity is separated from the abdominopelvic cavity by the diaphragm, the major muscle used in breathing.

RESPIRATORY FUNCTION

The physical process of respiration is so constant in a healthy person that he is seldom aware of his own breathing. The act of breathing is an *automatic function*. We can, for short periods, control the rate and depth of our breathing. However, most of the time breathing is *involuntary*, controlled by respiratory centers in the brain. The amount of carbon dioxide in our blood is constantly being monitored. If this level becomes too high, we automatically begin to breathe faster and deeper. A low level of oxygen also can be detected, which sets off a faster and

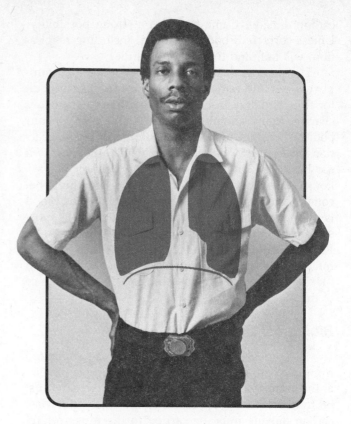

Figure 4-3: The thoracic cavity.

deeper breathing rate.

If you try to hold your breath, the respiratory centers in your brain will urge you to breathe. Should you try to run, taking very slow, shallow breaths, these centers would automatically adjust the rate, depth, and rhythm of breathing to suit the needs of your cells. Asleep, or even unconscious, if there is no damage to the respiratory centers and the heart continues circulating oxygenated blood to the brain, breathing will remain an involuntary, automatic function.

Breathing takes place due to changes in volume and pressure brought about as a result of the combined actions of the muscles attached to the rib cage and the diaphragm. An **inspiration** (the process of breathing in) takes place when these muscles contract. When the diaphragm and the muscles attached to the ribs relax, an **expiration** (the process of breathing out) takes place.

A basic law of physics governs breathing: AS VOLUME INCREASES, PRESSURE DECREASES. Consider the moment just before you begin an inspiration. The thoracic cavity has a certain volume and internal pressure. The lungs also have a certain volume and internal pressure. If the volume of the cavity is increased, the pressure within the cavity will decrease. If the volume of the lungs increases, the pressure within the lungs decreases. For an inspiration to take place, there must be a pressure decrease in the lungs to a point where it is less than the pressure of the atmosphere. Once this occurs, air

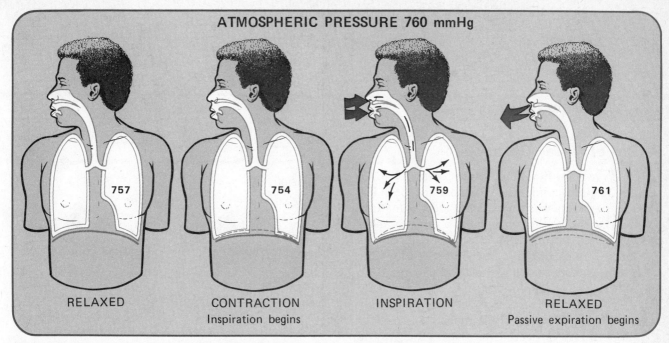

ATMOSPHERIC PRESSURE 760 mmHg

| 757 | 754 | 759 | 761 |

| RELAXED | CONTRACTION
Inspiration begins | INSPIRATION | RELAXED
Passive expiration begins |

Figure 4-4: Changes in volume and pressure produce inspirations and expirations.

will move from a place of high pressure, to one of low pressure.

NOTE: Do not think of the above as something entirely new. Relate it to the fact that the air taken out of a bicycle tire will not inflate a truck tire. There is a relationship between volume and pressure. You also know that air will move from an area of high pressure to one of low pressure. A punctured balloon or tire demonstrates this.

Inspiration and Expiration

You begin an inspiration by increasing the volume of the thoracic cavity. The muscles attached to the ribs contract and the ribs are pulled outward. The diaphragm flattens downward as it contracts, further increasing the volume in the chest cavity above its position. During this process the pressure on the outside of the lungs decreases and the lungs start to expand. This causes the volume of the lungs to increase. AS THE VOLUME OF THE LUNGS INCREASES, THE PRESSURE INSIDE THE LUNGS DECREASES. At a certain point, the pressure inside the lungs becomes less than atmospheric pressure. Air begins to flow from high to low pressure, or from the atmosphere into the lungs.

In the expiration phase, the diaphragm and the muscles attached to the ribs relax. The chest cavity and the lungs are reduced in volume. As the volume decreases, the pressure increases. At a certain point, the pressure within the lungs becomes greater than the pressure in the atmosphere. Air then moves from high to low pressure until the two pressures are equal.

The process of breathing is repeated 12 to 20 times each minute in the average adult male at rest. Each breath moves about one-half liter (500 cc or one pint) of air.

RESPIRATORY FAILURE

Simply stated, **respiratory failure** is either the cessation of normal breathing or the reduction of breathing to the point where oxygen intake is not sufficient to support life. When breathing stops completely, the patient is in **respiratory arrest**.

Diagnostic Signs

To determine SIGNS OF NORMAL BREATHING, you should:

- LOOK for the even rise and fall of the chest associated with breathing.
- LISTEN for air entering and leaving the nose or mouth. The sounds should be typical, free of gurgling, gasping, crowing, or wheezing.
- FEEL for air moving out of the nose or mouth.
- CHECK for typical skin coloration. There should be no blue or gray.
- NOTE that the rate and depth of breathing should be typical for a person at rest.

SIGNS OF INADEQUATE BREATHING include:

- No chest movement, or uneven chest movements
- No air can be felt or heard at the nose or mouth, or exchange is evaluated as below normal
- Noisy breathing
- The rate is too rapid or too slow

- Breathing is very shallow or very deep and labored
- The patient's skin is blue or gray. This is called **cyanosis** (sigh-ah-NO-sis).

AIRWAY OBSTRUCTION

Causes of Airway Obstruction

Every year in the United States, nearly 100,000 people die from accidents, and more than 600,000 die from heart attacks. Of the many deaths that annually occur away from hospitals, a large number probably could be prevented if modern resuscitative measures were used. Quite frequently, death is due to an airway obstruction. As noted in Chapter 3, in the ABC's of basic life support, the ''A'' stands for airway. As an EMT, you must be able to quickly detect and correct airway obstructions.

Many factors can cause the patient's airway to become partially or fully obstructed, including:

- OBSTRUCTION BY THE TONGUE—the tongue can fall back and block the pharynx (throat). This often occurs when a patient's head flexes forward and is allowed to remain in that position. This problem is most commonly seen with unconscious patients and patients who have abused alcohol or some other drug.
- FOREIGN OBJECTS—these can include pieces of food, ice, toys, dentures, broken teeth, vomitus, and liquids pooling in the back of the throat.
- TISSUE DAMAGE—these accident-related tissue problems can be caused by puncture wounds to the neck, crushing wounds to the face, breathing hot air (as in fires), poisons, and severe injury due to blows to the neck. Swelling (**edema,** e-DE-mah) presents a major problem in providing emergency care.
- DISEASES—respiratory infection, allergic reactions, and certain chronic illnesses such as asthma, can cause edema or bronchial spasms that will obstruct the airway.

Keep in mind the mechanisms of injury. Look over the scene. Together, such knowledge will tell you when to be alert for airway problems. Something as simple as noticing a half-eaten sandwich may make a difference.

Signs of Partial Airway Obstruction

Be alert for partial airway obstruction if you note:
- *Unusual breathing sounds*—Listen for:

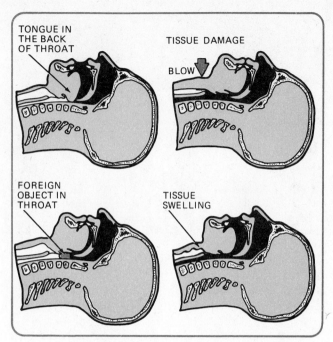

Figure 4-5: Four possible causes of airway obstruction.

SNORING—probably caused by the tongue obstructing the pharynx.
GURGLING—often due to a foreign object, or blood and other fluids in the trachea.
CROWING—probably caused by spasms in the larynx.
WHEEZING—this may not indicate any major problems along the airway. However, wheezing should not be treated lightly since it may be due to serious edema or spasms along the airway.
- *Skin discoloration*—The patient is breathing, but there is a noticeable blue or blue-gray color to the skin, lips, tongue, fingernail beds, or earlobes.
- *Changes in breathing*—The patient's breathing may keep changing from near normal to very labored.

A conscious patient will usually point to his mouth or hold his neck trying to indicate a problem. Many do this even when a partial obstruction does not prevent speech. For the conscious patient with an apparent partial airway obstruction, have him COUGH. A strong forceful cough indicates he is exchanging enough air. Continue to encourage the patient to cough. Such action may dislodge and expel the object.

WARNING: In cases where the patient has an apparent partial airway obstruction, but he cannot cough or has a very weak cough, begin to treat the patient AS IF THERE IS A COMPLETE AIRWAY OBSTRUCTION. This rule also applies to patients who are cyanotic.

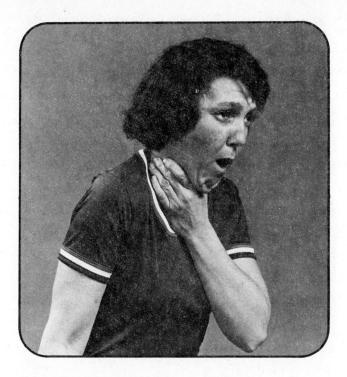

Figure 4-6: The distress signal for choking.

Signs of Complete Airway Obstruction

The *conscious* patient will try to speak, but he will not be able to do so, nor will he be able to cough. Usually, he will display the distress signal for choking, by clutching the neck between thumb and fingers. It will soon become apparent that he cannot breathe. The *unconscious* patient with a complete airway obstruction exhibits none of the usual signs of breathing, namely rhythmic chest movements and air exchange at the nose and mouth. We will study shock in Chapter 7. For now, keep in mind that the typical signs of shock can be seen in unconscious patients with full airway obstruction.

Opening the Airway

Many problems of partial airway obstruction, particularly those caused by the tongue, can be corrected by opening the patient's airway. This is the same procedure that you follow during the primary survey. There are several methods recommended for opening the airway.
WARNING: This procedure is NOT recommended for use on any patient with possible injuries to the neck or spine.
   Head-Tilt   The head-tilt procedure is a simple repositioning of the head. For cases where the patient is conscious and in a seated position, reposition the head so that it does not flex forward on the chest. Ask the patient if he can hold his head in a normal position. If he cannot, you should assist him. When the patient is lying down, place one of your hands on the forehead and apply gentle, firm, back-

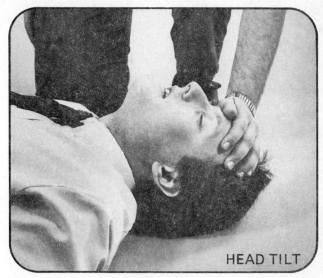

Figure 4-7: The Head-Tilt Maneuver.

ward pressure using the palm of your hand. This will tilt the patient's head backward.

In some cases, you will find a patient lying on several pillows, or with his head against some object. Repositioning of the head, or removal of these objects will prevent his head from flexing too far forward.

WARNING: This procedure is not recommended for use on any patient with possible neck or spinal injuries.
   Head-Tilt, Chin-lift Maneuver   This technique

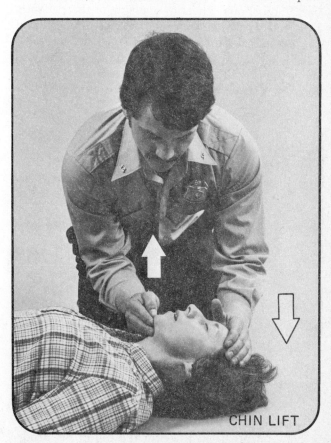

Figure 4-8: The Head-Tilt, Chin-Lift Maneuver.

is gaining in popularity, offering the maximum opening of the airway. It is useful on patients who are conscious and need assistance in breathing. Many rescuers have found that it works well for patients with loose dentures. The maneuver can be employed where the Head-Tilt, Neck-Lift maneuver is recommended in basic life support.

One hand is placed on the patient's forehead, while the fingertips of the other hand are placed under the chin. The fingertips are used to bring the chin forward and to support the jaw. This movement will also help to tilt the head. Most of the head-tilt is provided by pushing down on the patient's forehead. During the entire procedure, it is important that you do not compress the soft tissues under the lower jaw, and that you lift the chin and move it to a point where the lower teeth are almost touching the upper teeth. The patient's mouth is NOT to be closed. To provide an adequate opening at the mouth, you may find it necessary to use your thumb to pull back the patient's lower lip.

WARNING: This procedure is not recommended for use on any patient with possible neck or spinal injuries.

Head-Tilt, Neck-Lift Maneuver This is the same procedure described in Chapter 3 for use during the primary survey. This maneuver can be carried out on a seated patient; however, most agree that it is more effective if the patient is placed on his back. You should kneel to one side of the patient's head. Place one hand on the patient's forehead and the other hand under his neck. Lift the patient's neck while pushing down on the forehead. This will move the patient's tongue away from the back of the throat and provide an adequate airway opening.

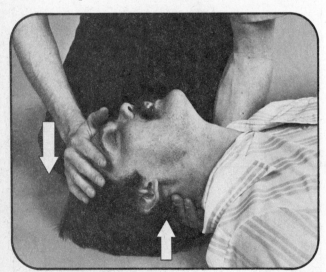

Figure 4-9: The Head-Tilt, Neck-Lift Maneuver.

The Modified Jaw-Thrust The patient should be lying on his back. Kneel at the top of his head, resting your elbows on the same surface on which

the patient is lying. Carefully reach forward and gently place one hand on each side of the patient's chin, at the angles of the lower jaw. Push the patient's jaw forward, applying most of the pressure with your index fingers. Do NOT tilt or rotate the patient's head.

NOTE: The modified jaw-thrust is the *only* widely recommended procedure for use on unconscious patients with possible neck or spinal injuries.

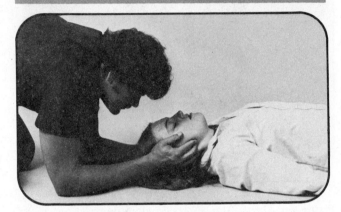

Figure 4-10: The Modified Jaw-Thrust.

Correcting Airway Obstructions

The conscious patient usually will be able to indicate that he is having problems with his airway. This will allow you to act swiftly to provide an adequate airway. However, if the patient is not able to communicate, or is unconscious, you must be able to determine quickly that the airway is obstructed, and take appropriate measures to clear it. Since so many obstructions are caused by the tongue, you should always make certain the airway is open. Once this is done, three maneuvers are recommended for removal of foreign materials. These are *back blows*, *manual thrusts*, and *finger sweeps*. On any given patient, you may have to use all three methods.

The techniques used in clearing the airway vary depending on whether the patient is conscious, loses consciousness while being treated, or is unconscious. We will begin by describing the techniques used to clear the airway, then we will apply specific procedures to each type of patient.

NOTE: If the cause of airway obstruction is blood, liquids, or vomitus pooling in the throat, you should consider the use of suctioning to clear the airway (see Chapter 6). Do NOT delay efforts to clear the airway in order to locate and set up suctioning equipment.

Back Blows With the conscious patient *sitting* or *standing*, position yourself at his side, slightly behind him. Place one hand high on his chest, around the clavicles, to provide support while you bend him over at the waist. The patient's head should be positioned at chest level or lower so that gravity will help to remove the obstruction. Use your free hand to rapidly deliver FOUR SHARP BLOWS to the spinal area between the shoulder blades. You are trying to cause pressure waves of air to leave the lungs with enough force to dislodge the foreign object. This will not occur if you just pat the patient. You

MUST deliver a rapid series of sharp blows, using common sense to vary the force of the blows in relation to the patient's size and age.

The unconscious patient should be positioned on his back. If the patient is conscious, but unable to sit or be seated with your assistance, he may be placed in a supine position. When the patient is *lying down*, kneel beside the patient and roll him onto his side, bringing his chest firmly against your knees. Support him with one hand. (Some systems are very specific about this hand placement, believing that it should be placed to provide protection for the patient's head). Use your other hand to rapidly deliver FOUR SHARP BLOWS to the area of the spine directly between the shoulder blades.

Back blows can be used when providing care for infants and small children. An **infant** is any patient between birth and one year of age. A **child** is any patient between the ages of one and eight. When the patient is an infant or small child, cradle the patient face down on your forearm, with the head lower than the trunk. Best results can be obtained if you are seated and rest this forearm on one of your thighs. You MUST support the patient's head by placing a hand around the lower jaw and chest. Use the heel of your free hand to rapidly deliver FOUR SHARP BLOWS to the spinal area between the shoulder blades.

NOTE: Do NOT place infants or small children into this head-down position if they have a partial obstruction and can breathe adequately in an upright

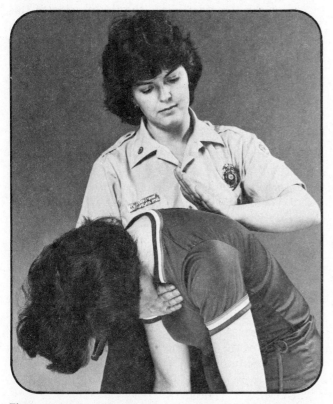

Figure 4-11: Rapidly deliver four sharp back blows.

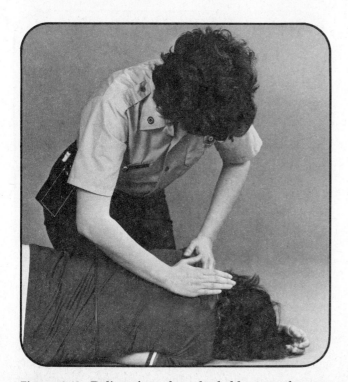

Figure 4-12: Deliver four sharp back blows to the area between the shoulder blades.

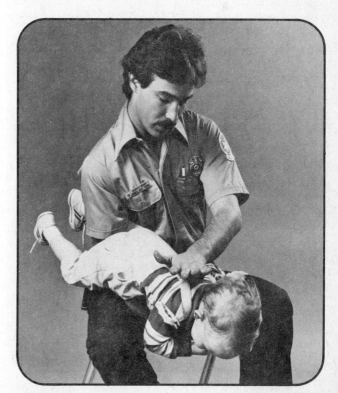

Figure 4-13: Cradle the infant or small child face down on your forearm.

position. Keep in mind that forceful coughing is a good sign in cases of partial airway obstruction.

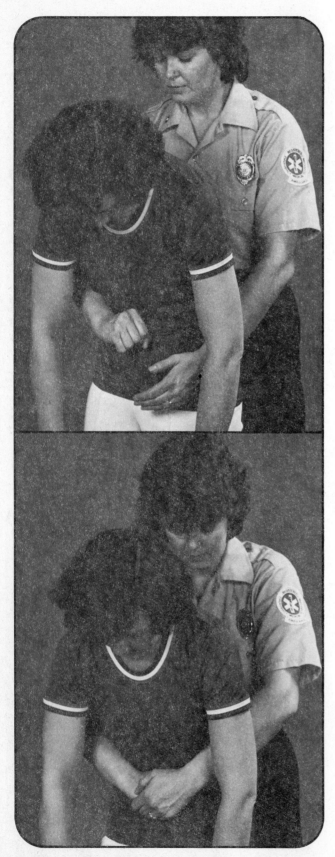

Figure 4-14: Place your fist on the patient's midline between the waist and rib cage. Grasp the fist and rapidly deliver four upward thrusts.

Manual Thrusts—Abdominal   Abdominal thrusts are used to force a burst of air from the lungs that will be sufficient to dislodge an obstructing object.

With the conscious patient *standing* or *sitting*, stand behind him and slide your arms under his armpits, wrapping both of your arms around his waist. Make a fist and place the thumb side of this fist against the midline of the patient's abdomen, between the waist and rib cage. Avoid touching the patient's chest, especially the area immediately below the sternum (the region of the xiphoid process). Grasp your properly positioned fist with your other hand and apply pressure as an upward thrust. This will cause your fist to press into the patient's abdomen. Deliver FOUR RAPID UPWARD THRUSTS.

Abdominal thrusts are best delivered to the unconscious patient when he is in a supine position. The same technique can be used for a conscious patient who cannot sit up or be seated with your assistance. When the patient is *lying down*, move him into a supine position. Kneel close to his side at hip level, facing his chest. Place the heel of your hand on the midline of his abdomen, slightly above the navel and below the rib cage. Now place your free hand over the positioned hand and lock your arms at the shoulders and elbows. Deliver compressions by rocking forward, pressing your hands inward and upward toward the patient's diaphragm. Stop your forward motion when your shoulders are directly over the patient's abdomen. Deliver FOUR RAPID ABDOMINAL THRUSTS.

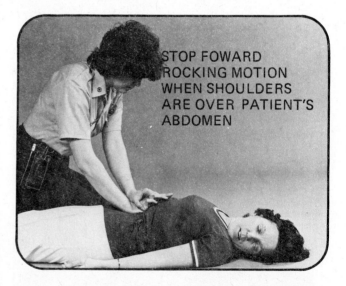

STOP FOWARD ROCKING MOTION WHEN SHOULDERS ARE OVER PATIENT'S ABDOMEN

Figure 4-15: Abdominal thrust technique used on a patient who is lying down.

If the patient is very large, or if you are a small individual, you can deliver more effective thrusts if you straddle one leg of the patient, or you straddle the entire patient at the level of the hips.

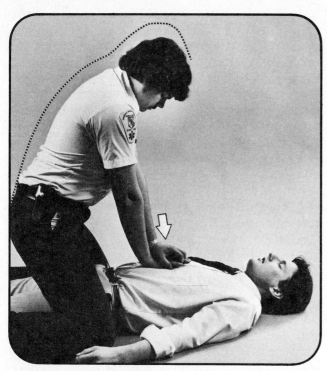

Figure 4-16: Your abdominal thrusts may be more effective if you straddle the patient.

WARNING: The American Heart Association (AHA) does NOT recommend abdominal thrusts for infants and children.

Manual Thrusts—Chest The chest thrust is an alternative method to the abdominal thrust. It is useful if the patient is an infant, small child, pregnant, or when the patient is too large for you to wrap your arms around his waist.

When the conscious patient is *standing or sitting*, position yourself behind the patient and slide your arms under his armpits, so that you encircle his chest. Form a fist with one hand and place the thumb side of this fist on the patient's sternum. You should make contact with the midline of the sternum, about two to three finger-widths above the lower tip of the sternum. Grasp the fist with your other hand and rapidly deliver FOUR QUICK THRUSTS directly backward. Do NOT exert this force in an upward or downward direction, or off to one side.

Again, the best procedure for an unconscious patient is carried out when the patient is in a *supine* position. Kneel beside the patient at the level of the chest. Have both of your knees facing the patient's chest. Position the heel of one hand on the midline of the sternum, two to three finger-widths from the lower tip (your fingers should be perpendicular to the sternum). Lift and spread your fingers to avoid applying too much pressure to the ribs. Place your other hand on top of the first, lock your elbows and lean forward until your shoulders are directly over the midline of the patient's chest. Rapidly deliver FOUR QUICK THRUSTS in a downward direction.

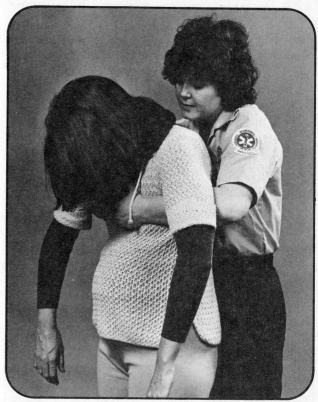

Figure 4-17: The chest thrust applied to a pregnant patient.

If you find it necessary to use the chest thrust procedure on an *infant* or *small child*, you should

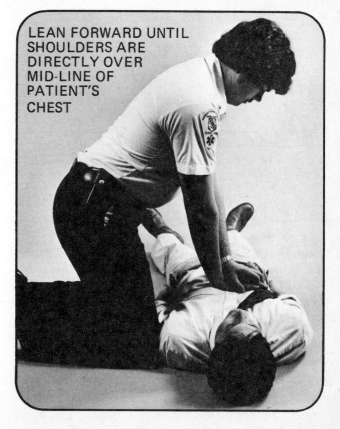

LEAN FORWARD UNTIL SHOULDERS ARE DIRECTLY OVER MID-LINE OF PATIENT'S CHEST

Figure 4-18: The chest thrust method can be used when the patient is lying on his back.

cradle the infant, face down, on your forearm and deliver FOUR BACK BLOWS. Sandwich the patient between your hands and turn him to a face up position on your thigh, making certain that you provide adequate support for the head throughout the turn. Reposition the patient so that the head is lower than the trunk. Deliver FOUR CHEST THRUSTS, using the tips of two or three fingers, applying pressure along the midline of the sternum, directly between the nipples.

If your patient is a child who is too large to hold on your forearm, kneel on one knee and drape the child across your thigh. Again, the head of the patient must be lower than his trunk. Rapidly deliver FOUR BACK BLOWS. Support the child's head and back and place him face up on the floor or ground. Apply FOUR CHEST THRUSTS to the sternum, between the nipples. If three fingertips do not produce results, use the heel of one hand.

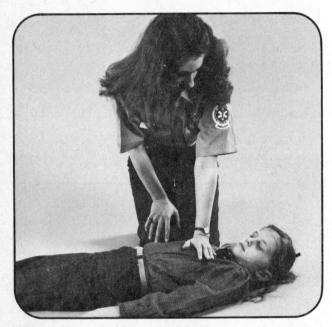

Figure 4-19: For infants and children, chest thrusts are applied to the midline of the sternum, directly between the nipples.

Finger Sweeps   Manual removal of an object can be tried if the object is dislodged or partially dislodged. Always take great care not to force the object further down the patient's throat. This is especially true in infants and small children. *Do NOT use "blind" finger sweeps and probes in infants and children.* You must *see* the object before trying to grasp it with your fingers.

You can open an unconscious patient's mouth and airway by using the tongue-jaw lift procedure. This requires you to grasp both tongue and lower jaw between your thumb and fingers and lift to move the tongue away from the back of the pharynx. This movement will also move the tongue away from any foreign object that might be lodged in the

back of the throat. This procedure may partially solve the problem of obstruction. However, it will be necessary to insert the index finger of your free hand into the patient's mouth and move this finger along the inside of the patient's cheek to the base of the tongue. Using your finger as a hook, attempt to dislodge the object and sweep it into the mouth so it can be removed.

In some cases, it may be necessary to use your index finger to push the foreign object against the opposite side of the patient's throat in order to dislodge and lift the object. During such a procedure, you must take extra care not to push the object further down the patient's throat.

CAUTION: A conscious patient has a gag reflex that can induce vomiting. Vomitus can be inhaled into the lungs. This is why some EMS Systems do not sanction the use of finger sweeps on conscious patients. Some localities believe that there are situations where aggressive actions must be taken during basic life support. If an obstructing object becomes visible, the EMT can use a finger sweep to dislodge and remove the object. If you are using a finger sweep method on a conscious patient, or you are trying to grasp a dislodged object, take great care not to induce vomiting or force the object further down the patient's airway.

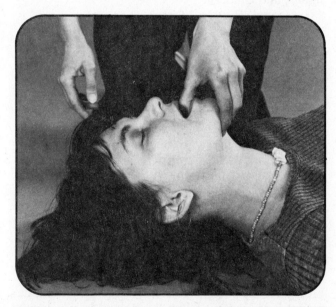

Figure 4-20: The tongue-jaw lift can be used to open the mouth and airway of an unconscious patient.

You can use the crossed-finger technique to open the mouth of an unconscious patient. Use one hand to steady the patient's forehead. Take your free hand and cross the thumb under the index finger. Place your thumb against the patient's lower lip and your index finger against his upper teeth. Uncrossing your fingers will force open the patient's mouth. Once the mouth is open, hold the lower jaw so that it cannot close.

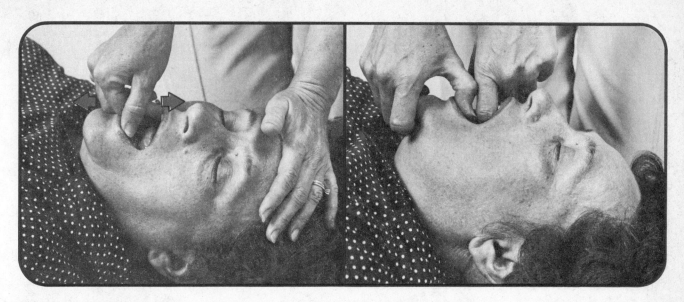

Figure 4-21: Open the patient's mouth using the crossed-fingers technique. Use finger sweeps to remove foreign objects from the airway and mouth.

Once you have opened the patient's mouth, release the patient's forehead and use the index finger of this hand as you would in the tongue-jaw lift procedure.

NOTE: When using the finger sweep technique, remember: If the object comes within reach, grasp the object and remove it. Be careful not to push it down the patient's airway.

Correcting Airway Obstructions—Combined Procedures If a person has only a partial airway obstruction and is still able to speak and cough forcefully, do not interfere with his attempts to expel the foreign body. Carefully watch him, however, so that you can immediately provide help if this partial obstruction becomes a complete one.

An unconscious patient or one with total airway obstruction will present the greatest problems. The combined procedures listed here for both conscious and unconscious patients are those recommended by American Heart Association research. The AHA has shown that a specific sequence of actions will provide the greatest chance for you to clear the patient's airway. The research is continuing, meaning that procedures may change in the future. You must keep up-to-date in basic life support techniques.

If the adult patient is conscious, you should:

1. Determine if there is a COMPLETE OBSTRUCTION. Look, listen and feel for the signs of complete obstruction. Be certain to ask, ''Can you speak?''

2. Deliver FOUR BACK BLOWS in rapid succession. If the object is not expelled. . .

3. Provide FOUR MANUAL THRUSTS (abdominal or chest) in rapid succession. If the manual thrusts do not expel the obstruction. . .

4. Alternate four back blows and four manual thrusts until you are successful or the patient loses consciousness.

If the patient loses consciousness, you should:

1. Protect the patient from possible injury due to falling.

2. Position the patient lying down on his back.

3. Attempt to open the patient's airway by the head-tilt, neck-lift; head-tilt, chin-lift; or modified jaw-thrust maneuver. Remember to look, listen, and feel for breathing.

4. Pinch the patient's nostrils closed. Typically, this is done with the hand used to hold the patient's forehead. Try to give FOUR QUICK VENTILATIONS as described in the section on mouth-to-mouth ventilation (p. 77). Do not allow the patient's lungs to deflate between ventilations. You can usually tell if ventilation will be successful after the first attempt. If your attempts to ventilate the patient fail, you should. . .

5. Administer four back blows in rapid succession. If this fails. . .

6. Provide four manual thrusts in rapid succession, keeping the patient's head to the side. If this fails. . .

7. Attempt finger sweeps. If you cannot find and remove the obstruction, you should. . .

8. Reposition the patient's head, attempt to create an open airway, and try to ventilate. If this fails. . .

9. Repeat the sequence of:

   A. Delivering four back blows;

   B. Providing four manual thrusts;

   C. Performing finger sweeps.

CLEARING AIRWAY OBSTRUCTIONS COMBINED PROCEDURES

CONSCIOUS PATIENT

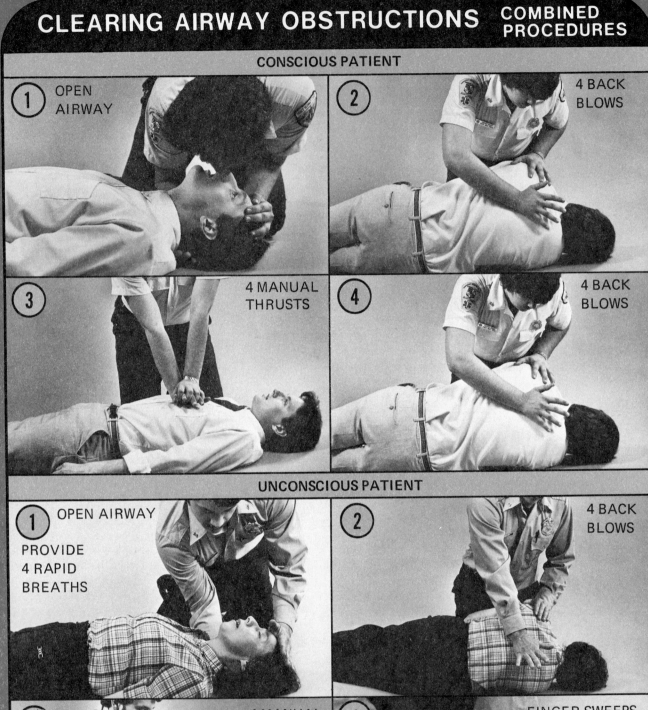

(1) OPEN AIRWAY

(2) 4 BACK BLOWS

(3) 4 MANUAL THRUSTS

(4) 4 BACK BLOWS

UNCONSCIOUS PATIENT

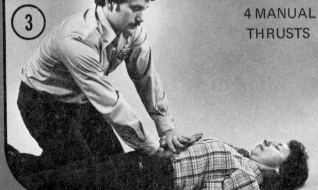
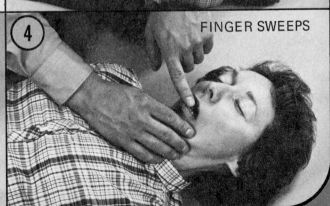

(1) OPEN AIRWAY

PROVIDE 4 RAPID BREATHS

(2) 4 BACK BLOWS

(3) 4 MANUAL THRUSTS

(4) FINGER SWEEPS

SCAN 4.1

If you are unable to dislodge the obstruction, you have a *true emergency* requiring transport to a medical facility without delay. You must continue efforts to clear the obstruction, even if you can do no more than partially dislodge the object. Once the object is partially dislodged, you should be able to keep the patient alive by mouth-to-mouth ventilations or other accepted techniques. Keep in mind that cardiopulmonary resuscitation may be necessary.

If the patient is unconscious when you arrive at the scene, you should:

1. Use the methods describe in Chapter 3 to see if the patient is unconscious. Gently tap the patient on the shoulders and ask, "Are you okay? Are you okay? Are you okay?" Avoid shaking the patient.
2. Establish an open airway and check for adequate breathing. If you believe the patient has an airway obstruction, or if the patient is not breathing, you should. . .
3. Attempt to provide the patient with FOUR QUICK VENTILATIONS. You will probably know if you are going to be successful on the first attempt. If you are not successful. . .
4. Reposition the patient's head and repeat your attempts to ventilate. If this second attempt fails, you should. . .
5. Deliver FOUR BACK BLOWS. Perform four manual thrusts. Attempt finger sweeps to clear the airway of foreign objects. If these attempts fail. . .
6. Try to ventilate the patient and repeat the sequence of back blows, manual thrusts, and finger sweeps. Once the airway is open, provide artificial ventilation or CPR as necessary.

REMEMBER: You must persist in your efforts until the airway is clear or until you have dislodged the object enough to allow for you to provide artificial ventilations. If the patient's brain cells do not receive oxygen, they will begin to die in ten minutes. Keep in mind that procedures used to clear the airway may at first fail, only to be successful later as muscles in the patient's body relax.

If the patient is a conscious INFANT or SMALL CHILD, you should:

1. Apply four sharp back blows.
2. Deliver four chest thrusts.
3. Alternate four back blows and four chest thrusts until the airway is cleared or until the patient becomes unconscious.

If the infant or child patient becomes unconscious, deliver four chest thrusts and then insert your thumb into his mouth, over the tongue. Wrap your finger around the lower jaw and lift the tongue and jaw forward, opening the patient's mouth. Look for any objects causing the obstruction. If you can see the object, remove it, but do NOT attempt "blind" finger sweeps. If you cannot see and remove an object, deliver four quick breaths by the mouth-to-mouth and nose technique (p. 79) and continue the cycle of back blows, chest thrusts, attempts to remove the object, and ventilations until the airway is cleared. Should the patient develop respiratory arrest and you have cleared enough of the obstruction to provide adequate mouth-to-mouth and nose ventilation, provide four breaths and check for heart action to see if you must initiate CPR (see Chapter 5).

PULMONARY RESUSCITATION

Rescue breathing, or artificial ventilation, is called **pulmonary resuscitation** (PUL-mo-ner-e re-SUS-si-TAY-shun). When you perform pulmonary resuscitation, you are providing artificial ventilations to the patient in an effort to restore normal lung function. The patient may not start breathing on his own (spontaneous breathing), but the procedure will allow oxygen to enter the bloodstream and carbon dioxide to be removed.

Many students wonder how artificial ventilations provide enough oxygen to the patient, since the air has already been in the rescuer's lungs. Atmospheric air contains 21% oxygen. The air you exhale contains 16% oxygen. This means that the air you provide for the nonbreathing patient still contains about three times the amount of oxygen that is normally removed by the lungs.

Mouth-to-Mouth Ventilation

This technique can be performed by one person, with no special equipment. It is the most efficient of the basic resuscitative techniques, and it is easy for the rescuer to tell if his efforts are effective. Primarily, this procedure is used when the patient is in **respiratory arrest,** that is, when he is no longer breathing.

Keep in mind that you may use the head-tilt, neck-lift maneuver, or the head-tilt, chin-lift maneuver. If there is a possibility of spinal injuries, the modified jaw-thrust should be used.

When providing mouth-to-mouth ventilations, you should:

1. Establish if the patient is responsive.
2. Open the patient's airway.
3. Determine if the patient is breathing and if the breathing is adequate.
   - LOOK for chest movements.
   - LISTEN for air flow (note any unusual sounds).

- FEEL for air exchange (against your cheek).
- NOTE anything that appears wrong, such as blue coloration of the skin.
  Take FIVE SECONDS to determine if the patient is breathing.
4. Maintain the patient in the optimum head-tilt position and pinch the nose closed with the thumb and forefinger of the hand you are using to hold the patient's forehead.
5. Open your mouth wide and take a deep breath.
6. Place your mouth around the patient's mouth and make a tight seal with your lips against the patient's face.
7. Quickly exhale into the patient's mouth until you see his chest rise and feel the resistance offered by his expanding lungs.
8. Break contact with the patient's mouth to allow him to passively exhale. Quickly take in another deep breath and exhale this air into the patient's airway BEFORE his lungs can deflate. Repeat this process two more times to give a total of FOUR QUICK BREATHS to the patient. Do NOT let his lungs deflate completely between these four ventilations.
9. If the patient does not begin spontaneous breathing, check for a carotid pulse (see Chapter 5). If there is a pulse, but no breathing, continue with the following cycle:
   - Take a deep breath and pinch the patient's nostrils closed.
   - Form a seal with the patient's mouth and quickly exhale air into the patient's airway.
   - Break contact with the patient's mouth and allow his nostrils to open. Air should be passively released from his lungs while you. . .
   - Turn your head to watch the patient's chest fall and listen and feel for the return of air.
   - Take another deep breath, close the patient's nostrils, and begin the cycle again.

IMPORTANT: For the mouth-to-mouth technique provided to the adult patient, you must deliver breaths to the patient **once every five seconds** to give a rate of **twelve breaths per minute.** To help establish this rate, count to yourself, ''One, one thousand; two, one thousand; three, one thousand; four, one thousand; B-R-E-A-T-H-E.''

Once you are breathing for the patient, you must continue to do so until he starts to breathe on his own, until you transfer the responsibility to another trained person, or until you detect cardiac arrest and must begin CPR.

You will know that you are following correct procedures and that you are *adequately ventilating* the patient if you:

- SEE the chest rise and fall.
- HEAR and FEEL air leaving the patient's lungs.
- FEEL resistance to your ventilations as the patient's lungs expand.
- NOTE if skin color improves or remains normal.
- NOTE the pupils of the eyes react to light.

The most common *problems* with the mouth-to-mouth technique include, in the following order, failure to:

- Form a tight seal over the patient's mouth
- Pinch the nose completely closed
- Establish an open airway because of inadequate head-tilt or head positioning
- Have the patient's mouth open wide enough to receive ventilations.

Mouth-To-Nose-Ventilation

Occasionally, you will not be able to ventilate a nonbreathing patient by the mouth-to-mouth technique. An accident victim may have severe injuries to the mouth and lower jaw. Patients lacking teeth or dentures may have pronounced receding chins. For such patients, you may have to use the mouth-to-nose technique. Most of the procedure is the same as mouth-to-mouth. The airway must be opened and the first four breaths are delivered without allowing the patient's lungs to deflate. As with the mouth-to-mouth procedure, breaths are delivered *once every five seconds* to equal *twelve breaths per minute.* The differences in the mouth-to-nose procedure include:

- You must keep one hand on the patient's forehead and use your other hand to close the patient's mouth.
- The patient's nose is left open.
- To provide breaths, you must seal your mouth around and deliver ventilations through the patient's nose. The patient's mouth must be kept closed during delivery of the ventilation.
- When allowing the patient to exhale passively, you must break contact with his nose and slightly open his mouth. Keep your hand on the patient's forehead to help keep his airway open as he exhales.

Ventilating Infants and Children

To provide ventilations to the infant or child, you should:

1. Establish whether the patient is responsive.
2. Lay the patient on a hard surface. When necessary, you can cradle an infant in your arms.
3. Open the airway and determine if the patient is breathing.
   CAUTION: A *slight* head-tilt is all that is required to open the airway of children. Almost no tilt is needed to open the airway of infants and small children. Too great a tilt could actually obstruct the airway of a young infant.
4. Take a breath and cover both the mouth and nose of the infant or small child patient (mouth-to-mouth and nose technique).
5. Use GENTLE BREATHS. Only SMALL PUFFS from your cheeks are needed to ventilate infants.
   CAUTION: You must stay alert for resistance to you ventilations and for chest movements. If you are too forceful with your ventilations, air will be forced into the patient's stomach.
6. When allowing the patient to exhale, uncover both mouth and nose.
7. Provide ventilations as one gentle puff or one small breath every three to four seconds. The ideal rate for *infants* is ONE PUFF EVERY THREE SECONDS. The ideal rate for *children* is ONE SMALL BREATH EVERY FOUR SECONDS.

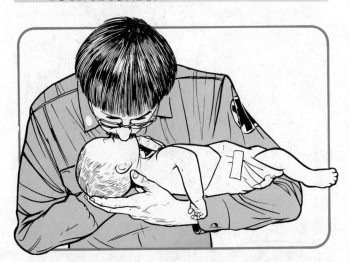

Figure 4-22: Ventilating infants and small children: Deliver one puff or small breath every 3 to 4 seconds. Do NOT hyperextend the neck.

Ventilating Neck Breathers

Although such occasions are rare, you may have to ventilate a neck breather, or laryngectomy (LAR-

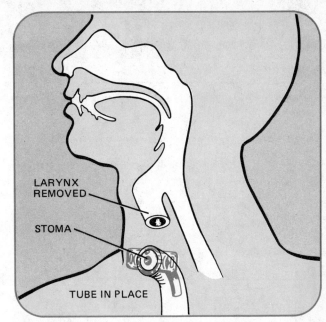

Figure 4-23: Anatomy of a laryngectomy patient.

in-JEK-to-me) patient. This is someone who has had a laryngectomy (surgical procedure in which part or all of the larynx has been removed). The trachea is shortened and usually brought to the front of the neck as a permanent opening called a stoma. The patient is called a laryngectomee (LAR-in-JEK-to-me).

A laryngectomy requires the construction of a permanent stoma. A tracheostomy (TRAY-ke-OS-to-me), the creation of an artificial opening into the trachea through the neck, may be temporary or permanent, depending upon the reason for the surgery. The opening of a tracheostomy is round and usually no more than several millimeters in diameter. The opening often contains two metal tubes, although some patients may have only one tube made of metal or plastic. When two tubes are used, there is an

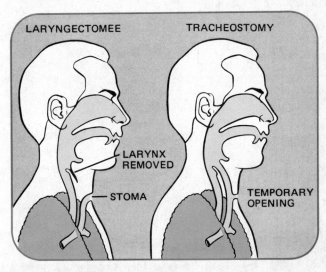

Figure 4-24: Differences between the laryngectomy and the tracheostomy.

RESCUE BREATHING

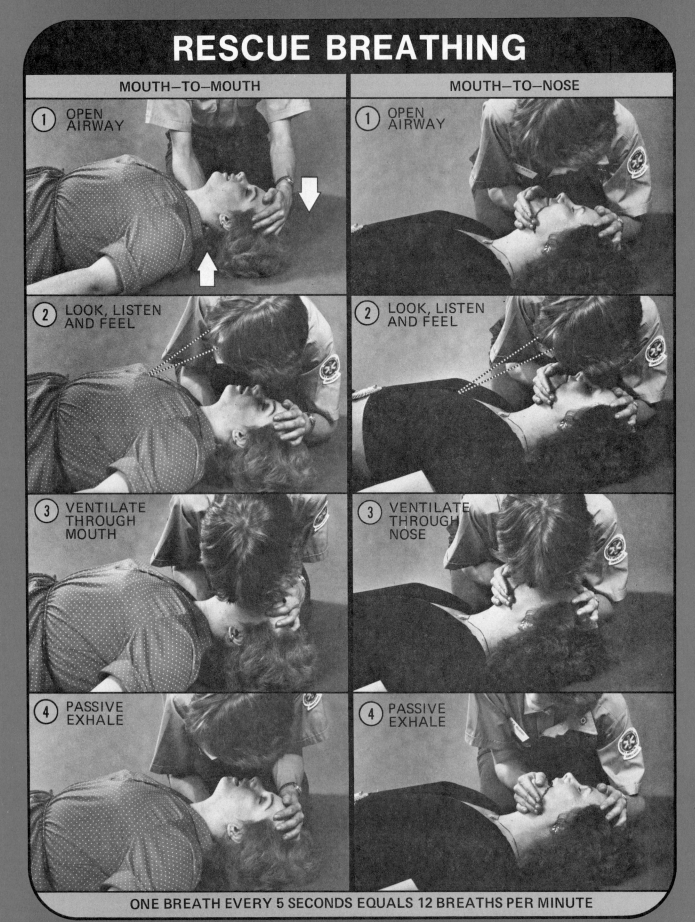

MOUTH—TO—MOUTH	MOUTH—TO—NOSE
① OPEN AIRWAY	① OPEN AIRWAY
② LOOK, LISTEN AND FEEL	② LOOK, LISTEN AND FEEL
③ VENTILATE THROUGH MOUTH	③ VENTILATE THROUGH NOSE
④ PASSIVE EXHALE	④ PASSIVE EXHALE

ONE BREATH EVERY 5 SECONDS EQUALS 12 BREATHS PER MINUTE

SCAN 4.2

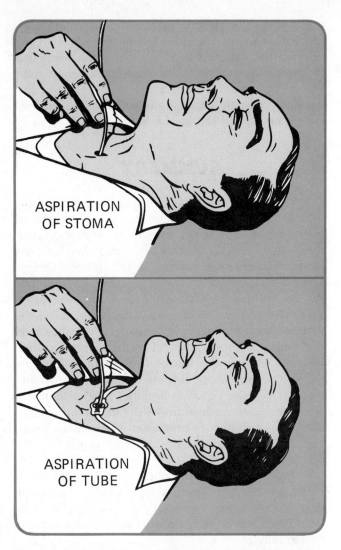

Figure 4-25: Suctioning techniques for the laryngectomee.

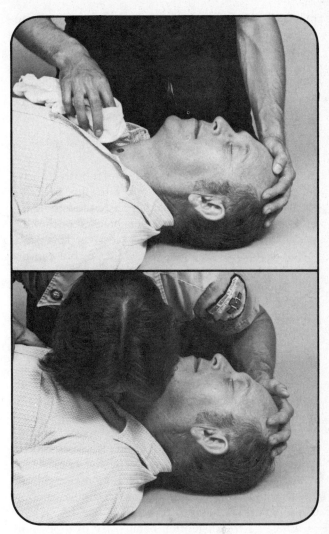

Figure 4-26: Mouth-to-stoma ventilations.

outer tube and an inner one connecting the skin to the trachea. In the laryngectomy, the opening is large and round, and the edge of the tracheal lining can be seen attached to the skin. There is no metal tube. The method of ventilation is the same for both types of patients.

When you examine a patient's stoma, you may find that there is a breathing tube (or tubes) in the opening. This tube may become clogged and need cleaning. Removal and cleaning of this tube create no problems for laryngectomees. The tube can be cleaned and replaced after it is moistened with the patient's saliva. However, in recent cases of tracheostomy, the tube should not be removed since the slit will close. The tube must be cleaned while in place.

Before you attempt any kind of resuscitative measures for the laryngectomee, first check for obstruction in the trachea. Clean the neck opening of encrusted mucus and foreign matter. Pass a suction catheter tube through the stoma and into the trachea while holding the tube pinched off (see Chapter 6). Do NOT insert the tube more than 2 or 3 inches into

the trachea. Release the pressure on the tube and withdraw it to allow suctioning to take place.

Keep in mind that a conscious patient may wish to do this for himself. Since he is trained in the procedure you should allow him to do so.

Since the patient's airway from throat to trachea has been interrupted, you will have to use the **mouth-to-stoma** technique on neck breathers. Use the same basic technique as for mouth-to-mouth ventilation, but do NOT tilt the head. Best results come from keeping the patient's head straight and his shoulders slightly elevated. Place your mouth directly on the patient's stoma rather than his mouth (mouth-to-stoma ventilation is actually cleaner than mouth-to-mouth ventilation). Use the same size breaths you normally would, and provide ventilations at the rate of ONE EVERY FIVE SECONDS. Make certain to watch for the patient's chest to rise and fall as you provide ventilations.

If the patient's chest does not rise, it may mean that the patient is a *partial neck breather*. This type of patient does take in and expel some air through the mouth and nose. In such cases, you will have to pinch closed the nose and seal the mouth with the palm of your hand.

NOTE: Other special patients, including the elderly, near-drowning victims, and accident victims will be covered in this text. The special problems of airway obstruction and artificial ventilation will be discussed when these cases are presented.

Gastric Distention

The mouth-to-mouth and the mouth-to-nose procedures can force some air into the patient's stomach. The stomach becomes distended (bulges), often indicating that the airway is blocked or that the ventilations being provided are excessive. This problem is seen most frequently in children, but can occur with any patient. A slight bulge is of little worry, but a major distention can cause two serious problems. First of all, the air-filled stomach reduces lung volume by forcing up the diaphragm. Secondly, vomiting is a strong possibility. This could lead to additional airway obstruction or the **aspiration** (breathing in) of vomitus into the patient's lungs.

The best way to avoid gastric distention is to properly position the patient and limit the volume of ventilations delivered. This is one reason why it is so important to watch the patient's chest rise as a ventilation is delivered. The volume delivered should be limited to that which causes the chest to rise.

WARNING: The AHA states that no attempt should be made to force air from the stomach unless suction equipment is on hand for immediate use.

Once gastric distention begins, try to reposition the patient's head to provide a better airway. Be prepared for vomiting, and turn the patient's head to the side should it occur. If suction equipment is

on hand and the patient has marked distention, you can turn him on his side, facing away from you. Support the patient's head with one hand and use the palm of your other hand to apply moderate pressure to the abdomen between the rib cage and the navel. Be prepared to use suction to clear the patient's mouth and throat of vomitus.

SUMMARY

We breathe to bring in oxygen, remove carbon dioxide, and to help regulate the acid-base balance of the blood. The major muscle of respiration, the diaphragm, and the muscles between the ribs contract to increase the volume in the thoracic cavity. The lungs expand, thus becoming greater in volume. As the volume increases, the pressure decreases. When the pressure in the lungs decreases to where it is less than atmospheric pressure, air rushes into the lungs (an inspiration). When the diaphragm and the muscles between the ribs relax, the volume in the lungs decreases, causing the pressure to increase. Once the pressure becomes greater than the atmosphere, air rushes out of the lungs (an expiration). All of this is an involuntary, automatic process, controlled mainly by respiratory centers in the brain.

Clinical death occurs when an individual stops breathing and the heart stops beating. Biological death occurs when the brain cells start to die. This takes place when the brain cells are without oxygen for ten minutes.

In addition to the respiratory centers in the brain, the diaphragm, and the muscles between the ribs, the respiratory system includes: the nose and mouth, the pharynx (throat), larynx (with the voicebox and the epiglottis), the trachea (windpipe), bronchial tree (from bronchi through the bronchioles), and the lungs with their alveoli.

Look for chest movements, listen and feel for air exchange, and note anything that may indicate problems with breathing (unusual rate, depth, and skin color changes).

A variety of problems can cause partial or full airway obstruction. These include the tongue, foreign objects, tissue damage, and disease. Listen for snoring, crowing, gurgling, and wheezing sounds that may indicate partial obstruction. In cases of total obstruction, there will be no chest movements typical of breathing, no sounds of respiration, and no air exchange felt at the nose and mouth.

Encourage patients with partial airway obstruction to cough. If they cannot cough, or their coughing is very weak, treat as if they had a complete airway obstruction.

Conscious patients with airway obstructions will often grasp the neck trying to communicate the

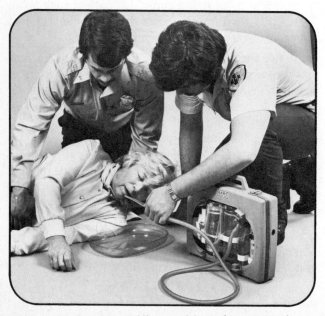

Figure 4-27: Be prepared for vomiting when attempting to relieve marked gastric distention.

problem. Be sure to ask patients, ''Can you talk?'' If they can, then the obstruction is partial.

Opening the airway can sometimes be done by simply repositioning the patient's head or performing a head-tilt maneuver. If the patient does not have spinal injuries, then the head-tilt, chin-lift or the head-tilt, neck-lift maneuver can be employed. If there is a possibility of spinal injury, the modified jaw-thrust should be used.

Correcting airway obstruction can be accomplished by using back blows, manual thrusts, and finger sweeps. It is sometimes necessary to use combined procedures on conscious patients:

- Opening the airway and providing four quick ventilations
- Four sharp back blows
- Four rapid manual thrusts (abdominal or chest)
- Finger sweeps

Remember that abdominal thrusts are not recommended for infants and children.

These various procedures are used in a very specific pattern. Before completing this chapter, make certain you can list the combined procedure steps for the conscious patient, the patient who becomes unconscious after care is started, and the unconscious patient.

Mouth-to-mouth ventilation is the most practical form of pulmonary resuscitation. There are no shortcuts to this procedure. Learn all the steps in this chapter, including the mouth-to-nose, mouth-to-stoma (for neck breathers), and the mouth-to-mouth and nose (for infants and children) techniques.

Remember that artificial ventilations for the adult are provided at the rate of one breath every five seconds to equal twelve breaths per minute. This is true for mouth-to-mouth, mouth-to-nose, and mouth-to-stoma techniques.

Infants receive a puff every three seconds, while children receive a gentle small breath every four seconds.

Be alert for gastric distention, where air is forced into the patient's stomach. Reposition the patient's head and be on the alert for vomiting. Do not attempt to force air from the patient's stomach unless you have suction equipment ready for immediate use.

5 basic life support ii: cpr—cardiopulmonary resuscitation

OBJECTIVES By the end of this chapter, you should be able to:

1. Locate the anatomical position of the heart. (p. 86)

2. Define clinical death and biological death. (p. 88)

3. Describe the relationship of heart, lung, and brain activity. (pp. 87-88)

4. Define cardiopulmonary resuscitation (CPR). (p. 88)

5. Describe, in terms of oxygen and circulation, how CPR keeps a patient alive. (p. 88)

6. Explain how CPR works. (p. 89)

7. List the signs of cardiac arrest. (p. 90)

8. Relate the starting of CPR to the results of the primary survey. (pp. 89-90)

9. Define CPR compression site and describe TWO ways to find this site on the adult patient. (pp. 90-91)

10. Describe how to deliver external chest compressions and interposed ventilations. (pp. 91-93)

11. List the rates of compressions and ventilations used during CPR on adults, children, and infants. (pp. 93, 97, 98)

12. State how the EMT can determine that CPR is effective. (p. 93)

13. List, step by step, the procedures for performing CPR on adults, children, and infants. (pp. 95-97)

14. Cite at least THREE complications that can occur during CPR. (p. 94)

15. State when an EMT can stop CPR. (p. 94)

16. List at least THREE advantages of two-rescuer CPR over one-rescuer CPR. (p. 97)

17. Compare one- and two-rescuer CPR in terms of rates of compression and rates of ventilations. (pp. 93, 98)

18. List, step by step, the procedures for two-rescuer CPR. (p. 99)

19. State how often you should check for a carotid pulse and breathing when performing two-rescuer CPR. (p. 98)

20. State how long compressions may be interrupted when checking for breathing and carotid pulse when performing two-rescuer CPR. (p. 98)

21. List, step by step, the sequence of procedures for changing positions during two-rescuer CPR. (p. 100)

22. State what the ventilator should do if he misses an interposed ventilation during two-rescuer CPR. (p. 98)

23. Describe, step by step, how to provide CPR when moving a patient. (p. 101)

SKILLS As an EMT, you should be able to:

1. Correctly evaluate a patient to detect cardiac arrest.

2. Perform CPR on adult patients, children, and infants.

3. Perform two-rescuer CPR, including the proper change of positions.

4. Perform CPR on a patient while he is being moved.

TERMS You may be using for the first time:

Cardiopulmonary Resuscitation (KAR-de-o-PUL-mo-ner-e re-SUS-ci-TA-shun), **CPR**—Heart-lung resuscitation. A combined effort to restore or maintain respiration and circulation.

Cardiac Arrest—when the heart stops beating, and no longer circulates blood.

Mediastinum (me-de-as-TI-num or me-de-ah-STI-num)—the central portion of the thoracic cavity, containing the heart, its greater blood vessels, part of the trachea, and part of the esophagus (e-SOF-ah-gus).

Pericardium (per-e-KAR-de-um)—the membranous sac that surrounds the heart, connecting to the base of the greater vessels superior to the heart.

Atrium (A-tree-um)—an upper chamber of the heart. There is a right atrium (receives blood returning from the body) and a left atrium (receives oxygenated blood from the lungs). The plural is atria.

Ventricle (VEN-tri-kl)—a lower chamber of the heart. There is a right ventricle (sends blood to the lungs) and a left ventricle (sends oxygenated blood to the body).

Pulmonary (PUL-mo-nar-e) **Artery**—the blood vessel that transports blood from the right ventricle to the lungs.

Aorta (a-OR-tah)—the artery that transports blood from the left ventricle to begin systemic circulation.

Conduction System—modified heart muscle that acts as nervous tissue to cause heart contraction.

Pulmonary Circulation—the transport of blood from the right atrium to the lungs where it is oxygenated, and then returned to the left atrium.

Pulmonary Veins—the vessels that transport oxygenated blood from the lungs to the left atrium.

Systemic (sis-TEM-ik) **Circulation**—the portion of the circulatory system that transports blood from the left ventricle out to the body's tissues and back to the heart.

Venae Cavae (VE-ne KA-ve)—the superior vena cava and the inferior vena cava. These two major veins return blood from the body to the right atrium.

CPR Compression Site—the sternal point approximately one finger-width superior to the substernal notch. The site is also defined as two finger-widths superior to the xiphoid process.

Substernal Notch—a general term for the lowest region on the sternum to which ribs attach.

Xiphoid (ZI-foyd) **Process**—a small projection at the inferior end of the sternum.

Sternum (STER-num)—the breastbone.

Clavicle (KLAV-i-kul)—the collarbone. There are two, one attached to the right side of the superior sternum, and one attached to the left side.

Interposed Ventilation—the artificial ventilation provided during CPR.

Brachial (BRAY-key-al) **Pulse**—the pulse measured by palpating the major artery (brachial artery) of the upper arm. This pulse is used to detect heart action and circulation in infants.

THE HEART

As you progress through this chapter, remember that uncorrected airway obstructions lead to respiratory arrest, and that respiratory arrest quickly leads to cardiac arrest. The process of dying can be reversed if resuscitative measures are initiated promptly and carried out effectively.

Anatomy of the Heart

The human heart is a muscular organ about the size of your fist. It is located in the center of the thoracic cavity, in an area called the mediastinum (me-de-as-TI-num or me-de-ah-STI-num). This portion of the thoracic cavity contains the heart, its large blood vessels, part of the trachea and part of the esophagus (e-SOF-ah-gus), the tube leading from throat to stomach. Go back to Chapter 2 and note the position of the heart as shown in Figure 2-7.

The heart is surrounded by a membranous sac called the pericardium (per-e-KAR-de-um) or peri-cardial sac. This sac protects the heart as it beats within the chest cavity.

There are two upper chambers of the heart called the left and right atria (A-tree-ah). The right atrium (A-tree-um) receives blood returning from the entire body. The left atrium receives oxygenated blood returning from the lungs. These two chambers are divided by a wall called the interatrial septum. When the right atrium is filling, so is the left atrium. When the right atrium is contracting, the left atrium is also.

There are two lower chambers of the heart called the left and right ventricles (VEN-tri-kls). The right ventricle receives blood from the right atrium and sends this blood to the lungs to be oxygenated. The left ventricle receives blood from the left atrium and pumps this blood out to the body. These two chambers are divided by the interventricular septum. Both ventricles fill and contract at the same time. Since it does more work, the left ventricle has the thickest muscle of the heart chambers.

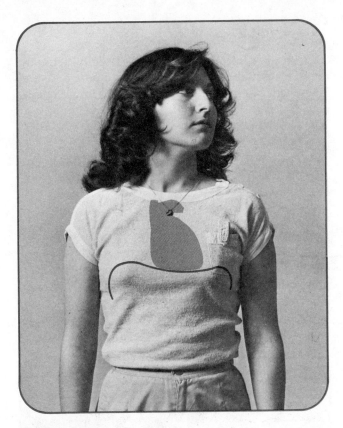

Figure 5-1: The mediastinum.

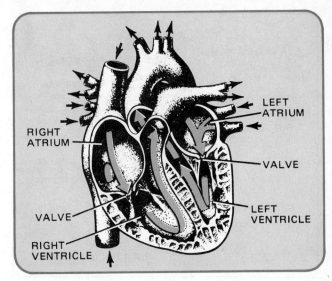

Figure 5-2: Structures of the heart.

Between each atrium and ventricle is a one-way valve to prevent blood in the ventricle from being forced back into the atrium. The major vessel leading from the heart to the lungs, the **pulmonary** (PUL-mo-nar-e) **artery,** also has a one-way valve so that blood does not return to the right ventricle. The major vessel leading out to the body, the **aorta** (a-OR-tah), has a one-way valve to keep blood from leaking back into the left ventricle. This system of one-way valves keeps blood moving in the proper direction as it comes from the body, goes to and from the lungs, and is circulated to the body's tissues.

The beating of the heart is an automatic, involuntary process. The heart has its own 'pacemaker' and a system of specialized muscle tissues that allow the heart to beat. This is called the **conduction system.** Regulation of rate, rhythm, and force of heartbeat comes from the cardiac centers of the brain. Nerve impulses from these centers are sent to the pacemaker of the heart. These nerve impulses and chemicals released into the blood (e.g., epinephrine) control heart action.

Heart Function

The heart may be compared to a pump—a very efficient pump. It moves more than 16,000 pints of blood each day. In an average lifetime, this human pump is required to beat over 2.5 billion times to move over 450 million pints of blood. Unlike a me-

chanical pump, the heart accomplishes this remarkable feat without interruption. The only care that is needed is to maintain a healthy body. Lack of exercise, poor diet, smoking, and stress are its greatest enemies.

Blood from the body returns to the heart by way of superior and inferior **venae cavae** (VE-ne KA-ve), to enter the right atrium. It is sent from this chamber into the right ventricle through a one-way valve that prevents return to the atrium. When the right ventricle contracts, it sends blood by way of the **pulmonary artery** to the lungs where carbon dioxide is given up and oxygen is taken from the alveoli. This oxygenated blood is sent by way of the **pulmonary veins** back to the heart to enter the left atrium, which sends this blood through a one-way valve into the left ventricle. The left ventricle contracts to send blood through the aorta, out to the body.

As you can see, there are really two circulatory systems functioning at the same time. One is called **pulmonary circulation,** where blood is sent from heart to lungs and back to the heart. The other is called **systemic** (sis-TEM-ik) **circulation.** This is the flow from the heart, out to the entire body and back to the heart. In its flow, the blood delivers oxygen to the tissues and picks up carbon dioxide.

The Heart-Lung-Brain Relationship

There is a close relationship between the functions of the heart, the lungs, and the brain. This relationship may be seen as follows:

- A patient develops respiratory arrest. The blood being pumped to the brain will not contain enough oxygen. The cardiac control centers will stop sending signals to the heart, causing it to beat improperly and then stop beating altogether. Without oxygen, the brain will die.

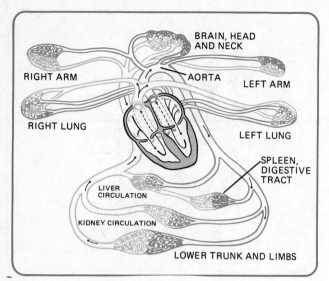

Figure 5-3: The heart pumps blood through pulmonary and systemic circulation.

- The patient is breathing, but his heart stops beating. Blood will not be sent to the lungs to pick up oxygen, nor will the blood be sent to the body's tissues. The respiratory centers of the brain will not receive oxygen. They will stop sending signals and the patient will stop breathing. Without oxygen, the brain will die.

- The patient's heart is beating and he is breathing, but the cardiac and respiratory centers of his brain are damaged. Soon, both heart and lung actions will cease. Without oxygen, the brain will die.

In Chapter 4 we defined clinical and biological death. Remember, when the patient stops breathing, soon his heart will stop beating. When the patient's heart is not beating and he is not breathing, this is **clinical death**. This condition may be reversed. Once the patient's brain cells begin to die, this is **biological death**, occurring about *ten minutes after clinical death*. This is not reversible. You will study how to try to prevent a patient in clinical death from reaching biological death. Later we will consider what factors may delay biological death and allow you to resuscitate a patient who has been clinically dead for more than ten minutes.

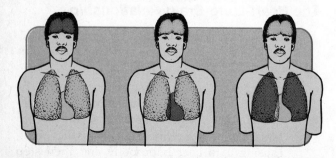

Figure 5-4: The actions of the heart, lungs, and brain are interdependent. If one fails, they all will fail.

CPR

CPR is **cardiopulmonary** (KAR-de-o-PUL-mo-ner-e) **resuscitation**. This basic life support measure is applied when a patient's heart and lung actions have stopped. During CPR, you will have to:

- Maintain an open airway
- Supply breaths to the patient
- Force the patient's heart to circulate blood

Remember, basic life support is concerned with the ABC's of emergency care:

A = Airway
B = Breathing
C = Circulation

CPR is a procedure involving the ABC's of emergency care. Artificial ventilations are not effective unless there is an open airway. Artificial ventilation is not effective unless the blood is circulating. Circulating blood will not be effective unless the blood is oxygenated.

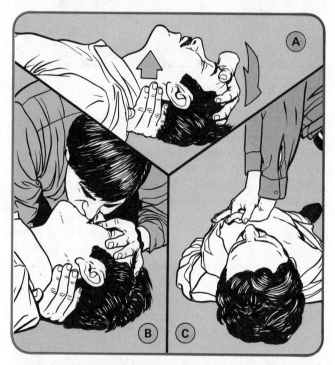

Figure 5-5: The ABC technique of CPR.

Remember that bleeding can prevent proper and adequate circulation. If a patient has lost too much blood, then CPR will not be effective. When bleeding is very profuse, as in the case of a severed major artery, CPR may speed up the patient's blood loss, causing biological death. Even though such a case is rare, you may have to stop or reduce this blood loss before effective CPR can be initiated.

How CPR Works

The heart is located in the mediastinum, between the sternum and the spinal column. Most of the ribs attach to the sternum. These, along with the clavicles (KLAV-i-kls), or collarbones, support the sternum over the heart.

In Chapter 4 we discussed rescue breathing (pulmonary resuscitation). Providing oxygen to the patient will do little good unless the blood is circulating. In CPR, the patient's heart is forced to circulate blood by the rescuer applying external chest compressions. This causes artificial circulation to take place.

Artificial circulation is produced when the chest is compressed along its midline. This action causes pressure changes to take place within the thoracic cavity, provided that the patient is lying on his back on a hard surface. During compression, blood is forced into both pulmonary circulation and systemic circulation. In other words, the blood leaves the right ventricle and flows to the lungs, while blood in the left ventricle side is sent out to the body. When pressure on the sternum is released, the elastic nature of the chest wall causes the sternum to return to its normal position. The release of excess pressure in the thorax results in a sucking action that draws blood from the body into the right side of the heart and blood from the lungs into the left side of the heart.

Simply stated, compress and blood is pumped from the heart; release and the heart fills with blood.

In one-rescuer CPR, a set number of external chest compressions are given to the patient, then breaths are provided. These breaths, known as **interposed ventilations,** provide the patient with oxygen.

When to Use CPR

First of all, the patient must be in **cardiac arrest.** This means that his heart has stopped beating com-

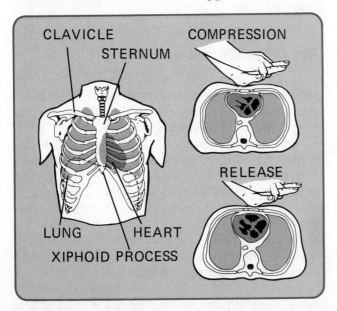

Figure 5-6: During CPR, blood is forced into circulation.

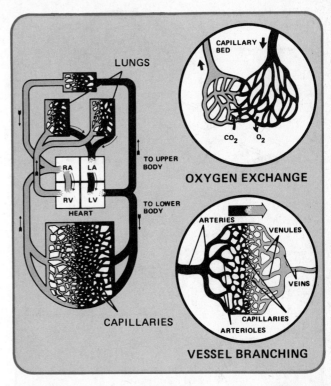

Figure 5-7: CPR provides the patient with oxygen and forces the heart to circulate blood.

pletely (cardiac standstill). Or, because of shock, severe bleeding, or certain drugs, the heart beats too weakly to circulate blood (cardiovascular collapse). Or, his heartbeats are so irregular and uncoordinated that there is no effective output (ventricular fibrillation).

Should the patient be breathing at the time of cardiac arrest, within 30 seconds he will go into **respiratory arrest.** A patient needing CPR will not be breathing and will have *no carotid pulse.* The signs of cardiac arrest are listed in Figure 5-8.

THE TECHNIQUES OF CPR

When to Begin CPR

The decision to begin CPR must come from the results of the primary survey. The events leading to the beginning of CPR should be:

1. ESTABLISH UNRESPONSIVENESS—Is the patient responsive? Gently tap the patient on the shoulders and shout, "ARE YOU OKAY?...ARE YOU OKAY?...ARE YOU OKAY?" Patients requiring immediate CPR will be unconscious.
2. ESTABLISH AN OPEN AIRWAY—This should be done by the head-tilt, neck-lift; head-tilt, chin-lift; or modified jaw-thrust. Usually at this time, you can easily check to see if the patient is a neck breather.
3. CHECK FOR BREATHING—Use the LOOK, LISTEN, and FEEL method, taking

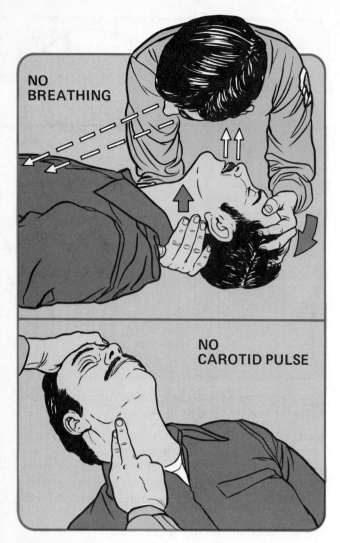

Figure 5-8: The signs of cardiac arrest.

five seconds to determine if the patient is
breathing. A patient who is breathing does
not need immediate CPR. If the patient is in
respiratory arrest, you should. . .
4. DELIVER FOUR QUICK BREATHS—Use
rescue breathing techniques, keeping the
patient's lungs from deflating between
breaths. If you note an airway obstruction,
clear the airway. If the patient's airway is
clear and he is in respiratory arrest. . .
5. CHECK FOR A CAROTID PULSE—If there
is *no* pulse after 5 seconds of palpating, the
patient is in *cardiac arrest* and you should. . .
6. BEGIN CPR.

Positioning the Patient

The cardiac arrest patient should be placed on a
hard surface, such as the floor or ground. If the
patient is in bed or on an ambulance stretcher, a
spine board, backboard, serving tray, or similar rigid
object should be placed under his back. CPR cannot
be delayed because of patient injury. Do NOT try to

immobilize the spine or splint fractures before initiating CPR.
    The patient must be placed in the supine posi-
tion. The American Heart Association suggests that
the patient's lower extremities be elevated to improve artificial circulation. In such a position, the
back of the patient must still be flat on a hard surface.

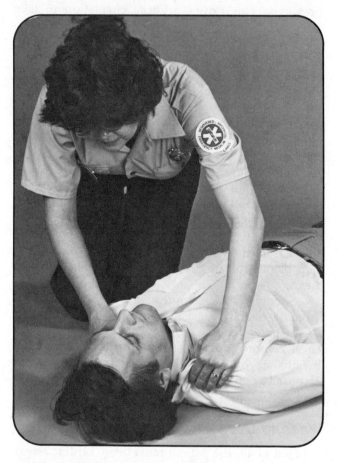

**Figure 5-9: Establish unresponsiveness and position the
patient for CPR.**

The CPR Compression Site

    To be effective and prevent serious injury to the
patient, external chest compressions MUST be delivered to the **CPR compression site.** There are two
accepted methods of finding this site.
    One way to locate the CPR compression site
does not require you to locate the xiphoid (ZI-foyd)
process at the inferior end of the sternum. This
method has recently been gaining popularity and is
now the more recommended of the two accepted
techniques.
    Begin by positioning yourself at the patient's
side, with your knees in toward the patient. Use the
index and middle fingers of your hand closest to the
patient's feet to locate the lower margin (border) of
the rib cage. Do this for the side of the chest closest
to your knees. Move your fingers along the rib cage

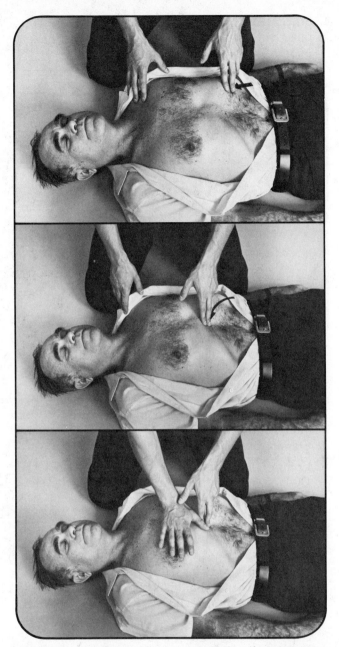

Figure 5-10: Finding the notch where the ribs connect to the sternum will enable you to locate the CPR compression site.

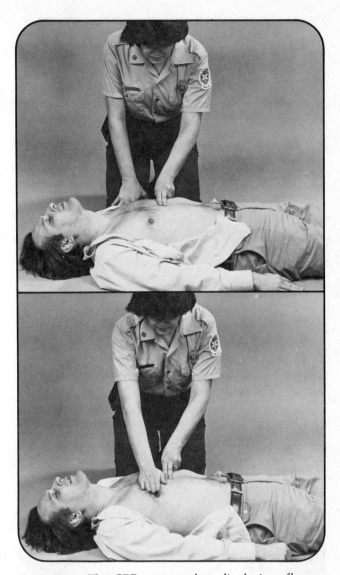

Figure 5-11: The CPR compression site is two finger-widths above the xiphoid process.

this region you will be able to feel a small projection extending down from the breastbone. This is the xiphoid process. The CPR compression site is found by measuring *two finger-widths* toward the patient's head along the midline of the sternum.

Providing Chest Compressions

Remember that the patient is lying on his back on a hard surface. You are kneeling beside the patient, with your knees in toward the patient. Your knees should be spread apart, about shoulder-width. Having found the CPR compression site, you should:

1. Place the hand that was closest to the patient's head directly on the CPR compression site.

2. Position the hand used to locate the substernal notch or xiphoid process directly over the first hand. The heels of both hands should be parallel to one another and the fingers of both hands must be pointing away from your body.

until you find the point where the ribs meet the sternum (lower center of the chest). This area is called the **substernal notch.** Keep your middle finger at this notch and your index finger resting over the lower end of the sternum. If you now move your other hand to the midline of the sternum and place the thumb side of this hand against the positioned index finger of your lower hand, you will be directly over the CPR compression site. The heel of your hand should be on the midline of the sternum.

The other accepted method for locating the CPR compression site requires you to find the xiphoid process. Position yourself at the patient's side with your knees in toward the patient. Find the inferior end of the sternum and feel for where the hard breastbone stops and the soft abdomen begins. In

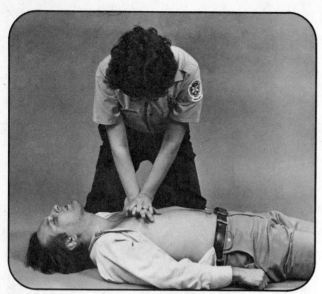

Figure 5-12: Positioning the hands for CPR.

3. Your fingers may be extended, or they may be interlaced—BUT—you must KEEP YOUR FINGERS OFF THE PATIENT'S CHEST to avoid injury to the patient. If you wish, you may grab the wrist of the hand placed on the CPR compression site with the hand that was used to locate the inferior sternum.

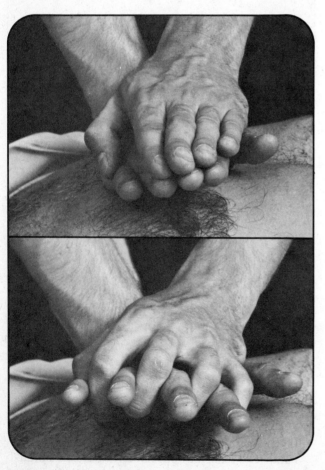

Figure 5-13: Two methods of positioning the hands to deliver external chest compressions.

4. Straighten your arms and lock the elbows. You must not bend the elbows when delivering or upon releasing compressions.

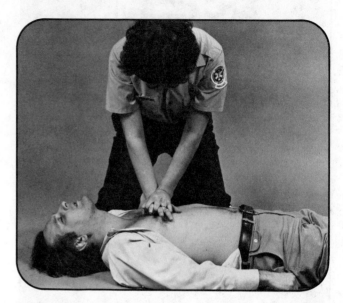

Figure 5-14: The arms must be straight, the elbows locked, and the shoulders directly over the site.

5. Make certain that your shoulders are directly over your hands. This will allow you to deliver compressions straight down onto the site.

6. Compressions are to be delivered STRAIGHT DOWN, with enough force to depress the sternum of an average adult *1½ to 2 inches* (4 to 5 cm).

7. Fully release pressure on the patient's sternum, but do NOT bend your elbows and do NOT lift your hands from the sternum. Make sure that you return your shoulders to their original position. RELEASE SHOULD TAKE AS MUCH TIME AS COMPRESSION.

Providing Interposed Ventilations

Ventilations are interposed (provided) after a set number of compressions. Use the same techniques that you learned for rescue breathing. The mouth-to-mouth, mouth-to-nose, or mouth-to-stoma methods can be used as needed. (In the mouth-to-mouth procedure, remember to pinch closed the patient's nostrils, form a tight seal with you mouth, and force air into the lungs until you see the chest rise and feel resistance from the patient's lungs).

Rates of Compressions and Ventilations

- Compressions are delivered at a rate of 80 PER MINUTE.
- Ventilations are delivered at 2 BREATHS AFTER EVERY 15 COMPRESSIONS.

- Once you begin, do NOT interrupt CPR for more than five seconds.

In one-rescuer CPR, the 15 compressions should be delivered in approximately 10 to 11 seconds. The interposed ventilations should be delivered in 4 to 5 seconds.

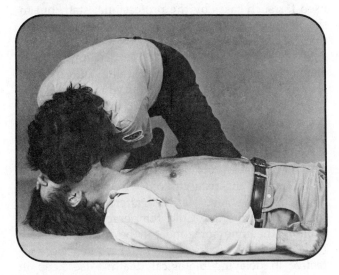

Figure 5-15: Providing interposed ventilations.

During one-rescuer CPR, time is taken away from compressions in order to provide ventilations. Even though you are delivering compressions at the rate of 80 per minute, only 60 compressions are delivered in one minute. To be certain that you are delivering compressions at the correct rate, you should say to yourself:

"One-and, two-and, three-and, four-and, five-and, . . " until you reach 15 compressions. At that point, you can deliver two quick interposed ventilations and begin the next set of 15 compressions.

Checking the Pulse

CPR should be carried out for ONE MINUTE. Then you should check for a carotid pulse. At the same time, you should determine if the patient is breathing. Do NOT stop CPR for more than five seconds. If the patient has a pulse, but is not breathing, begin pulmonary resuscitation, taking care to check every few minutes for a carotid pulse. If the patient is not breathing, and does not have a pulse, continue CPR, checking for a carotid pulse every few minutes.

Effective CPR

If CPR is effective the following MUST occur:
- The pupils constrict.
- The patient's color improves.
- Someone else can feel a carotid pulse each time you deliver a compression.

In addition, you may note any of the following:
- Spontaneous return of heartbeat
- Spontaneous gasping respirations

- Arm and leg movement
- Attempts to swallow
- Consciousness returns.

Keep in mind that you can provide effective CPR but the patient usually will not spontaneously regain heartbeat and breathing. The majority of patients who survive will require special advanced medical procedures before they can regain heart and lung function. As an EMT, you are providing CPR to keep a clinically dead patient biologically alive.

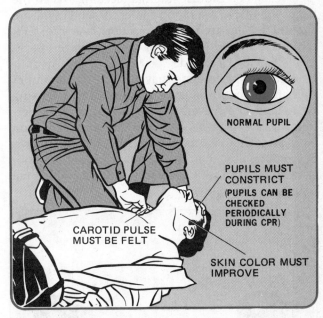

Figure 5-16: Indications of effective CPR.

Ineffective CPR

When CPR efforts are not effective, it is usually because of one or more of these problems:

- The patient's *head* is not placed in the proper head-tilt position for ventilations.
- The patient's *mouth* is not opened wide enough for air exchange.
- There is not an effective *seal* made against the patient's mouth or nose.
- The patient's *nose* is not pinched shut during mouth-to-mouth ventilations.
- The patient's *mouth* is not closed completely during mouth-to-nose ventilations.
- The patient is not lying on a *hard surface.*
- The rescuer's *hands* are incorrectly placed.
- There are prolonged (more than 5 seconds) *interruptions* of external chest compressions.
- The *chest* is not sufficiently compressed.
- The compression *rate* is too rapid or too slow.
- Compressions are *jerky*, not smooth with 50% of the cycle being compression and 50% being the release of compression.

Note that the first five problems relate to ventilation, as discussed in Chapter 4.

Complications of CPR

Injury to the rib cage is the most common complication of CPR. When the hands are placed too high on the sternum, fractures to the upper sternum and the clavicles may occur. If the hands are too low on the sternum, the xiphoid may be fractured or driven down into the liver, producing severe lacerations (cuts) and profuse internal bleeding. When the hands are placed too far off center, or when they are allowed to slip from their position over the CPR compression site, the ribs or their cartilage attachments may be fractured.

Other complications may result from improper CPR efforts, but most are easy to avoid by following AHA guidelines. Even when CPR is correctly performed, ribs may be fractured. In such cases, do NOT stop CPR. Far better that the patient suffer a few broken ribs, than die because you did not continue to perform CPR for fear of inflicting additional injury.

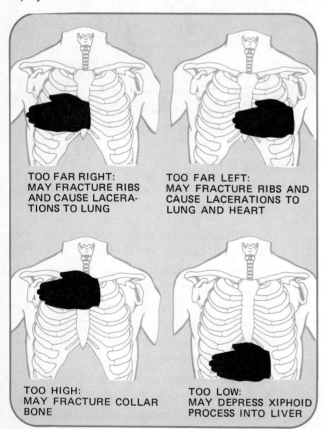

TOO FAR RIGHT:
MAY FRACTURE RIBS
AND CAUSE LACERA-
TIONS TO LUNG

TOO FAR LEFT:
MAY FRACTURE RIBS AND
CAUSE LACERATIONS TO
LUNG AND HEART

TOO HIGH:
MAY FRACTURE COLLAR
BONE

TOO LOW:
MAY DEPRESS XIPHOID
PROCESS INTO LIVER

Figure 5-17: Improper positioning of the hands during CPR can damage the rib cage and underlying organs.

BEGINNING AND TERMINATING CPR

When dealing with a patient in cardiac arrest, your duty as an EMT is to begin CPR *immediately*. Even though the patient may have a terminal illness, or he may be very old, you cannot decide to delay CPR. Bystanders may ask you not to begin CPR.

Family members may say that the patient would not want your help, but you have no proof of this. Even though some states now recognize that resuscitation may violate certain persons' rights to die with dignity, you cannot accept hearsay evidence. At the hospital, the physician's written order sheet can be used for such cases by the professional staff, but in the field, only a physician (with proper identification) at the scene may order you not to perform CPR. A few systems are currently deciding if radio communication of such orders is valid. Your instructor can inform you of the laws for your state.

CPR is most effective if started immediately after the beginning of cardiac arrest. If a patient has been in arrest for more than 10 minutes, resuscitation efforts usually are not effective. However, there are documented cases of adults in arrest for more than 10 minutes being resuscitated, with no major brain damage. Some have survived after being in arrest for over 30 minutes. Cold temperatures appear to prolong the time someone can be in arrest before biological death occurs. Cold water is even more effective in delaying biological death. Also keep in mind that children and infants may tolerate longer periods of cardiac arrest than adults.

Do not refuse to begin CPR because someone has been in cardiac arrest longer than 10 minutes. The moment the patient was seen to collapse and the moment of cardiac arrest are not usually the same. A patient can be unconscious with minimum effective lung and heart action for quite some time before actual cardiac arrest occurs.

Once you have started CPR, you MUST continue to provide CPR until:

- Spontaneous circulation occurs . . . then provide artificial respiration.
- Spontaneous circulation and breathing occur.
- Another trained rescuer can take over for you.
- You turn care of the patient over to a physician or a medical facility.
- You are too exhausted and cannot continue.

Many students have fears of having to stop CPR because of exhaustion. As a member of the EMS System, you have to be realistic about patient care and know when you have done all you can for a patient. If you are isolated and have provided CPR for 30 minutes to an hour and are too exhausted to go on, remember that there are physical limitations to the care you can provide. Few patients who received CPR for such a long period will survive. You will have done all you could for the patient and should not feel guilty about having to stop CPR.

You lessen the chances of physical exhaustion if you learn to control **rescuer hyperventilation.** When providing CPR, you establish an irregular pattern of breathing for yourself. This may cause you to begin

ONE RESCUER CPR

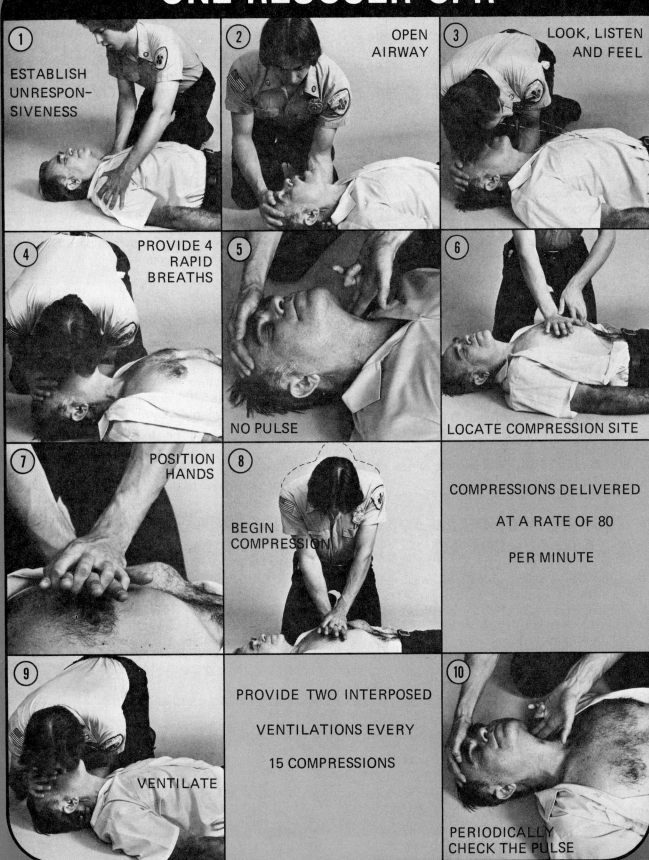

① ESTABLISH UNRESPONSIVENESS

② OPEN AIRWAY

③ LOOK, LISTEN AND FEEL

④ PROVIDE 4 RAPID BREATHS

⑤ NO PULSE

⑥ LOCATE COMPRESSION SITE

⑦ POSITION HANDS

⑧ BEGIN COMPRESSION

COMPRESSIONS DELIVERED AT A RATE OF 80 PER MINUTE

⑨ VENTILATE

PROVIDE TWO INTERPOSED VENTILATIONS EVERY 15 COMPRESSIONS

⑩ PERIODICALLY CHECK THE PULSE

SCAN 5.1

to breathe very quickly and deeply, unable to regain control. You may prevent this by keeping in good physical condition and learning not to try to take a breath with each compression. You have to learn to establish a normal breathing rate when delivering external chest compressions.

ONE-RESCUER CPR

Scansheet 5-1 shows all the techniques of one-rescuer CPR. Follow this page step by step as you practice on the adult manikins provided for your training.

There is one situation you should practice in addition to one-rescuer CPR as we have presented it here in this section. What if you are off duty and acting alone? The AHA states that the EMS System should be activated after a pulse check. Many EMS System guidelines call for activation when unresponsiveness is detected. Call out for help and have someone phone while you begin CPR. Direct the person to call 911 or the operator, depending on your location. Tell the person to state that it is an emergency, give the address, state CPR is being performed, and request an ambulance.

If there is no one on hand to help you, perform CPR for ONE MINUTE, quickly telephone for help, and return to providing CPR. Of couse, the telephone must be very close at hand. Interruption of CPR in complicated situations should not last longer than 30 seconds. If no telephone is near, perform CPR until someone can take over for you, or you are too exhausted to go on.

CPR TECHNIQUES FOR INFANTS AND CHILDREN

The techniques of CPR for infants and small children are essentially the same as those used for adults. You will have to:

1. Establish unresponsiveness.
2. Correctly position the patient.
3. Open the airway.
4. Establish respiratory arrest.
5. Provide artificial ventilations and clear the airway.
6. Establish the lack of pulse.
7. Provide external chest compressions and interposed ventilations.

Some procedures and rates differ when the patient is an infant or a child. If younger than one year of age, the patient is an infant. Between one and eight years of age, the patient is a child. Over the age of eight, adult procedures apply to the patient. Keep in mind that the size of the patient can also be

an important factor. A very small nine-year-old patient may have to be treated as a child.

Positioning the Patient

CPR is best performed when adults, children, and infants are placed on their back on a hard surface.

Opening the Airway

- INFANT—use the head-tilt, neck-lift technique, but apply only a *slight* tilt. Too great a tilt will close off the airway. Always be sure to support the infant's head.
- CHILD—The same caution applies to small children as to infants. Larger children can have their airways opened by standard head-tilt or jaw thrust techniques.

Establishing a Pulse

- INFANT—Do NOT use the carotid or radial pulse. For infants, you should use the **brachial** (BRAY-key-al) **pulse**. This is the pulse that can be felt when compressing the major artery of the upper arm, the brachial artery. You can find the brachial pulse by:
  1. Locating the point halfway between the infant's elbow and shoulder.
  2. Placing your thumb on the lateral side of the upper arm at this midway point.

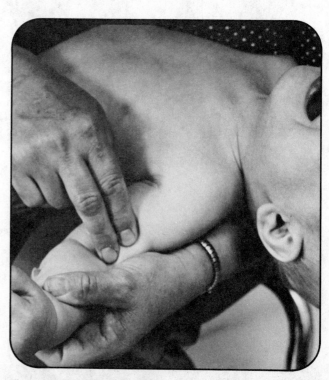

Figure 5-18: For infants, determine circulation by feeling for a brachial pulse.

3. Placing the tips of your index and middle fingers at the midway point on the medial surface of the infant's upper arm. You will feel a groove in the muscle at this location.

4. Pressing your index and middle fingers in toward the bone, taking care not to exert too much pressure. To do so will collapse the artery and stop circulation to the lower arm, and perhaps cause you to miss feeling the pulse.

- CHILD—determine circulation by finding a carotid pulse.

External Chest Compressions

- INFANT—apply compressions to the midline of the sternum, directly between the nipples.

  Use the tips of two or three fingers to deliver the compressions. The infant's breastbone should be depressed 1/2 to 1 inch (1.5 to 2.5 cm).

- CHILD—compressions are applied using the heel of one hand. The compression site is the midsternum, directly between the nipples. The child's breastbone should be depressed 1 to 1 1/2 inches (2.5 to 4 cm).

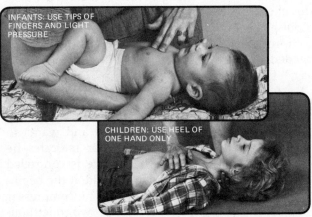

INFANTS: USE TIPS OF FINGERS AND LIGHT PRESSURE

CHILDREN: USE HEEL OF ONE HAND ONLY

Figure 5-19: External chest compressions for infants and children.

Interposed Ventilations

- INFANT—the rescuer should provide a *gentle breath* of air using the mouth-to-mouth and nose technique. This may be no more than a *puff* of air. It is essential to watch the rise and fall of the infant's chest. The rescuer should deliver just enough air to cause the infant's chest to rise.

- CHILD—a *gentle breath* is provided to the child patient. Again, only enough air is deliv-

ered to cause the patient's chest to rise. Mouth-to-mouth or mouth-to-nose techniques are usually employed. If the patient is a small child, you may have to use the mouth-to-mouth and nose method.

CPR Rates

- INFANT—deliver compressions at the rate of 100 per minute. Interpose a gentle breath every 5 compressions to give a ratio of 5:1.
- CHILD—deliver compressions at the rate of 80 per minute. Interpose a gentle breath every 5 compressions to give a ratio of 5:1.

NOTE: To establish the correct rate for infants, count to yourself: "One, two, three, four, five, breathe." Provide the interposed ventilation immediately after "five." For children, count: "One and two and three and four and five, breathe." Provide the interposed ventilation immediately after "five."

TWO-RESCUER CPR

Advantages

CPR efforts are more effective when two rescuers work together. The patient receives more oxygen, chest compressions are not interrupted, and the problem of rescuer fatigue is lessened.

Should you find yourself providing CPR while off duty, you may be able to have a bystander assist you in the two-rescuer method. However, be certain that the bystander has been trained by the American Heart Association or the American Red Cross in the two-rescuer procedure. Too often, people wish to help thinking they know the procedure based upon what they have seen on television, without the benefit of training in CPR. If you begin two-rescuer CPR with the aid of a bystander and find that the volunteer is unable to perform correctly, stop the two-rescuer procedure and begin one-rescuer CPR.

Compressions and Ventilations

For the two-rescuer method, the rate of compressions is *five compressions every five seconds*. This means that the EMT delivering compressions (the **compressor**) has to provide a full compression and release every second, thus providing 60 compressions per minute. The EMT delivering interposed ventilations (the **ventilator**) provides one full breath on the upstroke of every fifth compression, to provide a rate of 12 breaths per minute.

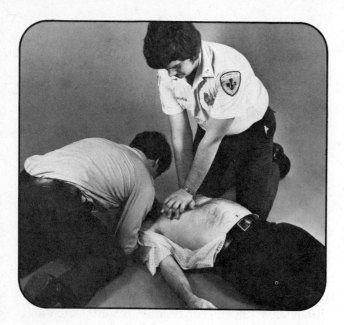

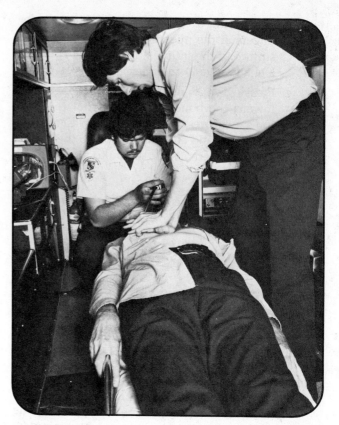

Figure 5-20: Opposite-side positioning in two-rescuer CPR.

COMPRESSIONS = 60 per minute, delivering 1 per second
VENTILATIONS = 12 per minute, delivering 1 per 5 compressions
RATIO = 5 compressions:1 ventilation

The compressor counts out loud saying, "one, one thousand; two, one thousand; three, one thousand; four, one thousand; five, BREATHE," starting the cycle again with, "one, one thousand; . . ." For each second counted, the compressor delivers a compression to the CPR compression site. The ventilator delivers a full breath on the upstroke of each fifth compression.

NOTE: If the ventilator misses a breath, he should not wait for the next fifth upstroke. The ventilation should be delivered on the upstroke of the next compression.

Though rare, two-rescuer CPR is sometimes performed on children. The ratio is 5:1, with a gentle breath provided on the upstroke of the fifth compression.

Two-Rescuer CPR Procedure

The complete procedure is shown in Scansheet 5-2. Both rescuers are shown on the same side of the patient to allow you to see what each person is doing. The procedure goes more smoothly if the rescuers are on *opposite* sides of the patient, as in Figure 5-20. This is particularly true when position changes are taking place. Once in the ambulance, the procedure will have to be done with both rescuers on the same side of the patient, as in Figure 5-21.

Every three to four minutes, the ventilator should check to see if the patient has a *carotid pulse* and note any *spontaneous breathing*. Since compressions cannot

Figure 5-21: Same-side positioning for two-rescuer CPR performed in the ambulance.

be delivered while trying to detect a carotid pulse, this check CANNOT last longer than five seconds. If a pulse is detected, the ventilator should say, "Stop compressions." Rescue breathing is provided if needed. If there is no pulse, the ventilator should say, "Continue CPR."

Changing Positions

If the compressor becomes tired and wants to change positions, or if the ventilator indicates he wishes a position change, the change is controlled by the *compressor*. The ventilator is told at the beginning of the next compression cycle. The compressor will say, "CHANGE, one thousand; two, one thousand; three, one thousand; four, one thousand; five, BREATHE." The ventilator will provide one full breath in $1/2$ second and the two rescuers will quickly change positions.

During the change, it is recommended that carotid pulse and breathing be checked by the compressor as he moves to the ventilator position. These checks should take *no more than* five seconds.

CPR: MOVING PATIENTS

Ideally, CPR should not be interrupted for more than five seconds. However, when CPR is being performed and the patient must be moved for safety reasons or transport, interruptions may be longer.

TWO RESCUER CPR

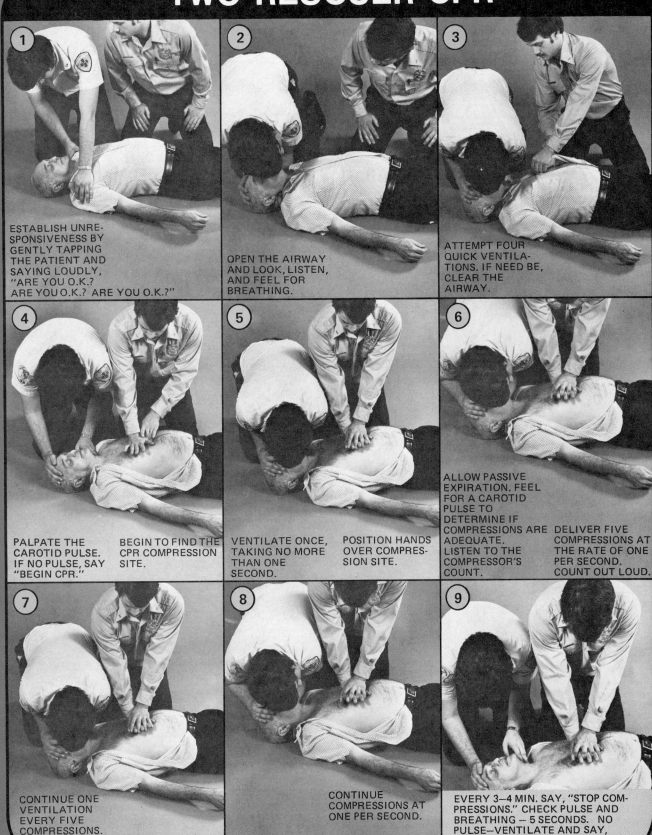

1 ESTABLISH UNRE-SPONSIVENESS BY GENTLY TAPPING THE PATIENT AND SAYING LOUDLY, "ARE YOU O.K.? ARE YOU O.K.? ARE YOU O.K.?"

2 OPEN THE AIRWAY AND LOOK, LISTEN, AND FEEL FOR BREATHING.

3 ATTEMPT FOUR QUICK VENTILA-TIONS. IF NEED BE, CLEAR THE AIRWAY.

4 PALPATE THE CAROTID PULSE. IF NO PULSE, SAY "BEGIN CPR." BEGIN TO FIND THE CPR COMPRESSION SITE.

5 VENTILATE ONCE, TAKING NO MORE THAN ONE SECOND. POSITION HANDS OVER COMPRES-SION SITE.

6 ALLOW PASSIVE EXPIRATION. FEEL FOR A CAROTID PULSE TO DETERMINE IF COMPRESSIONS ARE ADEQUATE. LISTEN TO THE COMPRESSOR'S COUNT. DELIVER FIVE COMPRESSIONS AT THE RATE OF ONE PER SECOND. COUNT OUT LOUD.

7 CONTINUE ONE VENTILATION EVERY FIVE COMPRESSIONS.

8 CONTINUE COMPRESSIONS AT ONE PER SECOND.

9 EVERY 3–4 MIN. SAY, "STOP COM-PRESSIONS." CHECK PULSE AND BREATHING – 5 SECONDS. NO PULSE—VENTILATE AND SAY, "CONTINUE CPR." PULSE – SAY, "STOP COMPRESSIONS."

CHANGING POSITIONS

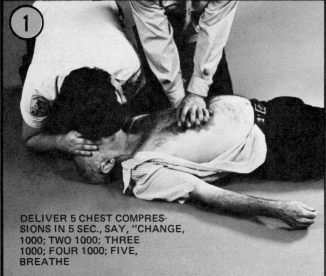

1 DELIVER 5 CHEST COMPRESSIONS IN 5 SEC., SAY, "CHANGE, 1000; TWO 1000; THREE 1000; FOUR 1000; FIVE, BREATHE

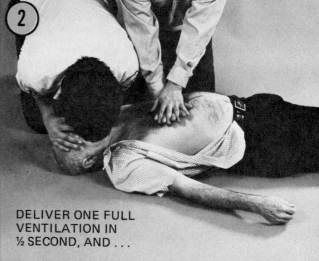

2 DELIVER ONE FULL VENTILATION IN ½ SECOND, AND . . .

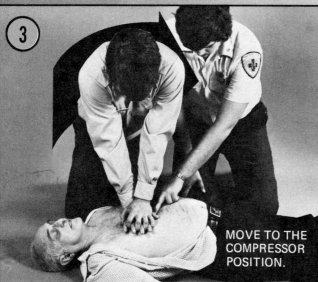

3 MOVE TO THE COMPRESSOR POSITION.

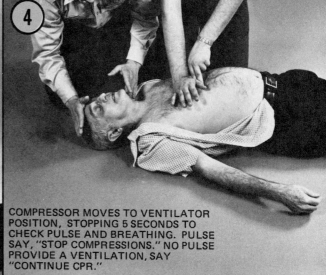

4 COMPRESSOR MOVES TO VENTILATOR POSITION, STOPPING 5 SECONDS TO CHECK PULSE AND BREATHING. PULSE SAY, "STOP COMPRESSIONS." NO PULSE PROVIDE A VENTILATION, SAY "CONTINUE CPR."

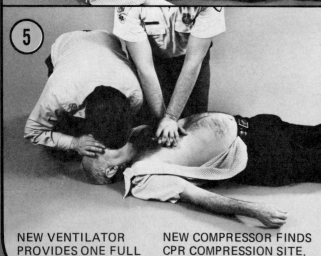

5 NEW VENTILATOR PROVIDES ONE FULL BREATH IN ½ SECOND.   NEW COMPRESSOR FINDS CPR COMPRESSION SITE.

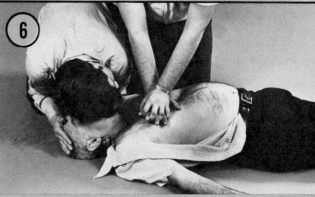

6 FEEL FOR A CAROTID PULSE TO DETERMINE IF COMPRESSIONS ARE EFFECTIVE.   DELIVER FIVE COMPRESSIONS AT THE RATE OF ONE PER SECOND.

CONTINUE CYCLE WITH 1 VENTILATION PROVIDED FOR EVERY 5 COMPRESSIONS.

SCAN 5-3

MOVING CPR

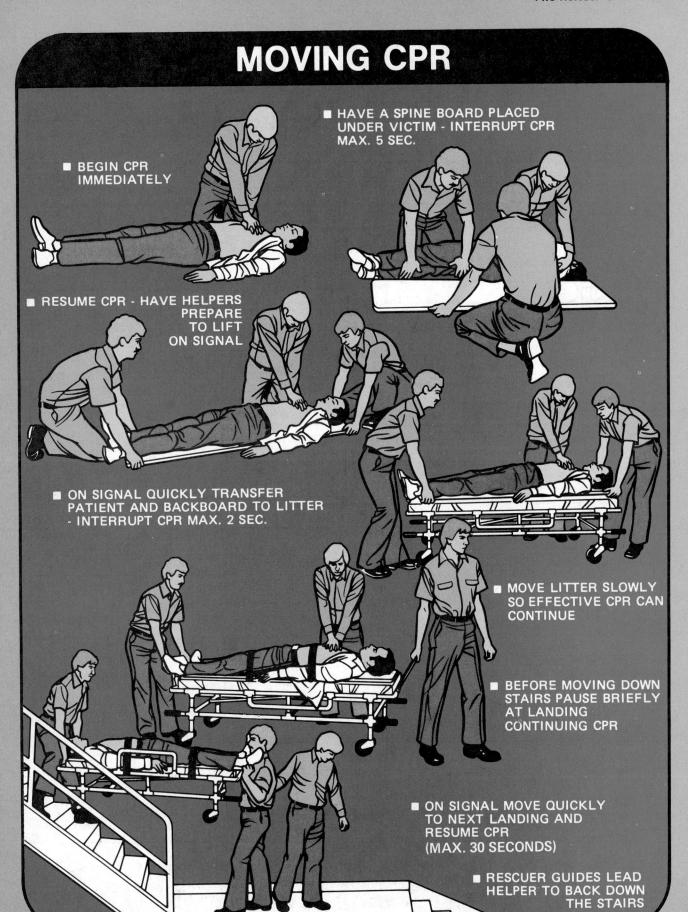

- BEGIN CPR IMMEDIATELY

- HAVE A SPINE BOARD PLACED UNDER VICTIM - INTERRUPT CPR MAX. 5 SEC.

- RESUME CPR - HAVE HELPERS PREPARE TO LIFT ON SIGNAL

- ON SIGNAL QUICKLY TRANSFER PATIENT AND BACKBOARD TO LITTER - INTERRUPT CPR MAX. 2 SEC.

- MOVE LITTER SLOWLY SO EFFECTIVE CPR CAN CONTINUE

- BEFORE MOVING DOWN STAIRS PAUSE BRIEFLY AT LANDING CONTINUING CPR

- ON SIGNAL MOVE QUICKLY TO NEXT LANDING AND RESUME CPR (MAX. 30 SECONDS)

- RESCUER GUIDES LEAD HELPER TO BACK DOWN THE STAIRS

SCAN 5-4

CPR SUMMARY

ONE RESCUER	FUNCTIONS	TWO RESCUER
	• ESTABLISH UNRESPONSIVE • OPEN AIRWAY • LOOK, LISTEN AND FEEL	
	• DELIVER 4 QUICK BREATHS	
	• CHECK CAROTID PULSE • BEGIN CPR	

	DELIVER COMPRESSION	
	80/MIN.	60/MIN.

	INTERPOSED VENTILATIONS	
	2/15	1/5

| | • PERIODICALLY CHECK PULSE
• NO PULSE CONTINUE CPR | |

CHANGING POSITIONS

COMPRESSOR: CHANGE—1000............5, BREATHE	CHECK PULSE "CONTINUE CPR" PROVIDE VENTILATION	CONTINUE CPR SEQUENCE

SCAN 5.5

Interruptions should last *no longer than 30 seconds.*

Major problems occur when moving a patient up or down a stairway, or along a narrow hallway. Provide the patient with effective CPR before the interruption. On signal, move the patient as quickly as possible and resume effective CPR at the next level, or at the end of the narrow hallway. Note that compressions can be delivered during the move.

CPR *must be continued* once the patient is loaded into the ambulance. The procedure should continue uninterrupted during transport. Only when the emergency department staff takes over CPR, or the physician on duty tells you to stop, can you stop CPR efforts.

NOTE: There are special situations where CPR and other basic life support measures must be taken. These include: drowning, electric shock, accidents producing crushing chest injuries, hangings, drug overdoses, and toxic gas inhalations. All of these will be covered later.

CAUTION: CPR skills can be quickly lost when not practiced on a regular basis. As an EMT, be certain to practice CPR on infant *and* adult manikins. You must be recertified in CPR at least once a year. One way to stay in practice is to become a CPR instructor for the AHA or the American Red Cross and teach CPR to the public.

SUMMARY

When someone stops breathing and the heart stops beating, clinical death occurs. Within ten minutes, biological death can result.

There is a vital relationship between breathing, circulation, and brain activities. If one function stops, all three will stop.

When a patient's heart stops beating, he is in cardiac arrest. He will be unconscious and have a "death-like" appearance. The major signs of cardiac arrest are no breathing and no pulse.

You should determine breathing by the LOOK, LISTEN, and FEEL method. Circulation is determined by feeling for a carotid pulse. If the patient is an infant (under one year of age), then feel for a brachial pulse.

If a patient is in cardiac arrest, you should take the ABC approach: A = Airway, B = Breathing, and C = Circulation. To perform CPR:

1. Establish the patient's unresponsiveness.
2. Correctly position the patient and open the airway CAUTION: Do NOT overextend the neck for infants and small children.
3. Determine that the patient is not breathing.
4. Provide four quick breaths and evaluate breathing. Clear the airway if necessary.

5. Determine that there is no breathing and no carotid (or brachial) pulse.
6. Find the CPR compression site:
   ADULT: one finger-width superior to the substernal notch or two finger-widths above the xiphoid process
   CHILD: along the midline of the sternum, between the nipples
   INFANT: along the midline of the sternum, between the nipples.
7. Correctly position your hands for compressions:
   ADULT: The heel of your hand closest to the patient's head is placed on the CPR compression site. Your other hand is placed on top of this hand so that the heels of both hands are parallel and the fingers are pointing away from your body. Your fingers can be extended or interlaced, but YOU MUST KEEP YOUR FINGERS OFF THE PATIENT'S RIBS.
   CHILD: Deliver compressions with the heel of one hand, positioned over the child's breastbone, between the nipples.
   INFANT: Deliver compressions with the tips of two or three fingers, positioned over the infant's sternum, between the nipples.
8. Provide external chest compressions:
   ADULT: Depth = 1½ to 2 inches (4 to 5 cm)
      Rate = 80/minute
   CHILD: Depth = 1 to 1½ inches (2.5 to 4 cm)
      Rate = 80/minute
   INFANT: Depth = ½ to 1 inch (1.5 to 2.5 cm)
      Rate = 100/minute
9. Provide interposed ventilations:
   ADULT: 2 rapid full breaths every 15 compressions
   CHILD: 1 small breath every 5 compressions
   INFANT: 1 gentle breath every 5 compressions
10. Check for a carotid pulse after one minute. Use the brachial pulse if the patient is an infant. If no pulse and no breathing, continue CPR, checking for a pulse every few minutes. If there is a pulse, but no breathing, stop compressions and provide rescue breathing. Continue to monitor pulse.

NOTE: The patient will not continue to breathe unless there is heart action.

You should not stop CPR for more than 5 seconds unless it is to move the patient. For such cases, do not stop CPR for more than 30 seconds. Continue CPR until heart or heart and lung functions start, until you are relieved by another trained person, care is given over to a physician or the staff of the emergency department, or you cannot continue due to exhaustion.

CPR is effective when the patient's skin color improves, the pupils constrict, and a carotid pulse can be felt with each external chest compression.

When a patient is in cardiac arrest, start CPR immediately, even if you worsen existing injuries, or cause injuries such as fractured ribs. Without CPR, the patient will go from clinical to biological death.

In two-rescuer CPR:

- Compressions = 1 per second (60 per minute)
- Ventilations = 1 per 5 seconds (12 per minute)

- Provide 1 ventilation every 5 compressions
- The compressor counts the 1 to 5 cycle.
- The compressor commands the change of positions.
- Check for a carotid pulse and spontaneous breathing every 3 to 4 minutes.
- Do not interrupt CPR for more than 5 seconds, except when moving the patient (30-second interruption is maximum).
- If you miss a breath, impose a ventilation on the upstroke of the next compression.

One- and two-rescuer CPR methods are compared in Scansheet 5-5.

6 breathing aids and oxygen therapy

TERMS you may be using for the first time:

Adjunct Airway—a device placed in a patient's mouth or nose to help maintain an open airway. Those inserted in the mouth help to hold the tongue in place.

Oropharyngeal (or-o-fah-RIN-je-al) **Airway**—a curved adjunct airway or S-tube inserted through the patient's mouth into the pharynx.

Nasopharyngeal (na-zo-fah-RIN-je-al) **Airway**—a flexible breathing tube inserted through the patient's nose into the pharynx.

Suction Device—a vacuum-, air-, or oxygen-powered device that is used to remove blood, secretions, or other fluids from a patient's mouth and throat. Electrical and hand-powered units are available.

Pocket Face Mask—a simple device to aid in mouth-to-mouth resuscitation that can be used with supplemental oxygen when fitted with an oxygen inlet.

Bag-Valve-Mask Ventilator—a hand-held unit with a self-refilling bag, directional valve system, and face mask. The bag is squeezed to deliver atmospheric air to the patient. This unit can be set up to deliver nearly 100% oxygen from an oxygen supply system.

Hypoxia (hi-POK-se-ah)—an inadequate supply of oxygen reaching the body's tissues.

Atelectasis (at-i-LEK-tah-sis)—complete or partial collapse of the alveoli of the lungs.

Oxygen Toxicity—uncommon, rarely fatal effect on a patient who has received too high a concentration of oxygen for too long.

Chronic Obstructive Pulmonary Disease (COPD)—a group of diseases and conditions, including emphysema, chronic bronchitis, and black lung. Delivery of more than 28% oxygen to such patients can lead to respiratory arrest. See Chapter 11 for more specifics.

D, E, and M Cylinders—the most commonly used oxygen cylinders. D cylinders contain 350 liters of oxygen, E cylinders contain 625 liters of oxygen, and M cylinders contain 3000 liters of oxygen.

Pressure Regulator—a device connected to an oxygen cylinder to reduce cylinder pressure to a safe working pressure.

Flowmeter—a Bourdon or pressure-compensated device used to regulate and measure the flow of oxygen.

Humidifier—a device connected to the flowmeter to add moisture to the dry oxygen coming from the cylinder.

Oxygen Delivery Device—typically, one of four face masks or a nasal cannula.

Positive Pressure Resuscitator—a manually triggered, oxygen-powered ventilating unit.

Demand Valve Resuscitator—a device that will deliver oxygen when the patient attempts an inspiration.

AIDS TO BREATHING

It is vitally important that the EMT know how to provide basic life support without using any special devices. Establishing and maintaining an open airway, providing artificial ventilation, and the technique of CPR can be accomplished without equipment. Initiating such basic life support is usually done without equipment. Should equipment not be on hand, or should equipment fail, the EMT can continue basic life support using the techniques presented in Chapters 4 and 5.

Even though basic life support can be provided without equipment, more effective emergency care is possible when devices are used to maintain an open airway, clear the airway, assist in ventilation, and provide oxygen. The use of such equipment provides more oxygen to the exchange levels of the patient's lungs and greatly reduces rescuer fatigue. It is critical that an EMT know how to use and maintain the aids to breathing and the oxygen delivery equipment carried on ambulances.

REMEMBER: NEVER delay resuscitation measures to locate, retrieve, and set up special equipment or oxygen delivery devices.

Keep in mind that new responsibilities come with the use of equipment in basic life support:

- YOU must be sure that the equipment is clean and that it is operational PRIOR TO USE.
- YOU must select the proper equipment for the patient receiving care.
- YOU must monitor the patient more closely once you begin to use any device or delivery system.
- YOU must make certain that the equipment is properly discarded, cleaned, or tested after its use.

Airways

WARNING: Oropharyngeal airways are only to be used on *unconscious* patients. These devices can induce vomiting in the conscious individual. This vomitus can be aspirated into the patient's lungs, causing serious airway obstruction and damage to the lungs. As little as two ounces of vomitus in the lungs can cause a fatal form of pneumonia. Also, oropharyngeal airways can induce some degree of bronchospasms in a conscious patient. NEVER use an oropharyngeal airway on a conscious patient.

NEVER practice the use of airways on anyone. Manikins should be used for developing skills with airways.

Once you gain access to a patient and begin the primary survey, your first course of action is to establish an open airway. This airway must be maintained throughout all care procedures. Once the airway has been opened by the head-tilt, neck-lift; head-tilt, chin-lift; or modified jaw-thrust, it can be kept open more easily by an adjunct airway. Keep in mind that you must guard against improper head movement if there is any chance of spinal injury. If the patient is unconscious, the EMT is to assume there is spinal injury.

Rules for Using Adjunct Airways

1. Open the patient's airway before use.
2. Use on non-breathing, unconscious patients. Any gagging by the patient indicates that the adjunct airway cannot be used.
3. Take great care not to push the patient's tongue back into the throat.
4. Constantly monitor the patient for spontaneous breathing or gag reflex.
5. Remove the device immediately if the patient begins spontaneous respirations or exhibits the gag reflex.

Oropharyngeal Airways

Once a patient's airway is opened, an oropharyngeal (or-o-fah-RIN-je-al) airway can be inserted to help keep the airway open. 'Oro' refers to the mouth. 'Pharyngeo' refers to the throat. An **oropharyngeal airway** is a curved device usually made of plastic, which can be inserted through the patient's mouth to extend back into the throat. The oropharyngeal airway has a flange that fits against the patient's lips. The rest of the airway holds down the patient's tongue as it curves back to the patient's throat. Thus, the oropharyngeal airway serves two purposes:

• To maintain an open airway
• To hold the tongue in place so that it cannot slip back and obstruct the throat.

When a patient becomes unconscious, the muscles relax. The tongue will slide back into the pharynx and obstruct the airway. Even though a head-tilt maneuver will help open the airway of a patient with no possible spinal injuries, the tongue may return to its obstructive position once the head-tilt is released. Sometimes, even when the head-tilt is maintained, the tongue will still "fall back" into the pharynx. The proper use of an oropharyngeal airway greatly reduces the chances of the patient's airway becoming obstructed.

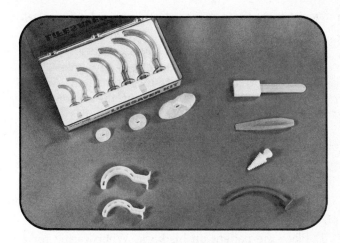

Figure 6-1: Various sizes of oropharyngeal airways.

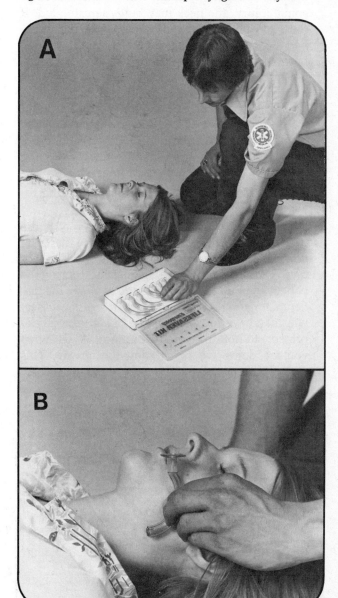

Figure 6-2: The airway is chosen and checked for correct size.

There are at least seven standard sizes of oropharyngeal airways. Many manufacturers make a complete line, ranging from sizes for infants to various sizes of adult airways. The entire set can be carried in one case to allow quick, proper selection. The device cannot be used effectively unless you select the correct airway size for the patient. An airway of proper size will extend from the center of the patient's mouth to the angle of the lower jaw (mandible). Before using an airway, hold the device against the patient's face to see if the airway extends from the mouth to the angle of the lower jaw. If the airway is not the correct size, do NOT use the airway on the patient.

Inserting the Airway

1. Place the patient on his back. When caring for a medical emergency patient with *no* indications of spinal injury, the neck may be hyperextended. If there are possible spinal injuries, use the modified jaw-thrust, moving the patient no more than necessary to assure an open airway (the airway takes priority over the spine). Extreme care must be taken.

2. Cross the thumb and forefinger of one hand and place them on the upper and lower teeth at the corner of the patient's mouth. Use a scissors motion to pry open the patient's jaws. Hold the mouth open with your crossed fingers.

3. Position the airway so that its tip is pointing toward the roof of the patient's mouth.

4. Insert the airway and slide it along the roof of the patient's mouth, past the soft tissue hanging down from the back of the mouth (the uvula), or until you meet resistance against the roof of the patient's mouth. Be certain not to push the patient's tongue back into the throat. In a few cases, you may have to use a tongue blade (tongue depressor) to hold the tongue in place. Watch what you are doing when inserting the airway. This procedure should not be performed by "feel" only.

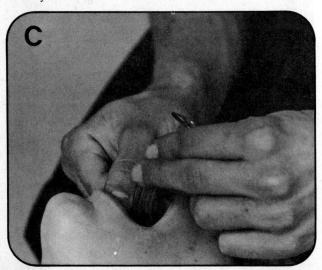

Figure 6-3: The airway is inserted with the tip pointing to the roof of the patient's mouth.

5. GENTLY rotate the airway 180 degrees. This will position the tip is so that it is pointing down the patient's throat.

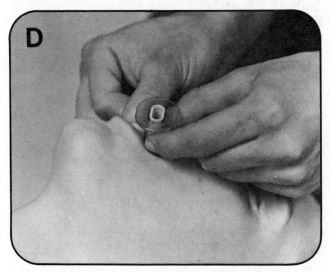

Figure 6-4: The airway is rotated into position.

6. Place the non-trauma patient in a maximum head-tilt position. Minimize all movements of the head if there are possible spinal injuries.

7. Check to see that the flange of the airway is against the patient's lips. If the airway is too long or too short, remove the airway and replace it with the correct size.

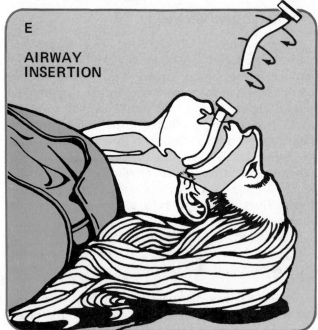

Figure 6-5: When positioned, the flange rests against the patient's lips.

8. Provide mouth-to-adjunct ventilation as you would provide mouth-to-mouth ventilation.

9. MONITOR the patient closely. If there is a gag reflex, remove the airway at once. Removal is accomplished by the reversal of the insertion procedures.

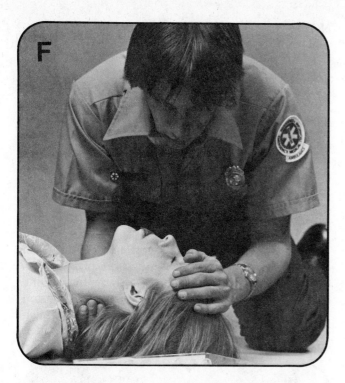

Figure 6-6: The patient is ready for ventilation.

A major disadvantage of the oropharyngeal airway is that it is not the perfect size for every patient. In some cases, the closest fit may be too small and partially block the airway. If the device is too large it may fall forward and push the tongue back into the pharynx, blocking the airway again. Too long a device may induce gagging, and may cause the patient to vomit.

S-Tube Airways

An **S-tube airway** is a special form of the oropharyngeal airway. In the past few years, this device has seen less use, with many systems utilizing other forms of oropharyngeal airways. The AHA no longer recommends this airway.

The S-tube's basic construction is the same as a standard oropharyngeal airway, except for an external tube that allows for the delivery of artificial ventilation without the rescuer having to make mouth-to-mouth contact with the patient. This can be an advantage in cases of facial injury. Since S-tubes have two curved airways giving them their "S" shape, they are often constructed with two different size curved tubes to give the rescuer a choice of two possible airways to insert through the patient's mouth. Some are made so that one tube can be removed and the unit can be used as a standard oropharyngeal airway.

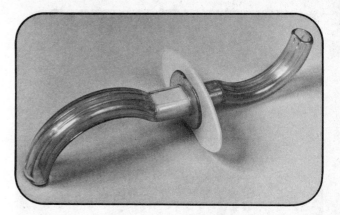

Figure 6-7: An S-tube adjunct airway.

The use of the S-tube is very similar to the use of a basic oropharyngeal airway. The tube to be inserted into the patient's mouth must be measured for size. Insertion and rotation are the same as for the oropharyngeal airway. When in place, the flange should rest against the patient's lips. If not, the S-tube is the wrong size and must be removed. When using an S-tube, the rescuer must hold the flange against the patient's lips to form a tight seal. Sometimes the seal is not very effective and a different adjunct airway must be selected.

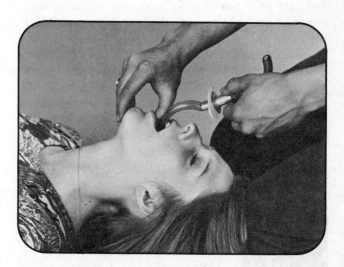

Figure 6-8: Inserting the S-tube.

Artificial ventilations are delivered through the external tube, following the same procedures used in mouth-to-mouth resuscitation. Gurgling respiration sounds indicate that the tube is the wrong size, or that there is an airway obstruction. When this occurs, you will have to remove the tube, suction the patient's airway, quickly determine the correct size tube, and reposition the tube.

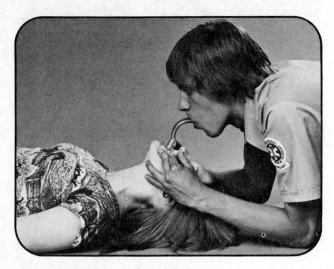

Figure 6-9: Mouth-to-adjunct ventilation.

Nasopharyngeal Airways

This type of airway is not used in all EMS Systems, but its popularity is growing. Many EMTs favor its use since the device does not tend to stimulate a gag reflex, thus making it a practical adjunct airway for conscious patients. The soft, flexible tube is inserted through the nose rather than the mouth. This allows the tube to be used in cases where there is oral cavity injury.

Keep in mind that you will have to lubricate this tube with a water-based lubricant before its insertion. Do NOT use a petroleum jelly or other such type of lubricant that may damage the tissue lining the nasal cavity and the pharynx. If there is resistance when inserting the nasopharyngeal tube, do NOT force the tube into the nose. Pull the tube out and try the other nostril. If the resistance is such that you cannot easily insert the tube, do not continue with your attempts. Once the airway is in place, the flange should rest firmly against the patient's nostril.

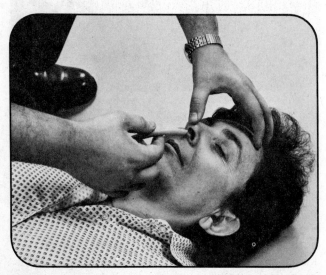

Figure 6-10: Inserting a lubricated nasopharyngeal airway.

NOTE: The esophageal obturator airway is presented in Appendix #4.

SUCTION DEVICES

To this point, we have discussed body positioning and finger sweeps as the primary techniques to remove blood, vomitus, phlegm, and other secretions from a sick or injured patient's throat. Fixed and portable mechanical suction devices are available to supplement these manual methods.

Fixed (Installed) Systems

A fixed or installed suction system should be in every ambulance (Fig. 6-11). This type of system is powered by the vacuum produced by the engine manifold, or by an electrically operated vacuum pump. To be effective, a fixed system must furnish an air intake of at least 30 liters/minute at the open end of a collection tube. This will occur if a vacuum

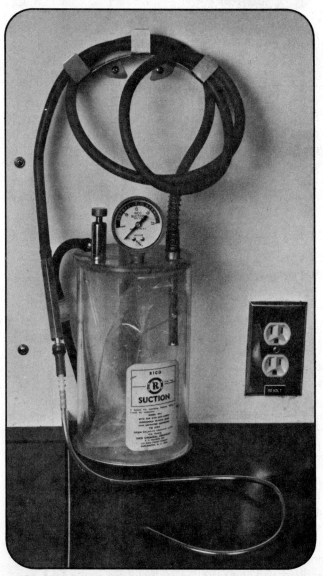

Figure 6-11: Fixed (installed) sunction unit for ambulance patient compartments.

of no less than 300 mmHg is produced when the collecting tube is clamped.

A fixed system should have a nonbreakable collection bottle, a large diameter, nonkinking, noncollapsing collection tube long enough to reach the patient, several rigid suction tips, a variety of catheters for clearing the throat, and water for rinsing the system. There should be some means for controlling the suction. To provide control, many systems have a ''Y'' or ''T'' placed in the line between the tip and the suction source.

Portable Suction Units

There are many different types of portable suction devices. The main difference among these units is the suction source.

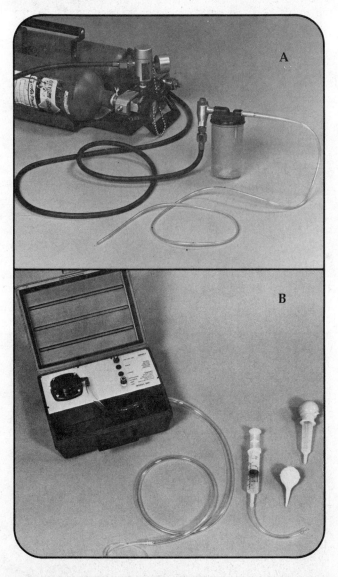

Figure 6-12. A. Oxygen-powered portable suction unit. B. Three types of portable suction units powered by electricity and hand.

- Oxygen- or air-powered units—Many oxygen-powered resuscitators are equipped with a venturi device that develops a vacuum for suctioning. Most of these units deplete oxygen at a great rate. Portable air-powered units are available. These devices may be more efficient than the oxygen-powered type, and are excellent for working in confined areas, such as vehicular wreckage. Some of these units are gas-powered and use freon as a source.
- Electrically powered units—These are highly efficient devices capable of developing a vacuum of up to 600 mmHg. Some units have a converter so that they can be operated by rechargeable battery or 110-volt sources.
- Hand-powered units—These have a simple rubber bulb aspirator or a hand- or foot-operated device to produce a vacuum for suctioning. These units are not as efficient as air- or electrically powered units.

Techniques of Suctioning

There are many variations in the technique of suctioning. A suggested procedure is presented in the next Scansheet.

REMEMBER: Use great care when suctioning a conscious patient. If you insert the catheter too deeply, it will trigger the gag reflex and the patient may vomit. Learn to protect your fingers in case the patient involuntarily bites down. Many squads carry a ''bite block'' made of several tongue depressors taped together. A bite block can be held between the patient's upper and lower teeth in cases where care requires you to insert your fingers into the patient's mouth.

Do NOT suction the nonbreathing patient for more than 15 seconds at a time before attempting to provide TWO ventilations. After the ventilations, suctioning may continue. If you suction for five seconds or less, provide one ventilation. NEVER suction longer than you can comfortably hold a normal breath.

VENTILATION-ASSIST DEVICES

Earlier, we discussed the S-tube and how it could be used to assist in the delivery of ventilations. Two other devices, the pocket face mask and the bag-valve-mask ventilator, also can be used to assist with ventilation.

The Pocket Face Mask

The **pocket face mask** is a modification of a resuscitator facepiece. It is made of soft collapsible material, and can be carried in the rescuer's pocket. The mask is available as shown, or can be fitted with an

TECHNIQUES OF SUCTIONING

POSITION YOURSELF AT THE PATIENT'S HEAD AND TURN HIS HEAD TO THE SIDE

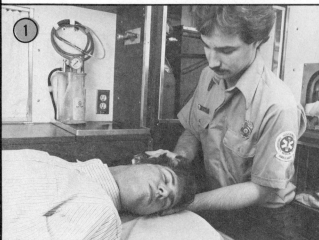

OPEN PATIENT'S MOUTH BY CROSS-FINGER TECHNIQUE AND CLEAR MOUTH

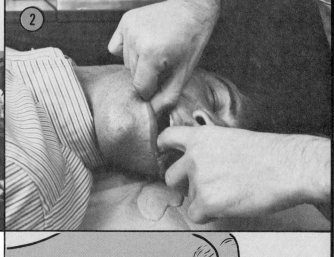

TURN UNIT ON AND CLAMP THE COLLECTION TUBE

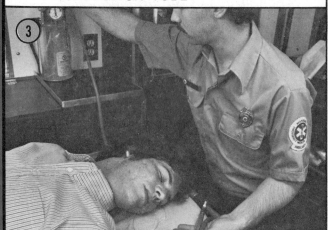

PLACE THE RIGID PHARYNGEAL TIP SO THAT THE CONVEX (BULGING OUT) SIDE IS AGAINST THE ROOF OF THE PATIENT'S MOUTH. INSERT THE TIP TO THE BEGINNING OF THE THROAT. DO NOT PUSH THE TIP DOWN INTO THE THROAT OR INTO THE LARYNX

MEASURING FLEXIBLE SUCTION CATHETER EQUAL DISTANCE BETWEEN PATIENT'S MOUTH AND EARLOBE

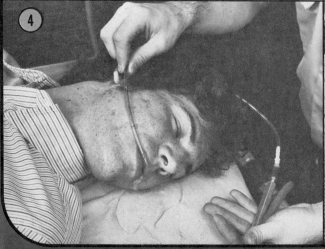

APPLY SUCTION AFTER THE TIP OF THE CATHETER, OR THE RIGID TIP, IS IN PLACE

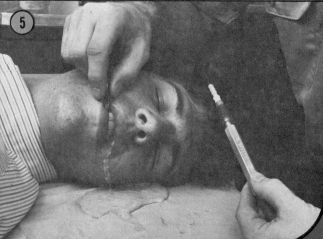

SCAN 6.1

oxygen inlet. Mouth-to-mask ventilations are provided through a chimney on the mask. If oxygen is being provided, the EMT can simultaneously ventilate the patient with air from his own lungs and the oxygen source. The oxygen delivered by this simultaneous method ranges from 40 to 45% at 10 liters per minute.

Table 6.1: Feasible Oxygen Concentrations*

O₂ Flow LPM	Inhalation (spontaneously breathing patient)	Ventilation (non-breathing patient)
5	50%	40%
10	68%	50%
30	90%	98% (with intermittent occlusion of mask)

* Safar/Lind: "Triple airway maneuver, artificial ventilation and Oxygen Inhalation by mouth-to-mask and bag-valve-mask techniques."—published in Procedings, National Conference on Standards for Cardiopulmonary Resuscitation (CPR) and Emergency Cardiac Care (ECC), 1973.

One distinct advantage of the pocket face mask is that it allows the rescuer to use both hands to maintain the proper head-tilt and to firmly hold the mask in place. The mask can also be used as a facemask for patients who do not require assistance with breathing.

To provide mouth-to-mask ventilation, you should:

1. Position yourself at the patient's head and open the airway. You may need to insert an oropharyngeal airway to keep the patient's airway open. If necessary, clear the airway, also.
2. Position the mask on the patient's face so that the apex is over the bridge of the nose and the base is between the lower lip and the prominence of the chin.
3. Hold the mask *firmly* in place while maintaining the proper head-tilt:
   • Both thumbs at the dome of the mask
   • First three fingers of each hand grasping the lower jaw on each side, between the angle of the jaw and the earlobe, to lift the jaw forward
4. Take a deep breath and exhale into the port of the mask chimney.
5. Remove your mouth from the chimney and allow for passive exhalation. Continue the cycle as you would for mouth-to-mouth ventilations, providing a breath every 5 SECONDS.

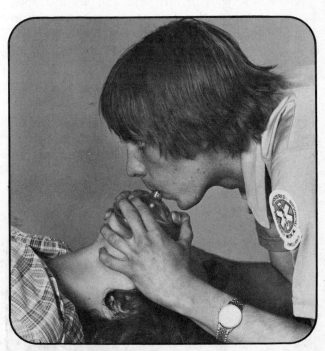

Figure 6-14: Providing mouth-to-mask ventilations. Note placement of the EMT's hands.

The Bag-Valve-Mask Ventilator

NOTE: Most EMS Systems recommend that you insert an oropharyngeal airway before attempting to ventilate the patient with a bag-valve-mask ventilator.

The hand-held unit most often used to ventilate a nonbreathing patient is the **bag-valve-mask ventilator,** commonly called a bag mask unit. The bag-valve-mask unit may be used to ventilate patients

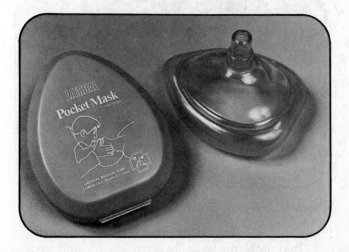

Figure 6-13: A pocket face mask. Note the chimney for mouth-to-mask ventilations.

with shallow and failing respirations (as in drug overdose). This device comes in infant, pediatric, and adult sizes.

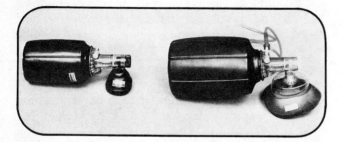

Figure 6-15: Pediatric and adult bag-valve-mask ventilators.

REMEMBER: When providing mouth-to-mouth ventilations you are delivering 16% oxygen to the patient. The bag-valve-mask unit will deliver 21% oxygen from the atmosphere and 50% to nearly 100% oxygen from an oxygen delivery source, depending on the type of device and the flow rate.

Numerous types of this ventilator are available; however, all have the same basic parts as shown in Figure 6-16. Most units have a 15/22 mm fitting to accept a variety of masks or endotracheal tubes for paramedic use.

WARNING: The facepiece used on a bag-valve-mask unit must be transparent so that the EMT can see the patient's mouth. This is required so that you can see any vomitus or dislodged airway obstructions. When a clear facepiece is used, the EMT can see cyanosis (blue coloring) at the lips, which indicates the patient needs oxygenation.

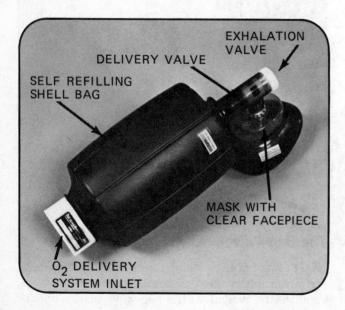

Figure 6-16: The typical bag-valve-mask ventilator.

The operation of a bag-valve-mask ventilator is simple to understand. When the bag is squeezed, air is delivered to the patient through a one-way valve.

The air inlet to the bag is closed during delivery. When the hand-squeeze on the bag is released, a passive exhalation occurs. This air from the patient's lungs cannot re-enter the bag. It passes through an exhalation valve into the atmosphere. While the patient is exhaling, air from the atmosphere refills the bag. Most adult unit bags will hold 1,000 to 1,200 ml of air.

When using the bag-valve-mask ventilator, you should:

1. Position yourself at the patient's head and provide an open airway. Clear the airway if necessary.
2. Insert an oropharyngeal airway.
3. Be certain to use the *correct size mask* for the patient. The apex or top of the triangular mask should be over the bridge of the nose (between the eyebrows). The base of the mask should rest between the patient's lower lip and the prominence of the chin.
4. Be certain to *hold the mask firmly* in position, with
   • the thumb holding the upper part of the mask;
   • the index finger between the valve and the lower cushion; and
   • the third, fourth, and fifth fingers on the lower jaw, between the chin and ear. With some units, you will have to hold your palm over the facepiece and hook your fingers under the patient's jaw.
5. With your other hand, squeeze the bag ONCE EVERY 5 SECONDS. The squeeze should be a full one, causing the patient's chest to rise.
6. Release pressure on the bag and let the patient passively exhale and the bag refill from the atmosphere or oxygen source.

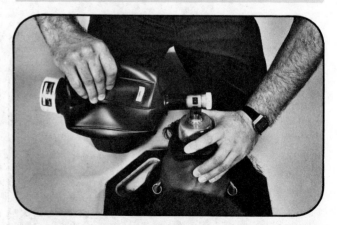

Figure 6-17: Hand positioning when using the bag-valve-mask.

Two problems typically occur when using a bag-valve-mask resuscitator. Sometimes the problem is due to an airway obstruction that must be cleared.

More often than not, the problem is caused by an improper seal between the patient's face and the mask. It should be rare for the bag, valve, or mask to be the problem. This is because a good EMT knows how to disassemble, clean, reassemble, and test the units before they need to be used in the field.

The bag-valve-mask ventilator can be used very effectively during two-rescuer CPR. The ventilator squeezes the bag quickly, but smoothly, on the compressor's fifth upstroke. Some EMS Systems now have the ventilator squeeze on the third upstroke, to oxygenate the patient better (not an AHA standard). A rescuer can easily meet this demand, whereas to increase mouth-to-mouth ventilation would be too taxing when providing ventilation during two-rescuer CPR.

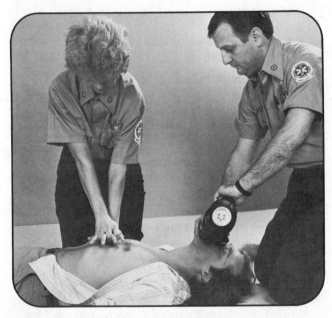

Figure 6-18: Two-rescuer CPR using a bag-valve-mask ventilator.

OXYGEN THERAPY

The Importance of Supplemental Oxygen

It is critical that an EMT know how to maintain oxygen equipment, how to administer oxygen to patients, and when to administer oxygen. Patients who receive oxygen during pulmonary resuscitation or CPR stand a much better chance of surviving. The same holds true for patients with internal bleeding, severe external blood loss, head injury, and major fractures. Heart attack and some stroke patients also do better when given high concentrations of oxygen. Administering oxygen may keep a patient from going into shock, or prevent the shock from worsening. Since shock is a real possibility with many trauma and medical emergency patients, providing oxygen therapy for patients is a major skill required of all EMTs.

A patient may require oxygen for a variety of reasons:

- Respiratory Arrest—failure to take oxygen into the lungs and rid the body of carbon dioxide.
- Cardiac Arrest—failure to pump blood to carry oxygen to the tissues. Keep in mind that respiratory arrest occurs along with cardiac arrest.
- Major Blood Loss—there is a reduction in the number of red blood cells required to carry oxygen, and the volume of blood is reduced, forcing the heart to work harder.
- Heart Attack and Heart Failure—the ability to pump oxygenated blood is greatly reduced.
- Lung Disease or Injury—the ability to take in and exchange oxygen is greatly reduced.
- Airway Obstruction—even partial obstruction causes the amount of oxygen reaching the lungs to be greatly reduced.
- Stroke—remember that the brain requires a constant supply of oxygen. If this supply is stopped or reduced, vessels in the brain can quickly constrict to cause an irreversible form of shock, and brain cells will start to die very quickly.
- Shock—since shock is a collapse of the cardiovascular system, all cases of shock can reduce the amount of oxygenated blood reaching the tissues.

When you are caring for a patient who is able to breathe, atmospheric air can provide no more than 21% oxygen to the patient. This is far more than the patient needs, provided that the airway is open, the exchange surfaces of the lungs are working properly, there is enough oxygen being carried by the blood, and the patient's cardiovascular system is properly circulating blood to all the body tissues. When any of these factors fails, a higher concentration of oxygen delivered to the patient's lungs may mean that the required level of oxygen will reach his body's tissues.

Providing oxygen to the nonbreathing patient by mouth-to-mouth techniques puts 16% oxygen into his lungs. This will be enough to keep the patient alive. Interposed ventilations provided by mouth-to-mouth techniques during CPR also deliver only 16% oxygen to the patient. CPR circulates the blood with less than a third of the efficiency of a healthy, beating heart. Body tissues thus receive only the minimum amount of oxygen required for short-term survival. Oxygen therapy, however, allows nearly 100% oxygen to reach the lungs. With more oxygen in the patient's blood, circulation efficiency is improved and the patient has a better chance for survival.

Always remember that oxygen is a medication. This means that you will have to decide if it is needed, how much to provide, what results are expected, and what harm may be done. The use of oxygen is a special responsibility that can be given only to someone of professional status.

Hypoxia

Hypoxia (hi-POK-se-ah) is a decrease in the supply of oxygen in the body tissues. Sometimes the term 'anoxia' is used to mean the same thing; however, this term means a *complete* lack of oxygen. There are several major causes of hypoxia, including:

- Respiratory insufficiency—too little oxygen is exchanged between the alveoli (al-VE-o-li), or microscopic airsacs of the lungs, and the blood (hypoxic hypoxia). This can be due to the air itself, as in cases of hypoxia produced by the rarefied air of high altitudes. The oxygen in the air can be reduced, as in fire. Breathing such air will lead to hypoxia.

  Damage to the lungs through injury (punctured lung), or disease (emphysema) may also prevent the proper amount of oxygen from reaching the blood. Chest injuries may produce this form of hypoxia.

- Circulatory insufficiency—a reduction of blood flow due to heart attack, heart failure, cardiovascular collapse, obstructed blood vessels, or blood loss can lower the amount of oxygen picked up from the lungs or circulated to the tissues (circulatory hypoxia).

- Hemoglobin insufficiency—when there is not enough hemoglobin in the red blood cells, if the hemoglobin is not free to pick up oxygen (as in carbon monoxide poisoning), or if the ability to pick up and carry oxygen is reduced (as with certain pain medications), hypoxia can occur (hemic hypoxia).

- Cellular exchange problems—even if a sufficient amount of oxygen is delivered to the tissues, it must be taken *into* the cells or hypoxia will occur (cellular hypoxia). Certain poisons such as cyanide can prevent oxygen exchange between the bloodstream and the cells. Drug and alcohol abuse also can cause this form of hypoxia.

As an EMT, your concern will not be *why* the hypoxia has occurred, but rather, how to prevent it from becoming worse and, when possible, to reduce the level of hypoxia. There are some cases of lung disease where you will have to modify the oxygen therapy delivered to the patient. However, in most cases where oxygen is required, you will be delivering the maximum oxygen needed to prevent or to control hypoxia. Remember, if hypoxia is allowed to continue, the patient may suffer brain damage or develop respiratory arrest.

The Disadvantages of Oxygen Therapy

There are certain hazards associated with the administration of oxygen. These hazards can be grouped as nonmedical and medical.

The nonmedical hazards of oxygen therapy include:

1. The oxygen used in emergency care is stored under pressure, usually 2000 to 2200 pounds per square inch (psi) or greater in a full cylinder. If the oxygen tank is punctured, or if a valve breaks off, the supply tank can become a missile. Damaged tanks have been able to penetrate concrete walls. Imagine what would happen in the passenger compartment of an ambulance if such an oxygen cylinder-related accident occurred.

2. Oxygen supports combustion, causing fire to burn more rapidly. It can saturate towels, sheets, and clothing and cause them to burn very rapidly.

3. Under pressure, oxygen and oil do not mix. When they come into contact with one another, a severe reaction occurs which, for our purposes, can be termed an explosion. This is seldom a problem, but it can easily occur if you try to lubricate a delivery system or gauge with petroleum products.

The *medical* hazards of oxygen therapy include:

1. Oxygen toxicity—destruction of lung tissue due to high concentrations of oxygen provided for a long period of time. This is extremely rare in EMT-level emergency care.

2. Airsac collapse—the alveoli of the lungs react to oxygen in a fashion similar to the way the pupils of the eyes react to light. If the concentration of oxygen is low, the alveoli expand. If the concentration of oxygen is high, the alveoli constrict. If too high a concentration of oxygen is given for too long a period of time, the alveoli may constrict and never be able to regain their normal size. This condition is known as **atelectasis** (at-i-LEK-tah-sis). In severe cases, whole sections of a lung may collapse. The condition can be fatal, but it is seldom a problem in emergency care.

3. Infant eye damage—seen when infants are given too much oxygen, particularly the premature infant. Scar tissue will form behind the lens of the eye (retrolental fibroplasia), leading to impaired vision or permanent blindness.

4. Respiratory arrest—this problem occurs in patients with chronic obstructive pulmonary disease

(COPD), including emphysema, chronic bronchitis, and black lung. When given oxygen in too high a dosage (about 28%), these patients can develop respiratory arrest.

As an EMT, you probably will not see oxygen toxicity or alveolar collapse. The time required for such conditions is too long to cause any problems during standard field emergency care. Damage to the eyes of a premature infant can be prevented by delivering oxygen to a tent of aluminum foil that has been placed over the patient's head. The amount of time the infant will be exposed to the oxygen is shorter than the time required to cause eye damage. In addition to the exposure time, most cases of eye damage are associated with concentrations of oxygen above 40%. The tent delivery of oxygen usually does not maintain this high a level of oxygen. For more on the delivery of oxygen to the infant patient, see Chapter 12, Section One.

The COPD patient is another matter. You can cause serious problems for such a patient if you deliver too high a concentration of oxygen. In healthy individuals, the primary control center for respiration is in the brain. This center reacts to the amount of carbon dioxide in the blood. The higher the concentration of carbon dioxide, the more rapid the ventilations. A patient with COPD has, *over a period of time*, an increase in blood carbon dioxide level. At a certain point, the primary center for respiration will no longer respond to the high carbon dioxide level in the blood. Secondary centers, located in the carotid arteries (*carotid bodies*) take over the major control of respiration. These centers react to the level of oxygen in the blood. If you provide too much oxygen quickly to the patient, the carotid centers will shut down. Since the primary center in the brain is not functioning normally, the patient will stop breathing. For more on COPD, see Chapter 11, Section One.

REMEMBER: Never deliver more than 28% oxygen to a COPD patient. Many EMS Systems recommend no more than 24%, with constant monitoring of the patient. The exception is when the patient is in respiratory arrest or cardiac arrest. Since the worst has already happened, there is no need to worry about too high an oxygen level stopping respirations. Resuscitation is best done with the highest concentration of oxygen available.

EQUIPMENT AND SUPPLIES FOR OXYGEN THERAPY

An oxygen delivery system for the breathing patient includes an oxygen source, pressure regulator, flowmeter, and a delivery device (face mask or cannula). When possible, a humidifier should be added to provide moisture to the dry oxygen. The delivery system is the same for a nonbreathing patient, but a device must be added to allow the EMT to force oxygen into the patient's lungs. This is known as positive pressure ventilation.

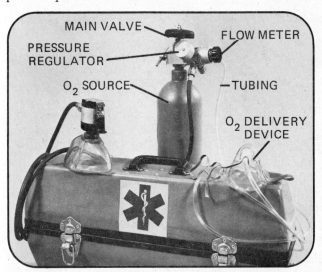

Figure 6-19: An oxygen delivery system.

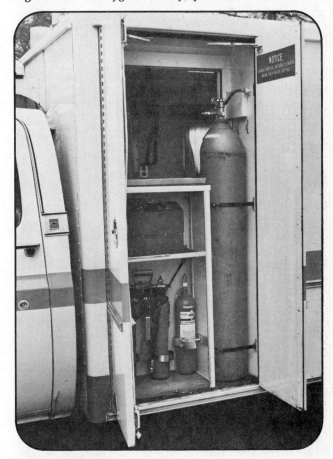

Figure 6-20: Larger cylinders are used for fixed systems on ambulances.

Oxygen Cylinders

Outside a medical facility, the standard source of oxygen is a seamless steel or lightweight alloy cylinder filled with oxygen under pressure, equal to 2000 to 2200 psi when the cylinders are full. Cylinders come in various sizes and are identified by letters. Those in common usage in emergency care include:

- D cylinder—contains about 350 liters of oxygen
- E cylinder—contains about 625 liters of oxygen
- M cylinder—contains about 3000 liters of oxygen

You cannot tell if an oxygen cylinder is full or empty by lifting or moving the cylinder. Part of your duty as an EMT is to make certain that the oxygen cylinders YOU will use are full and ready before they are needed to provide care. The length of time you can use an oxygen cylinder depends on the pressure in the cylinder and the flow rate. The method of calculating cylinder duration is shown in Table 6-2. Oxygen cylinders should NEVER be allowed to empty below the safe residual. The safe residual for an oxygen cylinder is determined when the pressure gauge reads 200 psi. At this point, you must switch to a fresh cylinder.

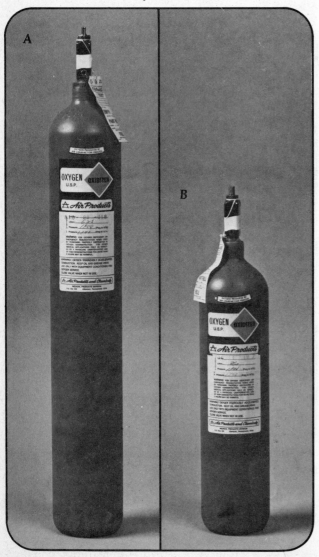

Figure 6-21: A. "E" size cylinder B. "D" size cylinder.

Table 6.2: Oxygen Cylinders: Duration of Flow

SIMPLE FORMULA

$$\frac{\text{Gauge pressure in psi - the safe residual pressure} \times \text{constant}}{\text{Flow rate in liters/minute}} = \begin{array}{l}\text{duration of} \\ \text{flow in} \\ \text{minutes}\end{array}$$

RESIDUAL PRESSURE = 200 psi

CYLINDER CONSTANT

D	= 0.16	G	= 2.41
E	= 0.28	H	= 3.14
M	= 1.56	K	= 3.14

Determine the life of an M cylinder that has a pressure of 2000 psi and a flow rate of 10 liters/minute.

$$\frac{(2000 - 200) \times 1.56}{10} = \frac{2808}{10} = \begin{array}{l}\text{281 minutes,} \\ \text{or 4 hours and} \\ \text{41 minutes}\end{array}$$

SAFETY is of prime importance when working with oxygen cylinders. You should:

- NEVER drop a cylinder or let it fall against an object. Make certain the cylinder is well secured, preferably in an upright position.
- NEVER allow smoking around oxygen equipment in use. Clearly mark the area of use with signs that read, "OXYGEN—NO SMOKING."
- NEVER use oxygen equipment around an open flame.
- NEVER use grease or oil on devices that will be attached to an oxygen supply cylinder. Take care not to handle these devices when your hands are greasy.
- NEVER try to move an oxygen cylinder by rolling it on its side or its bottom.
- ALWAYS use the pressure gauges and regulators that are intended for use with oxygen.
- ALWAYS assure that valve seat inserts and gaskets are in good condition. This prevents dangerous leaks.
- ALWAYS use medical-grade oxygen. Industrial oxygen contains impurities. The cylinder should be labeled, "OXYGEN U.S.P."
- ALWAYS open the valve of an oxygen cylinder fully, then close it half a turn to prevent someone else from thinking the valve is closed and trying to force the valve open.
- ALWAYS store reserve oxygen cylinders in a cool, ventilated room.
- ALWAYS have oxygen cylinders hydrostatically tested every TEN YEARS. The date a cylinder should be retested is stamped on the cylinder.

Pressure Regulators

The pressure in an oxygen cylinder is too high to be a safe working pressure. A pressure regulator must be connected to the cylinder to provide a safe working pressure of *30 to 70 psi.*

On cylinders of the E size or smaller, the pressure regulator is secured to the cylinder valve assembly (Figure 6-22) by a yoke assembly. The yoke is provided with pins that must mate with corresponding holes in the valve assembly. This is called a "pin-index safety system." Since the pin position varies for different gases, this prevents an oxygen delivery system from being connected to a cylinder of another gas.

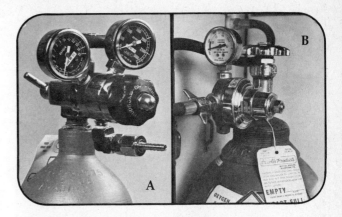

Figure 6-23: A. Two-stage regulator for "D" and "E" size cylinders; B. Single-stage regulator.

Before connecting the pressure regulator to an oxygen supply cylinder, *crack* the cylinder valve slightly for just a second to clear dirt and dust out of the delivery port or threaded outlet.

Flowmeters

A flowmeter allows control of the flow of oxygen in liters per minute. It is connected to the pressure regulator. Two types of flowmeters are available. In emergency care use in the field, the pressure compensated flowmeter is considered to be superior to the Bourdon gauge flowmeter.

- Pressure Compensated Flowmeter—This meter is gravity dependent and must be in an upright position to deliver an accurate reading. The unit has an upright, calibrated glass tube in which there is a ball float. The float rises and falls according to the amount of gas passing through the tube. This type of flowmeter indicates the actual flow at all times, even though there may be a partial obstruction to gas flow (as from a kinked delivery tube). If the tubing collapses, the ball will drop to show the lower delivery rate. This unit is not practical for many portable delivery systems.

- Bourdon Gauge Flowmeter—This unit is a pressure gauge calibrated to indicate flow in liters per minute. The meter is fairly inaccurate at low flow rates and has often been criticized as being unstable. However, it can be a useful gauge for some portable units.

The major fault with this type of flowmeter is its inability to compensate for back pressure. A partial obstruction (as from a kinked hose) will be reflected in a reading that is higher than the actual flow. The gauge may read 6 liters/minute and only be delivering 1 liter/minute. This type of gauge contains a filter that can become clogged and cause the gauge to read higher than the actual flow.

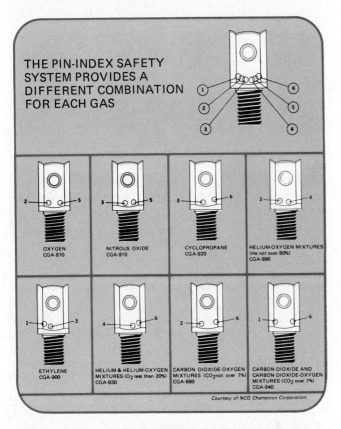

THE PIN-INDEX SAFETY SYSTEM PROVIDES A DIFFERENT COMBINATION FOR EACH GAS

OXYGEN
CGA-870

NITROUS OXIDE
CGA-910

CYCLOPROPANE
CGA-920

HELIUM-OXYGEN MIXTURES
(He not over 80%)
CGA-890

ETHYLENE
CGA-900

HELIUM & HELIUM-OXYGEN MIXTURES (O_2 less than 20%)
CGA-930

CARBON DIOXIDE-OXYGEN MIXTURES (CO_2 not over 7%)
CGA-880

CARBON DIOXIDE AND CARBON DIOXIDE-OXYGEN MIXTURES (CO_2 over 7%)
CGA-940

Courtesy of NCG Chemetron Corporation

Figure 6-22: The pin-index safety system.

Cylinders larger than the E size have a valve assembly with a threaded outlet. The inside and outside diameters of the threaded outlets vary in size according to the gas in the cylinder. This prevents an oxygen regulator from being connected to a cylinder containing another gas. In other words, a nitrogen regulator cannot be connected to an oxygen cylinder, and vice versa.

Cylinder pressure can be reduced in one or two steps. For a one-step reduction, a single-stage pressure regulator is used. A two-step reduction requires a two-stage regulator. Most regulators used in emergency care are the single-stage variety.

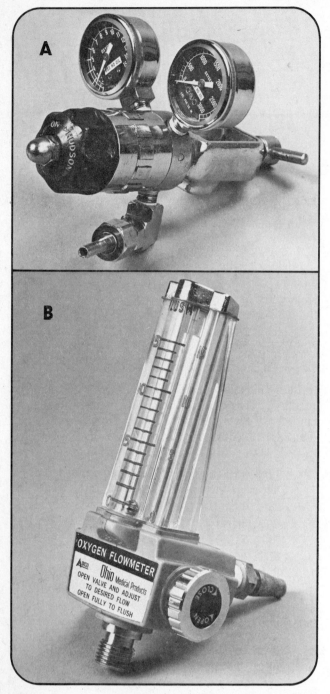

Figure 6-24: A. Bourdon gauge flowmeter (pressure gauge); B. Pressure compensated flowmeter.

Humidifiers

A humidifier can be connected to the flowmeter to provide moisture to the dry oxygen coming from the supply cylinder. Dry oxygen can quickly dehydrate the mucous membranes of the patient's airway and lungs. In most short-term usage (20 to 30 minutes), the dry nature of the oxygen being delivered is not a problem.

A humidifier is usually no more than a jar of water attached to the flowmeter. Oxygen passes through the water to become humidified. As with all oxygen delivery equipment, the humidifier must be kept clean. The water reservoir can become a breeding ground for algae, harmful bacteria, and dangerous fungal organisms. Always use *fresh* water in a clean reservoir for each patient.

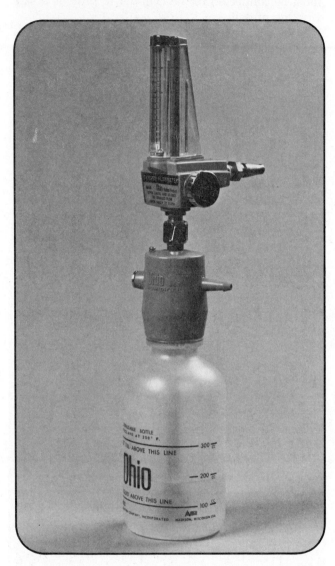

Figure 6-25: A simple oxygen humidifier.

Oxygen Delivery Devices

There are five oxygen delivery devices in common use for the emergency care of *breathing* patients. The nasal cannula and four types of face masks provide a wide selection of devices for oxygen delivery. Although it is not a standard, many EMS Systems are using the nasal cannula to start oxygen therapy on breathing medical emergency patients (The exception is the COPD patient.). If shock appears to be a problem, or if the patient is very cyanotic or has very labored breathing, a face mask is used. These same systems use one of the four types of face masks to begin oxygen therapy for breathing trauma patients.

A simple rule determines the percentage of oxygen being delivered to a patient:

For every 1 liter per minute increase in oxygen flow, you deliver a 4% increase in the concentration of oxygen.

If you know a particular device will give 24% oxygen at 4 liters per minute, an increase to 5 liters per minute will deliver a concentration of approximately 28% oxygen.

The five major oxygen delivery devices for breathing patients include:

- Nasal Cannula—There are two types, one with an elastic band for holding the device in place, and the newer design with a sliploop to secure around the patient's ears and chin. Both types deliver oxygen into the patient's nostrils through two small plastic prongs. The efficiency of the device is greatly reduced by nasal injuries, colds, and other types of nasal airway obstruction. In common usage, a flow rate of 4 to 8 liters per minute will provide the patient with 30% to 50% oxygen. The relationship of oxygen concentration to liter per minute flow is:

1 liter/minute	24% oxygen
2 liters/minute	28% oxygen
4 liters/minute	36% oxygen
8 liters/minute	52 to 54% oxygen

After 8 liters per minute, the device does not deliver any higher concentration of oxygen and proves to be very uncomfortable for most patients.

NOTE: The nasal cannula can be used for COPD patients if a flow rate no greater than 1 to 2 liters per minute is maintained. However, we do NOT recommend its use for such patients. There are too many variables to be considered. The venturi mask is the delivery device of choice for COPD patients. Follow your local guidelines.

- Simple Face Mask—This is a soft, clear plastic mask that will conform to the contours of the patient's face. There are small perforations in the mask to allow atmospheric air to enter and the patient's exhaled air to escape. The mask is used to deliver moderate concentrations of oxygen (35% to 60%) with a flow rate of 6 to 15 liters per minute. The practical maximum flow is considered to be 12 liters per minute.

CAUTION: Always start with 6 liters per minute flow when using this mask. If you start with less, carbon dioxide can build up in the mask. At a flow of 1 liter per minute, the patient is getting less oxygen than he would from atmospheric air.

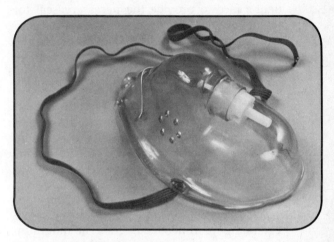

Figure 6-27: A simple face mask.

- Partial Rebreathing Mask—This device combines a face mask and a reservoir bag. The mask will only function properly if it is well fitted to the patient's face. Oxygen should be in the reservoir before you place the mask on the patient's face. The reservoir bag must be

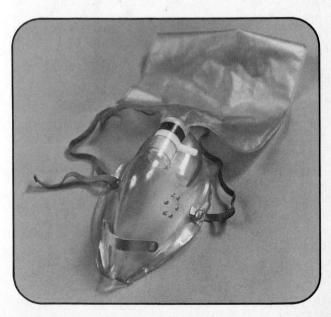

Figure 6-28: A partial rebreathing mask.

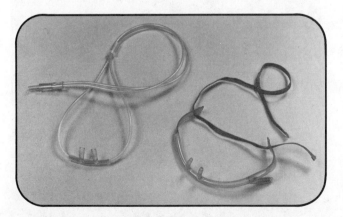

Figure 6-26: Two models of nasal cannula—loop type and elastic-held type.

filled with enough oxygen so that it does not collapse by more than one-third when the patient inhales. Part of the patient's exhaled air will enter the reservoir bag to be mixed with oxygen, the rest will escape through perforations in the mask. Concentrations of 35% to 60% can be delivered when flow rates are between 6 and 10 liters per minute.

- Non-rebreathing Mask—Excluding the bag-valve-mask resuscitator used with oxygen and the demand valve resuscitator, the non-rebreathing mask is the EMT's best way to deliver high concentrations of oxygen. This device MUST be placed properly on the patient's face to provide the necessary seal for the delivery of high concentrations of oxygen. The reservoir bag must be inflated before the mask is placed on the patient's face. To inflate the reservoir bag, use your hand to cover the exhaust portal. The reservoir must always contain enough oxygen so that it does not deflate by more than one-third when the patient takes his deepest inspiration. Air exhaled by the patient does not return to the reservoir. Instead, it escapes through a flutter valve in the facepiece.

This mask will provide concentrations of oxygen ranging from 80% to 95%. The minimum flow rate is 8 liters/minute. Depending on the manufacturer and the fit of the mask, the maximum flow can range from 10 to 15 liters/minute. New design features allow for one emergency port in the mask so that the patient can still receive atmospheric air should the oxygen supply fail. This feature prevents the mask from delivering 100% oxygen, but is a necessary safety feature. The mask is excellent for use in shock and for severely hypoxic patients who do not suffer from COPD.

NOTE: Some devices are made so that they can be rebreathing or non-rebreathing masks, depending upon a valve adjustment.

- Venturi Mask—This mask is used when low concentrations (24% to 40%) of oxygen are required. The oxygen is delivered into the mask by a jet that pulls in atmospheric air to mix with the oxygen. The flow is rapid enough to flush out carbon dioxide that tends to accumulate in a face mask.

Various size adaptors can be attached to the device to control the oxygen flow to the patient. Standard sizes include 3, 4, and 6 liter per minute adaptors. If a 4-liter adaptor is in place and you try to deliver 8 liters of oxygen per minute, the jet will draw in more atmospheric air to mix with the oxygen. This "venturi effect" draws in enough air so that only 4 liters of oxygen per minute reaches the patient (see Fig. 6-31).

NOTE: The venturi is the only face mask recommended for COPD patients. Delivery concentrations should begin at 24%.

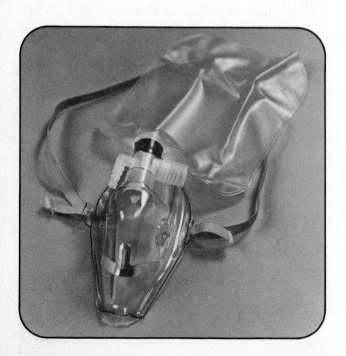

Figure 6-29: A non-rebreathing mask.

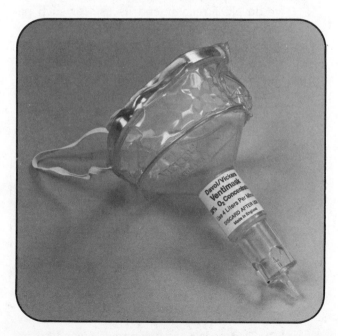

Figure 6-30: A venturi mask.

Table 6.3: Oxygen Delivery Devices

Oxygen Delivery Device	Flow Rate	% Oxygen Delivered	Special Use
Nasal cannula	1-8 LPM	24-52%	Most medical patients and COPD at low concentrations (when absolutely necessary)
Simple face mask	START at 6 LPM... can go as high as 15 LPM, but 12 LPM more practical	35-60%	Preferred on trauma patients
Partial rebreathing mask	6-10 LPM	35-60%	
Non-rebreathing mask	START with 8 LPM, practical high is 12 LPM	80-95%	Good for severe non-COPD, hypoxia, and shock patients. Provides high oxygen concentrations
Venturi mask	4-8 LPM	24-40% (Delivers as indicated on adaptor)	COPD patients and long-term use

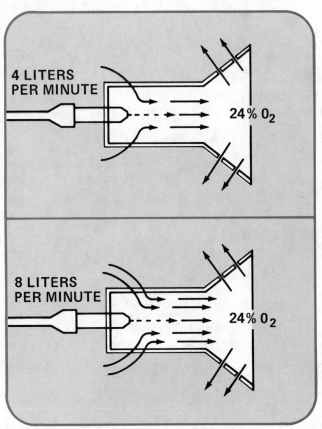

Figure 6-31: The venturi effect.

ADMINISTERING OXYGEN

The next Scansheets will take you step by step through the process of administering oxygen and discontinuing the administration of oxygen.

WARNING: Do NOT attempt to learn on your own how to use oxygen delivery systems. Work with your instructor and follow his directions for the specific equipment you will be using.

ADMINISTERING OXYGEN TO A NONBREATHING PATIENT

Remember that a pocket face mask with an oxygen inlet can be connected to a high flow oxygen source and used in combination with your own ventilations to deliver 40 to 45% oxygen to the patient.

Most EMS Systems currently use the bag-valve-mask resuscitator with 100% oxygen under pressure and the manually controlled demand valve resuscitator with 100% oxygen under pressure can be used in ventilating the nonbreathing patient.

NOTE: Before using either of these two devices, an oropharyngeal airway should be inserted.

WARNING: These devices can be used for two-rescuer CPR, but NOT for one-rescuer CPR. Even with face straps, the face mask will not remain in place and keep a tight seal. The delay between compressions and properly interposed ventilation will be too great for efficient one-rescuer CPR.

The Bag-Valve-Mask Ventilator and Oxygen

This device can be connected to an oxygen supply system by a hose that joins the oxygen inlet of the bag-valve-mask unit to the outlet of the flowmeter. Some devices have an oxygen reservoir attached to the bag to improve efficiency. The bag-valve-mask device used with oxygen will deliver from 50% to nearly 100% oxygen for pulmonary resuscitation and for interposed ventilations during two-rescuer CPR. Maintain a tight mask-to-face seal, squeeze the bag to deliver oxygen, and release the bag to allow for passive expiration. There is no need to remove the mask to allow for expirations. Keeping a proper seal

PREPARING THE O₂ DELIVERY SYSTEM

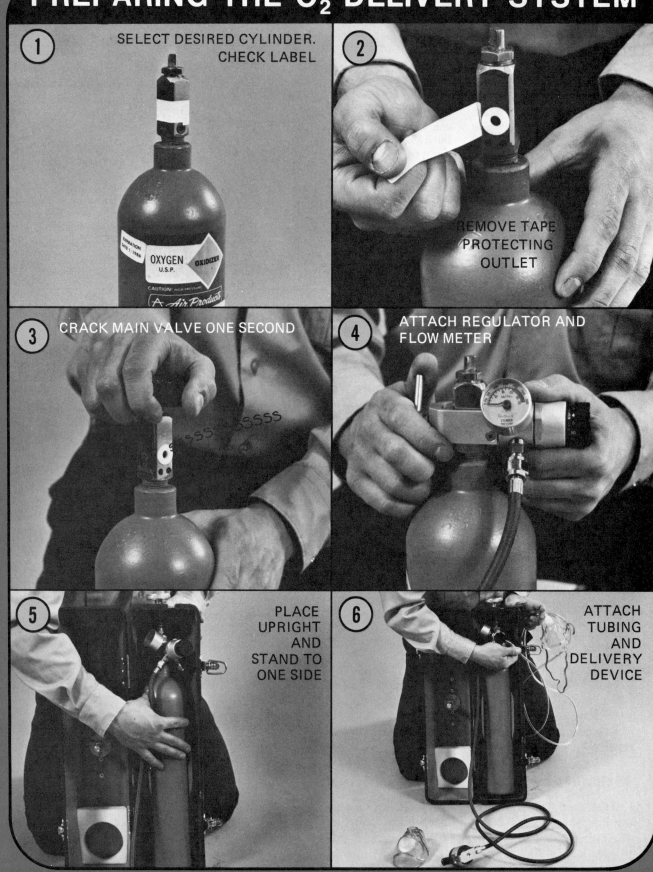

1 SELECT DESIRED CYLINDER. CHECK LABEL

2 REMOVE TAPE PROTECTING OUTLET

3 CRACK MAIN VALVE ONE SECOND

4 ATTACH REGULATOR AND FLOW METER

5 PLACE UPRIGHT AND STAND TO ONE SIDE

6 ATTACH TUBING AND DELIVERY DEVICE

SCAN 6.2

ADMINISTERING OXYGEN

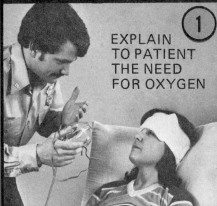

(1) EXPLAIN TO PATIENT THE NEED FOR OXYGEN

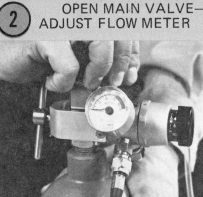

(2) OPEN MAIN VALVE— ADJUST FLOW METER

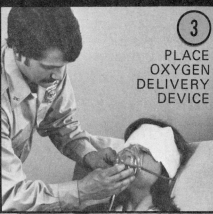

(3) PLACE OXYGEN DELIVERY DEVICE

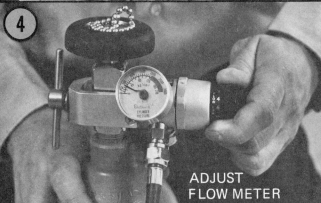

(4) ADJUST FLOW METER

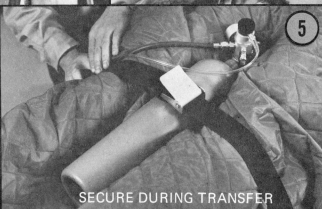

(5) SECURE DURING TRANSFER

DISCONTINUING OXYGEN

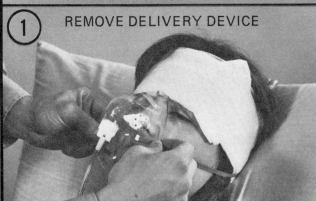

(1) REMOVE DELIVERY DEVICE

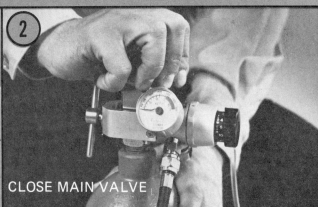

(2) CLOSE MAIN VALVE

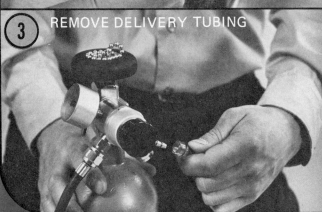

(3) REMOVE DELIVERY TUBING

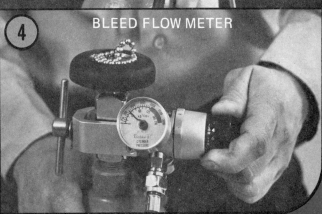

(4) BLEED FLOW METER

SCAN 6.3

requires special skills that you can only acquire through practice.

This device also can be used to assist the breathing efforts of a severely hypoxic patient, or one who has failing respirations (as in drug overdose).

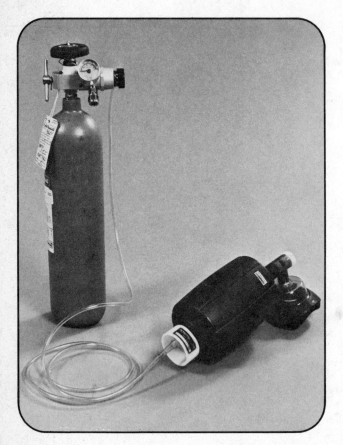

Figure 6-32: A bag-valve-mask ventilator connected to an oxygen supply.

The Positive Pressure Resuscitator

Most positive pressure resuscitators have a control button on top of the valve unit to which the facepiece is attached. When the EMT depresses the control button, oxygen flows into the face mask at a high rate (up to 150 liters per minute in some models). The patient's lungs will inflate until a preset back pressure is reached (about 40 mmHg), or until the control button is released. The EMT MUST keep one hand free to properly seal the mask to the patient's face. Stay alert for gastric distention.

The Demand Valve Resuscitator

Commonly called a "demand valve," the entire device is a demand valve resuscitator. It will deliver nearly 100% oxygen to the patient's lungs if the face mask is properly sealed to the patient's face. When an inspiration occurs, the device will deliver oxygen and then shut off flow as soon as an expiration begins.

Multiple Function Resuscitator

At present, federal regulations require resuscitators to have manual controls. Some resuscitators are made to function in the manually triggered positive pressure mode or the patient demand mode.

NOTE: For CPR, you should use a manually controlled resuscitator. During two-rescuer CPR, a ventilation can be provided on the fifth upstroke. Many systems are now providing this ventilation at the end of every third downstroke. Even though this is not the same as AHA guidelines for two-rescuer CPR, it must be remembered that these guidelines were originally developed for people working without positive pressure oxygen therapy equipment. To be effective in CPR, a demand valve resuscitator MUST deliver a flow rate of not less than 100 liters per minute, on demand.

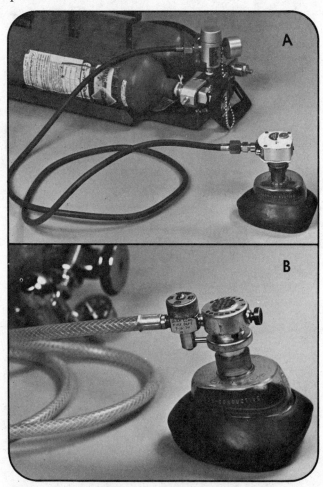

Figure 6-33: A. Manually triggered positive pressure demand valve resuscitator; B. Manually triggered positive pressure resuscitator with regulated oxygen inhalation.

SUMMARY

The EMT should *never* delay resuscitation measures to locate, retrieve, and set up special equipment or oxygen delivery systems.

Adjunct airways can be used to maintain an open airway. There are two major types, oropharyngeal and nasopharyngeal. The S-tube is a modification of the oropharyngeal airway.

Oropharyngeal airways also will help keep the tongue from slipping back into the throat. These airways are only to be used for unconscious patients who have no gag reflex. Before insertion, the adjunct airway must be measured to ensure it is the correct size. The airway is inserted with the tip toward the roof of the mouth and then rotated into position. Once inserted, the flange must be against the patient's lips.

Nasopharyngeal airways must be lubricated with a water-based lubricant. These devices can be used for a conscious patient. Before inserting the device, be sure to explain to the patient what you are going to do.

Fluids can be removed from a patient's mouth and throat using a fixed or portable suction system. Suction is not to begin until the rigid tip or catheter is in place, at the beginning of the throat. Do not suction the nonbreathing patient for more than 15 seconds before providing two ventilations.

There are two common ventilation-assist devices, the bag-valve-mask ventilator and the pocket face mask. When using the bag-valve-mask device, one hand must hold the facepiece firmly in place. Air is delivered by squeezing the bag. For the nonbreathing patient, the rate is once every 5 seconds. The pocket face mask has a chimney on the mask to allow for mouth-to-mask ventilations.

Oxygen administration is essential for patients in respiratory arrest and cardiac arrest. Realize that certain patients will do better if placed on oxygen, including patients suffering from blood loss, major fractures, head injury, shock, lung disease or injury, heart attack, stroke, and heart failure. Atmospheric air contains 21% oxygen. The air provided by mouth-to-mouth techniques only delivers 16% oxygen to the patient. REMEMBER, OXYGEN IS A MEDICATION.

Hypoxia is a low concentration of oxygen at the tissue level. This can be caused by respiratory insufficiency (hypoxic hypoxia) due to the air itself, lung disease, lung injury, or chest injury. Circulatory insufficiency (circulatory hypoxia) can be due to blood loss or problems with the heart and blood vessels. There may not be enough hemoglobin in the red blood cells (hemic hypoxia) to carry the required amount of oxygen. Problems with cellular exchange (cellular hypoxia) may prevent oxygen from entering the cells.

Oxygen can be dangerous because it is stored under pressure, it supports combustion, and it can detonate if mixed with oil. Prolonged used of high concentrations of oxygen can cause lung damage (oxygen toxicity), collapsed alveoli (atelectasis), and damage to a premature infant's eyes (retrolental fibroplasia).

Of major concern to the EMT is the effect of too much oxygen on chronic obstructive pulmonary disease patients (emphysema, chronic bronchitis, black lung). When given oxygen above 28% in concentration, such patients can develop respiratory arrest. Most systems recommend delivery of oxygen at 24% using a venturi face mask.

Three sizes of oxygen cylinders are commonly used: D, E, and M. Oxygen is kept under pressure equal to 2000 to 2200 psi. You can calculate the length of time you can use a cylinder. The formula, residual pressure and constants are given in Table 6-2 on page 118.

A pressure regulator is used to reduce the pressure in an oxygen cylinder to a safe working pressure (30 to 70 psi). E size and smaller cylinders use the pin-index safety system. Larger cylinders use threaded outlets to prevent the wrong regulator or gas being used. Remember to "crack" the cylinder valve before use to clear the delivery port or threaded outlet.

A flowmeter allows the control of oxygen flow in liters per minute. The gravity-dependent, ball float meter is a pressure-compensated flowmeter that measures actual flow. The Bourdon gauge flowmeter is a calibrated gauge that measures flow in liters per minute, but this gauge cannot compensate for back pressure.

Oxygen used for medical purposes is a dry gas. Moisture can be added by using a humidifier.

There are five commonly used oxygen delivery devices for the breathing patient, including:

- Nasal cannula—24% to 54% oxygen delivered.
- Simple face mask—35% to 60% oxygen delivered.
- Partial rebreathing mask—35% to 60% oxygen delivered.
- Non-rebreathing mask—80% to 95% oxygen delivered.
- Venturi mask—24% to 40% oxygen delivered.

If you begin with the minimum flow rate and concentration of oxygen delivered by a device, the oxygen delivered will increase 4% for every additional liter per minute flow.

The nasal cannula and venturi mask can be used for COPD patients if the concentration of oxygen delivered is approximately 24%. We do not recommend the cannula for COPD patients.

The simple face mask requires a flow rate of no less than 6 liters per minute. The minimum flow rate for the non-rebreathing mask is 8 liters per minute.

Oxygen can be administered to the nonbreathing patient by using a pocket face mask with the oxygen inlet connected to a high flow oxygen source. Most systems use a bag-valve-mask ventilator, a positive pressure resuscitator, or a demand valve resuscitator with oxygen under pressure. Before using any of these devices, insert an oropharyngeal airway. The bag-valve-mask or the positive pressure device can be used during two-rescuer CPR. The positive pressure resuscitator should be manually triggered.

7 basic life support iii: bleeding and shock

OBJECTIVES By the end of this chapter, you should be able to:

1. List the FIVE major functions of blood. (pp. 130-1)

2. List the THREE major types of blood vessels and describe the functions of each type of vessel. (p. 131)

3. Classify bleeding as external or internal and relate the types of blood vessels to the THREE kinds of external bleeding. (pp. 131-2)

4. Relate profuse bleeding to the primary survey and basic life support. (p. 132)

5. List the EIGHT methods to control external bleeding. (pp. 132-3)

6. Describe the direct pressure control of profuse and mild bleeding. (pp. 133-4)

7. Describe the application of a pressure dressing. (p. 134)

8. Describe the use of elevation in the control of external bleeding, listing when this procedure should NOT be used. (p. 134)

9. Define arterial pressure point, and list and locate the major pressure point sites used in EMT-level emergency care. (p. 135)

10. Describe, step by step, the use of pressure points to control bleeding from the upper limb, lower limb, and neck. (pp. 135-6)

11. Describe how a blood pressure cuff can be used to control bleeding. (p. 136)

12. Explain why tourniquets are used as a last resort only after other methods of controlling profuse bleeding have failed. (pp. 136-7)

13. Describe, step by step, the procedures for applying a tourniquet, including all precautions for the procedure. (p. 137)

14. List the symptoms and signs of internal bleeding and state FOUR factors that may cause difficulties when trying to detect this type of bleeding. (pp. 138-9)

15. List at least EIGHT conditions associated with internal bleeding. (p. 138)

16. Describe, step by step, the EMT-level procedures for controlling internal bleeding. (pp. 139-40)

17. Define shock and match the causes of shock to the types of shock. (pp. 140-2)

18. List the symptoms and signs of shock. (p. 142)

19. Describe, step by step, the procedures used in the prevention and treatment of shock. (pp. 142-4)

20. Describe anaphylactic shock in terms of what it is, how serious it is, and what causes it. (p. 144)

21. List the symptoms and signs of anaphylactic shock. (p. 145)

22. Compare the care provided in anaphylactic shock with the care provided for other types of shock. (pp. 142-4, 5)

23. Describe how to reduce a patient's chances of fainting. (p. 146)

SKILLS As an EMT, you should be able to:

1. Evaluate the seriousness of bleeding and the approximate blood loss.

2. Control external bleeding by:

    A. Direct pressure
    B. Direct pressure and elevation
    C. Arterial pressure point
    D. Splinting (including air splints)
    E. Blood pressure cuff
    F. Tourniquet

    Note: MAST garments may be part of your course. See Appendix #4.

3. Survey for internal bleeding and apply the measures required to control this type of bleeding.

4. Survey for shock and anaphylactic shock.

5. Apply the measures needed to prevent shock and to care for shock.

6. Apply the measures needed to care for anaphylactic shock.

7. Carry out the procedure used to help prevent fainting.

TERMS   you may be using for the first time:

Plasma (PLAZ-mah)—the fluid portion of the blood. It is the blood minus the formed elements.

Formed Elements—red blood cells, white blood cells, and platelets.

Platelet (PLATE-let)—the formed elements of the blood that release chemical factors needed to form blood clots.

Artery—any major blood vessel carrying blood away from the heart.

Vein—any major blood vessel returning blood to the heart.

Capillary—the thin-walled, microscopic blood vessels where oxygen/carbon dioxide and nutrient/waste exchange with the tissues takes place.

Perfusion—the constant flow of blood through capillaries.

Hemorrhage (HEM-o-rej)—internal or external bleeding.

Embolism (EM-bo-liz-m)—a blood clot or foreign body such as fat or an air bubble inside a blood vessel.

Liter (LE-ter)—metric measurement of liquid volume equal to 1.057 quarts. One pint is almost equal to ½ liter.

Facial Artery—a major artery supplying blood to the face. Some types of external facial bleeding can be controlled by applying pressure to the facial artery pressure point.

Femoral (FEM-o-ral) **Artery**—the major artery supplying the leg. Some types of external bleeding from the leg can be controlled by applying pressure to the femoral pressure point.

Subclavian (sub-CLA-vi-an) **Artery**—The major artery located under the clavicle. Some types of external bleeding of the upper trunk can be controlled by skillful application of pressure to the subclavian artery pressure point.

Temporal Artery—the major artery in the region of the temple. Some types of external scalp bleeding can be controlled by applying pressure to the temporal pressure point.

Shock—usually, but not always, the failure of the cardiovascular system to provide an adequate supply of blood to all parts of the body.

Anaphylactic (an-ah-fi-LAK-tik) **Shock**—allergy shock. The most severe type of allergic reaction in which a person develops shock when he encounters a substance to which he is allergic. This is a true emergency.

Cyanosis (sigh-ah-NO-sis)—when the skin, lips, tongue, ear lobes, nailbeds, and/or the mucous membranes turn blue or gray due to insufficient oxygen in the blood.

Coma—a state of complete unconsciousness, the depth of which may vary.

BLEEDING

The Blood

Blood is a living tissue made up of plasma (PLAZ-mah) and formed elements. Plasma is a watery, salty fluid that makes up over half the volume of the blood. The formed elements are:

• Red Blood Cells—also called RBC's, erythrocytes, and red corpuscles. Their primary function is to carry oxygen to the tissues and carbon dioxide away from the tissues.

• White Blood Cells—also called WBC's, leukocytes, and white corpuscles. They are involved in destroying microorganisms (germs) and producing substances called antibodies that help the body resist infection.

• Platelets (PLATE-lets)—membrane-enclosed fragments of specialized cells. When these fragments rupture, they release chemical factors needed to form blood clots.

The functions of blood are:

• TRANSPORTATION OF GASES—to carry oxygen from the lungs to the tissues and to carry carbon dioxide from the tissues to the lungs.

• NUTRITION—to carry food substances from the intestine or storage tissues (fatty tissue, the liver, and muscle cells) to the rest of the body tissues.

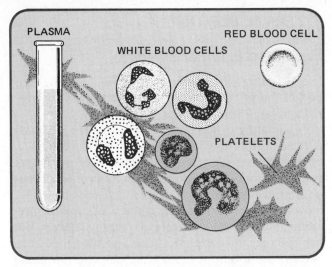

Figure 7-1: The major components of blood.

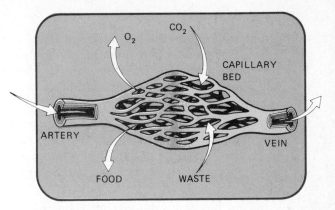

Figure 7-2: The blood vessels.

- EXCRETION—to carry wastes away from the tissues to the organs of excretion (kidneys, large intestine, skin, and lungs).
- PROTECTION—to defend against disease-causing organisms by engulfing and digesting (eating), or by producing antibodies against them (immunity).
- REGULATION—to carry hormones, water, salt, and other chemicals that control the functions of organs and glands. The regulation of body temperature is aided by the blood carrying excessive body heat to the lungs and skin surfaces.

'The volume of blood differs from person to person, depending on body size. The typical adult male has about 6 liters of blood, or slightly over 12 pints. The loss of blood volume is very significant, not only in terms of the loss of formed elements, but also in loss of plasma. Keep in mind that a minimum volume of blood is needed in circulation to keep the cardiovascular system working efficiently enough to maintain life.

Blood volume varies with size and age. An infant may have only 300 milliliters (ml) of blood (1 ml equals about 20 drops from a medicine dropper). Depending on size, children have from 1.5 to 2 liters of blood. Adolescents usually have from 4.5 to 5.5 liters of blood.

In the field, you will have to estimate the percentage of blood loss for patients. Since you will not have time to calculate a patient's approximate blood volume, you should begin to practice estimating people's weight and approximating their blood volume. Start with your family, friends, and fellow students. Once you find that you can estimate body weight, look at someone and guess his weight, then:

1. Divide the estimated weight by 2.2 to convert pounds to kilograms.

2. Multiply the kilogram weight by 6.5% (.065).

This will give you the approximate total blood volume for the individual. Through practice, you will be able to associate total blood volume with the size and weight of different people. Being able to do this will be of great value in estimating total blood loss.

Blood Vessels

The major types of blood vessels are:

- Arteries—carry blood away from the heart.
- Capillaries—where oxygen/carbon dioxide and nutrient/waste exchange takes place.
- Veins—carry blood back to the heart.

The heart beats, circulating blood. Except for a few special cases in the body, blood moves through arteries, to capillaries, to veins, and back to the heart. Most of the heart's beating action is noticed in the arteries. Blood travels at its greatest speed and under the greatest pressure in these vessels. Arterial blood is sent ultimately through the thin-walled, microscopic capillaries. While moving through capillaries, blood does not pulsate as in the arteries. The flow is constant, taking place when the heart is contracting and when it is relaxing. This constant flow is called **perfusion** and is essential for the life of all tissues.

NOTE: A reduction of blood volume greatly affects perfusion. The failure of this constant flow of blood can lead to tissue death. The brain and nerve cells are very sensitive to the failure of perfusion.

Classifying Bleeding

The term **hemorrhage** (HEM-o-rej) means bleeding. Bleeding can be classified as external or internal. In addition, bleeding can be classified as to the type of vessel losing the blood. At the EMT-level of care, this is done only for external bleeding.

External bleeding is classified as:

- Arterial Bleeding—the loss of blood from an artery. The blood loss is often rapid and profuse, as blood spurts from the wound. Usually, the blood spurts as the heart beats, and is bright red.
- Venous Bleeding—the loss of blood from a vein. The blood loss is a steady flow that can be profuse. The color of the blood is dark red, often appearing to be dark maroon or even blue.
- Capillary Bleeding—the loss of blood from a capillary bed. The flow is slow, often described as "oozing." The color of the blood is red, usually less bright than arterial blood.

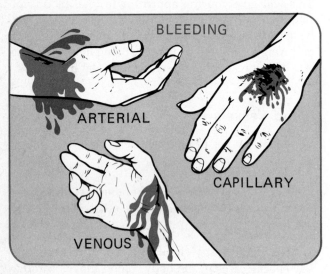

Figure 7-3: The three types of external bleeding.

Arterial bleeding is less likely to clot than other types of bleeding. When completely severed, arteries often constrict and seal themselves off. However, if an artery is not completely severed but is torn, or has a hole in its wall, it will probably continue to bleed.

Veins are usually located closer to the body surface than are arteries. Bleeding from surface veins is easier to control than arterial bleeding, even when the flow is profuse (a steady noticeable flow). Most veins will collapse when they are cut; however, bleeding from deep veins can be as profuse and as hard to control as arterial bleeding.

Open veins can suck in debris and air bubbles. This is sometimes the case with the major neck veins. When air is sucked in and forms an air bubble, known as an **air embolism** (EM-bo-liz-m), the bubble can be carried to the heart and interfere with or stop the heart's pumping action completely.

Bleeding from capillaries is slow, with clotting typically taking place in 6 to 8 minutes. This type of bleeding often involves a large area of injured skin, thus wound contamination and the chance of infection are problems.

EXTERNAL BLEEDING

Evaluating External Bleeding

Detecting and stopping profuse bleeding are part of the primary survey. Priority is given to arterial and large vein bleeding.

Estimating external blood loss requires some experience before the EMT can do so with confidence. Such estimates are important in terms of predicting possible shock, sorting patients for triage, and considering the seriousness of prolonged slow bleeding. Slow bleeding that normally could wait until the secondary survey may be a primary survey concern if it has been steady for a long time and blood loss has become significant. A rapid pulse rate and low blood pressure detected while taking vital signs are valuable indicators of possible significant blood loss.

To help form a concept of blood loss, pour a pint of water on the floor next to a fellow student or a manikin. Try soaking an article of clothing with a pint of water and note how much of the article is wet and how wet it feels to your touch.

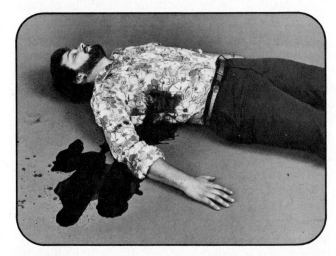

Figure 7-4: Estimating external blood loss; one-half liter (approx. 1 pint).

The amount of blood that can be lost before serious problems occur will vary from individual to individual. However, certain guidelines can be used. A loss of one liter of blood by an adult must be considered to be life-threatening. Depending on size, a loss of 1/4 to 1/2 liter of blood by a child will be life-threatening. For an infant, 25 ml of blood loss MUST be viewed as life-threatening.

Controlling External Bleeding

The eight methods used to control external bleeding are:

1. Direct pressure
2. Elevation

3. Pressure points
4. Splinting
5. Inflatable splints (air splints)
6. Blood pressure cuff
7. MAST garments (pneumatic counterpressure devices)
8. Applying a tourniquet.

Direct Pressure The most effective method of controlling external bleeding is by pressure applied directly to the wound. Direct pressure can be applied by your hand, a dressing and your hand, your fingers placed in a wound, or by a pressure dressing.

When bleeding is MILD, you should:

1. Apply pressure to the wound, preferably with a sterile dressing held against its surface. (A clean handkerchief or cloth can be used if a sterile dressing is not immediately available.)
2. Pressure held firmly on the wound for 10 to 30 minutes will usually stop the bleeding. Your role is to control the bleeding so that blood loss is not significant.
3. Once bleeding is controlled, hold the dressing in place with bandaging.
4. NEVER remove a dressing once it is in place. To do so may restart bleeding or cause additional injury to the site. Apply another dressing on top of the blood-soaked one and hold them both in place. Continue this procedure until bleeding is controlled, or until you deliver the patient to the staff of a medical facility.

If bleeding is PROFUSE, you should:

1. NOT waste time trying to find a dressing.
2. Place your hand directly on the wound and exert firm pressure.
3. Keep applying steady, firm pressure until the bleeding is controlled.
4. Once bleeding is controlled, a dressing can be bandaged into place to form a pressure dressing.

If bleeding remains uncontrolled, you should:

1. Insert your fingers directly into the wound and attempt to compress the vessel between your fingers.
2. If you cannot grasp the vessel, attempt to compress it between your fingers and a bony part of the patient's body.

NOTE: Results should be immediate. Do NOT waste valuable time trying to grasp a blood vessel.

A pressure dressing can be applied to establish enough direct pressure to control most bleeding.

DIRECT PRESSURE

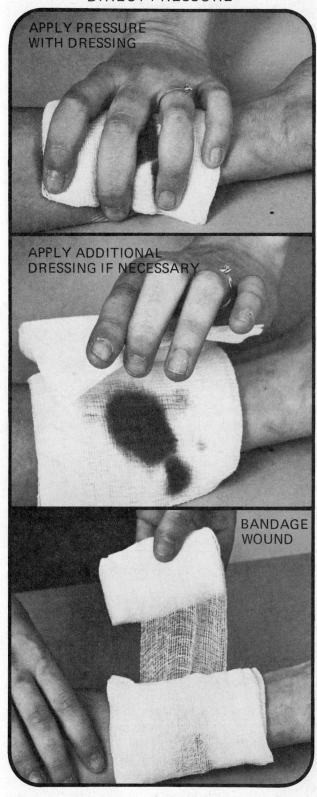

APPLY PRESSURE WITH DRESSING

APPLY ADDITIONAL DRESSING IF NECESSARY

BANDAGE WOUND

Figure 7-5: Direct pressure is applied until bleeding is controlled.

Several sterile gauze pad dressings are placed on the wound. A bulky dressing is placed over the gauze pads. An efficient bulky dressing for a severely bleeding wound is the combined or multitrauma dressing. Sanitary napkins also can be used. The

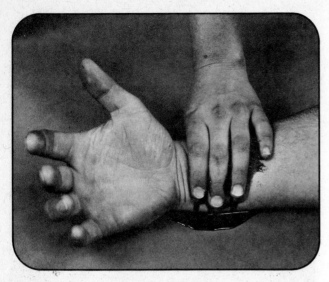

Figure 7-6: In cases of profuse bleeding, do NOT waste time hunting for a dressing.

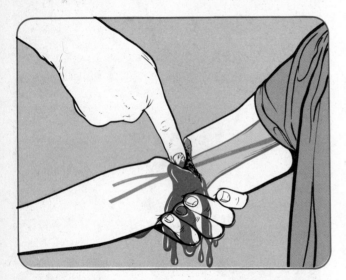

Figure 7-7: Insert your fingers directly into the wound.

dressings should be held in place with self-adherent roller bandage wrapped tightly over the dressing and above and below the wound site. Enough pressure must be created to control the bleeding.

The dressings should not be removed once they are applied. In cases where bleeding continues, more pressure can be added using the palm of your hand, or a tighter bandage can be applied. In rare cases, you may have to create more bulk by adding additional dressings.

A variety of dressings can be used in emergency situations. Some of these are shown in Figure 7-8.

Be aware that, in certain areas of the body, you may be unable to apply an effective pressure dressing, as when bleeding is from the armpit. You may have to maintain pressure by hand directly over the wound. Even though you may be contaminating the wound, the risk of uncontrolled bleeding far outweighs that of possible infection.

REMEMBER: Direct pressure is usually the quickest

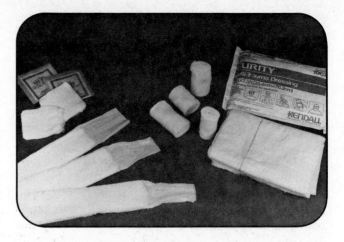

Figure 7-8: Dressings for use in emergencies.

and most efficient means of controlling external bleeding.

Elevation   When an injured extremity is elevated, gravity helps to reduce blood pressure, and thus slows bleeding. This method should NOT be used if there are possible fractures to the extremity, objects impaled in the extremity, or possible spinal injury. To use elevation, you should:

1. Elevate the injured extremity. If the forearm is bleeding, simply elevate the forearm. You do not have to elevate the entire arm.

2. Apply direct pressure to the site of bleeding.

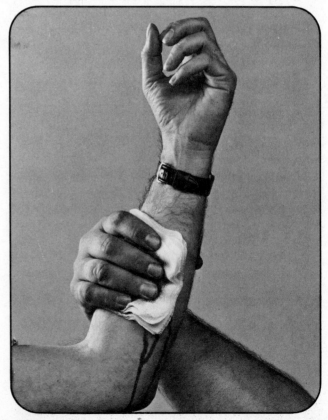

Figure 7-9: Combine elevation and direct pressure.

Pressure Points If direct pressure or direct pressure and elevation fail, your next approach may be the use of pressure points. A **pressure point** is a site where a main artery lies near the surface of the body, directly over a bone. There are 22 major pressure points (11 on each side of the body). Of these, 12 sites (6 on each side) are used to control profuse bleeding. These sites are:

- Brachial (BRAY-ke-al) Artery—for bleeding from the upper limb.
- Femoral (FEM-o-ral) Artery—for bleeding from the lower limb.
- Carotid Artery—for bleeding from the neck.
- Temporal Artery—for bleeding from the scalp.
- Facial Artery—for bleeding from the face.
- Subclavian (sub-CLA-vi-an) Artery—for bleeding from the chest wall or armpit.

The use of pressure points requires skill on the part of the rescuer. Unless you know the exact location of the point and how much pressure to apply, the pressure point technique is of no use. The subclavian pressure point is very difficult to use. In fact, some physicians believe it is only of use during surgery.

The temporal site is seldom used because direct pressure works so well. However, direct pressure can cause problems if there are injuries to the bones of the skull. For such cases, the temporal pressure point site can be used. If there is damage to the bone under the temporal artery site, do NOT apply pressure to this site.

Direct pressure is used more commonly than pressure points when caring for facial bleeding. If the facial artery pressure point is to be used, take care to do so *only* when there is no damage to the bones of the upper jaw.

REMEMBER: Pressure point techniques are to be used only after direct pressure or direct pressure and elevation have failed to control the bleeding.

Bleeding from the Upper Extremity. Apply pressure to a point over the brachial artery. To find the artery, hold the patient's arm out at a right angle to his body, with the palm facing up. (This angle will provide the best results, but may be reduced if a 90-degree extension is not possible.) Find the groove between the biceps muscle and the arm bone (humerus), about midway between the elbow and the armpit. Cradle the upper arm in the palm of your hand and position your fingers in this medial groove. You can now compress the brachial artery against the underlying bone by pressing your finger into this groove. If pressure is properly applied, you will not be able to feel a radial pulse. If the wound is to the distal end of the limb, bleeding may not be controlled by this method.

Bleeding from the Lower Extremity. Apply pressure to a point over the femoral artery. Locate this artery on the medial side of the leg where it joins the lower trunk. You should be able to feel

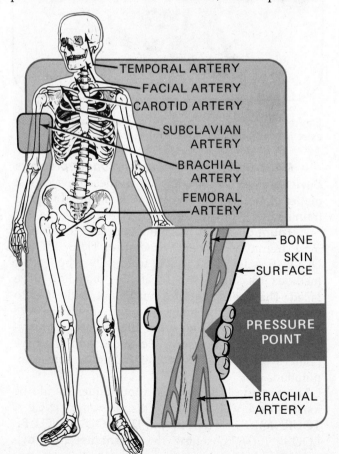

Figure 7-10: The six major pairs of arterial pressure points.

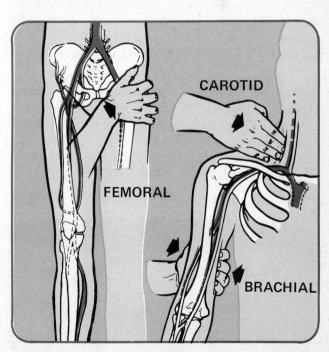

Figure 7-11: The use of pressure points to control profuse bleeding from the upper extremity, lower extremity, and neck.

pulsations at a point just below the groin. Place the heel of your hand over the site and exert pressure downward toward the bone until it is obvious that the bleeding has been controlled. You will need more pressure than that applied for the brachial artery pressure point. Considerable force must be exerted if the patient is very muscular or obese. If pressure is properly applied, the pedal pulse cannot be felt. This method may not control bleeding for distal wounds.

Bleeding from the Neck. Locate the trachea at the midline of the neck. Slide your fingers to the site of bleeding in the neck and feel for the pulsations of the carotid artery. Place your fingers over the artery, with your thumb behind the patient's neck. Apply pressure by squeezing your fingers toward your thumb. This action will compress the carotid artery as it is displaced against the spinal column.

WARNING: There are few occasions for using the carotid pressure point. Do NOT use this method unless it is a part of your training. If profuse bleeding from the neck is not controlled by direct pressure, you may have to use this technique. NEVER apply pressure to both sides of the neck at the same time. Take great care not to apply heavy pressure to the trachea. Stay alert for the patient may become faint or unconscious. Assume that the cervical spine has been injured and take all necessary steps to avoid excessive movement of the patient's head, neck, and back while you control profuse bleeding.

Splinting   The splinting of fractures will be covered in Chapters 9 and 10. Often, when a fracture is splinted, bleeding associated with the fracture is controlled. This occurs when the sharp ends of broken bones are stabilized, preventing additional damage to blood vessels at the injury site.

Inflatable Splints (Air Splints)   These devices may control bleeding from an extremity, even when there is no fracture. They are useful when a severe laceration or cut extends over the length of the extremity. The pressure produced by the splint is actually a form of direct pressure. The application of these splints will be covered in Chapter 9.

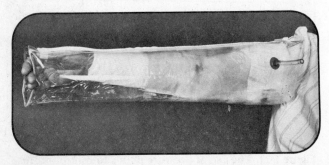

Figure 7-12: Air splints can be used to control bleeding from an extremity.

Blood Pressure Cuff   This device can be applied to control apparently life-threatening bleeding from an extremity. The cuff is placed above the wound (between the wound and the heart) and inflated to the pressure required to control the bleeding. This is usually in the 150-mmHg range. A dressing and bandage are secured after the bleeding is controlled. The cuff can safely be left inflated for 30 minutes; however, it must be monitored closely to make certain that pressure is not lost. Use of the blood pressure cuff may prove to be the only way to control bleeding for patients who are trapped in wreckage.

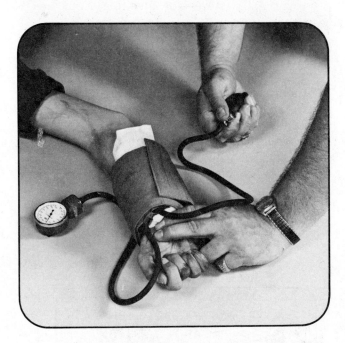

Figure 7-13: A blood pressure cuff may be applied to an extremity and inflated to control bleeding.

MAST Garments (Pneumatic Counterpressure Devices)   At present, the use of these devices is a matter of local policy. If their use is included in your training, see Appendix 4.

Tourniquet   A tourniquet applied to a bleeding extremity is an *extreme* measure. THIS PROCEDURE IS A LAST RESORT, used only when other methods to control life-threatening bleeding have failed. The application of a tourniquet could lead to eventual loss of the limb. An amputated extremity may leave you with no other choice than a tourniquet, but direct pressure, elevation, and pressure points work for most bleeding, including some amputations.

There is an old belief that a tourniquet should be loosened every 20 minutes. This is wrong. ONCE A TOURNIQUET IS IN PLACE, IT SHOULD NOT BE LOOSENED. Loosening the tourniquet may dislodge clots and precipitate enough additional bleeding to cause severe shock, which can then lead to death. A slowly developing form of **tourniquet** shock can occur due to harmful substances released by severely injured tissues. These substances are held back by the tourniquet, but are released in high concentration each time the tourniquet is loosened. The sudden release of blood can cause a such a pronounced variation in circulation that a rapidly developing form of tourniquet shock may develop. If you keep a tourniquet in place, the patient has a better chance for survival, even if it means the loss of a limb.

REMEMBER: A tourniquet is a last resort measure to be used for profuse bleeding of an extremity. Once a tourniquet has been applied, it should not be loosened.

NOTE: Many physicians recommend that the blood pressure cuff be used when direct pressure with bulky dressings does not control bleeding resulting from amputation.

If a commercially made tourniquet is not available, a makeshift one may be prepared from a cravat bandage, a stocking, a wide belt, or some other flat material. The ideal width for a tourniquet is 1½ to 2 inches. Among the items that should NOT be used are ropes, pieces of wire, or other small-diameter materials that could cut into the patient's skin and soft tissues.

To apply a tourniquet, you should:

1. Select a place between the heart and the wound, as close as possible to, but not flush with, the edge of the wound.

2. Place a pad made from a dressing or a folded handkerchief over the main supplying artery before applying the constricting band. This will help protect the site and will apply additional pressure over the artery.

3. If a commercial tourniquet is used, carefully place it around the limb at the site and pull the free end of the band through the buckle or friction catch and draw this end tightly over the pad. You should tighten the tourniquet to the point where bleeding is controlled. Do NOT tighten the tourniquet beyond this point.

   If you are using a cravat or other piece of material, carefully slip the material around the injured limb and tie a knot with the ends of the tourniquet. The knot should be over the pad. A stick, rod, or similar device should be inserted into the knot and used to tighten the tourniquet. Turn the device until bleeding is controlled. Do NOT tighten beyond this point. Tape or tie the tightening device in place.

4. KEEP THE TOURNIQUET IN PLACE. DO NOT LOOSEN.

5. Attach a notation to the patient to indicate that a tourniquet has been applied and the time of application. If a tag is not available, mark the pa-

tient's forehead in ink, or even blood if necessary. Write "TK" and the time of application. This notation MUST be written so that the tourniquet does not go unnoticed by the emergency department staff. Make certain that you do not cover the extremity to which the tourniquet has been applied.

NOTE: It is the EMT's responsibility to advise the emergency department staff of the application of a tourniquet.

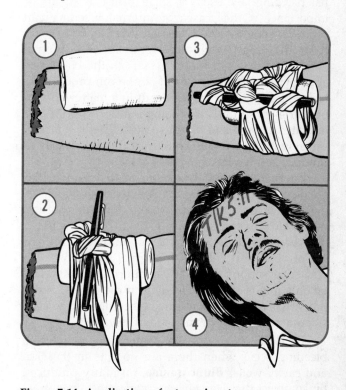

Figure 7-14: Application of a tourniquet.

There will be instances where you arrive at the scene and find that bystanders have applied a tourniquet. Most EMS Systems have standard operating procedures that MUST be followed in such cases. Usually, if the patient is responsive, he will be able to tell you if he thought the bleeding was serious. Since the bystanders applied the tourniquet, they may or may not be a good source of information. Obviously, they thought the bleeding was serious, but they may have applied the tourniquet thinking this is a proper procedure for all bleeding. If the EMT can judge that a tourniquet was not necessary, the tourniquet can be released slowly while applying direct pressure to the wound site. Remember, do this only if it is allowed in *your* EMS System. Check with your instructor.

Cryotherapy This is the treatment of an injury with cold, a basic technique used for centuries. Cold therapy is used for dislocations, sprains, burns, and minor bleeding. The application of cold will reduce pain, minimize swelling, and reduce bleeding by constricting blood vessels. Cryotherapy is not useful by itself, but it can be used in combination with other bleeding control techniques. Chemical cold packs and splints inflated with cryogenic liquids make cold therapy available in field situations.

INTERNAL BLEEDING

Significance of Internal Bleeding

A small *contusion* (bruise) is an example of internal bleeding. By itself, a small bruise is of minor importance. Other cases of internal bleeding can produce enough blood loss to bring about shock, heart and lung failure, and eventual death. Internal injury, rupturing of blood vessels in the chest and abdomen, and some types of stroke can produce internal bleeding that causes death in a matter of minutes or even seconds. Crushing injuries, ruptured or lacerated organs and blood vessels, bleeding ulcers, severely bruised tissues, and fractured bones can all produce serious internal blood loss.

Internal bleeding can occur with wounds that are deep enough to sever major arteries and veins. A deep chest or abdominal wound can cut through many blood vessels, causing blood to flow freely into the body cavity. Any cut into muscle or fracturing of bone also will cause internal blood loss. Often, such serious internal bleeding is accompanied by only minor external bleeding. If the patient is not properly assessed, the internal bleeding may be considered only minor or missed entirely.

Be alert to the fact that many cases of internal bleeding occur when there are no cuts in the skin and cavity walls. **Blunt trauma,** an injury produced by an object that was not sharp enough to penetrate the skin, often causes major internal bleeding. The force is carried into the body, rupturing vessels and organs. Patients who are thrown against dashboards, steering wheels, armrests, and other objects

in motor vehicle accidents can suffer from internal injuries that produce serious internal bleeding. Knowing the mechanism of injuries is important in detecting internal bleeding.

There may be life-theatening internal bleeding when there are no obvious signs of external injury. In blunt trauma situations, a minor bruise may be the *only* indication that an abdominal organ has ruptured. Also, a blow delivered to one side of the body may cause internal bleeding on the opposite side. For example, a blow to the right side of the abdomen may rupture the spleen (on the left side of the body) and release a liter (about a quart) of blood.

REMEMBER: The secondary survey is of major importance in detecting internal bleeding.

Detecting Internal Bleeding

Assume internal bleeding whenever you detect:

- Wounds that have penetrated the skull
- Blood in the ears or nose
- A patient vomiting or coughing up blood
- Wounds that have penetrated the chest or abdomen
- Large areas of bruised abdomen
- Abdominal tenderness, rigidity, or spasms (the patient may guard the abdomen)
- Blood in the urine
- Rectal or vaginal bleeding
- Bone fractures, especially the long bones of the arm and thigh

NOTE: These items follow the physical examination of the secondary survey.

As an EMT, you should learn to associate internal bleeding with the symptoms and signs of shock, which will be considered later in this chapter. For now, consider the patient assessment procedures. Related to internal bleeding, you will find certain symptoms of shock, including:

- Weakness
- Thirst
- Anxiety or restlessness

The signs of shock are closely associated with internal bleeding, including:

- RESTLESSNESS
- BODY—shaking and trembling
- BREATHING—shallow and rapid
- PULSE—rapid and weak
- BLOOD PRESSURE—drops, usually to 90/60 or lower
- SKIN—pale, cool, and clammy
- EYES—dilated pupils

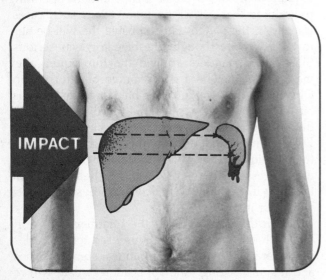

Figure 7-15: Blunt trauma injury can produce serious internal bleeding.

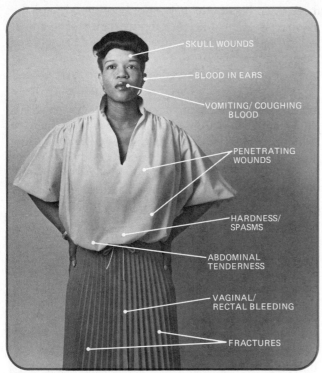

Figure 7-16: Symptoms and signs of internal bleeding.

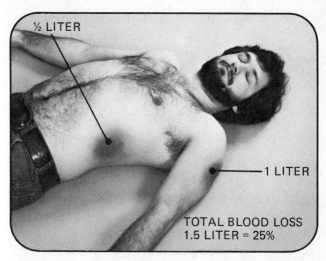

Figure 7-17: Estimating internal blood loss.

REMEMBER: You may detect internal bleeding by looking for mechanisms of injury, wounds and injuries that often produce internal bleeding, and the symptoms and signs of shock.

Evaluating Internal Blood Loss

Special tests and procedures are done at the hospital to determine the approximate amount of internal blood loss. At the scene, it is difficult for the EMT to know how serious internal bleeding may be. Consider internal bleeding to be severe if the patient is vomiting or coughing up blood that looks like coffee grounds. Rigidity or spasms of the abdomen also may indicate possible severe internal bleeding. If there is penetration of the chest cavity (over or superior to the heart), or if the region of the liver or spleen has been penetrated, consider internal bleeding to be an immediate threat to life. Blood loss of at least one liter (about a quart) must be considered anytime there is a fracture to the humerus (arm bone), femur (thigh bone), or pelvis.

Since it is very difficult to estimate internal blood loss, assume a 10% blood loss for every deep bruise found on the chest or abdomen that is the size of a man's fist. Even though this may not be true for a particular patient, it is better to overestimate the significance of possible internal bleeding.

Estimating internal blood loss will help you determine the possibilities of your patient developing severe shock, heart and lung failure, or cardiac arrest. Remember, when there is more than one patient, the order of care and transport may be affected by internal blood loss.

Controlling Internal Bleeding

Control of internal bleeding depends on the location of the injury and the cause of the bleeding. Internal bleeding related to a blunt injury to an extremity may be controlled by a pressure dressing and bandage. This pressure will tend to close off the ends of bleeding vessels. Extreme care must be taken, however, since the accident may have produced a fracture. Careless application of a pressure bandage to a closed fracture site may injure soft tissues or aggravate the fracture.

The application of a splint to an injured extremity often will help control internal bleeding related to fractures. Inflatable splints are useful for such cases.

Injury-related or illness-induced bleeding into the thoracic or the abdominopelvic cavity is not controllable at the accident scene using basic EMT-level skills. The use of pneumatic counterpressure devices other than air splints is considered by most EMS Systems to be an *intermediate* life support measure. This includes the use of medical anti-shock trousers (MAST garments). A MAST garment should only be applied by specially trained personnel who fully understand when and when not to use it. Appendix 4 includes a section on medical anti-shock trousers.

You must continue to assure an open airway and monitor vital signs. Patients with possible neck or spinal injuries must be given special care to avoid aggravation of these injuries. Profuse external bleeding must be cared for immediately.

When providing care for a patient with possible internal bleeding, you should:

1. Maintain an open airway.
2. Reassure the patient and provide emotional support throughout all aspects of care.
3. Keep the patient lying down and at rest.
4. Control all serious bleeding. If the bleeding is in an extremity, use a snug bandage over a bulky

pad applied directly over the injury site, and take care not to aggravate fractures. Remember, applying a splint serves both to immobilize an injured limb and to control bleeding.

5. Position and treat for shock, as described on page 143. You may have to immobilize fractures first before positioning for shock care.

6. Administer high concentrations of oxygen.

7. Loosen restrictive clothing at the neck and waist.

8. Provide appropriate care for fractures.

9. Give nothing to the patient by mouth. *Anticipate vomiting.*

10. Monitor vital signs every five minutes.

11. Transport as soon as possible to a medical facility. Avoid rough and excessive handling. Remember, patients with bleeding into the chest and abdominal cavities are HIGH-PRIORITY PATIENTS.

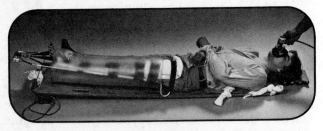

Figure 7-18: The control of bleeding and care for the patient with possible internal bleeding.

SHOCK

Defining Shock

The term shock has many meanings. In medicine, there are specific types of shock. In most cases, **shock** is the failure of the cardiovascular system to provide sufficient blood circulation to all parts of the body.

Shock can occur very rapidly, placing the patient in a critical condition long before you arrive at the scene. In other cases, the patient may develop shock slowly as you provide care. There is a saying used by EMS personnel: ''Patients can go into shock a little at a time.'' For such patients, you will have warning signs, but never assume a stable patient will not go into shock. Monitor your patients.

Figure 7-19 shows what occurs in the cardiovascular system when there is significant blood loss, or something alters the actions of the heart or blood vessels. The chambers of the heart and the blood vessels make up what is known as the **vascular container**. To function properly, this container must be filled with blood. Normally, there is enough blood to fill the vessels. The heart keeps pumping, circulating the blood to keep the vessels full. For the system to work, the heart must keep pumping adequately,

there must be an adequate supply of blood, and the blood vessels must keep changing diameter to adjust to different circulation patterns. If any of these three factors fail, perfusion in the brain, lungs, and other body organs will not be adequate.

Blood vessels can change their diameter. If an area of the body requires more blood because it is doing more work, the vessels in that area dilate to allow greater blood flow. At the same time, another area of the body may constrict its vessels to reduce blood flow to help keep the system filled with blood. If all the vessels in the body dilated at once, there would not be nearly enough blood to fill the entire system. If you are running, blood flow to the muscles increases through dilated arteries. At the same time, blood flow to the stomach and intestines lessens through constricted vessels.

At the onset of shock, the body tries to adjust to the loss of blood, improper heart activity, or the dilation of too many blood vessels. At a certain point in some types of shock, enough blood has been lost so that the system is no longer filled, no matter how hard the heart pumps or what diameter the vessels are. In other cases of shock, the heart becomes too inefficient in circulating blood and fails to keep the cardiovascular system full. There are also cases where there is no loss of blood volume and the heart is performing properly, but too many vessels are dilated. For these cases, there is too much volume (capacity) in the system to be filled by the available blood. Regardless of the mechanism, shock is the failure of the cardiovascular system to provide sufficient blood to every part of the body.

REMEMBER: Shock may develop if the heart fails as a pump, blood volume is lost, or blood vessels dilate to create a vascular container capacity too great to be filled by the blood available.

Types of Shock

Shock may accompany many emergency situations, thus treatment for it is included in emergency care procedures for virtually every serious injury and medical problem.

There is more than one type of shock. A patient may develop:

- Hemorrhagic (HEM-o-RIJ-ic) Shock— (bleeding shock) caused by blood loss or loss of plasma as seen in burns and crushing injuries. This type of shock is also called hypovolemic shock.

- Cardiogenic (KAR-di-o-jen-ic) Shock—(heart shock) caused by the heart failing to pump blood adequately to all parts of the body.

- Neurogenic (NU-ro-jen-ic) Shock—(nerve shock) caused by failure of the nervous system to control the diameter of blood vessels (seen with spinal injury). Once the blood ves-

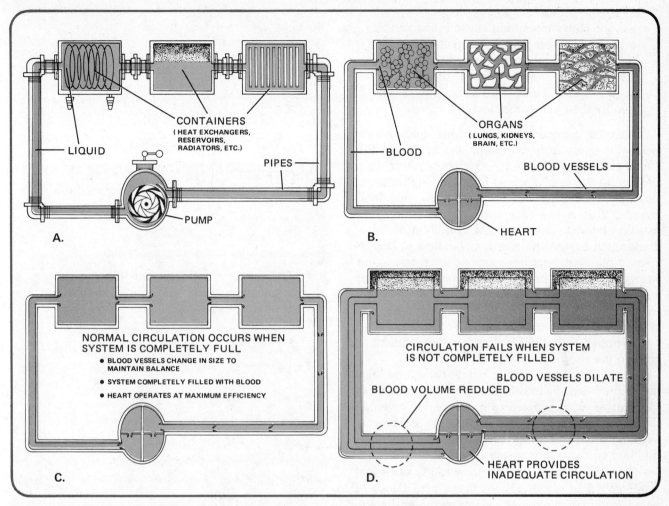

Figure 7-19: Shock is the failure of the cardiovascular system to provide sufficient blood to all parts of the body.

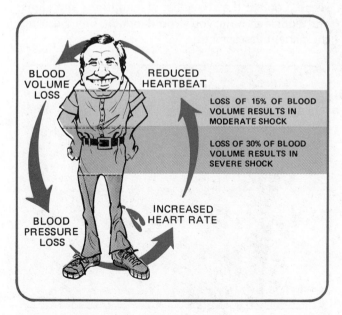

Figure 7-20: Blood loss and shock.

sels are dilated, there is not enough blood in circulation to fill this new volume, causing inadequate circulation of the blood.

• Anaphylactic (AN-ah-fi-LAK-tik) Shock— (allergy shock) a life-threatening reaction of the body to an allergen, something to which the patient is extremely allergic.

• Respiratory Shock—(lung shock) caused by too little oxygen in the blood, usually due to some sort of lung failure.

• Psychogenic (SI-ko-jen-ic) Shock—(fainting) often brought about by fear, bad news, the sight of blood, or a minor injury. This is a nervous system reaction, but it is not neurogenic shock. A sudden dilation of the blood vessels takes place and the proper blood flow to the brain is momentarily interrupted, causing the patient to faint. This is a temporary condition and is considered a self-correcting form of shock.

• Metabolic Shock—(body fluid shock) associated with diarrhea, vomiting, and polyuria (excessive urination). Such conditions cause loss of body fluids and changes in body chemistry, including salt balance and acid-base balance. This can be a form of hypovolemic shock as fluids are lost from the bloodstream.

• Septic Shock—(bloodstream shock) caused by

severe infection. Toxins (poisons) are released into the bloodstream and cause blood vessels to dilate, increasing the volume of the system beyond functional limits. In addition, plasma is lost through vessel walls causing a loss in blood volume. This type of shock is seldom seen by the EMT in the field.

The most common form of serious shock associated with injury is hemorrhagic shock, due to the loss of blood. Bleeding can be external or internal. In addition to the loss of whole blood, enough plasma also may be lost to cause a severe drop in blood volume. This is the case with serious burns and crushing injuries. A pre-existing condition of dehydration will hasten the reaction. Be alert to this in areas of high temperatures, such as warehouses and factories. This also can be a problem if the patient was sweating profusely prior to injury, as in sports and hunting accidents. Certain work situations such as those of dockworkers and steelworkers, may cause enough body fluid loss prior to the accident to quicken the effects of blood loss.

Cardiogenic shock can be brought about by injuries to the heart, heart attacks, and electrical shock. Many diseases, if allowed to go untreated, eventually may do enough heart damage to cause cardiogenic shock. Be on the alert for low blood pressure and edema of the ankles.

Neurogenic shock is sometimes called **vasovagal** (VAS-o-VA-gal) **shock.** There is no actual loss of blood, but dilation of blood vessels increases the volume of the system beyond the point where it can be filled. Blood no longer adequately fills the entire system, but pools in the blood vessels in certain areas of the body. Typically, this takes place in the muscles due to nerve paralysis caused by spinal cord or brain injuries. Severe blows to the abdomen also can disrupt nerves, bringing about neurogenic shock. This type of shock also is seen when circulation patterns change in cases of hypoglycemia (low blood sugar), overexertion, improper diet, or uncontrolled diabetes.

Respiratory shock is a failure of the lungs to provide enough oxygen for circulation to the tissues. Be alert for respiratory shock whenever you note long-term partial or full airway obstruction, penetrating chest wounds, fractured ribs or sternum, or any indications of neck or spinal cord injury. Since respiratory shock is not a collapse of the cardiovascular system, it is sometimes not listed in classifications of shock

Symptoms and Signs of Shock

The symptoms of shock can include:

- Weakness (the most significant symptom)
- Nausea
- Thirst
- Dizziness
- Coolness
- A feeling of impending doom. The patient may show fear and restlessness. Your observations of such can be included as signs of shock.

The signs of shock can include:

- ENTIRE BODY—look for evidence of:
  1. Restlessness
  2. Profuse external bleeding
  3. Vomiting
  4. Shaking and trembling (rare).
- STATE OF AWARENESS—the patient may become unresponsive, faint, or lose consciousness suddenly.
- PULSE—rapid and weak
- BREATHING—shallow and rapid
- BLOOD PRESSURE—marked drop (to 90/60 or lower)
- SKIN—pale, moist, and cool. Often profuse sweating and a clammy feel to the touch.
- EYES—lackluster, dilated pupils
- EYELIDS—pale inner surfaces
- FACE—pale, often with cyanosis at the lips and ear lobes

Imagine that you have just arrived at an accident scene. Look at the above list of symptoms and signs and consider how you would obtain them during the patient assessment.

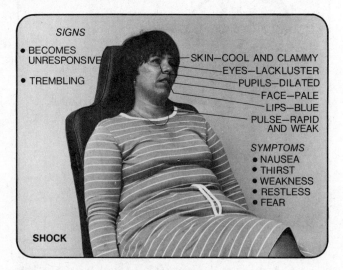

SIGNS
- BECOMES UNRESPONSIVE
- TREMBLING

SKIN—COOL AND CLAMMY
EYES—LACKLUSTER
PUPILS—DILATED
FACE—PALE
LIPS—BLUE
PULSE—RAPID AND WEAK

SYMPTOMS
- NAUSEA
- THIRST
- WEAKNESS
- RESTLESS
- FEAR

SHOCK

Figure 7-21: Symptoms and signs of shock.

Preventing and Treating Shock

The same basic care should be used both to keep a patient from *developing* shock and to treat a patient who is *in* shock. The basic difference is administering oxygen. In cases where you believe that shock is a distinct possibility, such as significant blood loss, provide the patient with oxygen. If the patient's vital signs and general condition are stable, you may decide to carry out all the steps except oxygen administration, according to local procedures, and monitor the patient in case oxygen is needed. When in doubt, treat for shock and provide oxygen.

Some specific measures must be added to our list of care procedures for the shock patient. These measures are:

- *Assure an adequate airway and breathing.* As in all cases, if the patient is breathing, maintain an adequate airway by properly positioning the patient's head. If the person is not breathing, establish an airway and provide pulmonary resuscitation. STAY ALERT FOR VOMITING. If both respiration and circulation have stopped, initiate CPR measures.

- *Control bleeding.* Use direct pressure, pressure points, splints, a blood pressure cuff, or a tourniquet as required. The loss of blood volume is life-threatening for the shock patient. Apply a MAST garment if needed, but do so only if you are trained in the procedure. Inflating the MAST usually requires an order by the emergency department physician.

- *Administer oxygen.* An oxygen deficiency will result from the reduced circulation taking place in shock. Provide a high concentration of oxygen in accordance with local policies. STAY ALERT FOR VOMITING.

- *Splint fractures.* Splinting slows bleeding and reduces pain, both of which aggravate shock. AVOID ROUGH HANDLING since body motion has a tendency to aggravate shock.

- *Position the patient.* You have four choices of patient position, depending on the patient's problem and local policies.

1. LOWER EXTREMITY ELEVATION: This is the most recommended position. Raise the patient's legs slightly, about 12 to 18 inches. If there are fractures of the lower extremities, they cannot be major and they MUST be splinted. Do NOT use this procedure if there are indications of neck or spinal injuries, head injuries, chest injuries, or abdominal injuries. Do NOT tilt the patient's entire body into a head down position. To do so will press the abdominal organs against the diaphragm.

2. SUPINE: The patient is placed flat on his back, with adequate padding to provide comfort to the patient. This position is of-ten used if there are serious injuries to the extremities.

3. SEMI-SEATED: This position is used for conscious patients with indications of respiratory or heart problems. The idea is to keep the patient as comfortable as possible and to allow the patient to find the position which provides for the easiest breathing.

4. COMA: This is a semiprone position that is used for the unconscious patient. It provides the best drainage in case of vomiting and provides the best positioning for many head and upper body wounds. Some EMS Systems do not use the coma position. Do NOT use it unless you are *trained* to do so and it is part of your local policy on EMT-level care.

WARNING: Regardless of the position used, be alert for vomiting.

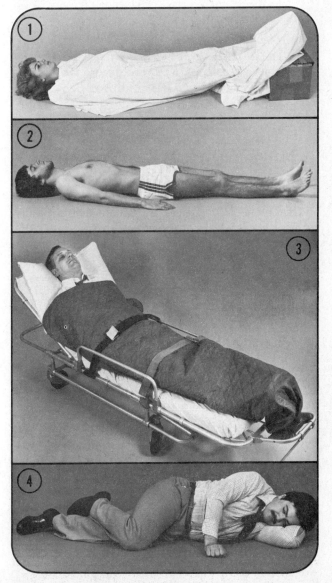

Figure 7-22: Positioning the shock patient.

- *REASSURE THE PATIENT.*

- *Keep the patient lying still.* The more at rest a shock patient remains, the better his chances for survival. Avoid excessive and rough handling.

- *Prevent loss of body heat.* You wish to keep the patient's body temperature as near normal as possible. Place a blanket under and over the patient (blanket placement is best done when positioning the patient so as not to increase body movement). Prevent heat loss, but *do not allow the patient to overheat.* When possible, remove any wet clothing. Do not move patients with head, neck, or spinal injury for the purpose of placing a blanket under them.

- *Give nothing by mouth.* Keep in mind that oxygen will dry the patient's oral and nasal pathways. If oxygen is to be used for long periods, the humidification of the oxygen should be considered. Do not give the patient anything to drink, including ice. Do not give any food or medications orally.

- *Monitor the patient.* You MUST take vital signs and record the results when you do the patient assessment. Read and record these signs EVERY FIVE MINUTES until you deliver both patient and information to a medical facility staff.

The use of MAST garments may be part of your EMS System's protocol for certain shock patients.

NOTE: The current trend is to provide conscious and unconscious severe shock patients with oxygen and ventilatory assistance on demand using the demand valve resuscitator (positive pressure resuscitator).

Anaphylactic Shock

This type of shock is a TRUE EMERGENCY and must be considered life-threatening whenever encountered. There is no way for you to predict what may happen to a patient in anaphylactic shock. A very mild allergic reaction may turn into serious anaphylactic shock in a matter of minutes.

Anaphylactic shock occurs when a person comes into contact with something to which he is extremely allergic. Causes of analphylactic reactions include:

- INSECT STINGS. Bees, yellow jackets, wasps, and hornets can cause a rapid and severe reaction.

- INGESTED SUBSTANCES. Foods such as spices, berries, fish and shellfish, and certain drugs can cause reactions. In most cases, the effect is slower than that seen with insect stings.

- INHALED SUBSTANCES. Dust, pollens, and chemical powders often can cause very rapid and severe reactions.

- INJECTED SUBSTANCES. Antitoxins and drugs like penicillin may cause severe reactions.

- ABSORBED SUBSTANCES. Certain chemicals, when in contact with the skin, produce severe reactions.

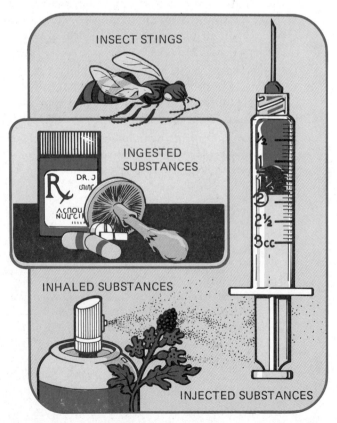

Figure 7-24: Substances that can cause anaphylactic shock.

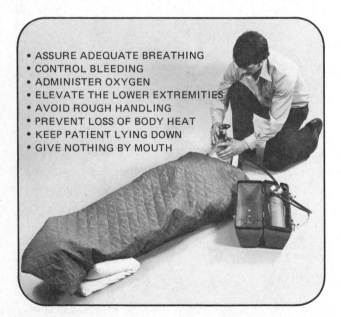

- ASSURE ADEQUATE BREATHING
- CONTROL BLEEDING
- ADMINISTER OXYGEN
- ELEVATE THE LOWER EXTREMITIES
- AVOID ROUGH HANDLING
- PREVENT LOSS OF BODY HEAT
- KEEP PATIENT LYING DOWN
- GIVE NOTHING BY MOUTH

Figure 7-23: Treating the shock patient.

The symptoms of anaphylactic shock can include:

- Itching and burning skin, especially about the face and chest
- Painful constriction of the chest with difficult breathing
- Dizziness
- Feelings of restlessness
- Nausea
- Headache
- Patient may report a temporary loss of consciousness

REMEMBER: When interviewing a patient, ask if he is allergic to anything. Check to see if that substance is at the scene, or is likely to be at the scene. If you are in the patient's residence, see if there is a ''Vial of Life'' sticker on the refrigerator. Patient information and medications can be found in such refrigerators. Look for medical identification devices to see if the patient has a known allergy.

The signs of anaphylactic shock can include:

- STATE OF CONSCIOUSNESS—restlessness, often followed by fainting or even coma
- BREATHING—difficult, sometimes with wheezing
- PULSE—very weak or imperceptible
- BLOOD PRESSURE—may drop to shock level
- SKIN—obvious irritation or blotches (such as hives)
- FACE—marked swelling of the face and tongue, often with cyanosis of lips
- VOMITING

Again, relate the above to the patient assessment.

Anaphylactic shock is a true emergency requiring the injection of medications to combat the allergic reaction. Initial emergency care efforts should be directed toward basic life support. As an EMT, you should:

1. PROVIDE LIFE SUPPORT MEASURES. Maintain an open airway and perform pulmonary resuscitation or CPR as required.
2. PROVIDE OXYGEN AND TREAT FOR SHOCK.
3. TRANSPORT TO A MEDICAL FACILITY IMMEDIATELY. Notify the facility by radio on the way. If the information is available, tell the staff the substance causing the reaction and the means of patient contact (sting, inhalation, etc.). Continue basic life support measures during transport.

NOTE: Some EMS Systems are now considering the problems faced by EMTs when asked by a patient to help in administering medications at the scene. These medications, usually epinephrine or antihistamines for cases of bee sting sensitivity, are provided by physicians to people with severe allergies. A more serious problem occurs when the patient is unconscious and the EMT finds a medical identification device and the medication is available at the scene. This text gives no recommendations. Your instructor will inform you of local policies for such cases.

Fainting

As noted in our classification of shock, fainting is a self-correcting form of shock. Usually, the serious problems related to fainting are injuries that occur during falls due to temporary loss of consciousness. Fainting may be caused by stressful situations. However, it may be an indication that the patient

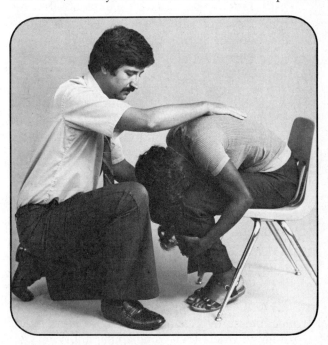

Figure 7-26: Protect the patient and try to prevent fainting.

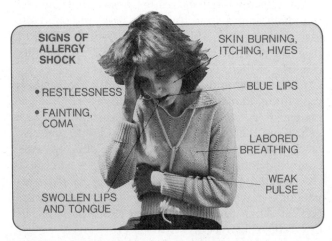

SIGNS OF ALLERGY SHOCK

SKIN BURNING, ITCHING, HIVES

BLUE LIPS

- RESTLESSNESS
- FAINTING, COMA

LABORED BREATHING

WEAK PULSE

SWOLLEN LIPS AND TONGUE

Figure 7-25: Signs of anaphylactic shock.

has blood pressure problems (sudden drop or elevation), or a serious medical problem. Brain tumors, undetected diabetes, and inner ear disorders are just a few medical conditions that may first present themselves through fainting. Take the blood pressure of ANYONE who faints. If you are called to the scene of a fainting and the patient refuses additional care, recommend that he see a physician as soon as possible. In a polite but firm manner, tell the patient not to drive or operate any machinery until he as been examined by a physician.

In all cases of fainting, protect the patient from injury and provide emotional support when the patient recovers. You can often prevent a patient from fainting by placing him in a seated position and lowering his head to a level between the knees. Do NOT do this for patients with fractures, possible neck or spinal injuries, or severe head injuries. This procedure is NOT RECOMMENDED for anyone having difficulty breathing or who has a known heart problem. Have these patients lie down with the feet slightly elevated and give emotional support. This will provide protection and may prevent fainting.

SUMMARY

Bleeding can be classified as external or internal and can range from minor to life-threatening.

External bleeding can be:

ARTERIAL—profuse loss of bright red blood spurting from an artery.

VENOUS—mild to profuse loss of dark red blood flowing steadily from a vein.

CAPILLARY—slow loss of red blood flowing from a bed of capillaries, as seen in minor scrapes of the skin.

The eight procedures for controlling external bleeding are:

1. DIRECT PRESSURE—where your hand, a sterile dressing, or a clean cloth can be used to apply pressure directly to a wound to stop bleeding. *Never* remove a dressing once it is in place. A pressure dressing can be applied to stop most cases of external bleeding from a limb. For severe profuse bleeding, you may have to insert your fingers directly into the wound to compress lacerated blood vessels.

REMEMBER: Direct pressure is the first choice in controlling bleeding.

2. ELEVATION—usually used in combination with direct pressure to control bleeding from an intact extremity, where there is no spinal injury.

3. PRESSURE POINTS—use of external hand pressure to compress an artery. This method most often is performed on the upper limb (brachial) and the thigh (femoral). The carotid point is a last resort for profuse neck bleeding. Do NOT apply pressure to both sides of the neck at once.

4. SPLINTING—stabilizing the ends of broken bones to prevent additional injury to blood vessels.

5. INFLATABLE SPLINTS—used even when there is no fracture. This method is useful for long cuts on an extremity.

6. BLOOD PRESSURE CUFF—used to control bleeding from an extremity.

7. MAST GARMENTS—pneumatic counterpressure devices useful for serious abdominal bleeding.

8. TOURNIQUET—a *last resort* measure to control bleeding from an extremity. The flat belt of a tourniquet is placed over a pad that has been set close to the wound, between the site of the wound and the patient's heart. The tourniquet belt is tightened to where the bleeding stops, and is fixed in place at this point. A plainly visible note stating that a tourniquet has been placed and the time of placement must accompany the patient. ONCE THE TOURNIQUET IS IN PLACE, DO NOT LOOSEN IT.

Internal bleeding can be very serious. Look for mechanisms of injury that may cause internal bleeding. Look for wounds associated with internal bleeding. Note that fractures may have caused internal bleeding, and examine the patient for the symptoms and signs of shock. Treatment for internal bleeding is basically the same as for shock. In addition, pressure dressings and splints can be applied for internal bleeding found in an extremity.

REMEMBER: Patients with serious blood loss will benefit from the administering of oxygen.

The symptoms of shock can include nausea, thirst, weakness, dizziness, coolness, and the feeling of impending doom.

The signs of shock can include the patient becoming unresponsive, restlessness, shaking and trembling, rapid weak pulse, shallow rapid breathing, marked drop in blood pressure, moist cool skin, pale face and inner eyelids, dilated lackluster pupils, cyanosis at the lips or ear lobes.

Prevention and treatment of shock are basically the same. Maintain an adequate airway, control major bleeding, and splint fractures. Administer oxygen. Keep the patient at rest, lying down, and covered to stay warm but not overheated. In most cases, the patient will benefit if the lower extremities are elevated. Give nothing by mouth, monitor the patient's vital signs, and provide emotional support.

NOTE: When providing care for shock patients, BE ON THE ALERT FOR VOMITING.

Anaphlactic shock (allergy shock) is a TRUE

EMERGENCY. This type of shock is brought about when the patient comes into contact with a substance to which he is allergic (bee stings, insect bites, chemicals, dust, pollens, drugs, foods).

The symptoms of anaphylactic shock include complaints of itching and burning skin, chest pains with difficult breathing, dizziness, restlessness, and nausea. The signs of anaphylactic shock can include restlessness, becoming unresponsive, difficult breathing, very weak pulse, hives or blotchy skin, swelling of the face and tongue, cyanosis, and vomiting.

The treatment for anaphylactic shock includes basic life support measures and the same care as for all shock patients. Transport the patient to a medical facility immediately.
REMEMBER: Ask the patient about allergies during the interview. Be certain to look for medical identification devices. If you are in the patient's residence, check the refrigerator door for a "Vial of Life" sticker.

Fainting is a mild form of self-correcting shock. Always look for injuries caused by falls due to fainting. Take the patient's blood pressure and provide emotional support. Discourage the patient from driving or operating machinery until he is examined by a physician. Urge the patient to see a physician.

Fainting can often be prevented by placing the patient in a seated position, protecting him from falling, and lowering his head to a level between the knees. Do NOT follow this procedure for patients with fractures, spinal injuries, heart problems, or difficult breathing.

Detection of bleeding and shock depends on the proper patient assessment procedures carried out by the EMT.

8 injuries i: soft tissues and internal organs

SECTION ONE: THE SOFT TISSUES

OBJECTIVES By the end of this section, you should be able to:

1. Define "soft tissues." (p. 150)
2. Define "closed" and "open wound." (p. 150-1)
3. Classify closed wounds as contusions, internal lacerations, internal punctures, crushing injuries, or ruptures. (p. 151-2)
4. Classify open wounds as abrasions, incisions, lacerations, punctures, avulsions, amputations, or crushing injuries. (p. 152-4)
5. Cite the basic procedures used in caring for a closed wound. (p. 154)
6. Cite the basic procedures used in caring for open wounds. (p. 154-7)
7. List the SEVEN steps used in caring for wounds having impaled objects. (p. 158)
8. Cite the basic procedures used in caring for avulsions, amputations, and crushing injuries. (p. 154-5)
9. Define dressing, multi-trauma dressing, occlusive dressing, and bandage. (p. 154)
10. State the FOUR basic rules that apply to the dressing of wounds. (p. 155-6)
11. State the FOUR basic rules that apply to bandaging. (p. 156)

SKILLS As an EMT, you should be able to:

1. Determine types of soft tissue injuries.
2. Control bleeding and provide the proper emergency care for open wounds.
3. Provide basic emergency care for closed wounds.

NOTE: Chapter 8 is divided into two sections so that you may study the types of soft tissue injuries before having to learn specific injuries. Do not try to learn this chapter in one long study session. Read through Section One, including the summary. Check the section objectives and be certain that you meet all of them. After you have met these objectives, go on with the second section, "SPECIFIC INJURIES."

TERMS you may be using for the first time:

Epidermis (ep-i-DER-mis)—the outer layer of skin.

Dermis (DER-mis)—the inner layer of skin found beneath the epidermis. It is rich in blood vessels and nerves.

Subcutaneous (SUB-ku-TA-ne-us) **Layers**—the layers of fat and soft tissues found below the dermis.

Contusion (kun-TU-zhun)—a bruise.

Abrasion (ab-RAY-shun)—scratches and scrapes.

Incision—a smooth cut.

Laceration—a jagged cut.

Avulsion (ah-VUL-shun)—the tearing away of skin and other soft tissues. This term may also be used for an eye pulled from its socket or a tooth knocked out of its socket.

Dressing—any material used to cover a wound that will help control bleeding and help prevent additional contamination.

Occlusive Dressing—dressing that forms an airtight seal.

Bandage—any material used to hold a dressing in place.

THE SOFT TISSUES

TYPES OF SOFT TISSUE INJURY

The soft tissues of the body include the skin, muscles, blood vessels, nerves, fatty tissues, and tissues that line or cover organs. The teeth, bones, and cartilage are considered hard tissues.

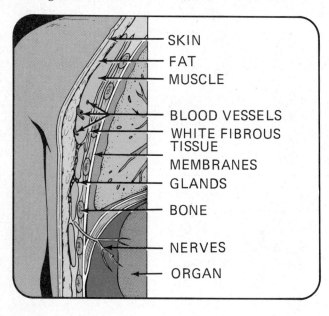

SKIN
FAT
MUSCLE
BLOOD VESSELS
WHITE FIBROUS TISSUE
MEMBRANES
GLANDS
BONE
NERVES
ORGAN

Figure 8-1: Soft tissues.

The most obvious soft tissue injuries involve the skin. The outer layer of the skin is called the **epidermis** (ep-i-DER-mis). This layer contains no blood vessels or nerves. Except for certain types of burns and injuries due to cold, injuries of the epidermis present few problems in EMT-level care.

The layer of skin below the epidermis is the **dermis** (DER-mis). This layer is rich with blood vessels, nerves, and specialized structures such as sweat glands and hair follicles. Once the dermis is opened to the outside world, contamination becomes a ma-

jor problem. The wound can be serious, accompanied by profuse bleeding and intense pain.

The layers of fat and soft tissue below the dermis are called the **subcutaneous** (SUB-ku-TA-ne-us) **layers.** Again, there are the problems of bloodstream contamination, bleeding, and pain when these tissues are injured.

There is little that the EMT can do for blood vessel and nerve damage, although additional injury can be prevented through prompt and efficient care. Controlling bleeding, protecting from additional contamination, and certain procedures to reduce pain are all that you can do in the field. This also is true of muscle injury. EMT-level care is limited to treating wounds and perhaps immobilizing the injured area. However, the control of bleeding and proper wound care are critical and may be the determining factor in patient survival.

The body's organs and glands are composed of soft tissues. Injuries to these structures can range from minor to immediate life-threatening problems. At the EMT-level of care, little can be done specifically for organ and gland injuries. Again, what *can* be done may be a major factor in patient survival.

The detection of organ and gland injury and how this knowledge affects care, order of care, and order of transport, are of great importance in emergency medicine. As an EMT, you must know the organs and major glands and where they are located. You must know which organs are solid and which are hollow so you can consider the possible types of injuries, extent of internal bleeding, and complications due to an organ rupturing. As you learn more about the body organs, remember to relate the organs of the abdominopelvic cavity to the abdominal quadrants (Chapter 2).

Closed Wounds

Closed Wounds   A general classification of soft tissue injuries includes closed wounds and open wounds. A **closed wound** is an internal injury.

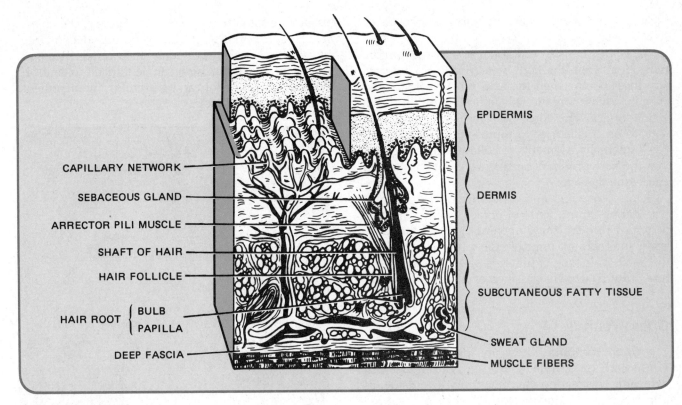

Figure 8-2: The skin.

There may or may not be damage to the skin; however, there is no open pathway from the outside to the injured site. These wounds usually result from the impact of a blunt object. Although the skin itself may not be broken, there may be extensive crushed tissues beneath it. Closed wounds can be simple bruises, internal lacerations (cuts), and internal punctures caused by fractured bones, crushing injuries, or the rupturing of internal organs. Bleeding can range from minor to life-threatening. As an EMT, you should always consider the possibility of soft tissue injuries when there are fractures and blunt trauma.

Contusions (kun-TU-zhun)—A **contusion** is a bruise. A variable amount of bleeding always occurs at the time of injury and may continue for a few hours after the trauma. Swelling may occur immediately, or it may be delayed as much as 24 to 48 hours. A blood clot almost always forms at the injury site as blood seeps into the surrounding tissues to form the characteristic "black and blue" mark. This process is called *ecchymosis* (EK-i-MO-sis). Many patients will show a bruise that is more a brownish yellow at the time you perform the patient assessment. Keep in mind that large bruises can mean serious blood loss and an indication of fractures or extensive tissue damage below the site of the bruise.

Internal Lacerations and Punctures—When bones are fractured, sharp ends can cut or puncture internal body structures. The lungs, heart, and liver can be lacerated by fractured ribs. Fractured ribs may even puncture a lung, allowing inspired air to flow

into the thoracic cavity. On rare occasions, the urinary bladder can be lacerated or punctured as a result of pelvic fractures. Realize that a fractured bone can damage muscles, blood vessels, nerves,

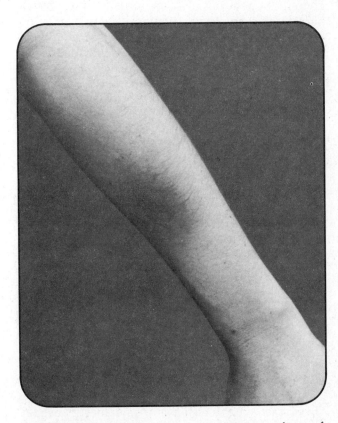

Figure 8-3: Contusions are the most common form of closed wound.

organs, glands and other structures composed of soft tissues.

Crushing Injuries and Ruptures—Force can be transmitted from the body's exterior to the internal structures, even when the skin remains intact and even in cases where the only indication of injury is a simple bruise. This force can cause the internal organs to be crushed, or to rupture (burst open) and bleed internally. Contents of hollow organs can leak into the body cavities, causing severe inflammation and tissue damage.

Organ coverings and cavity linings also can rupture during injury. Parts of organs or muscles may be forced through these openings, yet all the damage is internal, not directly visible on the outside of the body. This type of injury is often called a "rupture," but is actually classified as a hernia (her-NE-ah).

Open Wounds

Open Wounds   These are injuries where the skin is torn (interrupted), exposing the tissues underneath. This tearing can come from the outside, as a laceration, or from the inside when a fractured bone end tears outward, through the skin.

Abrasion (ab-RAY-shun)—This classification of wound includes simple scrapes and scratches where the outer layer of the skin is damaged, but all the layers are not penetrated. Skinned elbows and knees, "mat burns," "rug burns," and "brush burns" are examples of abrasions. There may be no detectable bleeding, or only the minor ooze of blood from capillary beds. Care should be provided to reduce wound contamination. The patient may experience great pain, even though the injury is minor.

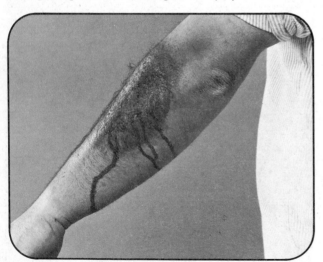

Figure 8-4: Abrasions are the least serious form of open wound.

Incisions—An **incision** is a smooth cut, usually made by a sharp object, such as a knife or razor blade. The edges of the cut skin and the underlying

tissues are smooth due to the sharpness of the object inflicting the injury. If the wound is deep, large blood vessels and nerves may be severed. Bleeding from a long, deep incision can be difficult to control. The air-inflated splint can be useful in the treatment of this type of wound.

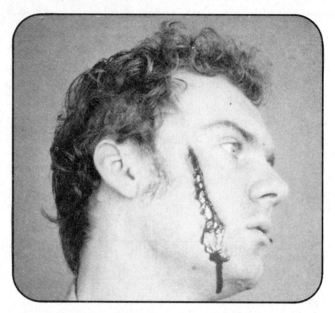

Figure 8-5: The edges of an incision wound are smooth.

Lacerations—A **laceration** is a jagged cut. The tissues are snagged and torn, forming a rough edge around the wound. Often, this type of wound is caused by objects having sharp, rough edges, such as broken glass or a jagged piece of metal. However, a laceration also can result from a severe blow or impact with a blunt object. The rough edges of a laceration tend to fall together and obstruct your view as you try to determine the wound depth. It is usually difficult to look at the outside of a laceration and determine the extent of the damage to underlying tissues. Do NOT pull apart the wound edges in an effort to see into the wound. If significant blood

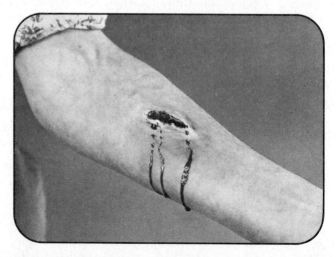

Figure 8-6: The edges of a laceration are jagged and rough.

vessels have been torn, bleeding will be considerable, but usually less than that seen with incisions. Remember, when blood vessels are stretched and torn, curling and folding of the cut ends aid in rapid clot formation.

Punctures—When an object passes through the skin and damages all the tissues in its path, a **puncture wound** has occurred. Typically, puncture wounds are caused by sharp pointed objects—nails, ice picks, splinters, or knives. Often, there is usually

no severe external bleeding problem, but internal bleeding may be profuse. There are two types of puncture wounds. A **penetrating puncture wound** can be shallow or deep. In either case, tissues and blood vessels are injured. A **perforating puncture wound** has both an *entrance wound* and an *exit wound*. The object causing the injury passes through the body and out to create an exit wound. In many cases, the exit wound is more serious than the entrance wound. A "through-and-through" gunshot wound is an example of the perforating puncture wound.

Avulsion (a-VUL-shun)—In this type of wound, large flaps of skin and tissues are torn loose or pulled off completely. When the tip of the nose is cut or torn off, this is an avulsion. The same applies to the external ear. A glove avulsion occurs when the hand is caught in a roller or other pinching hazard. In this type of accident, the skin is stripped off like a glove. An eye pulled from its socket is a form of avulsion. The term "avulsed" is used in reporting

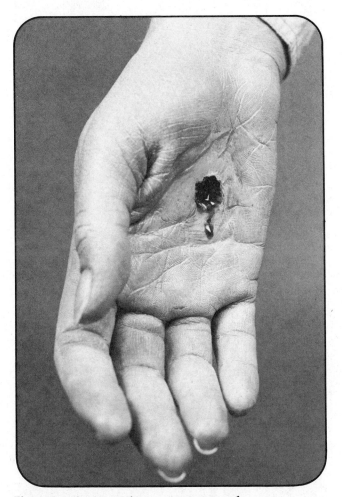

Figure 8-7: A penetrating puncture wound.

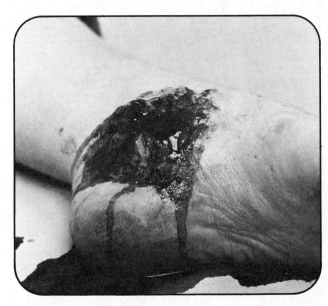

Figure 8-9: Avulsed skin.

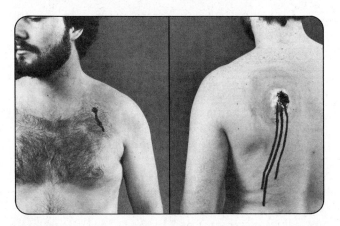

Figure 8-8: A perforating puncture wound has an entrance wound and an exit wound.

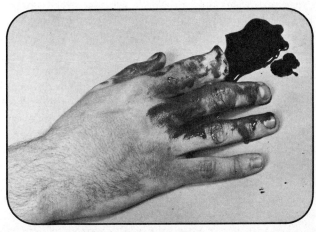

Figure 8-10: Amputation.

the wound, as in "an avulsed eye" or "an avulsed ear."

Amputation—These wounds involve the extremities. The fingers, toes, hands, feet, or limbs are completely cut through or torn off. Jagged skin and bone edges can be seen. There may be massive bleeding; however, the force that amputates a limb may close off torn blood vessels, limiting the amount of bleeding.

Crushing Injury—This type of injury can result when an extremity is caught between heavy items, such as pieces of machinery. Bones are fractured and may protrude through the wound site. Soft tissues and internal organs can be crushed, resulting in profuse external *and* internal bleeding.

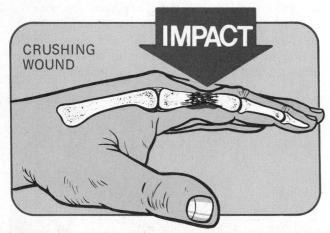

Figure 8-11: Both soft tissues and internal organs are damaged in crushing injuries.

SOFT TISSUE WOUND CARE

Closed Wounds

Contusions are the most frequently encountered closed wound. Most simple bruises will not require emergency care in the field; however, a bruise is an indication of possible internal injuries and related internal bleeding. Make certain you look for large areas of bruises and any large bruises directly over body organs, such as the spleen and liver. Swelling and deformity at the site of a bruise should warn you of possible underlying fractures.

If you find a contusion on the head or neck, search for blood in the mouth, nose, and ears. Should you find a bruise on the trunk of the body, find out if the patient is coughing up blood. Feel to determine if the patient's abdomen is rigid or tender. Each of these signs indicates serious internal injuries requiring special care. Later in this chapter, we will cover the care you need to render in specific cases of internal injuries to the soft tissues and body organs.

When the patient's injuries allow you to do so,

position the patient so that a minimum of weight is placed on a bruised area. If you believe there are internal injuries, TREAT AS IF THERE IS INTERNAL BLEEDING AND TREAT FOR SHOCK. Transport as soon as possible. Remember that most patients with internal injuries will benefit from the administration of oxygen.

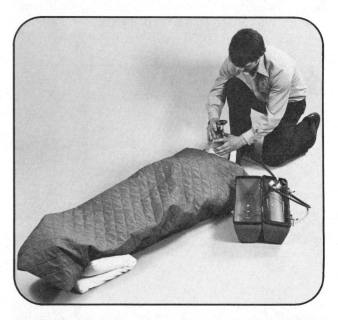

Figure 8-12: When caring for serious closed wounds, treat for internal bleeding and shock.

Open Wounds

There are few cases of open wound care that do not require the application of dressings and bandages. You should know the following definitions:

- DRESSING—Any material applied to a wound in an effort to control bleeding and prevent further contamination. Dressings should be sterile.
- BANDAGE—Any material used to hold a dressing in place. Bandages need not be sterile.

Dressings   Various dressings are carried in emergency care supplies. These dressings should be *sterile*, meaning that all microorganisms and spores that can grow into active organisms have been killed. Dressings also should be aseptic, meaning that all dirt and foreign debris have been removed. In emergency situations, when commercially prepared dressings are not available, clean cloth, towels, sheets, handkerchiefs, and other similar materials may have to be used.

The most popular dressings are individually wrapped sterile gauze pads, typically four inches square. A variety of sizes are available, referred to according to size such as 2 by 2's, 4 by 4's, and 4 by 8's.

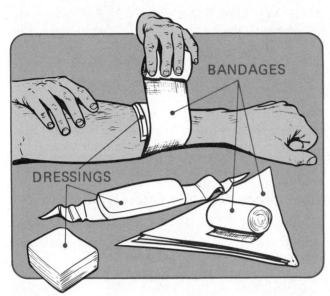

Figure 8-13: Dressings cover wounds, while bandages hold dressings in place.

Large bulky dressings, such as the multitrauma or universal dressings, are available when bulk is required for profuse bleeding, or a large wound must be covered. These dressings are especially useful for stabilizing impaled objects. Sanitary napkins can be used sometimes in place of the standard bulky dressings. While not sterile, they are separately wrapped and have very clean surfaces (avoid applying any adhesive surface directly to the wound). Of course, bulky dressings can be made by building up layers of gauze pads.

The **occlusive dressing** is used when it is necessary to form an air-tight seal. This is done when caring for open wounds to the abdomen, and for certain types of open wounds to the thorax. Sterile, commercially prepared occlusive dressings are available in three different forms. There are plastic wrap, aluminum foil, and petroleum gel-impregnated gauze occlusive dressings. Local protocols vary as to which form to use. Nonsterile wrap and foil also can be used in emergency situations. There are cases where EMTs have made their own emergency occlusive dressings from plastic credit cards and aluminum foil wrappers.

Large dressings are sometimes needed in emergency care. Bed sheets can be sterilized and kept in plastic wrappers to be later used as dressings. These can make effective burn dressings.

Bandaging Materials Bandages also are provided in a wide variety of types. The preferred bandage is the self-adhering, form-fitting roller bandage. It eliminates the need to know many specialized bandaging techniques developed for use with ordinary gauze roller bandages.

Dressings can be secured using adhering or nonadhering gauze roller bandage, triangular bandages, or strips of adhesive tape. When necessary, you can

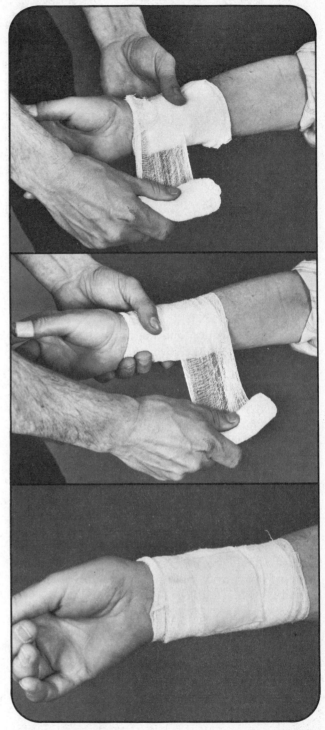

Figure 8-14: Applying a self-adhering roller bandage: 1. Secure with several overlying wraps. 2. Overlap the bandage, keeping it snug. 3. Cut and tape or tie into place.

use strips of cloth, handkerchiefs, and other such materials. Elastic bandages used in the care of strains and sprains should NOT be used to hold dressings in place. They can become constricting bands and interfere with circulation.

Dressing and Bandaging The following applies to the general dressing of wounds:

1. USE STERILE OR VERY CLEAN MATERIALS—

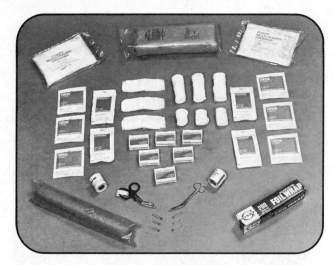

Figure 8-15: Materials used for dressings and bandages.

Avoid touching the dressing in the area that will come into contact with the wound.

2. COVER THE ENTIRE WOUND—The entire surface of the wound and the immediate surrounding areas should be covered.

3. CONTROL BLEEDING—With the exception of the pressure dressing, a dressing should not be bandaged into place if it has not controlled the bleeding. Continue to apply dressings and pressure as needed for the proper control of bleeding.

4. DO NOT REMOVE DRESSINGS—Once a dressing has been applied to a wound, it must *remain* in place. If bleeding continues, put new dressings over the blood-soaked ones.

The following applies to general bandaging:

1. DO NOT BANDAGE TOO TIGHTLY—All dressings should be held snugly in place, but they must not restrict the blood supply to the affected part.

2. DO NOT BANDAGE TOO LOOSELY—Hold the dressing by bandaging snugly, so the dressing does not move around, or slip from the wound. Loose bandaging is a common error in emergency care.

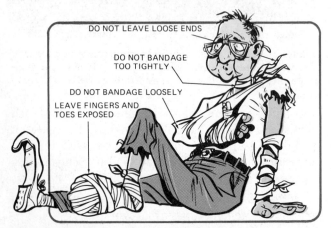

Figure 8-16: The rules of bandaging.

3. DO NOT LEAVE LOOSE ENDS—Any loose ends of gauze, tape, or cloth may get caught on objects when the patient is moved.

4. DO NOT COVER THE TIPS OF FINGERS AND TOES—When bandaging the extremities, leave the fingers and toes exposed whenever possible to observe skin color changes that indicate a change in circulation. Pain, pale or blue skin, cold skin, numbness, and tingling are all indications that a bandage is too tight.

Emergency Care For Open Wounds

Listed below are the general principles of emergency care that apply to the majority of open wounds:

1. EXPOSE THE WOUND—Clothing that covers a soft tissue injury must be lifted, cut, or split away. For some articles of clothing, this is best done with a seam cutter. Do NOT attempt to remove clothing in the usual manner. To do so may aggravate existing injuries and cause additional damage and pain.

2. CLEAR THE WOUND SURFACE—Do not waste time trying to pick out embedded particles and debris from the wound. Do not clean the wound; simply remove foreign matter from its surface. Proper wound cleaning must be done by a physician.

3. CONTROL BLEEDING—Start with direct pressure or direct pressure and elevation. When necessary, use pressure point procedures, apply an air-inflated splint, or use a blood pressure cuff. Remember, a tourniquet is used only as a last resort.

4. PREVENT FURTHER CONTAMINATION—Use a sterile dressing, if possible. When none is available, use the cleanest cloth material at the scene.

5. BANDAGE THE DRESSING IN PLACE.

6. KEEP THE PATIENT LYING STILL—Any patient movement will increase circulation, and could restart bleeding.

7. REASSURE THE PATIENT—This will help ease the patient's emotional response, thus lowering blood pressure and helping to reduce the bleeding rate.

8. For all serious wounds, treat for shock and administer oxygen.

NOTE: If serious bleeding originates from an extremity, or if the wound is a long laceration on an extremity, immobilize and elevate the injured part. An air-inflated splint serves to control bleeding.

Incisions and Lacerations Most incisions and lacerations can be cared for by bandaging a dressing in place. When bleeding is profuse, a pres-

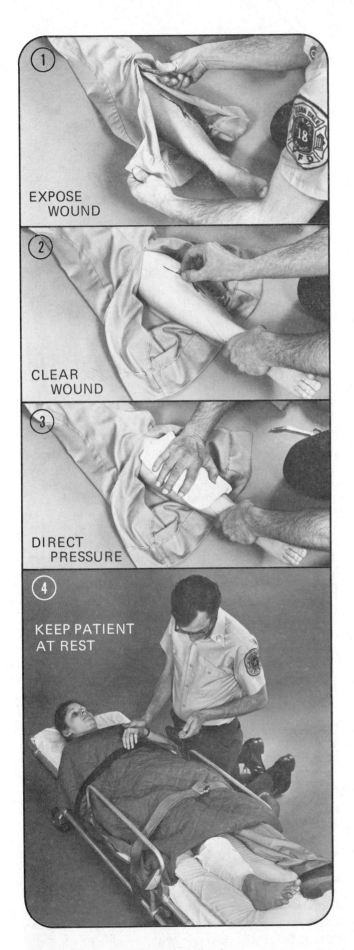

Figure 8-17: Care for open wounds.

sure dressing usually works well for these types of wounds. Some EMS Systems recommend a butterfly bandage for minor incisions and lacerations. The bandage strip can be made from adhesive tape and applied as shown in Figure 8-18. A gauze dressing should be bandaged over the butterfly strip.

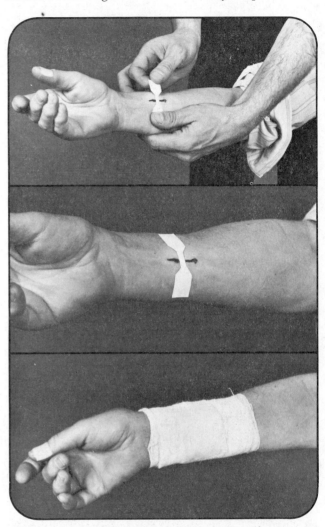

Figure 8-18: The application of a butterfly bandage.

Puncture Wounds Use caution when caring for puncture wounds. An object may appear to be embedded *only* in the skin, but actually goes all the way to the bone. In such cases, it is possible that the patient may not have any serious pain. A moderate puncture wound may cause extensive internal injury with serious internal bleeding. What appears to be a simple puncture wound may only be part of the problem. There also could be a severe exit wound that requires immediate care.

Gunshot wounds are puncture wounds that can fracture bones and cause intense injury to soft tissues and organs. As with all care, basic life support measures may be necessary. To ensure control of bleeding and adequate wound care, you must search for an exit wound.

Impaled Objects   As an EMT, you may have to care for patients with puncture wounds containing impaled objects. The object may be a knife, a steel rod, a shard of glass, or even a wooden stick, piercing any part of the body. In general, when caring for a patient with a puncture wound with an impaled object:

1. *DO NOT REMOVE THE IMPALED OBJECT.* To do so may cause severe bleeding when the pressure is released on any severed blood vessels. Removal of the object may cause further injury to nerves, muscles, and other soft tissues.

2. *Expose the wound area.* Cut away clothing to make the wound site accessible. Take great care not to disturb the object. Do not attempt to lift clothing over the object; you may accidentally move it.

3. *Control profuse bleeding by direct hand pressure if possible.* CAUTION: Position your hand so the fingers are on either side of the object and exert pressure downward. Do NOT put pressure on the object or the tissues directly adjacent to the object. Pressure must be applied with great care if the object has a cutting edge, such as a knife, or a shard of glass.

4. *Stabilize the impaled object with a bulky dressing.* Place several layers of bulky dressing over the injury site so that the dressings surround the object on all sides. It may be possible to cut a hole slightly larger than the object in a bulky dressing and *gently* pass the dressing over the object. Once bandaged into place, the dressings will stabilize the object and exert downward pressure on bleeding vessels. Adhesive strips serve well to hold the dressings in place. Some EMS System guidelines call for forming a "doughnut" ring from cravats to stabilize the impaled object.

5. Provide oxygen at a high concentration.

6. *Keep the patient at rest and provide emotional support.* Position the patient for minimum stress. If possible immobilize the affected area.

7. *Carefully transport the patient as soon as possible.* Avoid any movement that may jar, loosen, or dislodge the object.

NOTE: The above procedure may change as MAST garments become a greater part of EMT-level care. As an EMT, you must stay informed of care procedure changes. Special procedures are used when caring for objects impaled in the eye and in the cheek. These procedures will be covered in Section Two.

Avulsions   The emergency care for avulsions requires the application of large, bulky pressure dressings. In addition, you should make every effort to preserve any avulsed parts and transport them to the medical facility along with the patient. It may be possible to surgically restore the part or use it for skin grafts.

In cases where flaps of skin have been torn loose but not off:

1. Clear the wound surface;

2. As gently as possible, fold the skin back to its normal position; and

3. Control bleeding and dress the wound using bulky pressure dressings.

Should skin or another body part be torn from the body:

1. Control bleeding, dressing the wound with a bulky pressure dressing; and

2. Save the avulsed part in a plastic bag, plastic wrap, or aluminum foil, in accordance with local protocol. If none of these items is available at the scene, wrap the avulsed part in a lint-free, sterile dressing. Make certain you label the wrapped part as to what it is, and with the patient's name. The avulsed part should be kept as cool as possi-

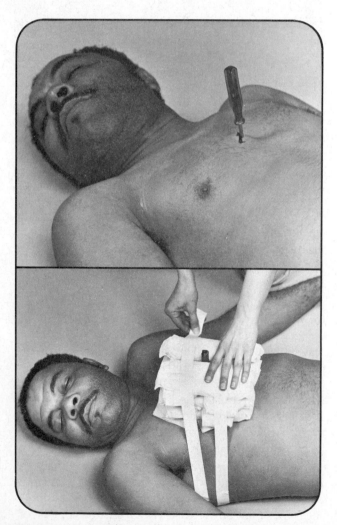

Figure 8-19: Impaled objects. Expose the wound, control bleeding, and stabilize the impaled object.

ble. Do NOT immerse the avulsed part in water or saline.

Amputations As in other external bleeding situations, the most effective method to control bleeding is a snug pressure dressing. This should be placed over the stump. Pressure point techniques or a blood pressure cuff also may be required to control bleeding. A tourniquet should not be applied unless the other methods used to control bleeding have failed. When possible, wrap or bag the amputated part in plastic and transport with the patient. It is best to keep the part cool, but not in direct contact with ice. Be sure to label the wrapped part, including what the part is and the name of the patient. Do NOT immerse the amputated part in water or saline.

Protruding Organs Open wounds of the abdomen may be so large and deep that organs protrude through the wound opening. In such cases:

1. Do NOT try to replace the organ.
2. Cover the exposed organ and wound opening with aluminum foil or plastic wrap in accordance with local protocol. Some systems use a sterile lint-free dressing soaked with sterile saline.
3. Apply a thick dressing pad or clean towel over the first dressing. This will help to preserve heat.
4. Treat for shock, positioning the patient to provide for a clear airway and minimum stress to the wound site. Administer oxygen in a high (50% or greater) concentration.

SUMMARY

Soft tissue damage may be classified as closed wounds and open wounds. Remember that body organs are composed of soft tissues. Contusions are the most common form of closed wound. Abrasions and lacerations are the most common forms of open wounds.

Puncture wounds are open wounds and classified as penetrating or perforating. Perforating wounds have both an entrance wound and an exit wound.

Avulsions occur when skin or a body part is torn loose or from the body. Amputation is the cutting or tearing off of a finger, hand, upper limb, toe, foot, or lower limb. Crushing injuries can create both external and internal injury with severe tissue damage.

Both internal and external bleeding are seen with such injuries.

Always treat closed wounds as if there is internal bleeding.

When treating an open wound, begin by exposing the wound. After clearing the wound surface, you should control bleeding.

Remember, when caring for a patient, your first priorities are airway, breathing, circulation, and control of profuse bleeding. Once this is done, continued control of bleeding and prevention of further wound contamination are achieved by dressing the wound.

If the patient has a puncture wound, assume there are serious internal injuries with bleeding. Look for an exit wound.

Keep in mind that patients suffering from blood loss do better when you administer oxygen and treat for shock. When dealing with an open or closed wound, keep the patient lying still and provide emotional support. Always be alert for vomiting in cases of internal injury.

Do NOT remove impaled objects. Control bleeding and stabilize the impaled object. Partially avulsed skin can be folded gently back to its normal position. If skin is torn off, preserve the part in aluminum foil or plastic. When confronted by an amputation, attempt to control bleeding by direct pressure applied to a bulky dressing held directly over the stump. If necessary, use pressure point techniques to help control bleeding. When an extremity is injured, the application of a blood pressure cuff may be the best way to control severe external bleeding. The *last* resort is a tourniquet.

Do NOT try to replace protruding organs. Control bleeding and cover with an occlusive dressing. Treat for shock.

Dressings cover wounds; bandages hold dressings in place. Dressings can be single-layered or built up into bulky dressings. Occlusive dressings are used to form air-tight seals.

The procedures for dressing a wound require you to control bleeding, use sterile or clean materials, and to cover the entire wound. Do NOT remove a dressing once it is in place.

The procedures for bandaging require you to adjust the bandage so that the dressing is neither too loose nor too tight, and to be sure that there are no loose ends. Remember, do NOT cover the patient's fingertips and toes.

SECTION TWO: SPECIFIC INJURIES

OBJECTIVES By the end of this section, you should be able to:

1. List the procedures for emergency care of scalp wounds. (p. 161-2)
2. List the procedures for emergency care of facial wounds. (p. 162-3)
3. Describe, step by step, the emergency care for a patient with an object impaled in the cheek. (p. 163-4)
4. Cite the procedures of care for cuts, burns, and foreign objects in the eye. (p. 166-7)
5. List the special care procedures for an object impaled in the eye. (p. 166)
6. Describe, step by step, the procedures for removing each of the three types of contact lenses. (p. 167-9)
7. Describe basic care for injuries to the external ear and what to do if you suspect internal injury. (p. 170)
8. Describe the emergency care procedures for nosebleeds and nonfracture injuries to the nose. (p. 171-2)
9. Describe the basic emergency care for injuries to the mouth. (p. 172-3)
10. List at least FOUR signs of blunt injury to the neck. (p. 173)
11. Contrast the procedures used to control arterial bleeding from the neck with those used to control venous bleeding from the neck. (p. 174)
12. List the types of nonpenetrating soft tissue injuries to the chest and the care for each type of injury. (p. 174)
13. List the major signs of abdominal injury and the symptoms associated with closed abdominal injury. (p. 174, 5-7)
14. State the procedures used to care for open and closed abdominal injuries. (p. 177)
15. Describe basic care for injuries to the genitalia. (p. 178-9)
16. Describe the basic care for inguinal hernia patients. (Note: local guidelines vary. Use those applying to your EMS System.) (p. 179)

SKILLS As an EMT, you should be able to:

1. Determine types of soft tissue injuries.
2. Control bleeding and apply the proper dressing and bandage for a given injury to the scalp, face, eye, ear, nose, mouth, neck, chest, abdomen, pelvis, and genitalia.
3. Demonstrate the special emergency care procedures for:

- Impaled object in the eye
- Severe bleeding from a neck vein
- Severe bleeding from a neck artery
- Impaled object in the cheek
- Nonpenetrating chest wounds
- Saving avulsed body parts
- Amputations

TERMS   you may be using for the first time:

Cornea (KOR-ne-ah)—the transparent covering over the iris and pupil of the eye.

Sclera (SKLE-rah)—the "whites of the eyes."

Iris—the colored portion of the anterior eye that adjusts the size of the pupil.

Pinna (PIN-nah)—the external ear. Also called the auricle (AW-re-kl).

External Auditory Canal—the opening of the external ear and pathway to the middle ear.

Epistaxis (ep-e-STAK-sis)—a nosebleed.

Maxilla (mak-SIL-ah)—refers to the upper jaw. Two maxillae (mak-SIL-e) bones join to form the upper jaw.

Mandible (MAN-di-bl)—the lower jaw bone.

Jugular (JUG-u-lar) **Veins**—the major neck veins that drain the head and face.

Eviscerate (e-VIS-er-ate)—usually applies to the intestine or other internal organ protruding through an incision or wound in the abdomen.

Genitalia (jen-i-TA-le-ah)—the external reproductive organs.

Inguinal (IN-gwin-al) **Hernia** (HER-ne-ah) or "**rupture**"—a soft tissue injury in which the lining of the abdominopelvic cavity ruptures and the intestine protrudes through the opening.

NOTE: Many new anatomical terms are used in this section. Those found in bold type should be used in communications.

SPECIFIC INJURIES

This section deals with specific injuries to soft tissues and to the organs of the abdominopelvic cavity. Injuries to bones and joints, brain injuries, and penetrating chest wounds will be covered in the next two chapters.

THE SCALP AND FACE

Of the many blood vessels in the scalp and face, quite a few are close to the skin surface. Wounds may bleed profusely even though a major vessel has not been severed. A minor laceration may initially bleed profusely. Usually, clotting is rapid and control is not a major problem. However, if an artery is cut, bleeding can be quickly fatal if no effort is made to control the flow of blood. Severe trauma to the face also may produce skull fractures and possible airway obstruction. Many patients with head injuries also have neck injuries that may involve the spinal cord.

Most soft tissue injuries of the scalp and face can be treated like any other soft tissue injury. There are three major EXCEPTIONS to the standard procedure:

1. Do NOT attempt to clear or clean the surface of a scalp wound. To do so may cause additional bleeding and may possibly cause great harm to the patient if there are skull fractures.
2. Do NOT apply finger pressure to the wound in an effort to control bleeding. There may be fractures to the skull.
3. DO remove objects impaled in the cheek if they penetrate the cheek and exit into the oral cavity.

Care of Scalp Wounds   Contamination occurs with every scalp wound. The hair may mat over the wound site. Foreign objects, such as glass fragments, pieces of metal, or bits of soil may be on the wound surface and in the wound itself. Dressing the wound will help prevent additional contamination. To care for a scalp wound:

1. Do NOT clear the wound surface. Do NOT try to clean the wound. Wiping actions or irrigation with water could cause objects to be driven through breaks in the skull and contaminate the brain.
2. Control bleeding with a sterile dressing carefully held in place with gentle pressure. Avoid finger pressure if there is any indication of skull fracture.
3. Strips of adhesive bandage do not work well in cases of scalp injury. Self-adherent roller bandage or gauze can be wrapped around the patient's head to hold the dressing in place. Remember that bleeding is to be controlled before a dressing is bandaged in place.

WARNING: Do NOT lift or attempt to wrap the patient's head if there are any signs of spinal injury, or the mechanism of injury indicates a possible spinal injury.

4. Keep the patient's head and shoulders raised to help control bleeding, if the patient survey, degree of trauma, and mechanism of injury do not indicate possible spinal injury, or injury to the chest or abdomen. Do NOT put the unconscious trauma patient into a head-raised position.

An effective way to hold a dressing on a scalp wound without applying excessive pressure is to use

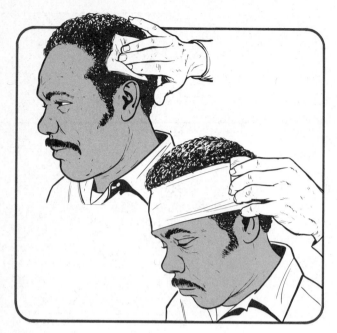

Figure 8-20: Caring for scalp wounds. Apply a sterile dressing, then bandage.

a triangular bandage. The steps for this process are shown in Figure 8-21.

Care of Facial Wounds   When treating a patient with facial injuries, keep in mind that there is likely to be a breathing problem associated with the wound and there also may be injury to the neck and spine. Monitor the patient to assure an open airway.

Check the patient's mouth for foreign matter as you assess the extent of oral cavity damage. Use your fingers to carefully sweep the inside of the person's mouth clean of broken dentures and teeth, gum, vomitus, or other obstructions. Look to see if an external injury to the cheek may have perforated the cheek wall, thus opening into the oral cavity.

If bleeding is profuse, position the patient so that drainage will be away from the throat. Suction away blood, mucus, and vomitus. Position the patient in the lateral recumbent (coma) position, with his head tilted back and turned so the mouth tilts downward. Should you suspect injury to the cervical spine, immobilize the patient's head, neck, and spine before moving him to a position for drainage (see Chapter 10).

Start artificial ventilation or CPR as required. Reposition the patient so that basic life support measures will be most effective. Facial damage may require you to use mouth-to-nose techniques, or, when injuries are slight, the bag-valve-mask unit. An adjunct airway may have to be inserted if injuries are severe (as long as the patient is unconscious, this airway can be left in place).

When caring for patients with facial injuries, you should:

1. Check for neck and spinal injuries, then correct any breathing problems.

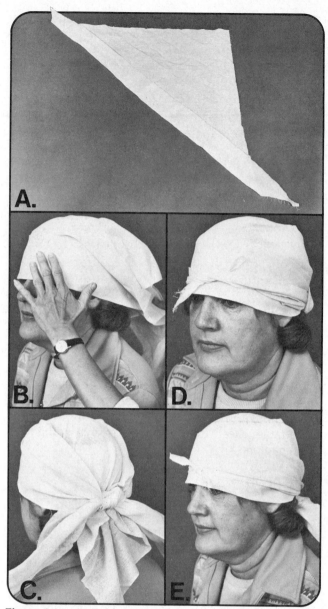

Figure 8-21: A. Fold a bandage several times to make a two-inch hem along its base. B. With the folded edge facing out, position the bandage on the patient's forehead, just above the eyes. The point of the bandage should hang down behind the head. C. Cross the front ends of the bandage behind the head, over the hanging point. D. Bring the ends to the front and tie them together. E. Draw the point of the bandage down and tuck it into the crossed folds.

2. Control bleeding by direct pressure on the wound, but use only enough pressure to stop the flow of blood. Remember, there may be facial fractures that are not obvious.

3. Apply a dressing and bandage.

You may need to use pressure point techniques to control bleeding. The temporal and the facial artery pressure point sites are useful (see Chapter 7), but take care not to apply pressure over possible fractures.

If blood vessels, nerves, tendons, or muscles have been exposed, they must be kept from drying

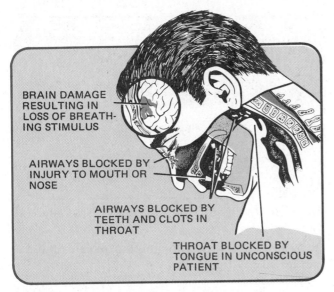

Figure 8-22: Injury-related breathing problems.

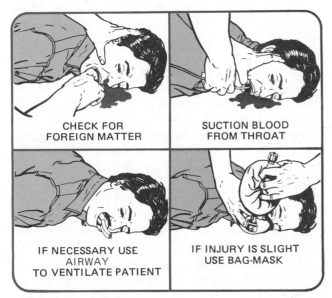

Figure 8-23: Correcting a breathing problem in a patient with facial injury.

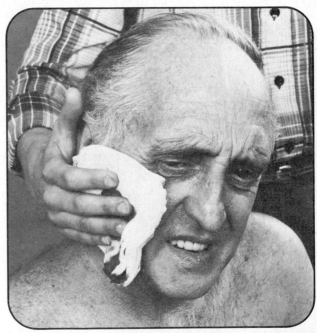

Figure 8-24: Care of soft tissue facial injury.

out. A sterile dressing, moistened with sterile saline (salt water made to equal the amount of salt in body fluids) can be used to dress this type of open wound. For short periods of time, sterile distilled water can be used. Distilled water is not sterile water. You must be certain that the water used is from a labeled, sterile source.

Partially avulsed facial skin can be returned to its normal position and dressings can be applied. Some systems use a sterile water wash of the wound before repositioning the flap. Your instructor will tell you if this is done in your area. Fully avulsed skin should be wrapped as described earlier, labeled, and transported with the patient.

A dangerous situation exists when the cheek has been penetrated by a foreign object. First of all, the object may go into the oral cavity and immediately become a possible airway obstruction, or it may stay

impaled in the wall, then work its way free and enter the oral cavity later. Secondly, when the cheek wall is perforated, bleeding into the mouth and throat may be profuse and interfere with breathing. Simple external wound care will not stop the flow of blood into the mouth.

If you find a patient with an object impaled in the cheek, you should:

1. Gently examine both the external cheek and the inside of the mouth. Carefully use your fingers to probe the inside cheek to determine if the object has passed through the cheek wall.

2. If the cheek is perforated, carefully *remove the impaled object* by pulling it out in the direction it entered the cheek. If this cannot be done easily, leave the object in place. Make certain that you position the patient's head for drainage. Spinal injuries may require you to immobilize the neck. Keep in mind that an object penetrating the cheek wall also may have broken teeth or dentures.

3. Once the object is removed, pack the inside of the cheek with rolled gauze between the cheek wall and the teeth. This also should be done in cases where the perforating object cannot be removed. Make sure you also stabilize the object on the external side of the cheek wall.

4. If the extent of injuries allow, keep the patient positioned for drainage. A lateral recumbent placement may be necessary during transport.

5. Dress the outside of the wound using a pressure dressing and bandage.

WARNING: Anytime you place something into a patient's mouth, you take on added responsibility for the patient. It is possible for objects such as

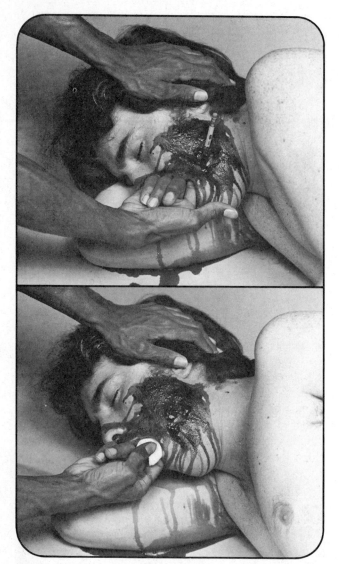

Figure 8-25: Procedure for removing an object impaled in the cheek.

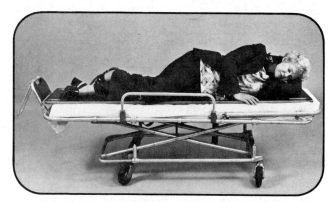

Figure 8-26: Transporting the patient with facial injuries.

on facial injury sites. Monitor the patient and be alert for airway problems.

Injuries to the Eye

Before considering the various types of eye injuries and their appropriate care, it is important to know the major structures of the eye and how it functions.

Structure and Function of the Eye   The eye is a globular structure, situated in a bony depression called the **orbit.** Each orbit is made up of parts of the bones of the forehead, temple, and upper jaw. Any serious blow to these bones may transfer the trauma to the eyes. The typical eye is almost one inch in diameter, with over 80% of the globe hidden within the orbit.

The white of the eye is the **sclera** (SKLE-rah). This is a semirigid capsule of fibrous tissue that helps to maintain the shape of the globe and contains the fluids found inside the eye.

The colored portion of the external eye is the **iris,** which has an adjustable opening called the **pupil.** In dim light, the pupil dilates to allow more light to enter, while in bright light, it constricts and restricts the amount of light entering the eye. Over the iris and pupil lies a clear portion of the sclera called the **cornea** (KOR-ne-ah). This structure protects the iris and pupil, and helps to keep fluids inside the eye. In addition, the cornea is highly involved with the eye's function of focusing light.

A thin delicate membrane called the **conjunctiva** (kon-junk-TI-vah) covers the sclera, the cornea, and the undersurfaces of the eyelids. When irritated, its tiny blood vessels become swollen with blood, giving the eye a "bloodshot" or pink appearance. This condition is know as conjunctivitis.

The internal eye is divided into an anterior and a posterior cavity. The anterior cavity exists between the cornea and the lens. The lens is located behind the iris and pupil. This cavity is filled with a clear, watery fluid known as **aqueous** (A-kwe-us) **humor** In some penetrating injuries, this fluid will leak from the eye, but with time and proper care, the body can

rolled gauze to become airway obstructions. Should the patient vomit, objects in the mouth can trap vomitus, which may be aspirated by the patient. This usually doesn't happen but the possibility exists. Keep close watch on any patient with anything placed into his mouth. Remember, too, that a conscious patient may not stay conscious.

Transportation of a Patient with Facial Injuries   Some facial injuries are relatively minor and require no special positioning of the patient. Patients with bleeding facial wounds should be transported in the lateral recumbent position with the head low to aid drainage. Since respiratory difficulty is often associated with this type of injury, this position is recommended, *provided* that spinal and neck injuries are properly cared for *before* positioning the patient, and that there are *no* indications of skull fracture. When the soft facial tissues are injured, there may be underlying bone fractures. Take care to transport the patient so that no unnecessary pressure is placed

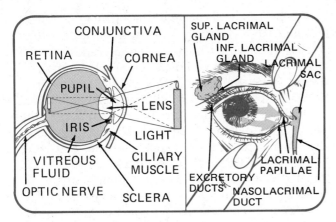

Figure 8-27: Anatomy of the eye.

replace it. The entire posterior cavity is located behind the lens. It is filled with a transparent jelly-like substance called the **vitreous** (VIT-re-us) **humor.** This substance is very important in maintaining the shape and length of the globe. Normal lens function takes place with a certain amount of pressure exerted on it by the vitreous humor. This gel *cannot* be replaced, and it *cannot* be restored by the body.

Light rays are bent when they pass through the cornea and the aqueous humor. This begins the focusing process. As light passes through the lens, muscular action changes the shape of the lens to focus the light on the **retina.** During this process, the image is inverted so that it focuses on the retina upside down (the brain reverts the image so that everything is seen in an upright position). The cells of the retina convert light into electrical impulses that are conducted through the optic nerve to the vision center of the brain. This is found at the back of the head in the **occipital** (ok-SIP-it-al) **lobe** of the brain.

The eye is protected by the eyelids. The inner surface of the eyelids and the surface of the eye are protected and moistened by tears produced by the **lacrimal** (tear) **gland.** Each time the eye blinks, the eyelids glide over the exposed surface, sweeping it clean of dust and other irritants. Tears are drained away through a lacrimal (tear) duct located in the medial corner of the eye, at the junction of the eyelids. This duct leads into the nasal cavity.

REMEMBER: It is important to keep the eyelids of an unconscious patient closed. An unconscious person has no involuntary blinking action to sweep tears across the exposed portions of the eyes. An unprotected eye will dry out quickly and become damaged. This damage may be permanent.

Types of Eye Injury Commonly seen eye injuries include:

- **Foreign Objects on the Eyes**—usually the patient complains of feeling the object and shows redness of the eye ("pink eye" or "bloodshot"). The eye often waters heavily with tears that may feel slippery.

- **Contusions**—these are closed wound injuries. There may or may not be damage to the eyelids. The patient usually complains of pain. If the patient says that he is having trouble seeing out of the injured eye, or if he reports double vision, then the damage may be very serious. The eye may appear reddened or swollen. Look at the iris. If it is not easily visible, or if you see blood between the cornea and the iris, the patient should be transported to a medical facility as soon as possible.

- **Abrasions**—minor scratches to the surface of the eye can be caused by foreign objects. Look for major scratches on the cornea. The cornea should appear clear, smooth, and wet. Do NOT touch the cornea or try to remove any foreign matter.

- **Lacerations**—look for cuts in the eyelids and the sclera. Consider a lacerated sclera to be a serious situation since a deep cut may allow vitreous humor to escape.

- **Puncture Wounds**—look for punctures, including eyelid perforations. Any puncture wound to the eye must be considered serious. Take great care to look for embedded and impaled objects.

- **Burns**—the patient and bystanders often are the source of information to tell you of a burn to eyes. The scene also may give clues. Look for highly irritated or damaged tissues. Burns to the eyelids indicate that there may be burns to the eyes.

- **Avulsions**—look to see if the eyelids are torn or torn away and if the eyeball protrudes or is pulled from its socket.

WARNING: Injury to the eye may mean that there are other head injuries, including brain damage. There also may be injuries to the cervical spine. Assume there are serious head injuries if: there are any indications of fractures around the orbit; the sclera is red due to bleeding; one or both eyes cannot be moved; one pupil is larger than the other; both pupils are unresponsive; one or both eyes protrude; or if the eyes cross or turn in different directions.

Emergency Care for Eye Injuries When caring for eye injuries, you will have to cover both eyes, even if only one eye is injured. Remember that when one eye moves, the other eye duplicates this movement. This action is called **sympathetic eye movement.** Explain to the patient why you must cover both eyes, and maintain contact with him to reduce his anxiety. If the patient is unconscious or has a low state of awareness, have someone with him at all times. This will help calm his fears should he regain consciousness or full awareness.

Foreign Objects—Some EMS Systems do not recommend that you wash a patient's eyes unless you are dealing with the problem of chemicals in the eye. If you are permitted to wash objects from the eye, be certain that the globe has not been deeply lacerated or penetrated. The steps for washing the eye are shown in Figure 8-28. If an object remains on the inner lid surface and will not wash away, use a sterile, moist applicator or gauze pad to *carefully remove this foreign body. NEVER ATTEMPT TO REMOVE AN OBJECT ON THE CORNEA. Do not try to probe into the eye socket or remove embedded objects.*

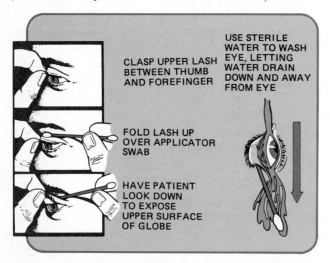

CLASP UPPER LASH BETWEEN THUMB AND FOREFINGER

USE STERILE WATER TO WASH EYE, LETTING WATER DRAIN DOWN AND AWAY FROM EYE

FOLD LASH UP OVER APPLICATOR SWAB

HAVE PATIENT LOOK DOWN TO EXPOSE UPPER SURFACE OF GLOBE

Figure 8-28: Washing a foreign object from the eye. Clasp upper lash between thumb and forefinger. Fold lash up over applicator swab. Have patient look down to expose upper surface of globe. Use sterile water (or saline) to wash eye, applying water at the medial corner of the eye socket.

Contusions—Some patients will request a cold pack or ice pack for bruised eyes. This may help relieve discomfort; however, this procedure should NOT be done if the patient shows any symptoms or signs of serious eye or head injury. You do not want to increase the risk of additional contamination, or cause rapid changes in circulation in the area of the injury.

Abrasions and Lacerations—If the eyelid is bleeding, do NOT apply a pressure dressing unless you are certain that there are no lacerations to the globe of the eye. Should the globe also have an open wound, cover the bleeding lid with loose dressings to aid clotting and prevent additional contamination.

In cases where there are no open wounds to the eyelid, but the globe of the eye is bleeding, or shows any other indication of an open wound, DO NOT APPLY PRESSURE. Use loose dressings.

REMEMBER: The jelly-like vitreous humor can be squeezed from an eye with an open wound. This substance cannot be replaced. Loss of vitreous humor can result in blindness.

Puncture Wounds—Use loose dressings for puncture wounds with no impaled objects. If you find an object impaled in the eye, you should:

1. Make a thick dressing with several layers of sterile gauze pads or multitrauma dressings.
2. Cut a hole in the center of this pad, approximately the size of the impaled object.
3. Carefully pass this dressing over the impaled object and position the pad so that the object is centered in the opening.
4. Fit a disposable drinking cup or paper cone over the impaled object and allow it to rest on the dressing pad. DO NOT allow it to touch the object. This will offer rigid protection and will call attention to the patient's problem.
5. Hold the rigid shield and cup in place with self-adherent roller bandage or with a wrapping of gauze.
6. The uninjured eye should be dressed and bandaged to reduce eye movement.
7. Reassure the patient and provide emotional support.

Burns—Burns to the eyes can be caused by chemicals, heat, or light.

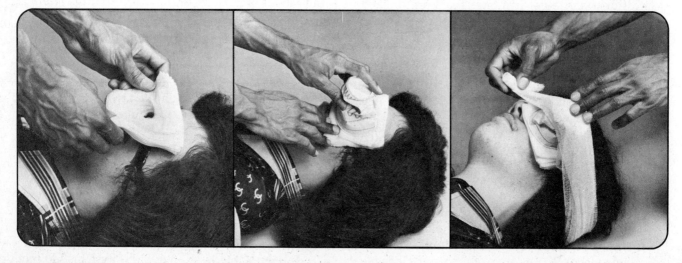

Figure 8-29: **Treating a patient with an object impaled in the eye.**

Chemical Burns—Flush the eyes with a steady stream of water, washing from the medial to the lateral corner. Use sterile water if it is available; otherwise, use tap water. Continue the wash for at *least* five minutes. If you know the chemical was an ALKALI, flush with water for at least fifteen minutes. Alkaline substances will continue to burn tissues even when diluted. For most chemical burns, it is best to irrigate the patient's eyes during transport to the medical facility, which means the patient receives care much sooner. If the ambulance does not carry special equipment for eye irrigation, use the rubber bulb syringe in the obstetrics kit. After washing, close the eyelid and apply a loose sterile dressing.

Heat Burns—In many cases, only the eyelids will be burned. Do NOT attempt to inspect the eyes if the eyelids are burned. With the patient's eyelids closed, apply a loose, moist dressing.

Light Burns—Light injuries can be caused by the flash from an arc welder or the extreme brightness of the sun as reflected off sand or snow. These burns are generally very painful, with many patients saying that it feels as if there is sand in the eyes. The onset is usually slow. In order to make the patient more comfortable, close his eyelids and apply dark patches over both eyes. If you do not have dark patches, ap-

ply a pad of dressings, followed with a layer of opaque material such as dark plastic.

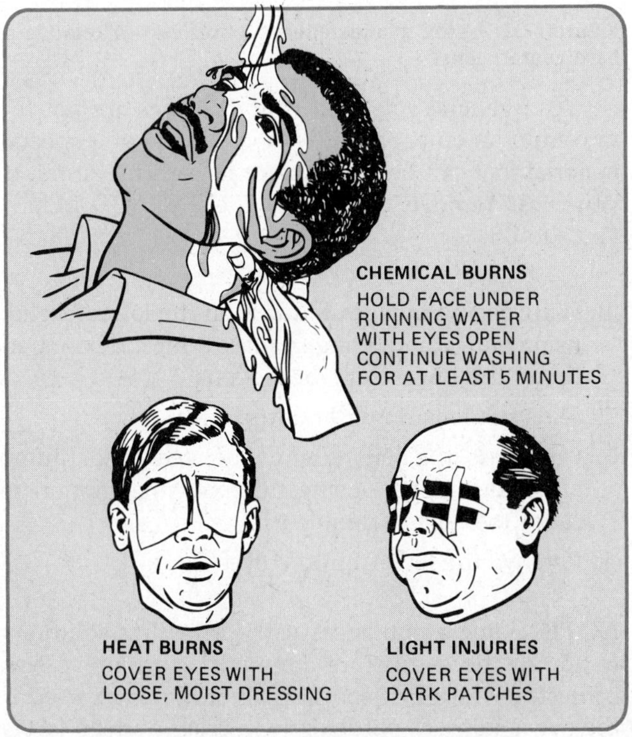

Avulsions—An avulsed eye is an eye pulled from its socket. This is a very rare occurrence. Do NOT try to force the eye back in. Treat an avulsed eye the same as you would an impaled object in the eye. Cut the dressing pad opening large enough so that the injured globe protudes through the hole. Wet the pad with sterile water or saline. Apply and secure in place a rigid protective device such as a disposable drinking cup.

Torn eyelids should be carefully covered with dressing materials. When the eyelid is torn off completely, the loose fragment should be recovered after proper wound care is completed on the remaining lid. Transport the avulsed part with the patient after wrapping the part in a moist sterile dressing and labeling appropriately.

Removing Contact Lenses   Care of eye injuries can be complicated by contact lenses. To avoid drying of the eyes and possible abrasive damage to the cornea, contact lenses should be removed from unconscious patients. Each contact lens is made to conform to the surface of the wearer's eye. Every time the person blinks, the lens moves. This movement is very important. The eye is a "breathing" organ, with gases being exchanged through the tissues. Since a contact lens shifts a little with each blink, gases cannot build up behind the lens to create pressure. An unconscious patient does not blink, so the lens will not move. Pressure can build quickly behind the lens causing what is known as a "blow out." The resulting damage to the cornea is permanent and may cause blindness.

It is not recommended that you remove contact lenses if there is obvious injury to the eye. To do so may cause additional damage. Some EMS Systems have guidelines as to *when* you can remove contact lenses. Follow the guidelines established in your area. Whenever you observe a patient wearing contact lenses, always report this fact to the medical facility staff.

Caring for patients with contact lenses is not as rare as you may think. Over 14 million people wear contact lenses, with the number of users growing at the rate of approximately 750,000 people per year. Four types of contact lenses are widely prescribed, the hard corneal, the flexible (soft lens), the "perma" lens, and the scleral lens.

- HARD CONTACT LENSES are the most common. When in position, this hard lens covers the cornea. It will appear to cover the entire iris. The typical size is about 0.3 inches in diameter (about the size of a shirt button).

- FLEXIBLE CONTACT LENSES are very popular. A flexible lens is slightly larger than a

CHEMICAL BURNS
HOLD FACE UNDER RUNNING WATER WITH EYES OPEN CONTINUE WASHING FOR AT LEAST 5 MINUTES

HEAT BURNS
COVER EYES WITH LOOSE, MOIST DRESSING

LIGHT INJURIES
COVER EYES WITH DARK PATCHES

Figure 8-30: Treating burns to the eyes.

dime—about 0.5 inches in diameter—and covers the entire cornea and part of the sclera.

- "PERMA" LENSES are long-term lenses worn by many postoperative cataract patients. These lenses are gaining in popularity with the general public, replacing flexible contact lenses. In the field, you will not be able to distinguish "perma" lenses from soft contact lenses.

- SCLERAL LENSES are the least common. About the size of a quarter, they cover the cornea and a large portion of the sclera.

To remove HARD CORNEAL LENSES, you should:

1. With clean hands, position one thumb on the upper eyelid and one thumb on the lower eyelid. Keep your thumbs near the margin (edge) of each lid.

2. Separate the eyelids and look for the lens over the cornea. The lens should slide easily with a gentle movement of the lids. If the lens is not directly over the cornea, slide it to that position with an appropriate movement of the eyelids.

3. Once the lens is over the cornea, open the eyelids further so that the margins of the lids are beyond the top and bottom edges of the lens (see Fig. 8-31). Maintain this opening.

4. Press both eyelids gently but firmly on the globe of the eye and move the lower lid so it is barely touching the edge of the lens.

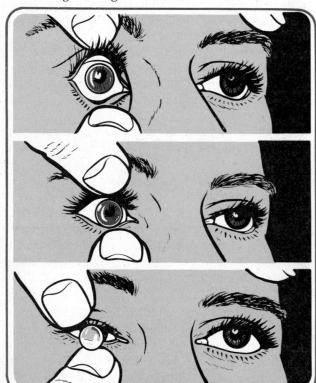

Figure 8-31: Removing a hard corneal contact lens.

5. Bring the upper lid margin close to the upper edge of the lens, keeping both lids pressed on the globe.

6. Press slightly harder on the lower lid, to move it under the bottom edge of the lens. This should cause the lens to tip outward from the eye.

7. When the lens has tipped sightly, begin to move the eyelids together. The lens should slide out between the eyelids where it can be removed.

REMEMBER: Never use force in removing a contact lens. If you see the lens but cannot remove it, gently slide it onto the sclera. The lens can remain there with greater safety until more experienced help is available.

NOTE: Special suction cups are available for the removal of hard contact lenses. They should be moistened with saline or sterile water before being brought into contact with the lens. The use of these cups is not recommended in cases of lacerated eyes.

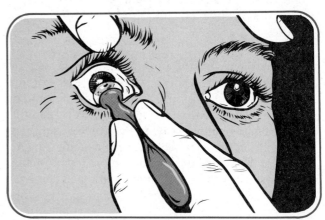

Figure 8-32: Using a moistened suction cup to remove a hard contact lens.

As a general rule, soft contact lenses are not removed in an emergency. They are made of a special material that can be left in place for several hours. If you *must* remove a FLEXIBLE CONTACT LENS, you should:

1. With clean hands, pull down on the lower eyelid, using your middle finger. Place your index fingertip on the lower edge of the lens.

2. Slide the lens down onto the sclera.

3. Compress the lens slightly between the thumb and index finger, using this pinching motion to cause the lens to double up.

4. Remove the lens from the eye.

NOTE: Some ambulances carry irrigating solutions to add to the eye before attempting to remove soft contact lenses. Such solutions should not be used if the eye is injured, particularly in cases of deep lacerations. Follow your local guidelines.

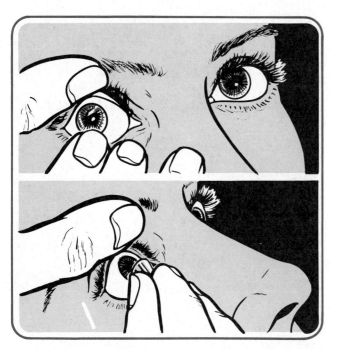

Figure 8-33: Removing flexible contact lenses.

To remove SCLERAL LENSES, you should:

1. With clean hands, position the index finger on the lower lid near the margin.
2. Slowly and carefully press the eyelid down until the bottom edge of the lens becomes visible. This requires more pressure than for the smaller corneal lenses, but avoid *excessive* pressure.

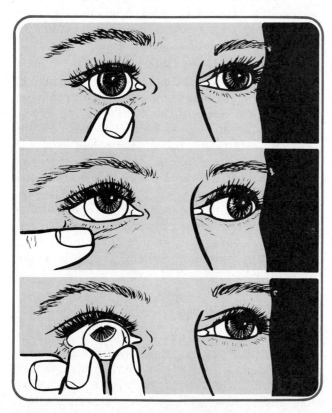

Figure 8-34: Removing a scleral lens.

3. Maintaining gentle but firm pressure on the eyelid, move your finger in a lateral direction to pull the eyelid taut.
4. The eyelid margin should slide under the lower edge of the lens, lifting the lens to a position where it can be grasped.

After the contact lenses have been removed, place them in a container with a little water or saline and label the container with the patient's name. The patient may have a contact lens case with him. Use this case when possible, making certain that is labeled with the patient's name.

For additional information, request a contact emergency care and instruction packet from the American Optometric Association, 7000 Chippewa Street, St. Louis, MO 63119.

Injuries to the Ear

Injuries to the ear often go undetected by the EMT, or, if detected, they are disregarded or treated lightly. Noting injury to the ear is very important since such an injury is a sign of more serious head injury. In addition, the internal structures of the ear may be damaged, leading to deafness and serious problems of balance.

Structure and Function of the Ears The ear is actually two important organs housed in one anatomical structure. One is the mechanism for *hearing*, in which sound waves are converted into nerve impulses. The other is a major part of our *sense of balance*, maintaining the proper relationship between head positioning and motion.

The ear is divided into three parts: the external ear, the middle ear, and the internal ear. Most of the ear's structures are hidden, housed in the temporal bone. This is the hardest bone in the human body.

The most prominent structure of the external ear is the **pinna** (PIN-nah) or **auricle** (AW-re-kl). Its shape is maintained by cartilage. The opening and the canal that runs from the pinna into the skull are called the **external auditory canal** (also called the external acoustic meatus, me-A-tus). This canal ends at the eardrum, the **tympanic** (TIM-pah-nik) **membrane**.

On the other side of the eardrum lies the middle ear, an air-filled chamber that connects with the nasal cavity by way of the internal auditory tube (eustachian tube). The middle ear contains three small bones, connected together to stretch from the drum to the inner ear. The inner ear is a maze of fluid-filled chambers hollowed out of bone. Sound waves cause the eardrum to vibrate. These vibrations, carried by the middle ear bones to the inner ear, cause the fluids to vibrate and stimulate special nerve endings. These nerves send impulses to the auditory center of the brain to be interpreted as specific sounds.

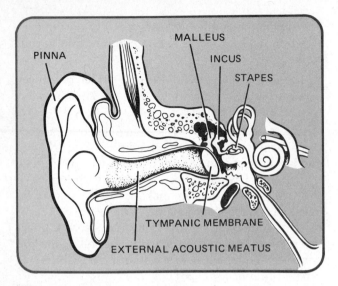

Figure 8-35: Anatomy of the ear.

The inner ear also has receptors that react to the motion of fluids each time the head or body changes position. Impulses are sent to the brain so that the body can make adjustments to stay balanced.

Types of Ear Injuries   All three parts of the ear can be injured. Contusions and crushing injuries to ear cartilage are closed wounds of the ear. Lacerations, abrasions, and avulsions can occur to the external ear. A ruptured eardrum is considered an external injury. You will not be able to tell if middle and inner ear structures are damaged, or if the symptoms and signs indicate an injury to the internal ear or the bones of the skull. Specific care procedures can be followed for external ear injuries, but the rest of the ear, if injured, must be cared for as if there is a skull fracture (see Chapter 10).

Patients may complain of ringing in the ears, internal ear pain, excessive wetness in their ears, and dizziness. You may observe blood or clear fluid coming from the ears, or a loss of balance as the patient attempts to reposition himself. Remember, ALL of these symptoms and signs may indicate a skull fracture. Clear or bloody fluids coming from the ear MUST be considered to be a sign of skull fracture.

Emergency Care for Ear Injuries

Abrasions and Lacerations—apply a sterile dressing and bandage in place.

Tears—apply bulky dressings so that the torn ear rests between layers of dressing. Bandage in place.

Avulsions—apply bulky dressings and bandage in place. If an avulsed part can be retrieved, place it in saline-soaked gauze in a plastic bag or wrap and transport the part with the patient. Keep the avulsed part cool. Make certain you label and wrap it.

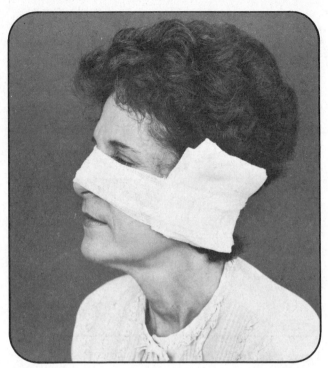

Figure 8-36: For external injuries to the ear, apply a dressing and bandage in place.

Bleeding from the Ears—Do NOT pack the external ear canal. To do so may cause additional injury and serious problems if there is a skull fracture. Loosely apply dressings to the external ear and bandage in place.

Clear Fluids Draining from the Ears—Do NOT pack the external ear canal. Apply loose external dressings. If possible, the dressings should be sterile. Bandage in place.

"Clogged" Ear and Objects in the Ear—When a patient complains of a clogged ear, this may be an indication that there is damage to the eardrum, fluids are in the middle ear, or foreign objects are in the ear canal. DO NOT PROBE INTO THE EARS. Prevent the patient from hitting the side of his head in an effort to free objects from the canal. Do NOT attempt to irrigate the canal with water if you cannot see the object or if there are indications of open wounds to the tissue. Some objects can be washed free using a rubber bulb syringe. Do so *only* if allowed in your EMS System. Transport all patients who complain of clogged ears.

Injuries to the Nose

The nasal cavity is divided into two chambers, right and left. Separating these two chambers is the **nasal septum.** It is made of cartilage that can be broken easily when struck by a blunt object. This can complicate soft tissue injury assessment and care. The nasal bones between the eyes also can be broken. Too often, assessment of the nose is made only in terms of the skin and the internal soft tissues.

We inhale primarily through the nose. Airway obstruction in the nasal cavity can occur with facial injury. Even though the mouth may be clear, blood and mucus released from nasal injuries can flow from the nose into the throat to cause a major airway obstruction. An open airway is your first priority in emergency care.

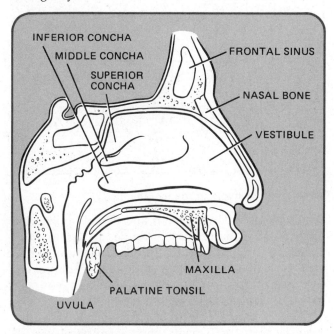

Figure 8-37: Anatomy of the nose.

Types of Nasal Injuries Contusions, abrasions, lacerations, puncture wounds, and avulsions can occur to the soft tissues of the nose. In addition, the EMT may have to treat problems caused by foreign objects in the nose.

When you see damage to the soft tissues of the nose, realize that other tissues also could be injured. The nasal septum or the nasal bones also may be damaged, increasing the chances of airway obstruction. The bones of the upper jaw, the **maxillae** (mak-SIL-e), and the lower jaw bone, the **mandible** (MAN-di-bl) may be fractured. The blow causing nasal damage may produce posterior head injuries in cases where the head is forced back against a hard object. Neck injuries also can be associated with nasal injuries.

Emergency Care of Nasal Soft Tissue Injuries Care for nasal injuries is usually conservative, directed toward maintaining an open airway, controlling bleeding, and positioning the patient so that blood does not drain into the throat.

Abrasions, Lacerations, Punctures—Control bleeding, apply a sterile dressing, then bandage in place.

Avulsions—Return any attached skin flaps to their normal position, then apply a pressure dressing and bandage. Fully avulsed skin and any avulsed portions of the external nose (usually the tip) should be recovered and wrapped in a sterile dressing moistened with sterile saline. This wrapped part should be labeled, kept cool, and transported along with the patient.

Foreign Objects—If the object protrudes, do NOT pull it free. It may have penetrated the septum or tissues high in the nose. Transport the patient without disturbing the object. If the object cannot be seen, do NOT probe for it. Have the patient gently blow his nose, keeping both nostrils open. Do not allow the patient to blow forcefully. If the object cannot be dislodged easily in this manner, transport the patient to a medical facility.

Nosebleeds—A nosebleed is called an **epistaxis** (ep-e-STAK-sis). In cases where there are no symptoms or signs of skull fracture, have the patient assume a seated position, leaning slightly forward. This position will provide better drainage for blood and mucus. If the patient is injured in such a way that a seated position is not practical, lay the patient back with the head elevated slightly, or simply turn the head to one side. Should the patient be unconscious, or if there are any indications of possible spinal damage, you will have to immobilize the neck and spine before positioning the patient for drainage. Suctioning may be required to keep the airway open.

When the patient can do so, have him pinch his nostrils shut to control bleeding. If the patient cannot, you will have to do so or have a

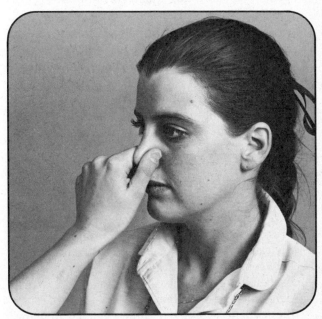

Figure 8-38: Treating a simple nosebleed.

bystander help to allow you to attend to other patients. Do NOT pack the patient's nostrils.

WARNING: If there is clear fluid coming from the nose or ears, clear fluid in the ears, or a mix of blood and clear fluids draining from the nose or ears, the patient probably has a skull fracture. Do NOT pinch the nostrils shut or attempt to stop the flow in any way.

Keep in mind that *all* nosebleeds are not the result of injuries related to accidents. High blood pressure can cause nosebleeds. So can infections and excessive sneezing. Such cases are usually easy to treat. Patients with bleeding diseases can have nosebleeds. Sometimes this type of bleeding can be difficult to control. Trauma-induced nosebleeds can range from minor to very serious. Prolonged or profuse nasal bleeding can cause a patient to develop shock.

Injuries to the Mouth

Injury to the soft tissues of the mouth generally results from blunt trauma, as when the lips are forcefully compressed against the teeth. Common injuries to the mouth include lacerations of the lips, inner cheek wall, or tongue. Avulsions of the lips and tongue also can occur. Often associated with soft tissue damage in the mouth is damage to the teeth. An open airway and proper drainage must be maintained throughout the care of the patient.

Emergency Care for Oral Injuries

Lacerated Lip or Gum—Control bleeding by placing a rolled or folded dressing between the lip and gum. If bleeding is profuse, position the patient to allow for drainage. Monitor so the patient does not swallow the dressing.

Lacerated or Avulsed Tongue—Do NOT pack the mouth with dressings. Position the patient for drainage. If the tongue is fully avulsed, (extremely rare), save and wrap the avulsed part and transport with the patient. You may find a portion of fully avulsed tissue still in the patient's mouth. Remove this tissue and wrap it for transport.

Avulsed Lip—Control bleeding with a pressure dressing and position for drainage. Save, wrap, and transport any fully avulsed tissues.

Lacerated or Perforated Inner Cheek—External pressure dressings will not control bleeding in the case of perforations. Rolled dressing, placed between the wound and the teeth, should be used for perforations and lacerations. The patient must be positioned for drainage. Monitor the patient to prevent him from swallowing dressing materials.

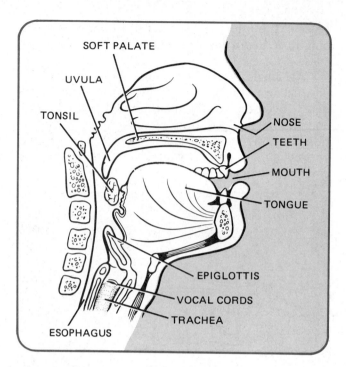

Figure 8-39: Anatomy of the mouth.

Problems involving teeth and dental appliances often occur with soft tissue injuries to the mouth. Search for and remove any dislodged teeth, crowns, or bridges. Remove dentures and the parts of broken dentures. Transport any dental appliance you remove, broken or intact, with the patient.

Take great care searching for dislodged teeth. Also, be alert for patients with a unilateral partial known as a Nesbit (commonly called a "spider"). This is typically a one- or two-tooth partial that is held in place at four points. People have been known to swallow such devices. If you find one in the mouth of an injured or an unconscious patient, remove it. You must take care not to drop the appliance down the patient's throat. When practical, position the patient with his head turned to the same side as the Nesbit. To avoid the problems caused by blood, mucus, and saliva, grasp the Nesbit with a piece of gauze dressing. Transport the device with the patient.

There will be bleeding from the socket of a dislodged tooth. To control this bleeding, have the conscious patient bite down on a pad of gauze placed over the socket. If the patient is unconscious you may have to place gauze into the socket. The less you disrupt the socket tissues, the better are the chances a dentist can replace the avulsed tooth successfully. Do NOT try to insert cotton packets into the socket.

Any avulsed tooth should be wrapped in moist dressings and transported with the patient. Do NOT rub the tooth to try to clean it. This will destroy microscopic structures needed to replant the tooth. Inform the emergency department staff that you have the avulsed tooth. The sooner a dentist or oral surgeon can replant the tooth, the better the chances of success. Best results are seen if the procedure is done within 30 minutes of the accident.

INJURIES TO THE SOFT TISSUES OF THE NECK

Injuries to the soft tissues of the neck can be classified as blunt or sharp. Either type can be so serious a life-threatening emergency that only immediate surgical intervention can save the patient.

Any injury to the neck must be considered serious until proven otherwise. The neck contains many vital structures, including the cervical portion of the spinal cord, the larynx and part of the trachea, a portion of the esophagus, the carotid arteries, and the jugular (JUG-u-lar) veins.

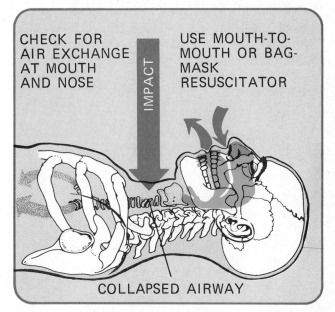

Figure 8-41: Blunt injuries to the neck.

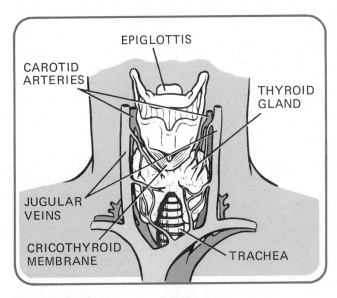

Figure 8-40: The anatomy of the neck.

Blunt Injuries

Blunt injuries to the neck can occur in a variety of accident situations. In a head-on vehicular accident, the driver may pitch forward and strike his neck against the steering wheel. Passengers often strike their necks on projections of the dashboard. The violent movements produced during an accident can throw people around inside the vehicle. Passengers may strike their necks on arm rests, seatbacks, and objects being carried in the passenger compartment. However, you should realize that a person may receive a serious neck injury in nothing more than a simple fall if his neck strikes some object.

Regardless of the cause, a major problem faced in blunt trauma to the neck is usually the collapse of the larynx or the trachea. These are rigid structures containing cartilage. Once they collapse or are crushed, they cannot spring back to their original shape and resume their normal function.

Symptoms and Signs of a Blunt Injury to the Neck For cases of blunt injury to the soft tissues of the neck, look for:

- The loss of voice.
- Signs of airway obstruction when the mouth and nose are clear and no foreign body can be dislodged from the airway.
- Contusions on or depressions in the neck.
- Deformities of the neck.
- Swelling or crackling sensations under the skin. This is known as **subcutaneous emphysema,** the result of air leaking into the soft tissues of the neck.
- Complaints of neck pain and tenderness.

Emergency Care for Blunt Trauma to the Neck Transport the patient to a medical facility without delay; emergency surgery may be needed to open the airway. Keep the patient calm and ask him to try to breathe slowly, if possible. Administer oxygen, using a bag-valve-mask unit, demand valve, or other form of ventilation-assist device if air must be forced past a complete obstruction.

REMEMBER: If the accident was serious enough to produce a blunt injury to the neck, it may have produced serious injury to the cervical spine. If basic life support measures must begin before immobilizing the neck, take *extreme care* to move the patient's head no more than absolutely necessary. Aggravation of cervical spine injuries can lead to permanent paralysis or death.

Sharp Injuries

The carotid arteries and the jugular veins pass through the neck relatively close to the body's surface. Sharp injuries to these vessels can produce catastrophic bleeding. Arterial bleeding will be profuse, with bright red blood spurting from the wound site. Venous bleeding can be profuse with a steady flow of dark red to maroon colored blood flowing steadily from the wound.

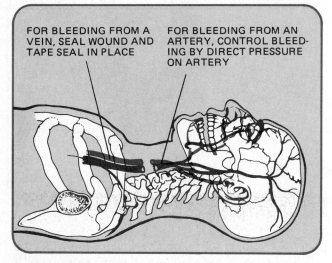

Figure 8-42: Sharp injuries to the neck.

Emergency Care for Severed Neck Artery

1. Apply direct pressure, using a sterile dressing, if one is available. Do NOT apply pressure over the airway, or to both sides of the neck at the same time. If this fails. . .
2. Attempt to control bleeding by utilizing the carotid artery pressure point technique. Simultaneous application of carotid artery pressure point techniques and direct pressure may improve your chance to control the bleeding.
3. Transport immediately, and administer a high concentration of oxygen.

Emergency Care for Severed Neck Vein Bleeding from a large neck vein usually cannot be controlled by direct pressure. Sometimes a large bulky dressing and firm hand pressure will control the bleeding, but usually the ends of the veins pull away from the wound site and bleed freely. In addition to loss of blood, there is the problem of air being sucked into the vein and carried to the heart as an air embolism. This is usually fatal. To control bleeding from a neck vein:

1. Apply an occlusive dressing or plastic wrap over the injury site.
2. Tape the dressing on all sides. The dressing must be *airtight*.
3. Transport immediately and administer a high concentration of oxygen.

INJURIES TO THE CHEST

Superficial open wounds to the chest include abrasions, lacerations, puncture wounds, and avulsions. You should treat these as you would any other superficial soft tissue injury. Deep wounds, crushing injury, severe blunt trauma, and impaled objects require special consideration because of the ribs, sternum, and organs of the thoracic cavity. Therefore, injuries to the chest will be covered in Chapter 10.

INJURIES TO THE ABDOMEN

The more you know about the structures of the abdomen and their positions the better you will be able to evaluate injuries in this region. Even with an EMT-level understanding of anatomy, it is difficult to be certain of many types of abdominal injury. **Referred pain** often occurs in the abdomen. This means that pain may be felt in an area other than the site of injury. Damage to the appendix may be expressed as pain below the xiphoid process. Injury to the gallbladder may be felt as pain on the back of the right shoulder. The head-to-toe survey is critical if you are to detect abdominal injuries.

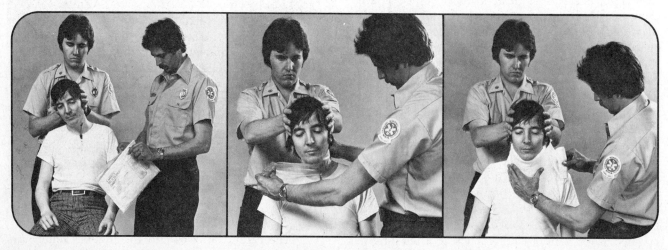

Figure 8-43: Apply an occlusive dressing in cases of severed neck veins.

In Chapter 2, the structures of the abdomen were named and related to the abdominal quadrants. Study this section again so that you can look at someone and know the approximate position for each major organ and gland, and relate these structures to the abdominal quadrants.

The abdominal organs can be classified as hollow or solid. The hollow organs are:

- *Stomach*—where the initial chemical breakdown of foods begins, producing a semisolid substance called **chyme** (kIm).

- *Small Intestine*—where chemical digestion is completed and absorption of foods takes place.

- *Large Intestine*—for the collection and removal of the wastes from digestion.

- *Appendix*—hollow finger-like tube located at the beginning of the large intestine. It has no proven function.

- *Gallbladder*—a pear-shaped reservoir for bile, located on the posterior undersurface of the liver.

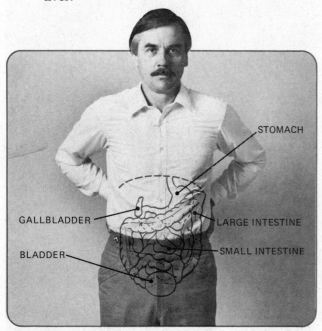

Figure 8-44: The hollow organs of the abdominopelvic cavity.

The solid organs are:

- *Liver*—large, multifunctional gland in the right upper quadrant, protected by the lower ribs. Its dome-shaped top presses against the diaphragm. Extremely vascular, the liver is a delicate gland that can be easily torn by blunt impact, or cut by penetrating objects. The resultant bleeding can be massive and quickly fatal. The liver is essential to life.

- *Spleen*—a highly vascular organ located behind the stomach and protected by the lower ribs on the left side of the body. The spleen is involved with blood storage and the removal of old blood cells. It is prone to rupture as a result of blunt trauma to the abdomen. A person can live without a spleen; however, when injured, the spleen can cause life-threatening bleeding.

- *Pancreas*—elongated, flat, triangular gland behind the stomach. It is involved with producing digestive juices and insulin. Serious injury to the pancreas is not common in accidents. When injured, as in abdominal gunshot wounds, the pancreas can bleed profusely. The pancreas is essential to life.

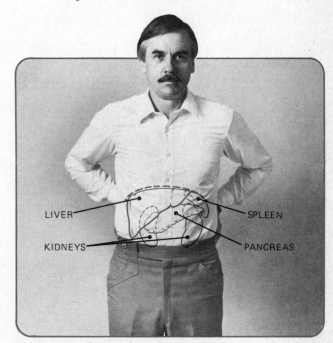

Figure 8-45: Solid organs of the abdomen.

Types of Abdominal Injury

Abdominal injuries can be open or closed, with closed injury usually due to blunt trauma. Internal bleeding can be severe if organs and major blood vessels are lacerated or ruptured. Very serious painful reactions can occur when the hollow organs are ruptured and their contents leak into the abdominal cavity.

Perforating wounds to the abdomen can be caused by objects such as knives, ice picks, arrows, and the broken glass and twisted metal of vehicle and structural accidents. Bullets can cause very serious perforating wounds, even when the bullet is of low caliber. Although some people believe otherwise, gunshot wounds without exit wounds can cause as much abdominal damage as those with exit wounds. Another misconception about bullet wounds is that it's easy to assess internal damage. Any projectile entering the body can be deflected, or it can explode and send out pieces in many directions. Do not believe that only the structures directly under the entrance wound have been injured. Also keep in mind that the pathway of a bullet between entrance wound and exit wound is seldom a straight line.

Complicating the problem even more is the fact that penetrating abdominal wounds can be associated with wounds in adjacent areas of the body. For example, a bullet can enter the thoracic cavity, pierce the diaphragm, and cause widespread damage in the abdomen. A complete patient survey is essential to determine the probable extent of injuries.

Symptoms and Signs of Injury

The symptoms of abdominal injury can include:

- Pain, often starting as mild pain then rapidly becoming intolerable.

- Cramps
- Nausea
- Weakness
- Thirst

The signs of abdominal injury can include:

- Rapid shallow breathing and a rapid pulse
- Low blood pressure (sometimes patients with abdominal injury who are in extreme pain show an initially elevated blood pressure)
- Obvious lacerations and puncture wounds to the abdomen
- Lacerations and puncture wounds to the pelvis, middle and lower back, or chest wounds near the diaphragm
- Coughing up blood

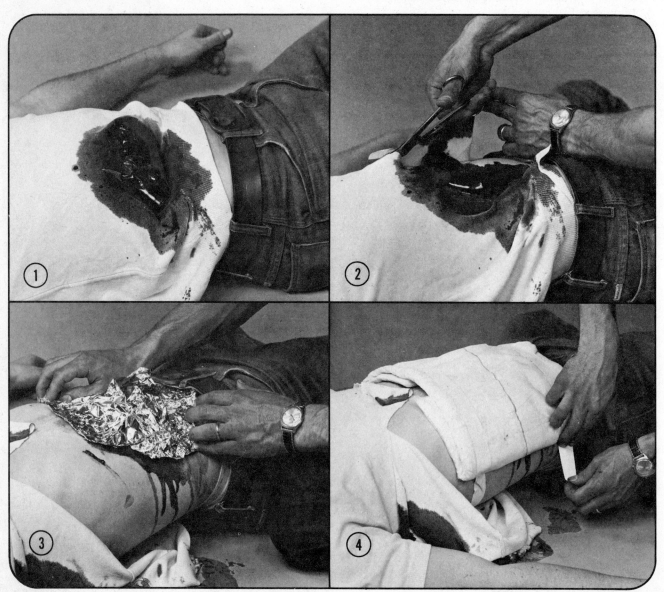

Figure 8-46: 1. Open abdominal wound with evisceration; 2. Cut away clothing from wound; 3. Apply an occlusive dressing; 4. Cover occlusive dressing to maintain warmth.

- Indications of blunt trauma, such as a large bruised area on the abdomen
- Rigid and/or tender abdomen
- The patient tries to protect his abdomen (guarded abdomen)
- The patient tries to lie very still, with his legs drawn up

Emergency Care for Abdominal Injuries

Care for open abdominal wounds by:

1. Controlling external bleeding and dressing all open wounds.
2. Laying the patient back, with the legs flexed to reduce pain by relaxing abdominal muscles.
3. Treating for shock and constantly monitoring vital signs (MAST garments may be required).
4. Being alert for vomiting.
5. Being certain not to touch any eviscerated (e-VIS-er-a-ted) or exposed organs. Cover such organs with an occlusive dressing (aluminum foil or plastic) and maintain warmth by placing dressings or a lint-free towel over top of the occlusive dressing.
6. Being certain NOT to remove any impaled objects. Remember to stabilize impaled objects with bulky dressings which are bandaged in place.
7. Transporting as soon as possible, while continuing to monitor vital signs. Administer oxygen and give nothing by mouth.

To care for closed abdominal injuries, you should:

1. Place the patient on his back with the legs flexed at the knees.
2. Treat for shock.
3. Apply a bulky pad held snugly in place with tape or bandage over the abdomen if there are any indications of internal bleeding or if the patient complains of extreme pain (see Fig. 8-47).
4. Keep alert for vomiting, making certain that the airway remains open.
5. Transport as soon as possible, administer oxygen, and give nothing by mouth. Monitor the patient's vital signs.

NOTE: Some patients show some relief of abdominal pain when allowed to hold a pillow or other soft, bulky object against the abdomen.

INJURIES TO THE PELVIS AND GROIN

The major structures housed in the pelvis include the urinary bladder, the end portions of the

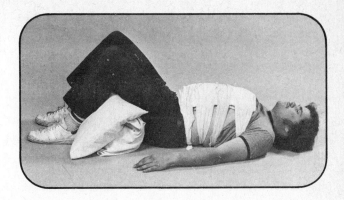

Figure 8-47: Treating a closed abdominal injury.

large intestine (including the rectum), and the internal reproductive organs. These structures are reasonably well protected, but they can be injured by intense blunt trauma, crushing injuries, and gunshot wounds.

The Urinary System

The urinary system includes the kidneys, which filter out wastes from the bloodstream and make urine; the ureters (u-RE-ter's), with one connecting each kidney to the urinary bladder; the urinary bladder, which serves as a reservoir for urine; and the urethra (u-RE-thrah), through which urine is expelled from the bladder.

The kidneys are not abdominal or pelvic organs. They are located behind the abdominal cavity. Severe blows to the back can cause kidney damage. Very often, kidney damage is not found by the EMT, even after a complete and proper patient survey. Likewise, damage to the urinary bladder, though severe, may not be evident to the EMT. Pain may not be felt *specifically* in the kidneys or the bladder.

NOTE: Consider back pain following blunt trauma to be an indication of possible kidney damage. If the patient has blood in his urine, assume that there are

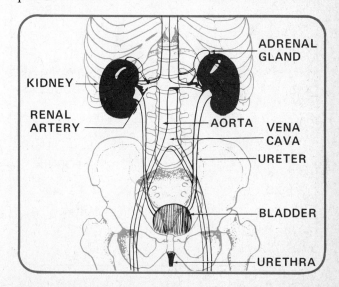

Figure 8-48: The urinary system.

serious problems within the urinary system. Treat as you would for internal abdominal organ injuries.

Reproductive System

Injury can occur to both the external and the internal reproductive organs. The external reproductive organs are often referred to as the external **genitalia** (jen-i-TA-le-ah). More injuries occur to these structures than to the internal reproductive organs, because of the protection offered by the bones of the pelvis. However, because of the locations of the external reproductive organs, injuries are not common. **NOTE:** Caring for genital injuries can be embarrassing for both patient and EMT. Approach the prob-

lem in a professional manner. Decide on a course of action and then act with authority as a member of the professional health care team. Timid, hesitant movements will only add to the patient's embarrassment. Explain what you are going to do and why, then provide care with no hesitation. Protect the patient from the stares of onlookers. When emergency care measures are completed, cover the patient with a sheet.

Table 8.1: The Reproductive Systems.

MALE		
STRUCTURE	INJURY	CARE
Scrotum (SKRO-tum) surrounds and protects the testes	Blunt trauma Lacerations and Avulsions (rare)	Ice pack, transport. Direct pressure, dressing, and triangular bandage applied like diaper. Keep avulsed parts moist and wrapped.
Testes (TES-tez) produce sperm cells and male hormone	Blunt Trauma Lacerations and Avulsions (rare)	Same as scrotum Same as scrotum
Spermatic (sper-MAT-ic) Cords suspend testes, each contains blood vessels, nerves, and vas deferens (vas DEF-er-en's) which transport sperm.	Blunt Trauma Lacerations (rare)	Same as scrotum Same as scrotum
Prostate (PROS-tat) Gland produces seminal fluids	Rare, usually gunshot wounds	Pressure dressing, treat for shock, oxygen.
Seminal Vesicles store seminal fluids	Rare, usually gunshot wounds	Same as prostate
Penis erectile organ containing the urethra	Blunt trauma Lacerations and Avulsions (also called amputation) Blunt trauma to an erect penis (known as "fracture")	Same as scrotum Same as scrotum Ice pack and transport

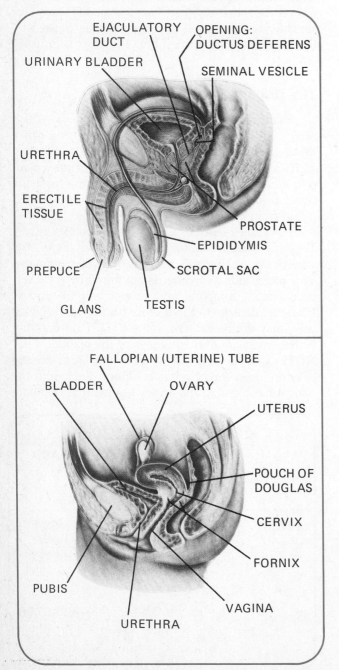

Figure 8-49: The male and female reproductive systems.

FEMALE

STRUCTURE	INJURY	CARE
Vulva (VUL-vah) external genitalia	Blunt Trauma	Ice pack, transport.
	Lacerations and Avulsions	Sanitary napkin and triangular bandage applied like diaper. Keep avulsed parts moist and wrapped.
Vagina birth canal	Lacerations (seen in rape and self-mutilation cases)	External application of sanitary napkin and triangular bandage.
Uterus (U-ter-us) womb for the developing fetus	Rupture due to extreme blunt trauma or crushing injury, especially during pregnancy	Unable to tell in field what organ is injured. Vaginal bleeding often profuse. Treat as internal injury with internal bleedng, apply sanitary napkin and triangular dressing over vaginal opening. This is a TRUE EMERGENCY.
	Lacerations (rare) usually due to gunshot or stab wound.	Treat as penetrating or perforating wound. Vaginal bleeding may or may not be seen.
Oviducts (O-vi-dukts) or Fallopian (fah-LO-pe-an) tubes carry egg (ovum) from the ovary to the uterus	Lacerations (rare) usually due to gunshot wound	Treat as penetrating or perforating wound Vaginal bleeding is usually not seen.
Ovaries (O-vah-res) produce female hormones and ova (O-vah) or eggs	Lacerations and puncture wounds (rare) usually due to gunshot or stab wounds	Treat as penetrating or perforating wound. Associated vaginal bleeding not likely.

Inguinal Hernia

Commonly called a "rupture," the **inguinal hernia** occurs when the intestine or bladder bulges into, or actually breaks through the inguinal canal. Typically, this is caused by pressure built up on the abdominopelvic cavity when a person attempts to lift a heavy object improperly. This also is seen when

someone tries to use his leg to slide a heavy object. Even small hernias can cause intense pain. A full herniation may have a significant portion of the intestine bulge into the scrotum, causing the patient to faint from pain.

Care for inguinal hernia varies from system to system. Since the blood supply to the intestine can be shut off due to constriction (strangulating hernia), transport is recommended. Patient positioning is important to reduce pain. Let the patient assume a position that is most comfortable. Suggest that he try lying on his back. Next, try to tilt the patient's body slightly so that he is in a head-low position. Should the pain remain too severe for the patient, try placing a pillow under his knees. If pain is still intense, have the patient turn over onto his stomach and assume a knee-chest position by drawing the knees up until they rest against the chest. Keep in mind that the most favorable position for the patient may not be possible during transport to assure patient safety. Most patients will be able to be transported in the supine position.

SUMMARY

The basic rules of open and closed injury care presented in Section One apply to specific areas of the body as covered in Section Two. You must know care procedures in an *exact* step-by-step fashion, so no attempt will be made to quickly review each procedure. Specific care procedures require you to remember certain rules and exceptions to rules. For example:

SCALP WOUNDS—Do NOT try to clear the surface of the scalp and do NOT apply finger pressure if there is any chance of skull fracture. Control bleeding with a dressing held in place by roller bandage or apply a triangular bandage.

FACIAL WOUNDS—Correct breathing problems, control bleeding, and dress and bandage the wound. *Position for drainage.* Remember, you can remove impaled objects from the cheek, provided that the object has passed through the cheek wall into the oral cavity.

EYE WOUNDS—You need to remember:

- Do NOT apply direct pressure to a lacerated eyeball.
- Do NOT attempt to remove foreign materials from the cornea.
- Do NOT remove impaled objects. Cover with a cut dressing pad and a rigid shield (e.g., paper cup), both bandaged into place.
- Do NOT try to replace an avulsed (extruded) eyeball. Treat as you would an impaled object, but moisten the dressing pad with *sterile* distilled water or saline.

- Do NOT open the eyes of a patient who has burns to the eyelids.

- DO remove contact lenses from unconscious patients with no serious eye injuries. Close the eyes of unconscious patients.

- According to your EMS System, wash foreign objects from eyes if there are no serious lacerations or puncture wounds.

- Treat chemical burns by washing the patient's eyes with flowing water. Hold the eyelids open for the wash to be effective.

- When you must cover a patient's eye, cover both eyes to reduce sympathetic movments.

EAR WOUNDS—Do NOT probe into the external ear canal and do NOT pack the canal with dressing or cotton. For lacerations and bleeding, apply dressings and bandage. Save avulsed parts in saline-soaked gauze wrapped in plastic or aluminum foil.

NOSE INJURIES—*Maintain an open airway*. Do NOT pack the nostrils. Bleeding from the nose (epistaxis) is best controlled by pinching the nostrils shut. Provide for proper drainage away from the throat. Keep avulsed parts moist.

INJURY TO THE MOUTH—*Maintain an open airway and allow for drainage*. Do NOT pack the mouth with dressing materials. If dressings are placed between cheek and gum, keep alert so they are not swallowed. Save all avulsed parts, including teeth. Avulsed teeth should be transported wrapped in moist dressings.

NECK WOUNDS—A neck wound indicates possible *spinal injury*. Treat arterial bleeding with pressure dressings. Venous bleeding from the neck will require the application of a bulky dressing and direct pressure. Treat serious venous bleeding with an occlusive dressing.

ABDOMINAL INJURIES—Look for the signs of abdominal injury and internal bleeding. Note if the patient's abdomen is rigid or tender. Treat for shock and be alert for vomiting. Flex the patient's legs to help reduce pain in cases of closed injury.

INJURIES TO THE GENITALIA—Conduct your examination and provide care in the strictest professional manner. Control bleeding by direct pressure and obey the general rules for open wound care. Remember that a sanitary napkin serves well as a bulky dressing and that a triangular bandage can be applied like a diaper.

9 injuries ii: the extremities

TERMS you may be using for the first time:

Axial (AK-si-al) **Skeleton**—the skull, spine, ribs, and sternum.

Appendicular (AP-en-DIK-u-ler) **Skeleton**—the upper and lower extremities.

Articulation (ar-TIK-u-LAY-shun)—formation of a joint where two or more bones come together.

Periosteum (per-e-OS-te-um)—the white fibrous membrane covering a bone.

Ligament—tissue that connects bone to bone.

Tendon—tissue that connects muscle to bone.

Open Fracture—either a broken bone with the ends or fragments tearing outward through the skin, or a penetrating wound with a fracture.

Closed Fracture—a broken bone with no soft tissue damage extending out through the skin.

Angulated Fracture—a break to a bone causing the limb or joint to take on an unnatural shape or bend.

Dislocation—injury causing the end of a bone to be pulled from its joint.

Sprain—partially torn ligament.

Strain—the overstretching or mild tearing of a muscle.

Crepitus (KREP-i-tus)—a grating sensation or sound made when fractured bone ends rub together.

Splinting—the process used to immobilize fractures and dislocations so that there is a minimum of movement to the bone and to the joints above and below the bone.

Traction—to pull gently along the length of an extremity prior to splinting.

Traction Splinting—to use a special splint to apply a constant pull along the length of a lower extremity. This helps to stabilize the fractured bone.

INTRODUCTION

Many students have an interest in extremity injuries and eagerly await the part of their training where they will study injuries to the bones and joints. A few hours of disciplined study enable them to learn the names and locations of the bones, how to classify and detect probable fractures, and how to apply splints to these injuries. However, while they are learning this new information, some students may forget what they have been taught about soft tissues. The muscles, nerves, connective tissues, and blood vessels are no longer considered as they should be in care procedures. This can carry over into the field; some EMTs become so concerned about detecting and caring for fractures that they fail to notice other injuries.

REMEMBER: When a bone is fractured, the damage to blood vessels, nerves, and other soft tissues is of greater significance than the fracture. Proper care of bone and joint injuries MUST include efficient soft tissue care.

Figure 9-1 shows the major blood vessels and muscles, along with a few of the major nerves found in the upper and lower limbs. As a EMT, you do not need to know *every* structure found in an extremity. However, you will need to remember how complex these structures are and consider the damage that may be done to soft tissues in cases of possible fracture or dislocation.

THE SKELETAL SYSTEM

The skeletal system is made up of all the bones and joints in the body. It is really only a part of a more complex system called the **musculoskeletal system.** This system is composed of all the bones, joints, muscles, tendons, ligaments, and cartilages in the body.

Bones are not simply mineral deposits that require less care than other living tissues of the body. If you do not realize that bones are hard yet somewhat flexible living structures, you may find yourself providing improper care.

Functions of the Skeletal System

The skeletal system provides the body with four major functions. The bones *support,* creating a framework to give the body form and to provide a rigid structure for the attachment of muscles and other body parts. Bones **articulate** (ar-TIK-u-lat) or connect to other bones to form joints, some of which are movable. Acting with muscles, bones and their joints allow for body *movement.* Bones also serve to provide *protection* for the vital organs. The skull protects the brain; the spinal column encloses and protects the spinal cord; the ribs protect the heart, lungs, liver, stomach, and spleen; and the bones of the pelvis protect the urinary bladder and the internal reproductive organs. Bones also protect a soft tissue called marrow that is found within them. Some bones have red bone marrow that contains cells involved in *blood cell production.*

The Anatomy of Bone

Bones are classified according to their appearance. There are long, short, flat, and irregular bones. The bones found in the arm and thigh are examples of **long bones.** The major **short bones** of the body

ANATOMY OF THE EXTREMITIES

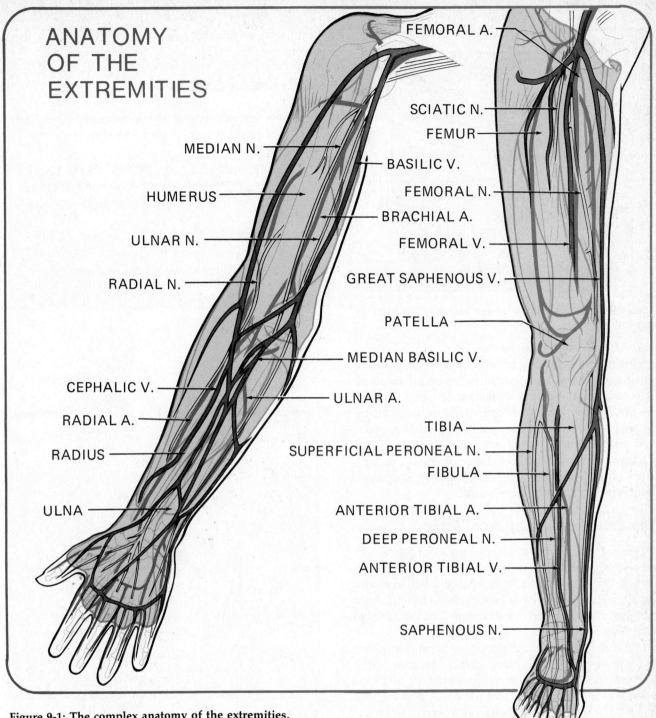

MEDIAN N.

HUMERUS

ULNAR N.

RADIAL N.

CEPHALIC V.

RADIAL A.

RADIUS

ULNA

FEMORAL A.

SCIATIC N.

FEMUR

BASILIC V.

FEMORAL N.

BRACHIAL A.

FEMORAL V.

GREAT SAPHENOUS V.

PATELLA

MEDIAN BASILIC V.

ULNAR A.

TIBIA

SUPERFICIAL PERONEAL N.

FIBULA

ANTERIOR TIBIAL A.

DEEP PERONEAL N.

ANTERIOR TIBIAL V.

SAPHENOUS N.

Figure 9-1: The complex anatomy of the extremities.

are in the hands and feet. Among the **flat bones** are the sternum, shoulder blades, and ribs. The vertebrae of the spinal column are examples of **irregular bones.**

The outward appearance of a typical long bone creates the impression that it is a simple, rigid structure, made of the same material throughout. Most people are aware that bone contains calcium, making it very hard. Bone also contains protein fibers that give it a degree of flexibility. The strength of our bones is a combination of this hardness and flexibility. As we age, there is less protein formed in the bones. As a result, they become brittle and fracture more easily than when we are young.

Bones are covered by a strong, white, fibrous material called the **periosteum** (per-e-OS-te-um). Blood vessels and nerves pass through this membrane as they enter and leave the bone. When bone is exposed as a result of injury, the periosteum becomes visible. You may see fragments of bones and foreign objects on this covering, but do not remove them. If they have pierced the tissue, the objects may offer a great deal of resistance to any pulling or sweeping efforts. In addition, you will not be able to tell if the object has entered the bone, or is impaled in an underlying blood vessel or nerve.

The typical long bone has a **shaft** that is cylindrical in shape. The shafts of bones appear to be

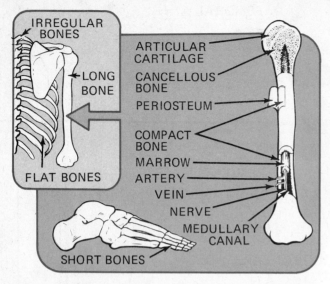

Figure 9-2: The anatomy of bone and classification by shape.

straight, but each bone has its own unique curvature. When the end of a bone is involved in forming a ball-and-socket joint, it will be rounded to allow for rotational movement. This rounded end is called the **head** of the bone. It is connected to the shaft by the **neck.** The ends of bones forming joints are covered with cartilage called **articular cartilage.** Bone marrow is contained in the center of bones. In long bones, this is found in a narrow cavity known as the **medullary** (MED-u-lar-e) **canal.**

The Self-Healing Nature of Bone

Before discussing fractures and emergency care procedures, let us examine how a broken bone repairs itself. Understanding this process will give you an appreciation of why a broken bone must be immobilized *quickly* and must *remain* immobilized to heal properly.

The first effect of an injury to a bone is swelling and the formation of a blood clot in the area of the fracture. Both are due to the destruction of blood vessels in the periosteum and the bone, and the loss of blood from adjacent damaged vessels. Interruption of the blood supply causes death to the cells at the injury site. Cells a little further from the fracture site remain intact and, within a few hours of the trauma, begin to divide rapidly to form a mass of new tissue. This mass grows together to form a collar of tissue that completely surrounds the fracture site. New bone is generated from this mass to eventually heal the damaged bone. The whole process can take weeks or months, depending on the bone that has been fractured, the type of fracture, and the health and age of the patient. Should the fractured bone be mishandled early in care, more soft tissues can be damaged, requiring a longer period for the formation of a tissue mass and replacement of the bone. If the bone ends are disturbed during regener-

ation, proper healing will not take place, and a disability results.

THE HUMAN SKELETON

There are 206 bones in the human body. Each bone is a part of one of the two major divisions of the skeletal system:

- AXIAL (AK-si-al) SKELETON: All the bones forming the upright axis of the body, including the skull, spinal column, sternum, and ribs.
- APPENDICULAR (AP-en-DIK-u-ler) SKELETON: All the bones forming the upper and lower extremities, including clavicles, scapulae, arms, forearms, wrists, hands, pelvis, thighs, legs, ankles, and feet.

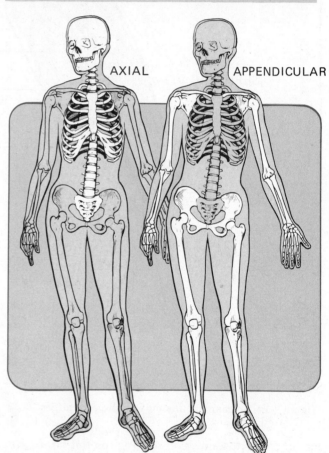

Figure 9-3: The major divisions of the skeletal system.

In this chapter, we will consider the structures making up the appendicular skeleton. The axial skeleton is covered in Chapter 10.

The Upper Extremities

As an EMT, you will be expected to know the medical names for the major bones in the body. This will allow you to communicate better with the other members of the patient care team and to utilize materials available for your continuing education.

Should you ever forget the medical name of a bone when presenting information to the emergency department staff, use the common name of the bone. The staff has been trained for such occasions.

NOTE: When a physician uses the term "arm," he is referring to the upper arm or humerus. The lower arm is the forearm. The entire structure, from shoulder to fingertips, is the upper extremity.

COMMON NAME	MEDICAL NAME
Shoulder girdle	Pectoral girdle (pek-TOR-al): clavicle, scapula, and head of humerus
Collarbone (1/side)	Clavicle (KLAV-i-kul)
Shoulder blade (1/side)	Scapula (SKAP-u-lah)
Arm bone (1/limb, from shoulder to elbow)	Humerus (HU-mer-us)
Forearm bones (2/limb, from elbow to wrist, 1 medial, 1 lateral)	Ulna (UL-nah)—medial Radius (RAY-de-us)—lateral
Wrist bones (8/wrist)	Carpals (KAR-pals)
Hand bones (palm bones, 5/palm)	Metacarpals (meta-KAR-pals)
Finger bones (14/hand)	Phalanges (fah-LAN-jez)

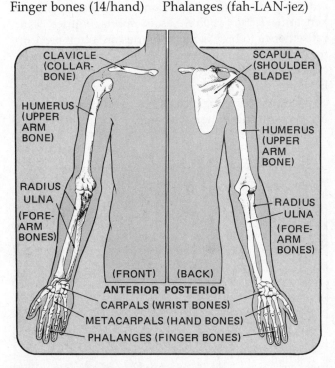

Figure 9-4: Bones of the upper extremity.

The Lower Extremities

NOTE: To a physician, the hip is the joint formed by the pelvis and the head of the femur. Many patients commonly refer to the lateral pelvis as their hip. The medical staff will call the upper leg the "thigh" and the lower leg the "leg." From pelvis to the tips of the toes is the lower extremity.

COMMON NAME	MEDICAL NAME
Pelvic girdle (pelvis or hips)	Os coxae (os KOK-se) or pelvis: on each side are the fused bones of the ilium, ischium, and pubis bone.
Thigh bone (1/limb)	Femur (FE-mer)
Kneecap (1/limb)	Patella (pah-TEL-lah)
Leg bones (shin bones, 2/leg, 1 medial, 1 lateral)	Tibia (TIB-e-ah)—medial Fibula (FIB-yo-lah)—lateral
Ankle bones (7/foot)	Tarsals (TAR-sals)
Foot bones (5/foot)	Metatarsals (meta-TAR-sals)
Toe bones (14/foot, some people have two bones in their little toe, others may have three)	Phalanges (Fah-LAN-jez)

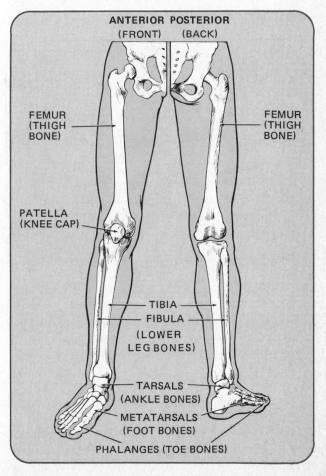

Figure 9-5: Bones of the lower extremity.

INJURIES TO BONES AND JOINTS

Structures of the musculoskeletal system are subject to injury from fractures, dislocations, sprains, and strains.

FRACTURES

By simple definition, a **fracture** is any break in a bone, including chips, cracks, splintering, and complete breaks. There are two basic types of fractures. A **closed fracture** (simple fracture) occurs when a bone is broken, but there is no penetration extending from the fracture through the skin. In other words, pieces of bone have not been forced outward to rip through the skin. In many cases of closed fracture, soft tissue damage is minor. In some cases, because of bone end displacement, soft tissue damage may be great with the damage being difficult to detect. Internal bleeding may be profuse.

An **open fracture** (compound fracture) can occur one of two ways. A bone can be fractured with soft tissues damaged from the fracture, outward through the skin. Pieces of bone may actually penetrate through the skin. In the other case, a penetrating wound can produce fractures. The wound is open from skin to the injured bone.

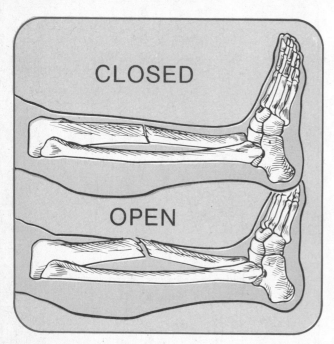

Figure 9-6: Basic types of fractures.

An **angulated fracture** involves a broken bone with the limb or joint taking on a new shape (the humerus may be bent or twisted between the shoulder and the elbow). Angulated fractures can be mild or very severe, occurring with both open and closed fractures.

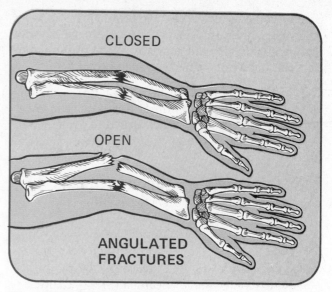

Figure 9-7: Angulated fractures.

Causes of Fractures

Enough force to fracture a bone can be applied in a variety of ways. *Direct violence* can fracture a bone at the point of contact. A person may be struck by the bumper of an automobile and suffer a fracture at the point where the leg was hit. *Indirect violence* also can fracture bones. This happens when forces are carried from the point of impact to the bone, as when a person falls on his hand and receives a broken arm. *Twisting forces,* as in sports injuries, can cause bones to break. Such injuries are often seen in football and skiing accidents where a person's foot is caught and twisted with enough force to fracture a leg bone. *Aging* and *bone disease* can increase the risk of fractures (pathologic fractures), with bones breaking even during minor accidents.

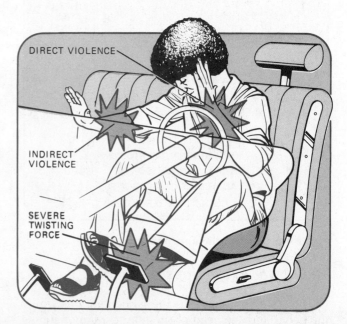

Figure 9-8: Bones may be fractured in a variety of ways.

Fractures may be hard to detect. When assessing a patient, you should always consider if the accident is of the type that might cause broken bones, the age of the patient, and the general health of the patient.

OTHER INJURIES

The most severe injuries to bones are fractures. Severe injuries to joints can be the result of fractures or dislocations. Joints occur wherever two or more bones articulate. The resulting joint can be immovable, as seen when two bones join together to form part of the cranium. Most joints are movable joints, such as the hinge joint of the elbow and the ball-and-socket joint of the hip.

A joint consists of the ends of the two joining bones, with these ends usually covered by articular cartilage. The highly movable joints in the body are **synovial joints.** They are surrounded by a fibrous **joint capsule** and contain membranes that produce a slippery fluid to lubricate joint movements. Injury to synovial joints can include injury to the capsule, the bone ends, and the ligaments that hold the bone ends in place.

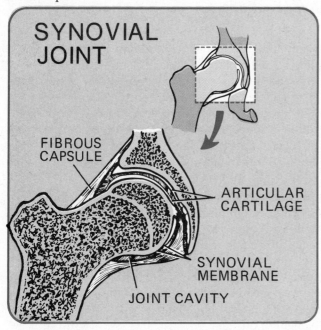

Figure 9-9: The anatomy of a synovial joint.

Dislocations occur when one end of a bone making up a joint is pulled out of place. Usually, the dislocated bone is pulled from its socket. Soft tissue injury can be very serious, including damage to blood vessels, nerves, and the joint capsule. Major blood vessels and nerves tend to be well protected in most parts of the body. However, in a movable joint, these structures lie close to the bones forming the joint.

Ligaments connect bone to bone, holding the ends in place to help form and strengthen joints. When ligaments are torn, **sprains** occur. These are

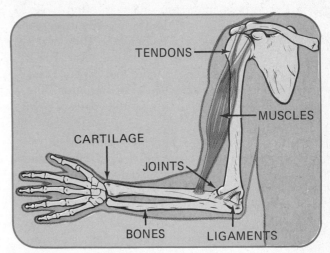

Figure 9-10: Ligaments, tendons, and joints.

different from **strains,** where muscles are stretched or where mild tearing of the muscle takes place.

NOTE: You will often have to treat injuries to the extremities as being fractures. Dislocations, sprains and some strains are difficult to distinguish from fractures. In certain cases, you will be able to tell that a dislocation has taken place. Most of the time, you will have to assume that any severe injury to an extremity has a possible fracture and treat accordingly.

SYMPTOMS AND SIGNS OF INJURY TO BONES AND JOINTS

The symptoms and signs of a fracture can include:

- The patient says that he felt a bone break or heard the bone snap.

- The patient tells you that he heard grating noises when he moved a limb. This sound is known as **crepitus** (KREP-i-tus). It is caused when the broken bone ends rub together. Do NOT ask him to move the limb so you can hear the noise.

- Deformity—If a part of a limb appears different in size, shape, or length than the same part on the opposite side of the patient's body, you must assume there is a fracture. Always compare both upper and lower limbs. If a bone or a joint appears to have an unusual angle, consider this deformity to be a reliable sign of fracture. Gently feel along the patient's limbs noting any lumps, fragments, or ends of fractured bones.

- Swelling and discoloration—These begin shortly after injury. Discoloration may start as a reddening of the skin. Black and blue bruises will not occur for several hours.

• Tenderness and pain—Pain is often severe and constant. The tissues directly over the fracture will be very tender. You should gently touch the area along the line of a bone in order to determine if there is a possible fracture and the exact location of the injury site. Do NOT probe into or near the edges of open fractures.

• Loss of function—The patient may not be able to move a limb or part of a limb. Sometimes he will be able to move a limb, but the movement will produce intense pain. If the patient can move the arm, but not the fingers, or if he can move the leg, but not the toes, there may be a fracture that has caused damage to adjoining nerves and blood vessels.

• Loss of radial or pedal pulse—The loss of a distal pulse is very serious.

• Crepitus (as a sign)—When the patient moves, the ends of the fractured bone rub together to produce a grating sound. If you hear this sound, do NOT ask the patient to move again so that you can confirm the sign.

• Exposed bone—Fragments or the ends of fractured bone may be visible where they break through the skin in some cases of open fractures.

• False motion—When the patient moves, the injured bone will display motion along the shaft, indicating that the bone has been fractured into separate segments.

• Major muscle spasms in the injured extremity.

NOTE: Any of the above symptoms or signs gives you enough evidence to assume there is a fracture.

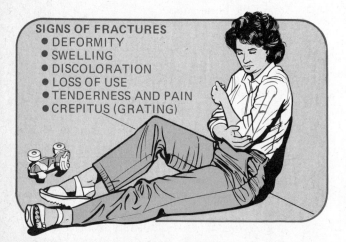

SIGNS OF FRACTURES
● DEFORMITY
● SWELLING
● DISCOLORATION
● LOSS OF USE
● TENDERNESS AND PAIN
● CREPITUS (GRATING)

Figure 9-11: Typical signs of a fracture.

Dislocations typically produce an obvious deformity of the joint. Swelling at the joint is a common sign. Usually there is pain, which increases with movement. The patient may lose use of the joint or may complain of a locked or "frozen" joint.

If the patient's only sign is deformity at a joint, a dislocation is more likely than a fracture. However, you MUST still consider a fracture to be a possibility. Even when you believe that a dislocation has occurred, you cannot rule out a *combined* injury of dislocation and fracture.

Sprains sometimes can be difficult to tell from fractures and dislocations. In most cases there is swelling, discoloration, and the patient complains of pain on movement. There may be considerable swelling and deformity associated with dislocations and fractures. A typical sprain should not have deformity, but may have swelling due to soft tissue injury.

The only sign of a strain will be pain. As an EMT, you should treat suspected sprains as if they were fractures. Even when you think you are dealing with an obvious strain, you should keep the patient at rest, and ask him not to move any part of the injured extremity. Remember, with the conditions at the accident scene, the diagnostic equipment you carry, and your level of training, you cannot rule out the possibility of fracture.

Complications

Muscle is often damaged when there are injuries to the joints and bones. In addition to this damage, injuries such as lacerations, punctures, impaled objects, and serious contusions can occur to muscle. The principles of soft tissue injury care must be applied to open wounds involving muscles. Splinting is often desirable even when there are no indications of fractures. Immobilizing the limb will help prevent additional injury to muscle tissue.

Fractures and dislocations can cause blood vessels to be lacerated or pinched shut. The major arteries of the extremities lie close to the bones. As part of the care provided, you should take a distal pulse (radial or pedal) when evaluating the extent of injury, and after you splint an extremity. No pulse indicates a lack of circulation below the injury site and may mean extensive tissue death will take place unless blood flow is re-established within a reasonable length of time.

Other signs can indicate impaired circulation. Carefully examine the skin at the distal end of the injured limb and compare what you find with the same area on the opposite side of the body. If the skin color has turned blue (cyanosis), pale (pallor) or cold, circulation is probably inadequate. Next, exert pressure over a nailbed on the injured limb, then release it. The nailbed should appear white for a brief moment, then regain its color as the capillaries refill. If **capillary refilling** does not take place within two seconds, there may be impaired circulation.

Just as blood vessels can become cut or have too much pressure placed on them, so too can the

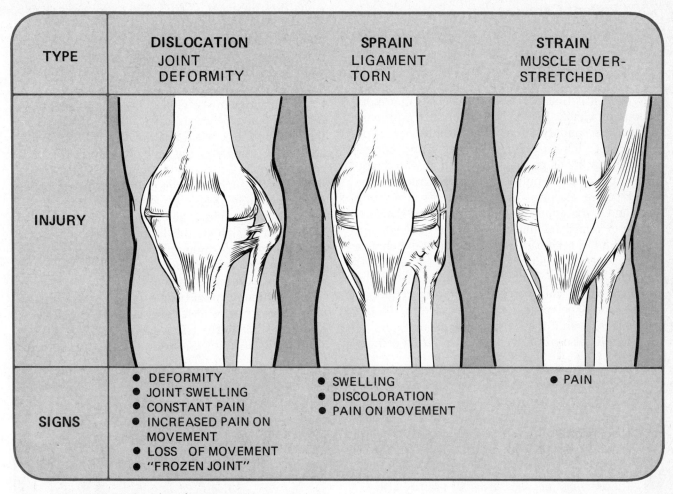

TYPE	DISLOCATION JOINT DEFORMITY	SPRAIN LIGAMENT TORN	STRAIN MUSCLE OVER- STRETCHED
INJURY			
SIGNS	• DEFORMITY • JOINT SWELLING • CONSTANT PAIN • INCREASED PAIN ON MOVEMENT • LOSS OF MOVEMENT • "FROZEN JOINT"	• SWELLING • DISCOLORATION • PAIN ON MOVEMENT	• PAIN

Figure 9-12: Injuries other than fractures.

nerves running through the extremities. When there is no spinal damage, the patient with nerve damage due to a fracture may be unable to move his fingers or toes, depending on the site of the injury. A fracture of the humeral shaft can interrupt the radial nerve, limiting the patient's ability to extend the hand at the wrist. Elbow injuries can damage the ulnar nerve, limiting muscular action of the hand, particularly in the fourth (ring) and fifth (little) fingers. Lack of movement at the ankles with no response to stimulus along the superior surface of the

NERVE INJURY
WOUND CONTAMINATION
SOFT TISSUE DAMAGE
BLOOD VESSEL DAMAGE
COMPLICATIONS ASSOCIATED WITH FRACTURES

Figure 9-13: Complications with fractures.

foot is seen in some cases of fibula fractures where nerves are damaged.

In the case of open fractures, a common complication is *contamination*. Do NOT reach into the wound, or try to clean the surface of the exposed bone. In long bone open fractures, contamination is a major problem in the long-term care of the patient. Improper initial care can lead to *serious infection*.

EMERGENCY CARE FOR INJURIES TO THE EXTREMITIES

While most fractures, especially open fractures, appear gruesome and very serious, few present a real threat to life. Your unhurried but efficient action may mean the difference between a rapid and complete recovery and a long, painful hospitalization and rehabilitation. When dealing with fractures, one of your main duties is to immobilize the injured limb. No matter how near the medical facility, fractures and dislocations should be immobilized to prevent aggravation of the injury. Of course, basic life support situations may necessitate transport before such care can be rendered.

Total Patient Care

Many untrained personnel arrive at the scene of an accident and try to start treating fractures. This is not the proper procedure for an EMT. When caring for a person with an injury to the bone or joint of an extremity, it is first necessary to resolve other more serious problems. Remember to conduct a primary survey, a secondary survey and an interview. You must detect life-threatening problems and correct these as quickly as possible. An open airway, respiration, pulse, and control of bleeding must be assured before starting care of fractures. Detecting neck and spinal injuries is more important than detecting extremity fractures. As with all patients, you must take the necessary steps to reduce the chance of the patient developing shock. Both open chest wounds and open abdominal wounds should be cared for before you worry about fractures. Serious burns should be cared for before fractures to the extremities, even if the fractures are major.

There is also an order of care in terms of fractures:

1. First Priority—fractures of the spine.
2. Second Priority—fractures to the head and rib cage.
3. Lowest Priority—fractures of the extremities. In most cases, pelvic fractures have the potential to be the most serious. Fractures of the lower limbs are cared for before those to the upper limbs. The order of priority after the pelvis is femurs, joints, other long bones.

Provide emotional support to patients with possible fractures. You may need to remind the patient that fractured bones will heal. Tell the patient that new techniques reduce the time a patient spends wearing a cast and receiving rehabilitative therapy. Your emotional support will help keep the patient at rest, and help to lower his blood pressure, pulse, and breathing rate.

GENERAL CARE FOR SKELETAL INJURIES

The proper time to care for a specific bone or joint injury is when the patient is *reasonably stable.* Care procedures are shown on Scansheet 9-1.

Straightening Angulated Fractures

Slightly angulated closed fractures of the extremities usually can be straightened and immobilized with few problems. However, severely angulated fractures pose serious problems. Angulations make splinting and transport more difficult. They can pinch or cut through nerves and blood vessels, and usually are painful for the patient.

WARNING: DO NOT ATTEMPT TO STRAIGHTEN

ANGULATED FRACTURES AND DISLOCATIONS OF THE SHOULDER OR WRIST. Major nerves and blood vessels pass through these joints, close to the major bones. Attempts to straighten fractures and dislocations may cause serious, even permanent damage.

Angulations of the elbow, knee, and ankle may be straightened if there is *no distal pulse.* Do not force the limb into its normal anatomical position. *Gently* attempt to straighten the limb, but stop if there is any resistance. Once a distal pulse is established, do not move the limb until the injured joint and bones have been immobilized.

If your first effort fails, do not make a second attempt to straighten the limb. If the joint shows evidence of a crushing injury, do not attempt to straighten the limb. Whenever there is no distal pulse, transport immediately.

Straightening angulations of *closed* fractures is within the scope of EMT-level care. YOU SHOULD NOT ATTEMPT TO STRAIGHTEN *OPEN* FRACTURE ANGULATIONS. To do so will cause greater

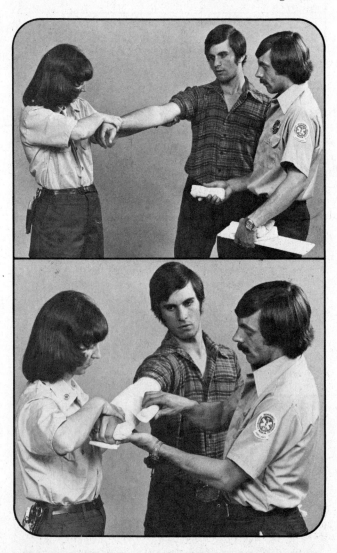

Figure 9-14: Procedure for straightening an angulated closed fracture.

GENERAL CARE FOR SKELETAL INJURIES

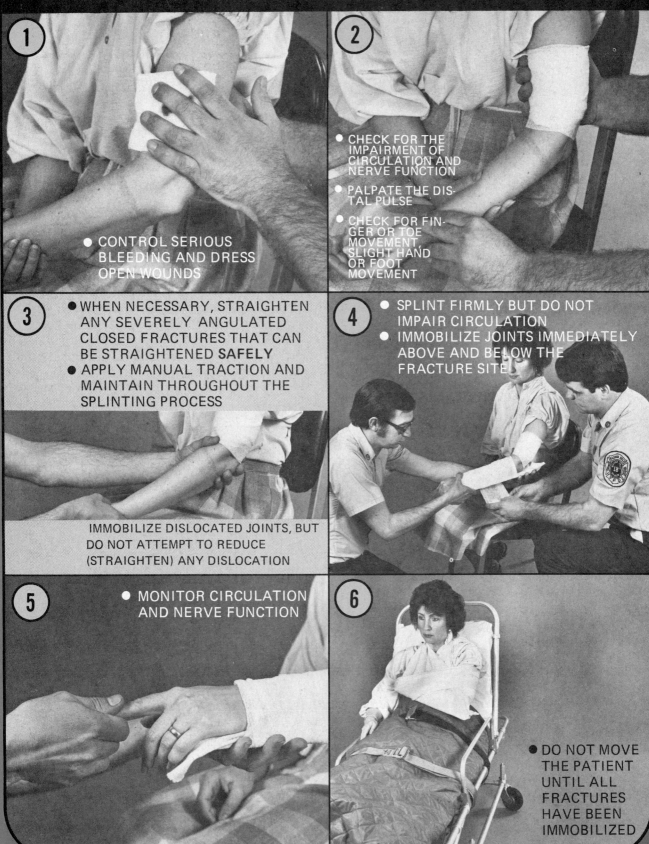

1
- CONTROL SERIOUS BLEEDING AND DRESS OPEN WOUNDS

2
- CHECK FOR THE IMPAIRMENT OF CIRCULATION AND NERVE FUNCTION
- PALPATE THE DISTAL PULSE
- CHECK FOR FINGER OR TOE MOVEMENT, SLIGHT HAND OR FOOT MOVEMENT

3
- WHEN NECESSARY, STRAIGHTEN ANY SEVERELY ANGULATED CLOSED FRACTURES THAT CAN BE STRAIGHTENED **SAFELY**
- APPLY MANUAL TRACTION AND MAINTAIN THROUGHOUT THE SPLINTING PROCESS

IMMOBILIZE DISLOCATED JOINTS, BUT DO NOT ATTEMPT TO REDUCE (STRAIGHTEN) ANY DISLOCATION

4
- SPLINT FIRMLY BUT DO NOT IMPAIR CIRCULATION
- IMMOBILIZE JOINTS IMMEDIATELY ABOVE AND BELOW THE FRACTURE SITE

5
- MONITOR CIRCULATION AND NERVE FUNCTION

6
- DO NOT MOVE THE PATIENT UNTIL ALL FRACTURES HAVE BEEN IMMOBILIZED

SCAN 9.1

damage to the lacerated tissue bed, blood vessels, and nerves.

The patient's pain will increase during the process of straightening an angulation. This will be temporary; the pain lessens as splinting is completed. The procedure for straightening closed angulated fractures *other* than those to the shoulders, elbows, wrists, or knees is as follows:

1. CAREFULLY cut away clothing that lies over the fracture site.
2. Upper Limb: Grasp the limb above and below the fracture site and apply smooth, steady tension along the long axis of the limb. Hold the limb until your partner can apply a splint.
   Lower Limb: Have your partner hold the limb firmly in place while you apply tension below the break. Maintain tension until a splint has been applied. If the limb must be lifted, the fracture site must be supported.

NOTE: If firm resistance is felt while applying tension, do NOT forcibly try to correct the angulation. Attempt to correct the angulation only once.

Splinting

A bone is a supporting structure. When it is broken, some substitute must be provided to prevent further injury. **Splinting** is the process used to *immobilize* fractures and dislocations. Any item that will immobilize a fracture or a dislocation is called a **splint.**

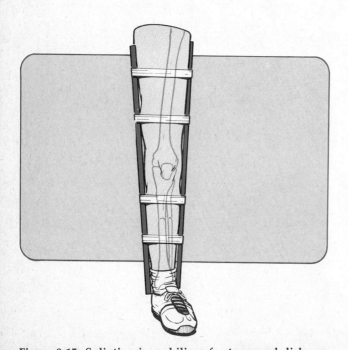

Figure 9-15: Splinting immobilizes fractures and dislocations.

The Reasons for Splinting

In addition to immobilizing the injured extremity, splinting helps to prevent or reduce the severity of the complications that accompany fractures and dislocations. These complications include:

1. Pain—much of the pain experienced by the patient is associated with the unrestricted movement of bone ends and fragments. In cases of dislocation, splinting may prevent bone ends from placing pressure on nerves, blood vessels, and sensitive tissues.
2. Damage to Soft Tissues—The processes of fracturing and dislocation cause soft tissue injuries that will be aggravated if the extremity is not immobilized.
3. Bleeding—Dislocated bones, the ends of fractured bones, and bone fragments can damage blood vessels.
4. Restricted Blood Flow—Dislocated bones, the ends of fractured bones, and bone fragments can press against blood vessels, reducing or shutting off the flow of blood.
5. Closed Fractures Becoming Open Fractures—The sharp edges of fractured bones may tear through the patient's skin to produce an open fracture.

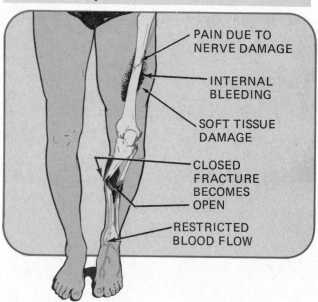

Figure 9-16: Splinting can prevent or lessen the complications associated with bone and joint injury.

Types of Splints

There are three types of splints: rigid splints, soft splints, and traction splints.

The process of splinting is easier to understand if you consider **rigid splints.** As the name implies, these splints are stiff, with very little flexibility. When applied along an injured bone, they serve to immobilize the bone and the joints immediately above and below the injury site, preventing the movement of the injured bone. A rigid splint also will allow for repositioning and transfer of the patient with a minimum of movement of the injured extremity.

There are many types of commercial rigid splints, including those made of wood, aluminum, compressed wood fibers, wire, and plastic. Some come with their own washable pads, others require padding to be applied before being secured to the patient. Most ambulances carry short padded board splints (18 inches long), medium padded board splints (3 feet long), and long padded board splints (at least 4 1/2 feet long).

Soft splints can be of two types. One type is the **air-inflatable splint.** This splint is classified as a soft splint even though it is rigid when finally applied to the site of injury (a Scansheet on air-inflated splints appears later in this chapter). Typically, soft splints consist of items such as pillows, blankets, towels, and dressings. Soft splinting usually is NOT the most effective form of splinting, but it does help to immobilize fractures and dislocations. In cases such as fractures to the foot, the soft splint is preferred over the rigid splint. One of the most useful soft splinting techniques is the application of a sling and swathe (a Scansheet on the sling and swathe appears later in this chapter).

Traction splints are used to immobilize broken bone ends so that further damage is avoided. **Traction** is the application of just enough force to stabilize the broken bone. It is not the stretching or moving of the fractured bone until the ends are aligned. When a bone breaks completely, the normal tendency of the muscles to contract often causes bone ends to slip past one another, or "override." When muscles are large and powerful, as in the thigh, the tendency is more pronounced. Patient movement and the movement necessary during transport can increase the override and cause serious soft tissue damage, including a closed fracture becoming an open fracture (a Scansheet on traction splinting appears later in this chapter).

There will be times when you do not have enough splints at the scene of an accident, or you respond while you are off duty and do not have any commercial splints. You will have to make your own splints from materials at the scene. Emergency splints may be soft splints such as pillows or rolled blankets, or they may be rigid splints made from a variety of materials. You can use lumber, plywood, compressed wood products, cardboard, rolled newspapers or magazines, umbrellas, canes, broom handles, shovel handles, sporting equipment (catcher's or hockey goalie's shin guards have been used), or tongue depressors (for fractured fingers). Some of these items can be found at the scene of a typical accident. Ask bystanders at the scene to help you find something that can be used as a splint. Give them suggestions and ASK if they have any ideas. Having bystanders check the trunks of their cars usually produces results. Tell them you are looking for something rigid and long enough to hold the fractured bone and the joints immediately above and below this bone.

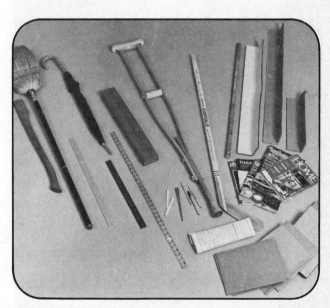

Figure 9-18: You must know how to make emergency splints.

SPLINTING THE UPPER EXTREMITIES

There are four basic rules you must keep in mind as you apply splints for injuries to the extremities:

- When in doubt, splint.
- Always be sure that a rigid splint is padded before it is applied to a patient.

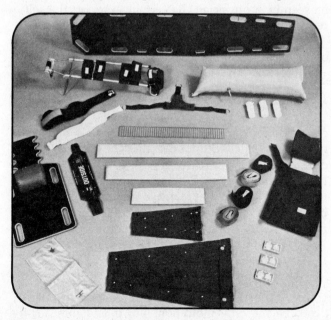

Figure 9-17: Types of splints include rigid, soft, and traction.

- Be certain you have not disrupted vascular or nerve function during the splinting process.
- Continue to check air-inflated splints to be certain that they have not lost or gained pressure. Altitude or temperature changes will affect splint pressure. Leaks may occur from punctures or the deterioration of valves or zippers.

The Shoulder Girdle

Symptoms and Signs

1. Pain in the shoulder may indicate several types of injury. Look for specific signs.
2. A "dropped" shoulder, with the patient holding the arm of the injured side against the chest, often indicates a fracture of the clavicle or scapula.
3. All the bones of the shoulder girdle can be felt except the scapula. Only the superior ridge called the spine can be easily palpated. Injury to the scapula is rare, but must be considered if there are indications of a severe blow striking the back over this bone.

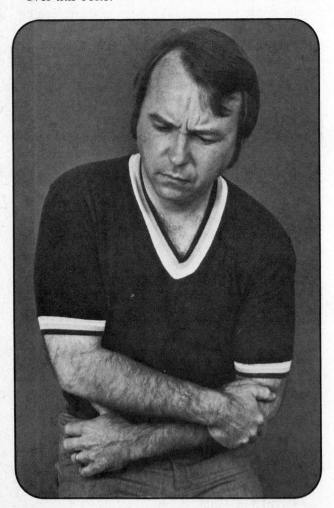

Figure 9-19: Fractured clavicle, noted by "dropped" shoulder.

4. Check the entire shoulder girdle:
   - Check for deformity where the clavicle attaches to the sternum—possible fracture or dislocation.
   - Feel for deformity where the clavicle joins the scapula—possible dislocation.
   - Feel and look along the entire clavicle for deformity—possible fracture.
   - Note if the head of the humerus can be felt or moves in front of the shoulder—possible anterior dislocation. This displacement also may be due to a fracture.

Emergency Care

1. Check for a radial pulse on the injured side. If there is no pulse, transport as soon as possible.
2. Check for nerve function by checking for feeling and movement of the fingers on the injured side. If there is possible nerve damage, transport as soon as possible.
3. It is not practical to use a rigid splint for injuries to the clavicle, scapula, or the head of the humerus. Use a sling and swathe (see Scansheet 9-2).
4. If there is evidence of a possible anterior dislocation of the head of the humerus, place a thin pillow between the patient's arm and chest before applying the sling and swathe.
5. Do NOT attempt to straighten angulations or reset any dislocations.

NOTE: Sometimes a dislocated shoulder will reduce itself. When this happens, you should check for a distal pulse and nerve function. Apply a sling and swathe and transport the patient. The patient must be seen by a physician. Be certain to report the self-reduction to the emergency department staff.

Scansheets 9-2 through 9-7 complete your study of the upper extremities.

SPLINTING THE LOWER EXTREMITIES
The Pelvis

Fractures of the pelvis occur in falls, motor vehicle accidents, or when a person is crushed between two objects. Pelvic fractures may be the result of direct or indirect violence.

NOTE: Indications of pelvic fractures mean that there may be serious damage to internal organs, blood vessels, and nerves. Internal bleeding may be profuse. Treat for shock and monitor vital signs. Any force strong enough to fracture the pelvis also can cause injury to the spine.

Symptoms and Signs

- Complaint of pain in pelvis or hips. This may be the only indication, but it is significant if the mechanism of injury indicates possible fracture.

SLING AND SWATHE

A SLING IS A TRIANGULAR BANDAGE USED TO SUPPORT THE SHOULDER AND ARM. ONCE THE PATIENT'S ARM IS PLACED IN A SLING, A SWATHE CAN BE USED TO HOLD THE PATIENT'S ARM AGAINST THE SIDE OF THE CHEST. COMMERCIAL SLINGS ARE AVAILABLE. ROLLER BANDAGE CAN BE USED TO FORM A SLING AND SWATHE. VELCRO STRAPS CAN BE USED TO FORM A SWATHE. USE WHATEVER MATERIALS YOU HAVE ON HAND, PROVIDED THAT THEY WILL NOT CUT INTO THE PATIENT. REMEMBER, SHIRTS, TIES, AND WIDE BELTS CAN BE USED TO MAKE BOTH SLING AND SWATHE.

(1) 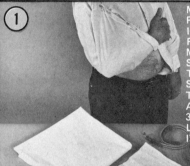 MAKE A SLING FROM A PIECE OF CLOTH, CLOTHING, TOWEL, OR SHEET. FOLD OR CUT THIS MATERIAL INTO THE SHAPE OF A TRIANGLE. THE IDEAL SLING SHOULD BE ABOUT 50 TO 60 INCHES LONG AT ITS BASE AND 36 TO 40 INCHES LONG ON EACH OF ITS SIDES.

(2) 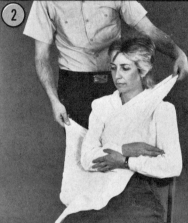 POSITION THE TRIANGULAR MATERIAL OVER TOP OF THE PATIENT'S INJURED CHEST AS SHOWN IN THE FIGURE. FOLD THE PATIENT'S ARM ACROSS THE CHEST. IF THE PATIENT CANNOT HOLD HIS OWN ARM, HAVE SOMEONE ASSIST YOU, OR PROVIDE SUPPORT FOR THE PATIENT'S ARM UNTIL YOU ARE READY TO TIE THE SLING. NOTE THAT ONE POINT OF THE TRIANGLE SHOULD EXTEND BEHIND THE PATIENT'S ELBOW ON THE INJURED SIDE.

(3) 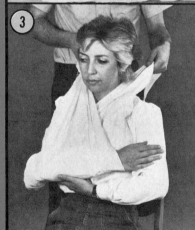 TAKE THE BOTTOM POINT OF THE TRIANGLE AND BRING THIS END UP OVER THE PATIENT'S ARM. WHEN YOU ARE FINISHED, THIS BOTTOM POINT SHOULD BE TAKEN OVER TOP OF THE PATIENT'S INJURED SHOULDER.

(4) 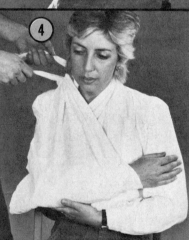 DRAW UP ON THE ENDS OF THE SLING SO THAT THE PATIENT'S HAND IS ABOUT FOUR INCHES ABOVE THE ELBOW (EXCEPTIONS ARE DISCUSSED LATER). TIE THE TWO ENDS OF THE SLING TOGETHER, MAKING SURE THAT THE KNOT DOES NOT PRESS AGAINST THE BACK OF THE PATIENT'S NECK. LEAVE THE PATIENT'S FINGERTIPS EXPOSED TO SEE ANY COLOR CHANGES THAT INDICATE LACK OF CIRCULATION. CHECK FOR A RADIAL PULSE. IF THE PULSE HAS BEEN LOST, TAKE OFF THE SLING AND REPEAT THE PROCEDURE.

(5) 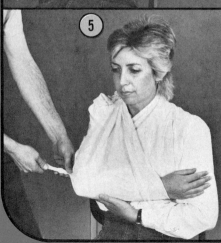 TAKE THE POINT OF MATERIAL AT THE PATIENT'S ELBOW AND FOLD IT FORWARD, PINNING IT TO THE FRONT OF THE SLING. THIS FORMS A POCKET FOR THE PATIENT'S ELBOW. IF YOU DO NOT HAVE A PIN, TWIST THE EXCESS MATERIAL AND TIE A KNOT IN THE POINT. THIS WILL PROVIDE A SHALLOW POCKET FOR THE PATIENT'S ELBOW.

(6) A SWATHE CAN BE FORMED FROM A SECOND PIECE OF TRIANGULAR MATERIAL. THIS SWATHE IS TIED AROUND THE CHEST AND THE INJURED ARM OF THE PATIENT, OVER THE SLING. DO NOT PLACE THIS SWATHE OVER THE PATIENT'S ARM ON THE UNINJURED SIDE.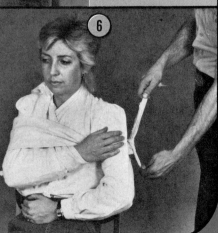

SCAN 9.2

INJURIES TO THE HUMERUS

SIGNS: INJURY OF THE HUMERUS CAN TAKE PLACE AT THE PROXIMAL END (SHOULDER), ALONG THE SHAFT OF THE BONE, OR AT THE DISTAL END (ELBOW). DEFORMITY IS THE KEY SIGN USED TO DETECT FRACTURES TO THIS BONE IN ANY OF THESE LOCATIONS.

①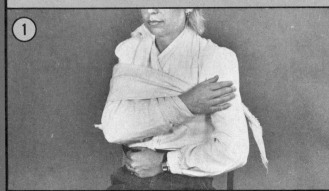

FRACTURE AT PROXIMAL END GENTLY APPLY A SLING AND SWATHE. IF YOU HAVE ONLY ENOUGH MATERIAL FOR A SWATHE, BIND THE PATIENT'S UPPER ARM TO HIS BODY, TAKING GREAT CARE NOT TO CUT OFF CIRCULATION TO THE FOREARM.

②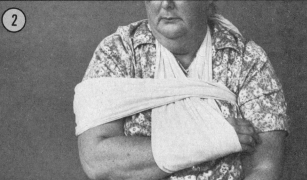

FRACTURE OF THE SHAFT   GENTLY APPLY A SLING AND SWATHE. THE SLING SHOULD BE MODIFIED SO THAT IT SUPPORTS ONLY THE WRIST.

③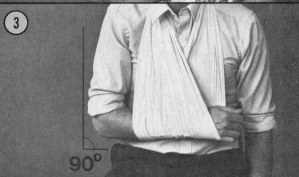

90°

FRACTURE AT DISTAL END   GENTLY APPLY A FULL SLING AND SWATHE. DO NOT DRAW THE HAND UPWARD TO A POSITION FOUR INCHES ABOVE THE ELBOW. INSTEAD, KEEP ELBOW FLEXION AS CLOSE TO 90° ANGLE AS POSSIBLE.

WARNING!

BEFORE APPLYING A SLING AND SWATHE TO CARE FOR INJURIES TO THE HUMERUS, CHECK FOR NERVE FUNCTION AND CIRCULATION. IF YOU DO NOT FEEL A PULSE, ATTEMPT TO STRAIGHTEN ANY SLIGHT ANGULATION IF THE PATIENT HAS A CLOSED FRACTURE. OTHERWISE, PREPARE FOR IMMEDIATE TRANSPORT. SHOULD STRAIGHTENING OF THE ANGULATION FAIL TO RESTORE FUNCTION, SPLINT WITH A LONG BOARD SPLINT. IF THERE IS NO SIGN OF CIRCULATION OR NERVE FUNCTION, YOU WILL HAVE TO ATTEMPT A SECOND SPLINTING. IF THIS FAILS TO RESTORE CIRCULATION AND NERVE FUNCTION, TRANSPORT IMMEDIATELY. DO NOT TRY TO STRAIGHTEN ANGULATION OF THE HUMERUS IF THERE ARE ANY SIGNS OF FRACTURE OR DISLOCATION OF THE SHOULDER OR ELBOW.

SCAN 9.3

INJURIES TO THE DISTAL HUMERUS

DISTAL HUMERUS: THE CLOSER A FRACTURE OF THE HUMERUS IS TO THE ELBOW, THE STRONGER THE RECOMMENDATION TO APPLY A RIGID SPLINT, RATHER THAN A SLING AND SWATHE. DEFORMITY AND SENSITIVITY TO TOUCH WILL HELP YOU LOCATE THE INJURY SITE. IF THE ELBOW ITSELF SHOWS NO OBVIOUS INJURY, YOU SHOULD:

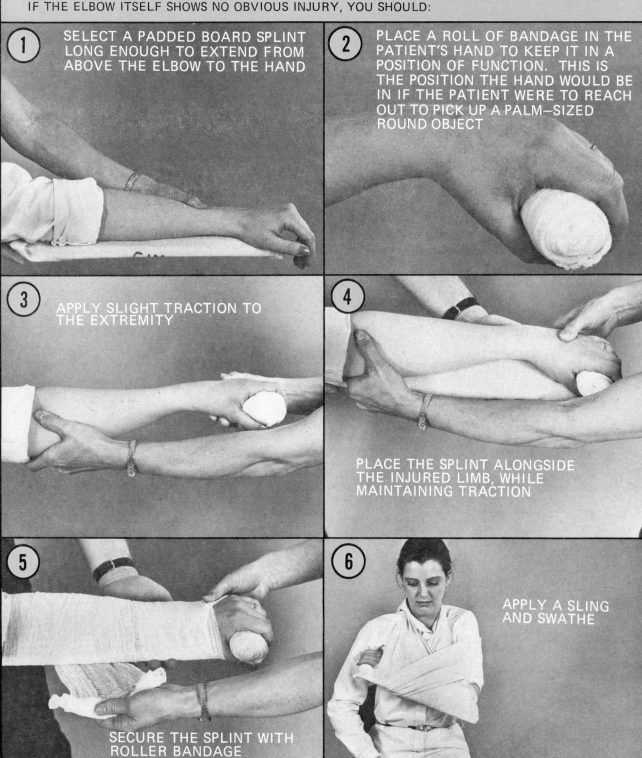

1 SELECT A PADDED BOARD SPLINT LONG ENOUGH TO EXTEND FROM ABOVE THE ELBOW TO THE HAND

2 PLACE A ROLL OF BANDAGE IN THE PATIENT'S HAND TO KEEP IT IN A POSITION OF FUNCTION. THIS IS THE POSITION THE HAND WOULD BE IN IF THE PATIENT WERE TO REACH OUT TO PICK UP A PALM—SIZED ROUND OBJECT

3 APPLY SLIGHT TRACTION TO THE EXTREMITY

4 PLACE THE SPLINT ALONGSIDE THE INJURED LIMB, WHILE MAINTAINING TRACTION

5 SECURE THE SPLINT WITH ROLLER BANDAGE

6 APPLY A SLING AND SWATHE

SCAN 9.4

ELBOW FRACTURES and DISLOCATIONS

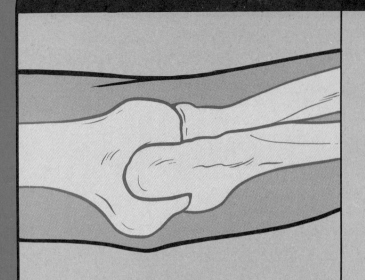

SIGNS THE ELBOW IS A JOINT AND NOT A BONE. IT IS COMPOSED OF THE DISTAL HUMERUS, AND THE PROXIMAL ULNA AND RADIUS FORMING A HINGE JOINT. YOU WILL HAVE TO DECIDE IF THE INJURY IS TRULY TO THE ELBOW. DEFORMITY AND SENSITIVITY WILL DIRECT YOU TO THE INJURY SITE.

CARE IF THERE IS A DISTAL PULSE, THE ELBOW SHOULD BE IMMOBILIZED IN THE POSITION IN WHICH IT IS FOUND. THE JOINT HAS TOO MANY NERVES AND BLOOD VESSELS TO RISK MOVEMENT. BE CERTAIN TO CHECK FOR CIRCULATION AND NERVE IMPAIRMENT BEFORE AND AFTER SPLINTING. WHEN A DISTAL PULSE IS ABSENT, MAKE ONE ATTEMPT TO GENTLY STRAIGHTEN THE LIMB. DO NOT FORCE THE LIMB INTO ITS NORMAL ANATOMICAL POSITION.

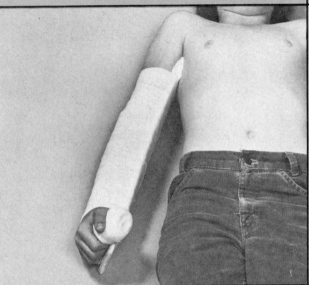

ELBOW IN STRAIGHT POSITION: USE A PADDED BOARD SPLINT THAT EXTENDS FROM UNDER THE ARMPIT TO A POINT PAST THE FINGERTIPS. PAD THE ARMPIT, AND PLACE A ROLL OF BANDAGE IN THE PATIENT'S HAND TO HELP MAINTAIN POSITION OF FUNCTION.

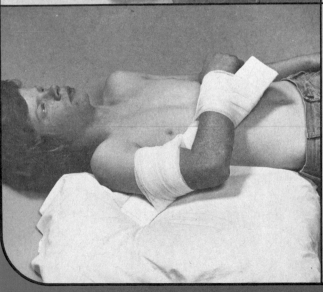

ELBOW IN BENT POSITION: IF THERE IS A DISTAL PULSE, DO NOT CHANGE POSITION. USE A SHORT PADDED BOARD SPLINT THAT CAN BE SECURED TO THE WRIST AND ARM TO IMMOBILIZE THE JOINT. A WRIST SLING CAN BE APPLIED TO SUPPORT THE LIMB.

SCAN 9.5

INJURIES — FOREARM, WRIST and HAND

SIGNS

- FOREARM — DEFORMITY AND TENDERNESS. IF ONLY ONE BONE IS BROKEN, DEFORMITY MAY BE MINOR.
- WRIST — DEFORMITY AND TENDERNESS, WITH THE POSSIBILITY OF A COLLES [KOL-EZ] FRACTURE THAT GIVES A "SILVER-FORK" APPEARANCE TO THE WRIST.
- HAND — DEFORMITY AND PAIN. DISLOCATED FINGERS ARE OBVIOUS.

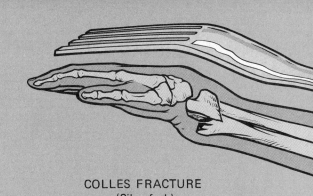

COLLES FRACTURE
(Silverfork)

CARE CHECK FOR CIRCULATION AND NERVE IMPAIRMENT. FRACTURES OCCURRING TO THE FOREARM, WRIST, OR HAND CAN BE SPLINTED WITH A PADDED RIGID SPLINT THAT EXTENDS FROM THE ELBOW, PAST THE FINGERTIPS. THE PATIENT'S ELBOW, FOREARM, WRIST, AND HAND ALL NEED THE SUPPORT OF THE SPLINT. ROLLER BANDAGE SHOULD BE PLACED IN THE HAND TO ASSURE THE POSITION OF FUNCTION. AFTER RIGID SPLINTING, APPLY A SLING AND SWATHE.

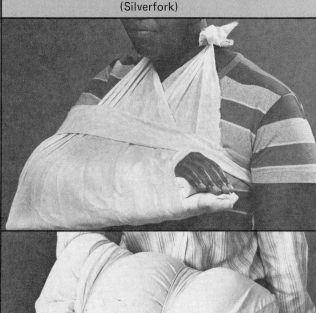

FRACTURES OF THE HAND AND DISLOCATIONS OF THE WRIST CAN BE CARED FOR WITH SOFT SPLINTING BY PLACING THE HAND IN THE POSITION OF FUNCTION AND TYING THE FOREARM, WRIST AND HAND BETWEEN THE FOLD OF ONE PILLOW OR BETWEEN TWO PILLOWS. AN INJURED FINGER CAN BE TAPED TO AN ADJACENT UNINJURED FINGER, OR SPLINTED WITH A TONGUE DEPRESSOR. DO NOT TRY TO "POP" DISLOCATED FINGERS BACK INTO PLACE.

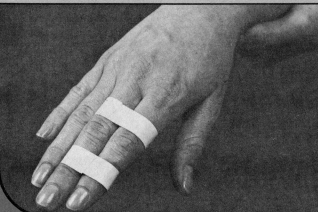

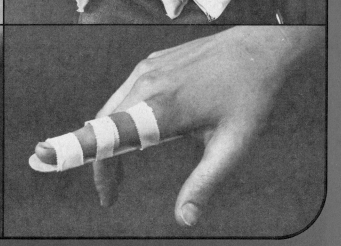

SCAN 9.6

AIR-INFLATED SPLINTS

WARNING!

WHEN APPLIED IN COLD WEATHER, AN INFLATABLE SPLINT WILL EXPAND WHEN THE PATIENT IS MOVED TO A WARMER PLACE. VARIATIONS IN PRESSURE ALSO OCCUR IF THE PATIENT IS MOVED TO A DIFFERENT ALTITUDE. OCCASIONALLY MONITOR THE PRESSURE IN THE SPLINT WITH YOUR FINGERTIP.

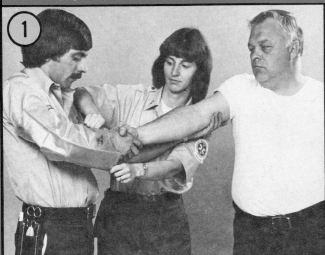

SLIDE THE UNINFLATED SPLINT UP YOUR FOREARM, WELL ABOVE THE WRIST. USE THIS SAME HAND TO GRASP THE HAND OF THE PATIENT'S INJURED LIMB AS THOUGH YOU WERE GOING TO SHAKE HANDS.

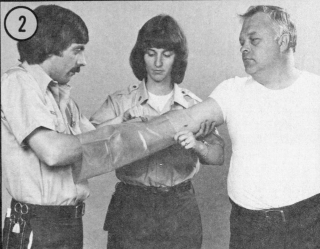

WHILE HOLDING HIS HAND IN THIS FASHION, GENTLY SLIDE THE SPLINT OVER YOUR HAND AND ONTO HIS LIMB. THE LOWER EDGE OF THE SPLINT SHOULD BE JUST ABOVE HIS KNUCKLES. MAKE SURE THE SPLINT IS PROPERLY PLACED AND FREE OF WRINKLES.

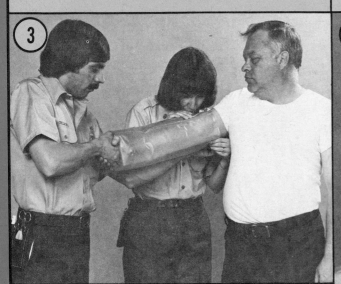

CONTINUE TO HOLD THE PATIENT'S HAND WHILE YOU HAVE YOUR PARTNER INFLATE THE SPLINT BY MOUTH TO A POINT WHERE YOU CAN MAKE A SLIGHT DENT IN THE PLASTIC WHEN YOU PRESS YOUR THUMB AGAINST THE SPLINT SURFACE.

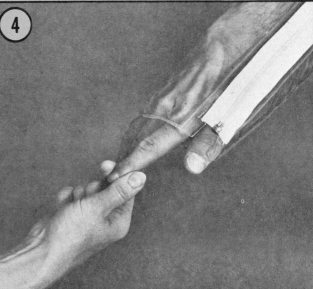

MONITOR THE PATIENT'S FINGERNAIL BEDS AND FINGERTIPS FOR INDICATIONS OF CIRCULATION IMPAIRMENT.

SCAN 9.7

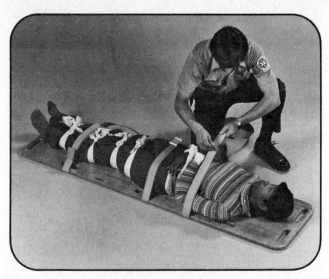

Figure 9-20: Immobilizing a patient with a pelvic injury on a long spine board.

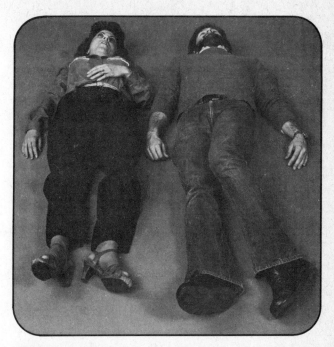

Figure 9-21: Signs of anterior and posterior hip dislocation.

- Painful reaction when pressure is applied to wings of pelvis (iliac crest) or to the pubic bones (symphysis pubis).
- Patient says that he cannot lift legs when lying on his back.
- The foot on the injured side usually turns outward.

Emergency Care

1. MOVE THE PATIENT AS LITTLE AS POSSIBLE. Any moves or rolls should be done so that the patient moves as a unit. Never lift the patient with the pelvis unsupported.
2. Place a folded blanket between the patient's legs and bind them together with wide cravats. Thin rigid splints are useful to push cravats under the patient at the knee void. The cravats can then be adjusted for proper placement.
3. Immobilize the patient on a long spine board, or use a scoop-style stretcher.

Hip Dislocation

It is difficult to tell a hip dislocation from a fracture to the proximal femur. Conscious patients will complain of intense pain.

Signs

- Anterior hip dislocation—the patient's entire lower limb is rotated outward.
- Posterior hip dislocation (most common)—the patient's leg is rotated inward and the knee is bent. The foot may hang loose ("foot drop") and the patient is unable to flex the foot or lift the toes. Often, there is a lack of sensation in the limb. These signs indicate possible damage to the sciatic (si-AT-ik) nerve caused by a dislocated femoral head.

Emergency Care

1. Check for circulation and nerve impairment.
2. Move patient onto a long back board (some systems use a scoop-style stretcher).
3. Immobilize the limb with pillows or rolled blankets.
4. Secure the patient to the board with straps or cravats.
5. Transport carefully, monitor vital signs, and continue to check for nerve and circulation impairment.

NOTE: If the head of the femur slides or pops back into place, report this to the emergency department staff so that the dislocation does not go unnoticed.

Hip Fractures

This is a fracture to the head of the femur, not to the pelvis. The fracture can occur to the head, neck, or at the proximal end of the femur, just below the neck of the bone. Direct violence (motor vehicle accidents) and twisting forces (falls) can cause a hip fracture. Elderly people are more susceptible to this type of injury.

Symptoms and Signs

- Localized pain, but some patients complain of pain in the knee.
- Sometimes the patient is sensitive to pressure exerted on the lateral prominence of the hip (greater trochanter).
- Discoloration of surrounding tissues
- Swelling
- Patient unable to move limb while on his back

- Foot on injured side usually turns outward
- Injured leg may appear shorter

Emergency Care   Be certain to check for nerve and circulatory impairment. This must be continued during transport.

- Binding the legs together: Place a folded blanket between the patient's legs and bind the legs together with wide straps, velcro-equipped straps, or wide cravats. Carefully place the patient on a long spine board and use pillows to support the lower limbs. Secure the patient to the board. A scoop-style stretcher can be used in place of the long spine board.

- Padded boards: Push cravats or straps under the patient at the natural voids so they will pass across the chest, the abdomen, just below the belt, below the crotch, above and below the knee, and at the ankle. Use thin splints to push the cravats or straps to avoid moving the patient.

  Splint with two long padded boards. Ideally, one board should be long enough to extend from the patient's armpit to beyond the foot. Splint with another padded board that is long enough to extend from the armpit to beyond the foot. Cushion with padding in the armpit and crotch and pad all voids created at the ankle and knee. Secure the boards with the cravats or straps.

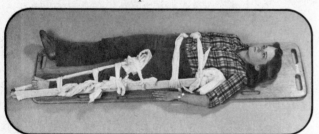

Figure 9-22: Long board splinting for a fractured hip.

- Traction splinting (see Scansheet 9-8): This procedure is recommended for most patients, but do not use it for the elderly. Many systems recommend this method for elderly patients only if transport will take more than 30 minutes or will be very rough. Traction splinting usually reduces patient pain.

Femoral Shaft Injuries

Symptoms and Signs

- Pain, often intense
- Often there will be an open fracture, sometimes with end of bone protruding through wound. When the injury is a closed fracture,

there will be deformity with possible severe angulation.

- The injured limb may appear shortened.

Emergency Care   Check circulatory and nerve impairment, then APPLY A TRACTION SPLINT.

Knee Injuries

The knee is a joint and not a single bone. Fractures can occur to the distal femur, to the proximal tibia and fibula, and to the patella (kneecap). What may appear to be a dislocation may be a fracture or a fracture and dislocation combined. Even if you believe that the patient has suffered only a dislocated patella and the kneecap has repositioned itself, other damage may be hidden. Always treat and transport.

Symptoms and Signs

- Pain and tenderness
- Deformity with obvious swelling

Emergency Care   If there is a distal pulse, DO NOT ATTEMPT TO STRAIGHTEN ANGULATIONS. Remember to check for circulatory and nerve impairment. If there is no distal pulse, you can try to move the leg gently to a straight anatomical position. DO NOT FORCE THE LEG. Stop if there is any resistance. Make only one attempt to straighten the leg.

Once splinting is done, monitor the patient. If there is a loss of distal pulse, a loss of sensation, or the foot becomes discolored (white or blue) and turns cold, transport without delay.

- Leg Straight—Immobilize with an air-inflated splint or a padded board splint. Applying two padded boards (one medial and one lateral)

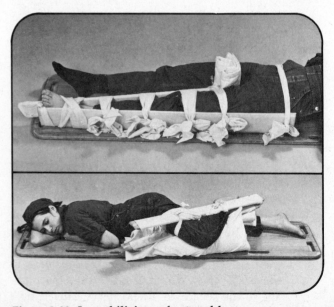

Figure 9-23: Immobilizing a fractured knee.

TRACTION SPLINTING

NOTE: TRACTION SPLINTS VARY DEPENDING UPON THE MANUFACTURER. LEARN TO USE THE EQUIPMENT SUPPLIED IN YOUR AREA AND KEEP UP TO DATE WITH NEW EQUIPMENT AS IT IS APPROVED FOR USE.

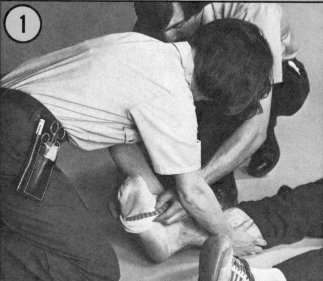

THE SPLINT IS ADJUSTED FOR LENGTH, TYPICALLY WITH THE RING PLACED AT THE LEVEL OF THE BONY PROMINENCE THAT CAN BE FELT IN THE MIDDLE OF EACH BUTTOCK (ISCHIAL IS—KE—AL TUBEROSITY) AND THE DISTAL END OF THE SPLINT EXTENDED TO 12 INCHES BEYOND THE FOOT. WITH SOME SPLINTS, THE RING IS PLACED AT THE LEVEL OF THE ILIAC CREST AND THE SPLINT IS EXTENDED 8 TO 10 INCHES BEYOND THE FOOT. ALL OF THE STRAPS ARE OPENED AND POSITIONED. THEY SHOULD BE PLACED TO BE APPLIED MID–THIGH, ABOVE AND BELOW THE KNEE, AND ABOVE THE ANKLE. EMT 1 REMOVES THE PATIENT'S SHOE AND SOCK WHILE EMT 2 STABILIZES THE LIMB. THE LIMB SHOULD NOT BE LIFTED. SOME EMS SYSTEMS LEAVE THE SHOE ON THE FOOT.

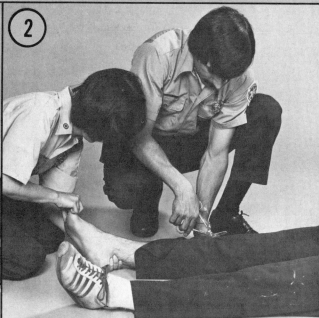

EMT 1 CUTS THE TROUSER LEG TO EXPOSE THE INJURY SITE WHILE EMT 2 STABILIZES THE LIMB AND PALPATES THE DISTAL PULSE. OPEN WOUNDS ARE DRESSED.

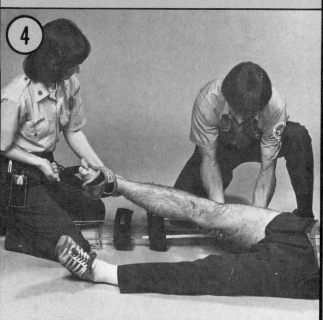

EMT 1 WRAPS THE ANKLE HITCH AROUND THE PATIENT'S FOOT WHILE EMT 2 APPLIES MANUAL TRACTION TO THE LIMB.

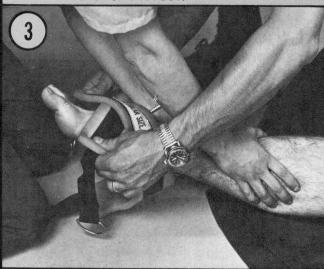

EMT 1 POSITIONS THE SPLINT WHILE EMT 2 MAINTAINS TRACTION TO THE ANKLE HITCH AND FOOT, AND SUPPORTS THE LIMB.

SCAN 9.8A

TRACTION SPLINTING (cont'd.)

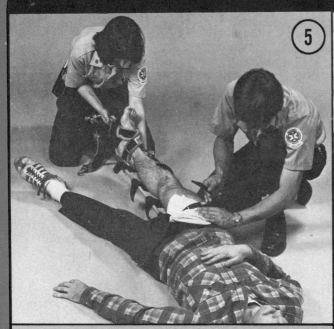

⑤

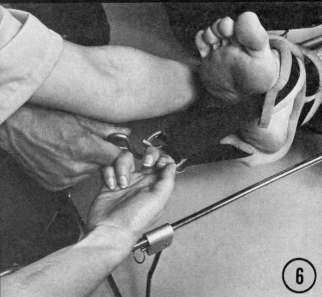

⑥

EMT 1 ATTACHES THE ISCHIAL STRAP. EMT 2 CONTINUES TO MAINTAIN TRACTION.

EMT 1 ATTACHES S—HOOK OF THE WINDLASS STRAP TO THE D—RINGS OR LOOPS OF THE ANKLE HITCH. EMT 2 MAINTAINS TRACTION.

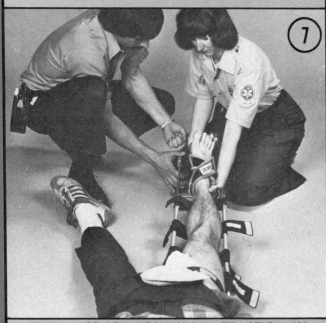

⑦

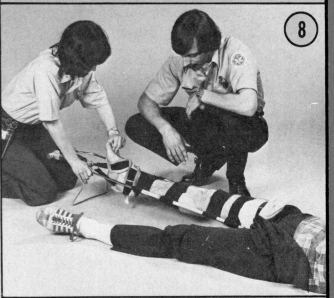

⑧

EMT 1 APPLIES MECHANICAL TRACTION BY TURNING THE KNURLED KNOB UNTIL IT WILL NO LONGER TURN MANUALLY.

THE REMAINING STRAPS ARE SNUGLY APPLIED (NOT OVER THE KNEE) AND THE DISTAL PULSE IS CHECKED TO SEE THAT CIRCULATION HAS NOT BEEN IMPAIRED. THE PATIENT IS TRANSPORTED WITH THE INJURED LIMB ELEVATED BY A SPLINT STAND.

WARNING!

NEVER ATTEMPT TO CORRECT ANGULATED FRACTURES OF THE FEMUR IF THERE ARE INDICATIONS OF HIP DISLOCATION.

SCAN 9.8B

offers the best support. Remember to pad the voids created at the knee and ankle.

- Leg Bent—Immobilize in the position in which the leg is found, unless there is no distal pulse. Tie a padded board splint to the thigh and above the ankle so the knee is held in position. A pillow can be used to support the leg.

Leg Injuries

Symptoms and Signs

- Pain and tenderness
- Swelling (other deformity is often absent)

Emergency Care

1. Check for circulatory and nerve impairment.
2. Apply an air-inflated splint. Slide the uninflated splint over your hand and gather it in place until the lower edge clears your wrist. Grasp the patient's foot with one hand and his leg just above the injury site using your free hand. While maintaining manual traction, have your partner slide the splint over your hand and onto the injured leg. Your partner must make sure that the splint is wrinkle free and that it covers the injury site. Continue to maintain traction while your partner inflates the splint. Test to see if you can cause a slight dent in the plastic with fingertip pressure. Remember to check periodically that the pressure in the splint has remained adequate.

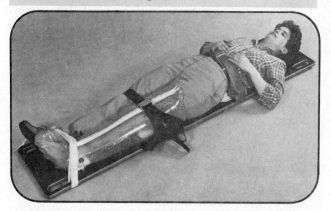

Figure 9-24: Using an air-inflated splint for leg fractures.

You can immobilize the fracture by using two rigid board splints. Apply one medial and one lateral, being certain to immobilize the leg, the knee, and the ankle. Be certain the splints are padded and that you pad any voids created at the knee and ankle.

Regardless of the technique used, you MUST check for circulation and nerve function after immobilization is completed.

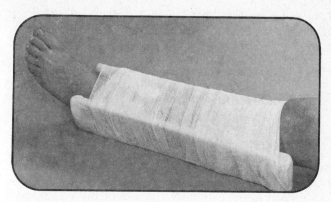

Figure 9-25: Using rigid board splints for leg fractures.

Ankle and Foot Injuries

Symptoms and Signs   It is often difficult to distinguish between fractures and sprains to the foot or ankle. Pain and swelling characterize both injuries.

Care   Long splints, extending from above the knee to beyond the foot, can be used. However, soft splinting is recommended. Mold a pillow around the foot and ankle. Secure by wrapping bandaging material around the pillow.

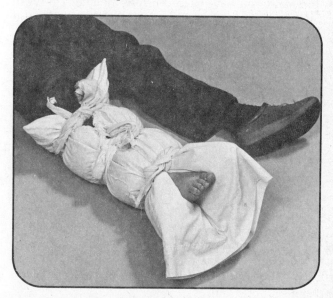

Figure 9-26: Pillow splinting a fractured ankle.

NOTE: Take care not to change the position of the ankle if there is a distal pulse.

SUMMARY

As an EMT, you should never become so preoccupied with fractures that you forget to conduct a primary survey, secondary survey, and an interview. Remember that an open airway, breathing, circulation, and bleeding are your first priorities. Neck, spinal, chest, abdominal, and head injuries, shock, and serious burns all are to be treated before fractures.

Remember, soft tissues are damaged when bones are injured.

The skeletal system is involved with body support, body movement, organ protection and certain aspects of blood cell production. There are two major divisions to the skeletal system, the axial skeleton and the appendicular skeleton. The upper and lower extremities are part of the appendicular skeleton.

Each upper extremity consists of the scapula, clavicle, humerus, ulna, radius, carpals, metacarpals, and phalanges.

Each lower extremity consists of the femur, patella, fibula, tibia, tarsals, metatarsals, and phalanges. Each femur joins with the pelvis.

If a part of a fractured bone tears through the patient's skin, the injury is an open fracture. This is also the case when a penetrating wound accompanies a fracture. If the fractured bones do not tear through the patient's skin, the injury is a closed fracture. You should apply sterile dressings, when possible, to all open fractures of the extremities.

When a bone is broken, it will often bend or twist to form an angulated fracture. Angulations can be straightened by grasping the limb above and below the site of the fracture and gently pulling with the hand you have placed below the site. Do NOT attempt to straighten angulations of or near the shoulders or wrists. Make one gentle attempt to straighten angulations of the elbow or knee only if there is no distal pulse. Do NOT attempt to straighten an angulation of the ankle if there is a distal pulse.

Any break of a bone is a fracture. A dislocation occurs when a bone is pulled out from a joint. Partially torn ligaments produce sprains. Stretching or minor tearing of muscles produce strains.

The symptoms and signs of fracture include deformity, swelling, discoloration, tenderness, pain, loss of function, loss of distal pulse, crepitus, the sound of breaking bone, and exposed bone. Dislocation usually has pain, deformity, swelling, and loss of function. Sprains normally have swelling, discoloration and pain on movement. Pain is usually the only sign of strain.

There are some special signs you need to know including:

- "Dropped' shoulder = clavicular fracture.
- Head of humerus bone out of socket = anterior dislocation of the shoulder.
- Pelvic pain when you compress the patient's hips = pelvic fracture.
- Pelvic injury with patient's foot turning outward = pelvic fracture.
- Lower limb rotates outward = possible anterior hip dislocation or pelvic fracture.
- Lower limb rotates inward and knee is bent = possible posterior hip dislocation.

Splinting is used to immobilize fractures. The process can be carried out using rigid splints, soft splints, or traction splints.

The application of a splint can help to prevent or reduce the severity of complications such as pain, soft tissue damage, bleeding, restricted blood flow, and closed fractures becoming open fractures.

When in doubt, splint.

Remember to cut away, remove, or lift away the patient's clothing over the injury site before splinting. Control bleeding and dress open wounds. Check for a distal pulse to determine nerve or circulatory impairment before and after splinting. When possible, straighten closed fracture angulations. All rigid splints should be padded before they are secured to the patient.

A rigid splint should immobilize the injured bone and the joints directly above and below the bone.

Whenever possible, immobilize all fractures and dislocations before moving the patient.

Traction is applied by pulling gently on an injured limb in the same way you would straighten an angulated fracture.

As an EMT, you must be able to use noncommercial splints. Consider lumber, plywood, rolled newspapers and magazines, compressed wood products, sporting equipment, canes, umbrellas, cardboard, and tool handles to make an emergency splint.

Rigid, soft, and traction splinting for various injuries to the extremities is summarized in Scansheet 9-9.

SPLINTING - EXTREMITIES

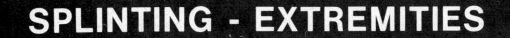

SLING AND SWATHE OR PAD, SLING, AND SWATHE

SLING AND SWATHE

WRIST SLING AND SWATHE OR RIGID SPLINT AND SLING

RIGID SPLINT AND SLING

SOFT SPLINT OR RIGID SPLINT (SECURED TO FOREARM AND UPPER ARM BONE)

SOFT SPLINT WITH SLING AND SWATHE, OR RIGID SPLINT AND SLING

RIGID SPLINT AND SLING

SOFT SPLINTING OR RIGID SPLINT AND SLING

RIGID SPLINT AND SLING OR PILLOW SPLINTS

TIE LOWER LIMBS AND SECURE TO LONG SPINE BOARD

DISLOCATION: SECURE TO LONG SPINE BOARD AND IMMOBILIZE LIMB
OBVIOUS FRACTURES: TIE PATIENT'S LOWER LIMBS TOGETHER AND SECURE TO LONG SPINE BOARD.....OR USE A LONG BOARD SPLINT..... OR TRACTION SPLINT (NOT FOR ELDERLY)

TRACTION SPLINT OR LONG BOARD SPLINTS

SOFT SPLINT OR USE RIGID SPLINT

RIGID SPLINTS OR AIR-INFLATED SPLINT

SOFT PILLOW OR SHORT RIGID SPLINT

10 injuries iii: the skull, spine, and chest

OBJECTIVES By the end of this chapter, you should be able to:

1. Define axial skeleton. (p. 210)

2. Distinguish between cranium and face. (p. 211)

3. Define suture, cranial floor, temporal bone, mandible, maxillae, and temporomandibular joint. (pp. 210, 1)

4. Name and label the FIVE major divisions of the spinal column. (p. 212)

5. Label the components of the rib cage. (p. 212)

6. Define central nervous system. (p. 213)

7. Define "open head injury," "closed head injury," "direct brain injury," and "indirect brain injury." (pp. 213-4)

8. List the basic symptoms and signs of possible skull fracture, facial fracture, and brain injury. (pp. 214-6)

9. List, step by step, the care for injury to the cranium and for injury to the facial bones. (pp. 216-9)

10. List the types of injuries to the spine and relate these injuries to mechanisms of injury. (pp. 219-20)

11. State how to determine possible spinal injury in the conscious patient. (p. 220-1)

12. State how to determine possible spinal injury in the unconscious patient. (p. 223)

13. Describe how to apply an extrication collar. (p. 224)

14. Describe and compare the four-rescuer and the two-rescuer log roll for transferring a patient to a long spine board. (p. 224-5)

15. Describe how a patient should be secured to a long spine board. (p. 224-5)

16. Describe how to remove a helmet from the head of an injured patient. (p. 221, 6)

17. Classify chest injuries and describe the general symptoms and signs associated with open and closed chest wounds. (p. 226)

18. Describe how to determine and care for possible sucking chest wounds, objects impaled in the chest, possible rib fractures, and flail chest. (pp. 226-9)

19. List and describe the common complications associated with injuries to the chest. (p. 229-31)

SKILLS As an EMT, you should be able to:

1. Apply patient assessment techniques to detect possible:
   - cranial fractures
   - facial fractures
   - brain injury
   - spinal injury
   - blunt trauma to the chest
   - fractured ribs
   - flail chest
   - sucking chest wounds

2. Provide emergency care for patients with possible fractured skulls or facial injuries.

3. Provide emergency care for patients with possible brain injury.

4. Apply an extrication collar, transfer and secure a patient to a long spine board.

5. Apply cravats for cases of possible rib fracture.

6. Care for a patient with a flail chest, including

the steps needed to correct paradoxical respirations.

7. Care for patients with objects impaled in the chest.

8. Care for sucking chest wounds and correct problems of tension pneumothorax associated with this care.

9. Detect possible hemothorax, pneumothorax, hemo-pneumothorax, cardiac tamponade, and traumatic asphyxia.

10. Provide proper EMT-level care for complications due to injuries to the chest.

TERMS   you may be using for the first time:

Cranium (KRAY-ni-um)—the bones forming the braincase of the skull.

Suture—where two bones of the skull articulate (join) to form an immovable joint.

Malar (MA-lar) or **Zygomatic** (zi-go-MAT-ik) **Bone**—the cheek bone.

Mandible (MAN-di-bl)—the lower jaw bone.

Maxillae (mak-SIL-e)—the two fused bones forming the upper jaw.

Temporomandibular (TEM-po-ro-man-DIB-u-lar) **joint**—the movable joint formed between mandible and temporal bone.

Spinous Processes—the bony extensions of the posterior vertebrae.

Cervical (SER-ve-kal)—relating to the 7 vertebrae in the neck.

Thoracic (tho-RAS-ik)—relating to the 12 vertebrae to which the ribs attach.

Lumbar (LUM-bar)—relating to the 5 vertebrae of the midback.

Sacral (SA-kral)—the 5 fused vertebrae of the lower back.

Coccyx (KOK-siks)—the 4 fused vertebrae that form the terminal bone of the spine.

Costal Arch—the anatomical landmark formed by the anterior cartilage of the ribs.

Jugular or **Suprasternal Notch**—the visible depression formed at the superior end of the sternum.

Central Nervous System—the brain and spinal cord.

Concussion—mild closed head injury without detectable damage to the brain. Complete recovery is usually expected.

Extrication Collar—a rigid device applied around the neck to help immobilize the head and neck.

Flail Chest—injury where usually three or more consecutive ribs on the same side of the chest are fractured, each in at least two locations. A flail chest can occur when the sternum is fractured loose from its attachments with the ribs.

Paradoxical Respiration—movement of a flailed section of chest in the opposite direction to the rest of the chest during respirations.

Pneumothorax (NU-mo-THO-raks)—condition resulting when air enters the chest cavity and is trapped in the pleural space.

Sucking Chest Wound—an open wound to the chest that draws air from the atmosphere into the chest cavity. This is a form of pneumothorax.

Tension Pneumothorax—condition where air escapes from a punctured lung and is trapped in the thoracic cavity.

Traumatic Asphyxia—a group of symptoms and signs associated with sudden severe compression of the chest.

THE AXIAL SKELETON

In Chapter 9, we divided the skeleton into two subdivisions; the *axial skeleton* and the *appendicular skeleton*. The axial skeleton is composed of the skull, the vertebral (VER-te-bral) column or spinal column, the ribs, and the sternum. It makes up the longitudinal axis of the human body.

The Skull

The skull is made up of 22 bones that form the cranium (KRAY-ni-um) and the face. The eight bones of the cranium are classified as flat bones, irregular in shape. These bones fuse together to produce immovable joints, forming the rigid braincase surrounding the cranial cavity (see Chapter 2). The point at which two bones of the cranium articulate (join together) is known as a suture. The fusion is not complete in infants, causing "soft spots" in a baby's cranium. This is why one must be careful in applying any pressure to the skull of an infant. Whenever care procedures call for you to support the head of a baby, spread your fingers to reduce pressure, avoiding these "soft spots."

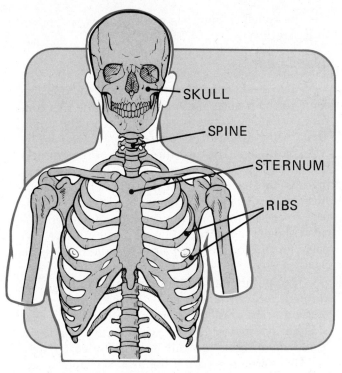

Figure 10-1: The axial skeleton.

The cranium forms the forehead and upper orbits, the top and back of the skull, and the sides of the upper skull. In addition, its bones fuse to form an internal structure called the **cranial floor.** This is the inferior wall of the braincase, containing numerous small openings to provide passageways for nerves and blood vessels that lead to and from the brain.

NOTE: Many people use the term ''skull'' to mean cranium. In most cases, when you hear that a patient has a skull fracture, you can be certain that the cranium is the injury site.

The remaining 14 bones of the skull form the face. These bones are very irregular, but when fused together, they give the face its characteristic shape. As in the case of the cranium, the facial bones are fused into immovable joints, except for the **mandible** (MAN-di-bl). It joins on each side of the cranium

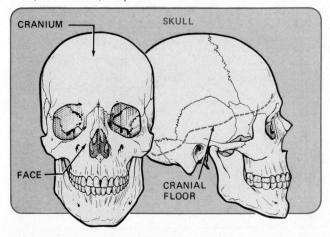

Figure 10-2: Divisions of the skull.

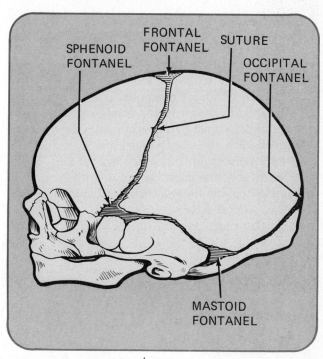

Figure 10-3: The infant skull.

with a **temporal** (TEM-por-al) **bone** to form the **temporomandibular** (TEM-po-ro-man-DIB-u-lar) joint.

The upper jaw is made up of two fused bones called the **maxillae** (mak-SIL-e). Each is known as a maxilla (mak-SIL-ah). The upper third, or bridge of the nose, contains two **nasal bones**. There is a cheek bone on each side of the skull. The cheek bone can be called the **malar** (MA-lar) or the **zygomatic** (zi-go-MAT-ik) **bone**. The malars and the maxillae form a portion of the **orbits** of the eyes.

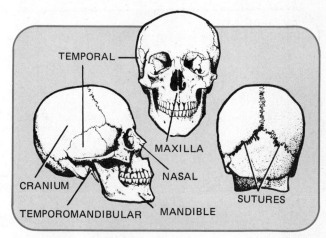

The Spinal Column

The spinal column is made up of 33 irregularly-shaped bones known as **vertebrae** (VER-te-bre). This column of bones gives support to the head and upper body, provides a point of attachment for the pelvis, and protectively houses the spinal cord within the spinal cavity (see Chapter 2). Each bone has a posterior **spinous process,** many of which can be felt along the midline of a person's back.

The vertebrae are connected by ligaments. Located between each two vertebrae is a **disc** of cartilage, hard enough in composition to prevent collapse, yet soft enough to serve as a cushion. Since the spinal cord must be protected, spinal movement is limited. The discs and ligaments in conjunction allow for movement, but excessive bending is not possible at any one particular joint. Any bending is accomplished by the restricted combined movements of several vertebrae.

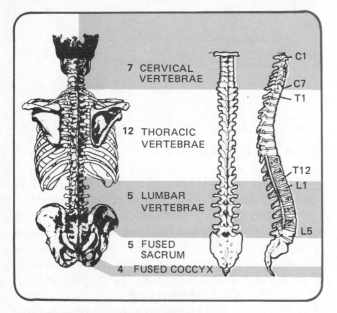

Figure 10-5: Anatomy of the spine.

The spinal column has five divisions, as shown in Figure 10-5.

The Chest

There are 12 pairs of ribs in the human body, the same for both male and female. All of the ribs connect posteriorly to the thoracic vertebrae. The upper seven pairs of ribs attach directly to the sternum by way of cartilage. The next three pairs of ribs connect to the cartilage of the seventh ribs. The term "floating ribs" is given to the last two pairs of ribs. These ribs are connected to the spine, but they do not attach to the sternum or the cartilage of the ribs located above them. Anteriorly, all of the ribs are palpable, except for the first pair, which lie behind the clavicles.

The points of attachment for rib pairs six through ten can be felt easily on each side of the sternum. The cartilage attachment points on each side are referred to as the **costal** (KOS-tal) **margin.** The costal margins combine to form the **costal arch.**

The **sternum** is part of the axial skeleton. In addition to the attachment of the ribs, the sternum also articulates with the clavicles. A visible depression occurs at this point, known as the **jugular** or **suprasternal notch.** The lower extension of the sternum is the **xiphoid process.**

The chest surrounds and protects the lungs and the pleura, the heart and the pericardial sac, part of the trachea, part of the esophagus, and the great blood vessels (aorta and venae cavae). The rib cage extends downward to offer protection to portions of the liver, gallbladder, stomach, and spleen.

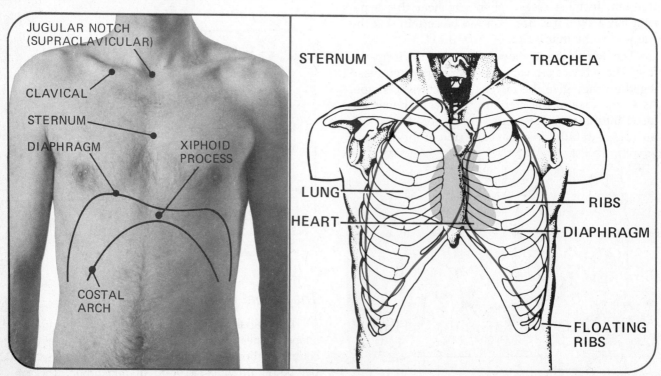

Figure 10-6: The anatomy of the chest.

THE NERVOUS SYSTEM

When evaluating a patient for injuries to the head and spine, always consider the possibility of nervous system damage. The same holds true for many types of chest injuries, since the thoracic spine also may have been injured. Of course, injury to the chest can damage the chest nerves.

Anatomically, the nervous system is divided into two systems: the central nervous system (CNS), and the peripheral nervous system (PNS). The central nervous system consists of the brain and the spinal cord. The peripheral nervous system includes the nerves that enter and leave the spinal cord and those nerves that travel between the brain and organs without passing through the spinal cord (e.g., the optic nerve between the eye and brain).

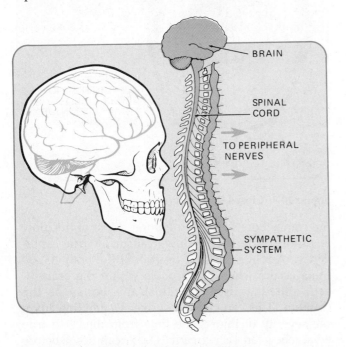

Figure 10-7: Anatomy of the nervous system.

The brain is the master organ of life, the center of consciousness, self-awareness, and thought. It controls basic functions, including breathing and, to some degree, heart activity. Messages from all over the body are received by the brain, which decides how to respond to changing conditions both inside and outside the body. The brain sends messages to the muscles so that they can move, or to a particular organ so that it will carry out a desired function. Any major skull injury can cause damage to the brain, causing vital body functions to fail.

The spinal cord is a relay between most of the body and the brain. A large number of the messages to and from the brain are sent through the spinal cord. Damage to the cord can isolate a part of the body from the brain. Function of this part can be lost, possibly forever.

Reflexes allow us to react quickly to such things as pain and excessive heat without the brain having to send orders. The spinal cord is the center of reflex activity. Damage to the cord can destroy reflex function in certain areas of the body.

The healing power of the brain and nerve tissue is limited. Once damaged to a certain point, function is lost and cannot be restored. As an EMT, your initial care will often prevent additional damage to the brain, spinal cord, and major nerves of the body.

INJURIES TO THE SKULL AND BRAIN

NOTE: Indications of possible injury to the skull or brain should alert you to the possibility of cervical spine injury.

TYPES OF INJURIES

Skull injuries include fractures to the cranium and to the face. If severe enough, these injuries can include direct and indirect injuries to the brain. In addition, there can be cuts to the scalp and other soft tissue injuries as covered in Chapter 8.

A practical classification of injuries to the skull corresponds to the classification of fractures and wounds, namely, either open or closed. When the bones of the cranium are fractured, even if the scalp is not broken, the patient has an open head injury. The word "closed" relates to the skull bones. In a closed head injury, there may be a laceration of the scalp. However, if the cranium is intact, or free of fractures, the term closed head injury is used since there is no opening to the brain.

There are four types of skull fractures. A linear skull fracture is a thin line crack in the cranium. A comminuted (KOM-i-nu-ted) skull fracture has cracks radiating out from the center of the point of impact. A depressed skull fracture is one in which bone fragments are separated from the skull and driven inward by the object that struck the head. Fractures to the cranial floor are called basal skull fractures. Analysis by a physician is needed to detect these fractures; however, clear fluid in the nose and ears suggests a basal skull fracture.

Facial fractures are usually impact-produced, as when a child is struck in the face by a baseball bat, or when someone is thrown against the windshield during a motor vehicle accident. These fractures can be so simple that they go undetected, or they may produce serious, grotesque injury. Of primary concern is the state of the patient's airway. Bone fragments may lodge in the back of the throat, causing airway obstruction. Blood, blood clots, and dislodged teeth also may cause partial or total airway obstruction. A condition that is sometimes missed with facial fractures is the possibility of fractures to the cranial floor.

Brain injuries can be classified as direct or indirect. *Direct* injuries can occur in open head injuries, with the brain being lacerated, punctured, or bruised by the broken bones of the skull, bone fragments, or by foreign objects.

In cases of closed head injuries and certain types of open head injuries, damage to the brain can be indirect. The shock of impact is transferred to the brain. Like any other mass of tissue, the brain swells when it is injured. This swelling is serious since there is little room for expansion within the cranium. *Indirect* injuries to the brain include:

- **Concussion**—A concussion may be so mild that the patient is unaware of his injury. When a person strikes his head in a fall, or is struck by a blunt object, a certain amount of the force is transferred through the skull to the brain. Usually there is no detectable damage to the brain and the patient may or may not become unconscious. Most patients with a concussion will feel a little "groggy" after receiving a blow to the head. Headache is common. If there is a loss of consciousness, it usually lasts only a short time and does not tend to recur. Some loss of memory (**amnesia**) of the events surrounding the accident is fairly common. Long-term memory loss associated with concussion is rare.

- **Contusion**—A bruised brain can occur with closed head injuries, when the force of the blow is great enough to rupture blood vessels found on the surface of, or deep within the brain. Often, this bruise or contusion takes place on the side of the brain *opposite* the point of impact.

With time, as you practice emergency care, you will hear of a patient with a **subdural hematoma** (sub-DU-ral he-mah-TO-mah). When the brain is bruised, lacerated, or punctured, blood from ruptured vessels can flow between the brain and its protective covering, the **meninges** (me-NIN-jez). The thick outer layer of the meninges is known as the dura mater. A subdural hematoma is situated between the dura mater and the brain.

Often, this bleeding is a slow venous flow. Even when the bleeding stops, the hematoma will continue to grow in size as it absorbs tissue fluids. Since there is no room for expansion in the cranium, severe pressure can be placed on the brain. Death can occur if vital brain centers are damaged. This type of hematoma may occur rapidly, or take a prolonged period of time to develop.

Two other types of hematoma are related to head injuries. The **epidural** (ep-i-DU-ral) **hematoma** occurs when blood flows between the meninges and

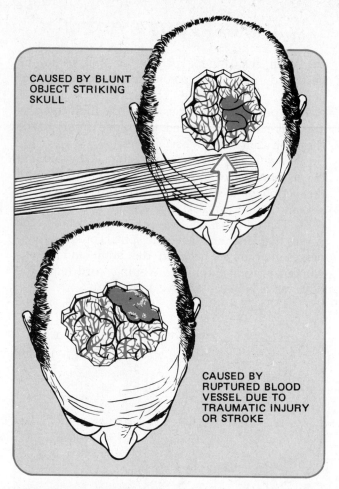

CAUSED BY BLUNT OBJECT STRIKING SKULL

CAUSED BY RUPTURED BLOOD VESSEL DUE TO TRAUMATIC INJURY OR STROKE

Figure 10-8: Closed head injuries.

the cranial bones (above the dura). Most of this flow is profuse arterial bleeding, causing a true emergency. An **intracerebral** (in-trah-SER-e-bral) **hematoma** occurs when blood pools within the brain itself, pushing tissues against the bones of the cranium. This can cause a stroke. Depending upon the severity of injury, the time from injury to true emergency can vary greatly. Death can occur before transport.

Lacerations can occur to the brain as a result of penetrating and perforating wounds of the cranium. Not only is there the problem of direct injury, but there may be severe indirect injury due to hematoma formation.

SIGNS AND SYMPTOMS OF SKULL INJURY

NOTE: If you have reason to believe there is injury to the skull, you must assume possible cervical spine injury.

Skull Fracture

Visible bone fragments and perhaps even bits of brain tissue are the most obvious signs of skull frac-

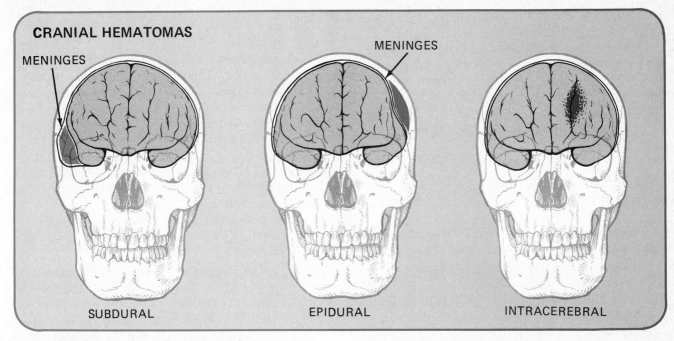

CRANIAL HEMATOMAS

MENINGES

MENINGES

SUBDURAL

EPIDURAL

INTRACEREBRAL

Figure 10-9: Hematomas within the cranium.

ture. You should consider the possibility of a skull fracture whenever you note:

- The patient is unconscious after injury or displays a decreased level of consciousness
- An injury that has produced a deep laceration or severe bruise to the scalp or forehead. Do NOT probe into the wound or separate the wound opening to determine wound depth.
- Any severe pain or swelling at the site of a head injury. Pain is a symptom of skull injury. Do NOT palpate the injury site.
- Deformity of the skull—depressions in the cranium, large swellings ("goose eggs"), or anything that looks unusual about the shape of the cranium.
- Any bruise or swelling behind the ear (Battle's sign). This is sometimes missed.
- Unequal pupils

- Black eyes or discoloration of the soft tissues under both eyes (raccoon's eyes)
- One eye appears to be sunken
- Bleeding from the ears and/or the nose
- Clear fluid flowing from the ears and/or the nose—This could be **cerebrospinal fluid** (ser-e-bro-SPI-nal), also called CSF. This fluid surrounds the brain and spinal cord. It cannot come out through the ears or nose unless the cranium has been fractured.

If fluids coming from the ears or nose are bloody, you will not be able to tell if they contain CSF unless you gently absorb some fluid onto a gauze dressing and see the clear fluid separate out from the spot of blood ("targeting").

Facial Fractures

Consider the possibility of facial fractures when you note:

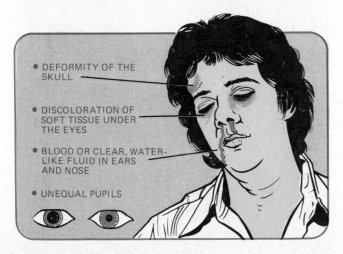

- DEFORMITY OF THE SKULL
- DISCOLORATION OF SOFT TISSUE UNDER THE EYES
- BLOOD OR CLEAR, WATER-LIKE FLUID IN EARS AND NOSE
- UNEQUAL PUPILS

Figure 10-10: Signs of skull fracture.

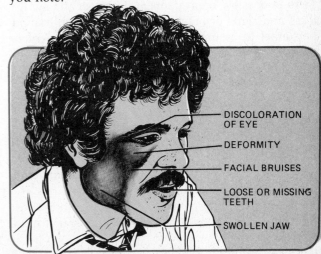

- DISCOLORATION OF EYE
- DEFORMITY
- FACIAL BRUISES
- LOOSE OR MISSING TEETH
- SWOLLEN JAW

Figure 10-11: Signs of facial fracture.

- Blood in the airway
- Facial deformities
- Black eyes or discoloration below the eyes
- A swollen lower jaw or poor jaw function
- Teeth that are loose or have been knocked out, or broken dentures
- Large facial bruises
- Any other indications of a severe blow to the face

SYMPTOMS AND SIGNS OF BRAIN INJURY

In cases of head injury, you should consider the possibility of a brain injury if you note:

- Pain, ranging from simple headache to severe discomfort
- Loss of consciousness or altered state of consciousness
- Confusion, usually increasing as time passes
- Personality changes, ranging from irritable to irrational behavior (major sign)
- Heart rate begins slow and full, then becomes fast and weak
- Respirations may change patterns, becoming labored, then rapid, and then stopping for a few seconds
- Temperature may increase
- Unequal or unresponsive pupils
- Vision impaired in one or both eyes
- Hearing may be impaired
- Equilibrium—May be unable to stand still with eyes closed, or stumbles when attempting to walk (do NOT test for this)
- Paralysis, often to one side of the body
- Any signs of a skull fracture

With so many factors to consider, the mechanism of injury and the location of the injury site become very important when trying to determine if there is possible brain damage. Some of the symptoms and signs of brain injury can cause untrained personnel to assume that a brain injury patient is merely intoxicated or abusing other drugs. Never assume intoxication or drug abuse.

CARE FOR HEAD INJURIES

Injuries to the Cranium

The following procedures apply to patients with or without possible brain damage.

When caring for patients with injuries to the cranium, you should assume that neck or spinal injuries also exist and:

1. Assure an open airway—careful handling is essential since there may be associated spinal injury. For such cases, the AHA guidelines call for the use of the modified jaw-thrust. If there are open injuries to the skull, or if skull fracture is obvious, always use the modified jaw-thrust technique.
2. Maintain an open airway—Monitor the conscious patient for changes in breathing. For the unconscious patient, an oropharyngeal airway may have to be inserted. This must be done *without* hyperextending the neck. Have suctioning equipment ready for immediate use.
3. Provide resuscitative measures if needed.
4. Keep the patient at rest. This can be a critical factor.
5. Control bleeding—Do not apply pressure if the injury site shows bone fragments, depression of the bone, or if the brain is exposed. Do NOT attempt to stop the flow of blood or CSF from the ears or the nose. If the skull is fractured, you may increase intracranial pressure and may also increase the risk of infection.
6. Administer oxygen—This is critical should there be brain damage.
7. Monitor vital signs.
8. Talk to the conscious patient to try to keep him alert. This may keep a patient from becoming unconscious. Ask him questions so that he will have to concentrate.
9. Dress and bandage open wounds, stabilizing any penetrating objects. (Do NOT remove any objects or fragments of bone.)
10. Treat the patient for shock—Avoid overheating.
11. Provide emotional support.
12. Position the patient properly (see below).

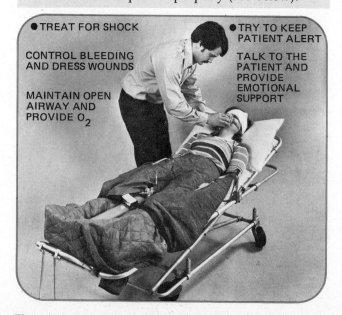

Figure 10-12: Care for cranial injuries.

WARNING: If an unconscious patient regains consciousness, only to lose consciousness again, you MUST report this to the emergency department staff. This is a strong indication of possible life-threatening brain injury.

ALL patients with head injury or suspected brain damage must be carefully monitored during transport. What you observe and report can have a great bearing on the initial actions taken by the emergency department staff. Since a number of observations must be made at relatively close intervals, many ambulances are provided with neurological observation forms. Proper use of these forms will allow you to provide emergency department personnel with an accurate record of your observations.

NEUROLOGICAL ASSESSMENT FORM			
TIME	INITIAL ASSESS-MENT_____		
CONSCIOUS	YES/NO	YES/NO	YES/NO
ORIENTED	YES/NO	YES/NO	YES/NO
RESPONSIVE TO VOICE	YES/NO	YES/NO	YES/NO
RESPONSIVE TO COMMAND	YES/NO	YES/NO	YES/NO
TALKS	YES/NO	YES/NO	YES/NO
REACTS TO PAIN	YES/NO/NA	YES/NO/NA	YES/NO/NA
ABILITY TO MOVE ● LEFT LEG ● RIGHT LEG ● LEFT ARM ● RIGHT ARM			
PUPILS ● REACTIVITY ● SIZE	L R	L R	L R

Figure 10-13: Neurological observation form.

Positioning the Patient with Cranial Injury

Proper patient positioning is important in caring for patients with head injuries. Conscious patients with apparently mild closed head injuries and *absolutely no signs of neck or spinal injuries* can be positioned in one of three ways:

1. Upper Body Elevated—Elevate the entire upper body, or slant the entire body to a head elevated position. Do NOT simply elevate the patient's head and neck. To do so may partially obstruct the airway. Placing the upper body at an angle gives better control should the patient vomit.

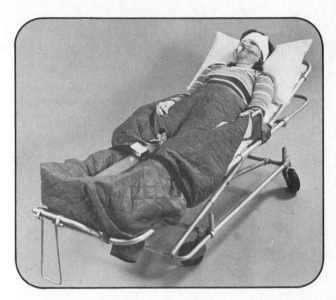

Figure 10-14: Head-elevated position for conscious patients with mild closed head injury but *no signs of spinal injury*.

2. Lateral recumbent—the patient with a mild closed head injury free of spinal involvement can be placed in a lateral recumbent position to improve drainage from any facial injuries. This offers greater airway protection in case of vomiting than does simple spine positioning.

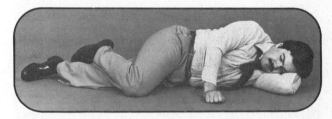

Figure 10-15: Side positioning for patients with mild closed head wounds.

3. Supine—Some systems have adopted positioning that places the patient flat on his back. They feel that there is little risk of intracranial pressure build-up in this position and that it helps to prevent shock. If you use this position you MUST have suction equipment ready and monitor continuously for vomiting.

If you are not certain as to the severity of the patient's injuries, if there is evidence of cervical spine injury, or if the head injury patient is unconscious, then special positioning is required. Blood and mucus must drain freely, and if the patient vomits—as brain-injured patients are likely to do—the vomitus must not be allowed to cause an airway obstruction or be aspirated. Provide careful support to the entire body, but in such a manner that will not require repositioning in case of sudden vomiting. Some head injury patients will vomit without warning. Many vomit without first experiencing nausea.

The traumatic coma position is a modification of the lateral recumbent position used for patients with mild head injuries. It is best to position the patient using four rescuers. If only two rescuers are present, the procedure for placement is as follows:

1. EMT 1 kneels behind the patient's head and establishes an open airway by modified jaw-thrust.

2. EMT 2 gently fastens an extrication collar or rigid "Philadelphia" type collar around the patient's neck with a minimum of neck movement. EMT 1 should be stabilizing the patient's head and neck.

3. Once the rigid collar is in place, EMT 2 places a long spine board next to the patient's left side and takes up a position next to the board.

4. EMT 1 continues to support the patient's head, while EMT 2 extends the patient's arm so that it does not interfere with log-rolling, and then flexes the patient's right leg.

5. EMT 2 places one hand on the flexed knee of the patient and his other hand across the patient's waist. On a signal from the EMT 1, the patient is log-rolled onto the board.

6. EMT 2 places a small folded blanket between the patient's head and his bent arm. The patient's spine is now maintained in a straight line while the mouth is tilted downward.

7. EMT 1 re-establishes the airway by modified jaw-thrust, if necessary.

8. The EMTs position the patient's right arm, secure the patient to the board (head first, then chest, hips, and knees). Patient and board are moved as a unit to the wheeled ambulance stretcher.

NOTE: Do not use this technique until you have mastered the skill of log rolling a patient with possible spinal injury. See page 224.

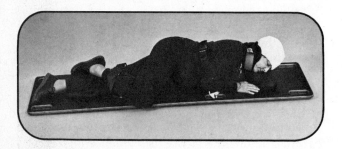

Figure 10-16: The traumatic coma position.

The traumatic coma position is not accepted in all jurisdictions. It is not presented here as a standard of care. Unless there is local EMS System approval for this technique, do NOT use the traumatic coma position. Where this positioning is not used, an extrication collar is attached and the patient is placed in a supine position on a spine board. Constant monitoring of the patient, with suction equipment ready for use, is recommended when you

transport an unconscious patient or a patient with severe head injury.

The patient secured properly in a supine position to a long spine board can be positioned for drainage if the patient and the board are rotated. You must be able to secure the patient and board in this position on the ambulance.

Cranial Injuries with Impaled Objects

If there is an object impaled in the patient's cranium or face, do NOT remove it. Instead, stabilize the object in place with bulky dressings. This, plus care in handling, minimizes accidental movement of the object during the remainder of care and transport. The exception to this procedure occurs when the object is impaled in the soft tissues of the cheek and has entered the oral cavity. Care for such cases was presented in Chapter 8.

In some situations you may be confronted with a patient whose skull has been impaled by a long object. This can make transporting of the patient impossible until the object is cut or shortened. Pad around the object with bulky dressings, then carefully—and rigidly—stabilize the object on both sides of where the cut will be made. Cutting should be done with a tool that will not cause the object to move or vibrate when it is finally severed. Often, a hand hacksaw is the best tool to use because it can be carefully controlled. In any case where you have to cut a long impaled object, call for advice from the emergency department physician.

Facial Bones

When confronted with a patient who has possible facial fractures, your principle concerns are to keep the airway open and to stop profuse bleeding. Direct pressure is the usual method used to control bleeding, but care must be exercised not to apply pressure directly over a probable fracture site.

During care at the scene and during transport, positioning for drainage is essential. If the patient is unconscious, or there are indications of possible facial fractures, application of an extrication collar is recommended. Such patients must be transported with support provided to the entire spine. This means that you will have to immobilize the spine by securing the patient to a long spine board. The board will have to be rotated to allow for drainage. If the traumatic coma position is used by your EMS System, you will have to position the patient so the *uninjured* side of the face is placed downward.

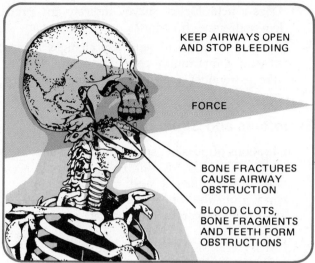

Figure 10-17: Potential complications from facial fractures.

INJURIES TO THE SPINE

TYPES OF INJURIES

Injuries to the spine must be considered anytime you find serious injury to the body. Remember that spinal injury can be associated with head, neck, and back injuries. Don't overlook the possibility of spinal injury when dealing with chest, abdominal, and pelvic injuries. Even injuries to the upper and lower extremities can be caused by forces intense enough to also produce spinal injury. Remember, you must always do a *complete* patient survey. Failure to do so will reduce your chances of detecting possible spinal injury.

Injuries to the spinal column include:
- Fractures, with and without bone displacement
- Dislocations
- Ligament sprains
- Disc injury, including compression

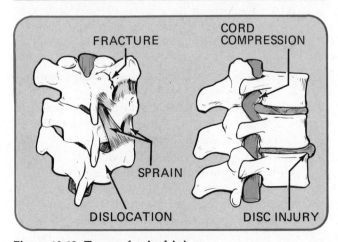

Figure 10-18: Types of spinal injury.

There may not be any damage to the spinal cord or spinal nerves with some types of injury. A fractured coccyx is a nondisplaced fracture below the level of the cord. Ligament sprains are relatively simple injuries. However, when displaced fractures and dislocations occur, the cord, disc, and spinal nerves may be severely injured. Serious contusions and lacerations, accompanied by pressure-producing swelling, can take place. The entire column can become unstable, leading to cord compression that may produce paralysis or death.

Mechanisms of Injury

NOTE: There is a simple rule you can follow. If there is any soft tissue damage to the head, face, or neck due to a sudden deceleration injury (e.g.: being thrown against a dashboard), then assume cervical spine injury. Any blunt trauma above the clavicles may damage the cervical spine.

Some parts of the spine are more susceptible to injury than others. Because they are somewhat splinted by the attached ribs, the segments of the thoracic spine are not usually damaged except in the most violent accidents, or in gunshot wounds. The pelvic-sacral spine articulation helps to protect the sacrum in the same way. On the other hand, the cervical and lumbar vertebrae are susceptible to injury because they are not supported by other bony structures. The cervical spine can be damaged in "whiplash" accidents, and the lumbar spine can become injured when a person tries to lift a heavy load improperly.

A common injury in vehicle accidents is "whiplash." When one vehicle strikes another vehicle or a fixed object head on, the neck can whip quickly back and forth. This neck movement is usually far in excess of the normal range of motion. Virtually the same thing occurs when a vehicle is struck from behind.

A fall can produce spinal injury as the victim strikes his head upon an object, the ground, or the floor. The force generated during a fall may be enough to fracture or crush vertebrae as the person strikes the ground. Cases of improper care have been reported where the head injuries were noted and cared for, but spinal injuries were overlooked.

Many sporting activities can lead to accidents that can cause spinal injury. Sledding and skiing accidents can hurl a person into trees or other fixed objects, twisting the spinal column in the process. In many of these accidents, there are no serious open wounds and the extremities are not fractured, yet spinal injury has occurred. The body of the victim is usually covered by bulky clothing, leaving no obvious signs of injury for the untrained rescuer. As a result, the victim may be placed on a stretcher without adequate examination and immobilization.

Diving board and diving accidents often produce injury to the cervical spine. When the victim strikes the board, the side or bottom of the pool, or an underwater object, the head can be severely forced beyond its normal limits of motion.

Football and other contact sports can have accidents severe enough to produce possible spinal injury. Whenever the game involves player contact or falling to the ground, be on the alert for spinal injury.

REMEMBER: Any violent accident and any falling accident can produce spinal injury. You must do a complete survey of the patient.

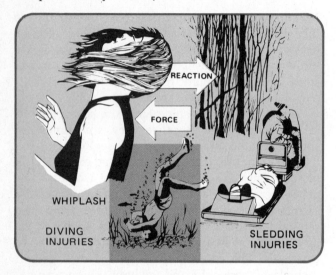

Figure 10-19: Mechanisms of neck injury.

DETERMINING POSSIBLE SPINAL INJURY

REMEMBER: You *must* assume that any unconscious patient who is the victim of an accident has spinal injury.

Spinal injuries can be difficult to detect. Your chances of finding possible spinal injury will increase if you:

1. Consider the mechanism of injury—Is the accident the type that can produce spinal injury? Serious falls, motor vehicle accidents, diving accidents, and cave-ins often cause spinal damage.

2. Observe the position of the patient—The patient in a supine position may have his arms stretched out above the head.

3. Question the patient and bystanders about the accident—They may be able to report something that is not obvious.

4. Do a head-to-toe-examination:
   - Are there injuries you can associate with spinal injuries? Facial injury, head wounds and fractures, neck wounds, blunt trauma to the back and chest, pelvic fractures and hip dislocations indicate a mechanism of injury that may have produced damage to the spine.
   - Are there symptoms and signs indicating possible spinal injury?

   - Does a neurological survey indicate any problem with nerve function?

5. Monitor the patient to note any changes associated with spinal injury—Numbness and tingling in the extremities may begin, or paralysis may occur.

Symptoms and Signs of Spinal Injury

Indications of possible spinal injury include:

- **PAIN WITHOUT MOVEMENT**—The pain is not always constant and may occur anywhere from the top of the head to the buttocks. Other painful injuries can mask out this symptom.
- **PAIN WITH MOVEMENT**—The patient normally tries to lie perfectly still to prevent pain upon movement. You should not request the patient to move just to determine if pain is present. However, if the patient complains of pain in the neck or back upon voluntary movements, you MUST consider this to be a symptom of possible spinal injury. Do NOT have the patient attempt hand and foot waves as part of your assessment if he reports that he has pain with movement.
- **TENDERNESS**—Gentle palpating of the injury site, when accessible, may reveal point tenderness.
- **DEFORMITY**—The removal of clothing to check the back for deformity is not recommended. OBVIOUS SPINAL DEFORMITIES ARE RARE. If you note a gap between the spinous processes of the vertebrae or if you can feel a broken spinous process, you MUST consider the patient to have spinal injuries.
- **IMPAIRED BREATHING**—Neck injury can impair nerve function to the chest muscles. Watch the patient breathe. If there is only a slight movement of the abdomen, with little or no movement of the chest, it is safe to assume that the patient is breathing with his diaphragm alone. Panting due to respiratory insufficiency may develop.
- **PRIAPISM**—Persistent erection of the penis is a reliable sign of spinal injury affecting nerves to the external genitalia.
- **CHARACTERISTIC POSITIONING OF THE ARMS**—In some cases of spinal injury, motor nerve pathways to the muscles that extend the arm can be interrupted, but those leading to the muscles that bend the elbow and lift the arm remain functional. The patient may be found on his back, with the arms extended above the head.
- **INVOLUNTARY LOSS OF BOWEL AND BLADDER CONTROL**

• NERVE IMPAIRMENT TO THE EXTREM-ITIES—The patient may have loss of use, weakness, numbness, tingling, or loss of feeling in the upper and/or lower extremities. PARALYSIS OF THE EXTREMITIES IS PROBABLY THE MOST RELIABLE SIGN OF SPINAL INJURY IN CONSCIOUS PATIENTS.

NOTE: Pain, pain on movement, and tenderness anywhere along the spine are reliable indicators of possible spinal injury in the conscious patient. If these are present, you have sufficient reason to rigidly immobilize him before proceeding with the survey. If immediate immobilization is not possible, use extreme care in handling the patient. In the field, it is not possible to completely rule out spinal injury even in cases where the patient has no pain and is able to move his limbs.

The next Scansheet reviews the elements of patient assessment that apply to spinal injuries.

CARE FOR SPINAL INJURIES

Regardless of where the apparent spinal injury is located on the cord, care is the same. For all patients with possible spinal injury, and for all accident victims where there is doubt as to the extent of injury, you should:

1. Provide manual traction for the head and neck.
2. Apply an extrication or rigid collar and continue to maintain manual traction.
3. Secure the patient to a long spine board.
4. Administer oxygen in high concentration. Edema to the cord may impair oxygen delivery to the cord. When this occurs, cell death can take place.

In some cases, it will be necessary to secure the patient to a short spine board prior to securing him to a long one. This is the case for patients found seated in motor vehicles and for patients found in locations where physical use of a long board is too restricted or impossible. The procedures to follow for difficult-to-reach patients, including those found in automobiles, will be covered later in Chapter 18. This chapter will present other devices, such as the Kendrick extrication device (K.E.D.) and the scoop-style stretcher. For now, master the skills of the extrication collar and the long spine board.

The next Scansheet presents the techniques for applying an extrication collar, placing a patient on a long spine board, and securing a patient to a long spine board. Before you study the Scansheet, consider the following:

• Most authorities no longer recommend the use of a soft cervical collar. An extrication collar or rigid-type collar provides better support.

• You must measure the collar to be certain that you apply the correct size to the patient. A large patient may not take a large collar. A small patient with a long neck may take your largest collar. The front width of the collar should fit between the point of the chin and the chest at the jugular notch.

• Once the head and neck are immobilized by hand, this immobilization must be maintained until an extrication or rigid collar is applied and the patient is secured to a long spine board.

• When a patient is secured to a long spine board, the order of ties goes from head to foot. The head is to be secured first, using 3-inch tape or a cravat. The tape offers more support, especially if the patient and board are to be tilted to allow for drainage. However, blood on the patient's skin and hair may make using tape impractical. You should learn both methods.

Care for Patients Wearing Helmets

Helmets are worn in many sporting events and by many motorcycle riders. Neck injury and spinal injury care may call for the removal of the helmet. The helmet should not prevent you from reaching the patient's mouth or nose if resuscitation efforts are needed. Protection shields can be lifted, and face guards can be cut away. If the face guard is to be cut away, one EMT must steady the patient's head and neck with manual traction. The other EMT should place *protective coverings* (towels or folded blankets) directly over the patient's face and the anterior neck. This EMT can now use a bolt cutter or other such suitable cutting device to remove the face guard.

When a helmet must be removed, it is a two rescuer situation. After fully explaining to the patient what you are going to do, the procedure is as follows:

1. EMT 1 maintains manual traction with a hand on each side of the lower jaw. The construction of the helmet may require the traction to be applied with the fingers, while the rest of the hand is placed on the side of the helmet.

2. EMT 2 opens, cuts, or removes the chin strap, then places one hand on the patient's chin (see Fig. 10-20) and, using the other hand, applies traction at the occipital region.

3. EMT 1 can now release manual traction and slowly remove the helmet. The lower sides of the helmet will have to be gently pulled out to clear the ears. Eyeglasses may have to be removed.

ASSESSING PATIENTS FOR SPINAL INJURIES

SYMPTOMS AND SIGNS

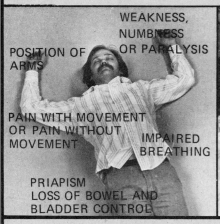

POSITION OF ARMS

WEAKNESS, NUMBNESS OR PARALYSIS

PAIN WITH MOVEMENT OR PAIN WITHOUT MOVEMENT

IMPAIRED BREATHING

PRIAPISM LOSS OF BOWEL AND BLADDER CONTROL

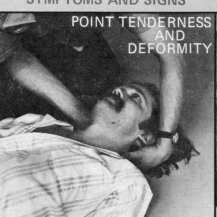

POINT TENDERNESS AND DEFORMITY

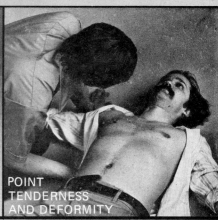

POINT TENDERNESS AND DEFORMITY

CONSCIOUS — LOWER EXTREMITIES ASSESSMENT

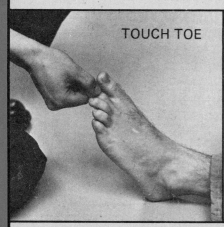

TOUCH TOE

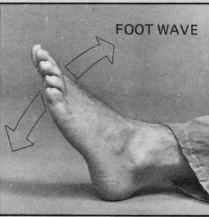

FOOT WAVE

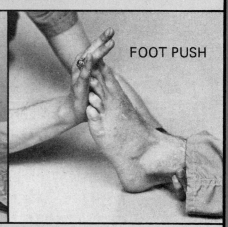

FOOT PUSH

RESULTS: IF THE PATIENT CAN PERFORM THESE TASKS, THERE IS LITTLE CHANCE OF SEVERE INJURY TO THE CORD ANYWHERE ALONG ITS LENGTH. IF THE TESTS CAN ONLY BE PERFORMED TO A LIMITED DEGREE AND WITH PAIN, THERE MAY BE PRESSURE SOMEWHERE ALONG THE CORD. WHEN A PATIENT IS NOT ABLE TO PERFORM ANY OF THE TESTS, YOU MUST ASSUME THERE IS SPINAL DAMAGE.

CONSCIOUS — UPPER EXTREMITIES ASSESSMENT

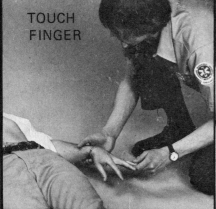

TOUCH FINGER

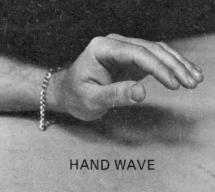

HAND WAVE

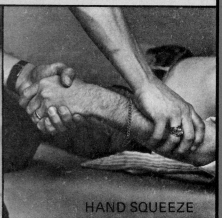

HAND SQUEEZE

RESULTS: PERFORMANCE OF ALL TESTS, NO INDICATION OF DAMAGE IN THE CERVICAL AREA.
LIMITED PERFORMANCE AND PAIN, PRESSURE ON CORD IN CERVICAL AREA.
FAILURE TO PERFORM ANY TEST AND NEGATIVE LOWER EXTREMITY RESULTS, CORD INJURY IN NECK.

SCAN 10.1A

ASSESSING PATIENTS FOR SPINAL INJURY (cont'd)

UNCONSCIOUS PATIENTS: TEST THE RESPONSES TO PAINFUL STIMULI APPLIED TO THE SOLES OF THE FEET AND THE PALMS OF THE HANDS. IF REMOVAL OF SHOES MAY AGGRAVATE EXISTING INJURIES, APPLY THE STIMULI TO THE SKIN AROUND THE ANKLES.

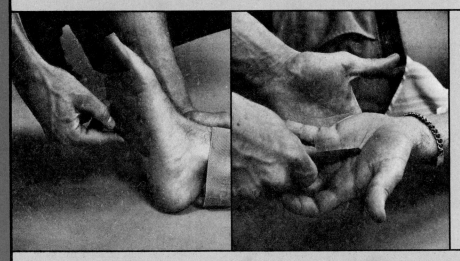

REMEMBER:

IT IS DIFFICULT TO SURVEY THE UNCONSCIOUS PATIENT WITH ACCURACY. A DEEPLY UNCONSCIOUS PATIENT WILL NOT PULL BACK FROM A PAINFUL STIMULUS. SHOULD THE MECHANISM OF INJURY INDICATE POSSIBLE SPINAL DAMAGE, BUT SURE SIGNS ARE NOT OBTAINABLE, ASSUME SPINAL INJURY IS PRESENT.

RESULTS: SLIGHT PULLING BACK OF FOOT—CORD INTACT
NO FOOT REACTION—POSSIBLE DAMAGE ANYWHERE ALONG THE CORD.
HAND OR FINGER REACTION—NO DAMAGE TO CERVICAL CORD.
NO HAND OR FINGER REACTION—POSSIBLE DAMAGE TO THE CERVICAL CORD

SUMMARY OF OBSERVATIONS AND CONCLUSIONS

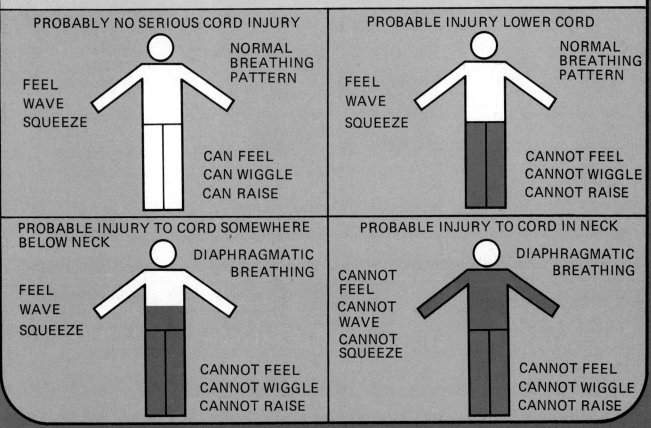

PROBABLY NO SERIOUS CORD INJURY
FEEL WAVE SQUEEZE
NORMAL BREATHING PATTERN
CAN FEEL CAN WIGGLE CAN RAISE

PROBABLE INJURY LOWER CORD
FEEL WAVE SQUEEZE
NORMAL BREATHING PATTERN
CANNOT FEEL CANNOT WIGGLE CANNOT RAISE

PROBABLE INJURY TO CORD SOMEWHERE BELOW NECK
FEEL WAVE SQUEEZE
DIAPHRAGMATIC BREATHING
CANNOT FEEL CANNOT WIGGLE CANNOT RAISE

PROBABLE INJURY TO CORD IN NECK
CANNOT FEEL CANNOT WAVE CANNOT SQUEEZE
DIAPHRAGMATIC BREATHING
CANNOT FEEL CANNOT WIGGLE CANNOT RAISE

SCAN 10.1B

CARING FOR SPINAL INJURIES

APPLYING AN EXTRICATION OR RIGID COLLAR

(1) APPLY STEADY, BUT GENTLE MANUAL TRACTION TO THE HEAD AND NECK

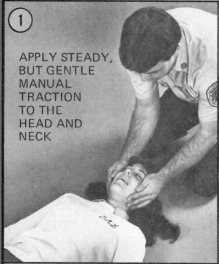

(2) PLACE AN EXTRICATION OR RIGID COLLAR AROUND THE PATIENT'S NECK

FASTEN THE COLLAR IN PLACE. MANUAL TRACTION MUST BE MAINTAINED UNTIL THE PATIENT IS SECURED TO A LONG SPINE BOARD

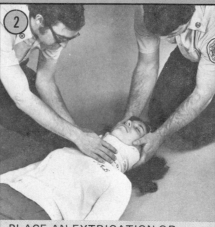

(3)

TRANSFERRING A GROUND—LEVEL PATIENT — FOUR RESCUER LOG ROLL

(1) ACTIVITY AROUND THE PT. IS RE-STRICTED

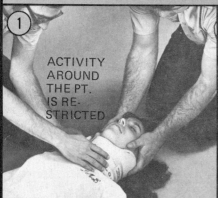

EMT 1 APPLIES MANUAL TRACTION AND AIRWAY IS OPENED BY THE MODIFIED JAW-THRUST. EMT 2 PLACES AN EXTRICATION COLLAR AROUND THE PATIENT'S NECK. EMT 1 MAINTAINS MANUAL TRACTION

(2) THE BOARD IS PLACED PARALLEL TO THE PT. WHEN POSSIBLE, PADDING IS PROVIDED AT THE LEVEL OF THE NECK, WAIST, KNEES AND ANKLES TO HELP FILL VOIDS BETWEEN BODY AND BOARD

(3)

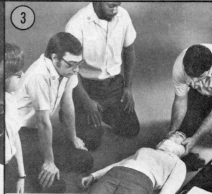

3 RESCUERS KNEEL AT PT.'S SIDE OPPOSITE BOARD, LEAVING ROOM TO ROLL PT. TOWARDS THEM. ONE RESCUER AT SHOULDER, ONE AT WAIST, ONE AT KNEE. EMT 1 MAINTAINS TRACTION

EMT 1 CONTROLS MOVE. THE SHOULDER LEVEL RESCUER IS DIRECTED TO EXTEND ARM OF PT. OVER THE HEAD OF THE SIDE ON WHICH THE PT. WILL BE ROLLED

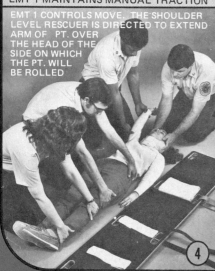

(4)

EMT 1 ORDERS RESCUERS TO REACH ACROSS PT. AND TAKE PROPER HAND PLACEMENTS.

- SHOULDER LEVEL RESCUER—ONE HAND UNDER PT.'S SHOULDER, OTHER HAND UNDER PT.'S UPPER ARM
- WAIST LEVEL RESCUER—ONE HAND ON PT.'S WAIST, OTHER UNDER PT.'S BUTTOCKS
- KNEE LEVEL RESCUER—ONE HAND UNDER PT.'S LOWER THIGH—OTHER UNDER THE MIDCALF

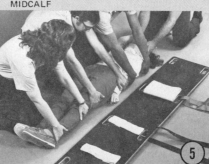

(5)

EMT 1 MAINTAINS MANUAL TRACTION TO HEAD & NECK—DIRECTS OTHERS TO ROLL PT. ON TO SIDE, MOVING PT. AS A UNIT

(6)

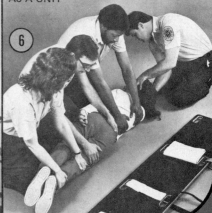

SCAN 10.2A

CARING FOR SPINAL INJURIES (cont'd.)

FOUR RESCUER LOG ROLL — CONTINUED

(7) EMT 1 DIRECTS WAIST-LEVEL RESCUER TO FREE HAND TO ADJUST PADS, GRIP SPINE BOARD, AND PULL INTO POSITION AGAINST PATIENT.

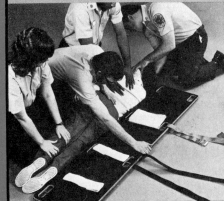

(8) EMT 1 ORDERS THE RESCUERS TO ROLL PT. ONTO BOARD

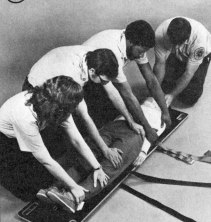

THE PT.'S HEAD IS SECURED TO BOARD WITH CRAVAT OR 3" TAPE. PLACE ROLLED BLANKETS BESIDE HEAD & NECK FOR ADDITIONAL PROTECTION. THESE MUST BE SECURED BY A CRAVAT OVER FOREHEAD AND TIED TO SIDES OF BOARD

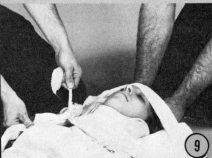

(9)

(10) PT. IS SECURED TO BOARD BY 3 ADDITIONAL STRAPS. ONE IS PLACED ACROSS CHEST, ONE ABOVE HIPS, ONE ABOVE THE KNEE. EMT 1 MAINTAINS TRACTION. TIE WRISTS LOOSELY TOGETHER

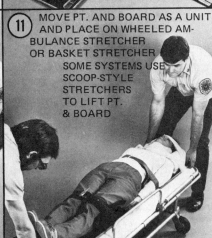

(11) MOVE PT. AND BOARD AS A UNIT AND PLACE ON WHEELED AMBULANCE STRETCHER OR BASKET STRETCHER. SOME SYSTEMS USE SCOOP-STYLE STRETCHERS TO LIFT PT. & BOARD

(12)

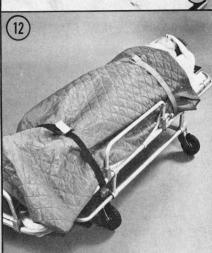

TWO RESCUER LOG ROLL

NOTE: USE EXTREME CARE. THIS METHOD SHOULD BE USED ONLY WHEN DANGERS AT THE SCENE THREATEN PATIENT AND RESCUERS.

(1) EMT 1 MAINTAINS OPEN AIRWAY & MANUAL TRACTION BY THE MODIFIED JAW-THRUST, WHILE EMT 2 APPLIES EXTRICATION COLLAR. EMT 1 MAINTAINS TRACTION—EMT 2 PLACES PADS & BOARD PARALLEL & CLOSE TO PT. CRAVATS ARE TIED AROUND FEET AND CALVES

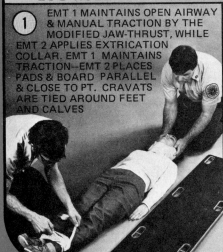

EMT 2 EXTENDS PT.'S ARM OVER HEAD, KNEELS AT PT.'S HIPS. EMT 1 ORDERS THE ROLL, MAINTAINING TRACTION. ROLL PATIENT AS A UNIT. AFTER COMPLETING ROLL, EMT 2 PULLS BOARD AGAINST THE PATIENT'S BACK

(2)

(3) THE PT. IS GENTLY ROLLED ONTO BOARD—SECURED TO BOARD BY STRAPS ACROSS CHEST, ABOVE WAIST, ABOVE KNEES. HANDS ARE LOOSELY TIED TOGETHER. STOP MANUAL TRACTION WHEN PT. SECURED

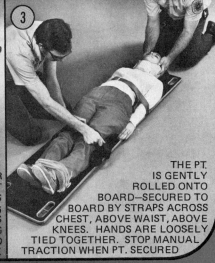

SCAN 10.2B

4. EMT 1, after removing the helmet, re-establishes manual traction and an open airway by using the modified jaw-thrust.

5. EMT 2 can release traction and apply an extrication or rigid collar. The patient should then be secured to a long spine board.

NOTE: This method has not been adopted in all EMS Systems. Your instructor will inform you of local policies.

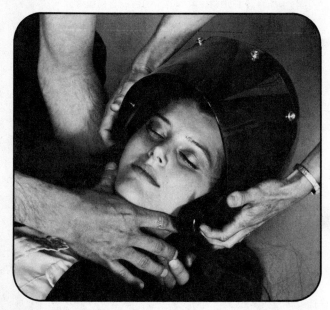

Figure 10-20: Maintaining traction when removing helmets.

INJURIES TO THE CHEST

TYPES OF CHEST INJURIES

The chest can be injured in a number of ways, including:

- *Blunt trauma.* A blow to the chest can fracture the ribs, the sternum, and the costal cartilage. Whole sections of the chest may collapse. With severe blunt trauma, the lungs and airway can be damaged, and the heart may be seriously injured.

- *Penetrating objects.* Bullets, knives, pieces of metal or glass, steel rods, pipes, and various other objects can penetrate the chest wall, damaging internal organs and impairing respiration.

- *Compression.* This is a severe form of blunt trauma where the chest is rapidly compressed, as when the driver of a motor vehicle pitches forward in a head-on collision and strikes his chest on the steering column. The heart can be severely squeezed, and the sternum and ribs fractured.

Injuries to the chest also may injure the lungs, heart, or great blood vessels. Basic life support may be the only course of action for the EMT. However, there are other care procedures that can undoubtedly save the patient's life.

Chest injuries can be classified as *open* or *closed*.

- *Open.* When the skin is broken, the patient has an open wound. However, most people use the term "open chest wound" to mean that the chest wall is penetrated, as, for example, by a bullet or a knife blade. An object can pass through the wall from the outside, or a fractured and displaced rib can penetrate the chest wall from within. The heart, lungs, and great vessels can be injured at the same time the chest wall is penetrated.

- *Closed.* The skin is not broken with a closed chest injury, leading some people to think that the damage is not serious. Such injuries, sustained through blunt trauma and compression accidents, can cause contusions and lacerations of the heart, lungs, and great vessels.

General Symptoms and Signs of Chest Injury

An obvious wound is the most reliable sign of chest injury. When there is no such wound, check for the following:

- Pain at the injury site
- Painful breathing
- Difficult breathing
- Rapid and weak pulse, indicating shock from blood loss or respiratory shock
- Low blood pressure
- Cyanosis, indicating oxygen deficiency
- Coughing up bright red frothy blood, indicating a punctured lung
- Distended neck veins
- Failure of the chest wall to expand and contract normally
- Pain upon compression of the lateral chest wall
- Unequal air entry

Note how the above can be determined from a complete and proper patient assessment.

Specific Open Chest Wounds

Puncture wounds can range from minor to life-threatening. The object producing the wound may remain impaled in the chest, or the wound may be completely open. Penetrating chest wounds occur when an object tears or punctures the chest wall, opening the thoracic cavity to the atmosphere. If there is an exit wound, then penetration is easy to determine. Otherwise, you will be able to tell if a puncture wound is a penetrating wound by noting:

- A severe chest wound where the chest wall is torn or punctured
- A sucking sound each time the patient breathes. These wounds are sometimes called "sucking" chest wounds.

Pneumothorax occurs when the pleural sac is punctured and air enters the thoracic cavity. The air can come through the external wound opening, or it may come out of a punctured lung. In pneumothorax, the lung collapses. Air accumulates on the injured side and can force the heart against the uninjured lung. The term "sucking chest wound" is used when the thoracic cavity is open to the atmosphere. Each time the patient breathes, air can be sucked into the opening. Along with the characteristic sucking sound, you will hear the patient gasp as he makes a desperate attempt to fill his lungs with air. This patient will develop severe dyspnea (difficult breathing). The delicate pressure balance within the thoracic cavity is destroyed and the lung on the injured side can collapse.

The object penetrating the chest wall may have seriously damaged a lung, major blood vessel, or the heart itself. This type of injury is a TRUE EMERGENCY that requires immediate initial care and transport to a medical facility as soon as possible.

Care for Pneumothorax

1. Maintain an open airway. Provide basic life support if necessary.
2. Apply an occlusive dressing and seal all four edges with tape. The last edge should be sealed when the patient forcefully exhales. If the seal is effective, respirations will be partially stabilized. If there is an exit wound in the chest you will have to apply an occlusive dressing over this wound.
3. Treat for shock.
4. Administer a high concentration of oxygen.
5. Transport as soon as possible, keeping the patient positioned on the injured side.
6. Monitor the patient and be prepared to suction blood from the oral cavity. Call ahead to alert the emergency department staff.

A complication can develop with pneumothorax that is caused by the application of a sealed occlusive dressing. This complication is called tension pneumothorax. If a patient has a penetrating chest wound with a punctured lung, air will enter the thoracic cavity through the open wound in the chest wall and through the opening in the lung. If you seal off the chest wall opening, air will still flow into the cavity with each breath. Pressure will build in the cavity. The signs of tension pneumothorax include:

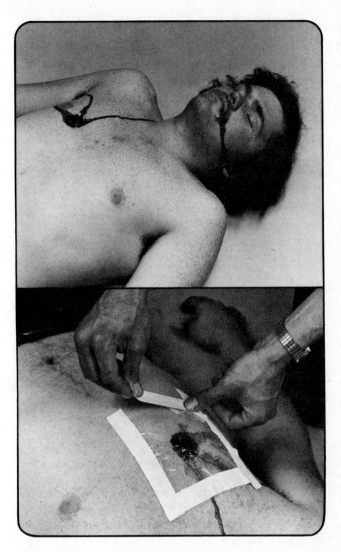

Figure 10-21: Applying an occlusive dressing for pneumothorax.

- Increasing respiratory difficulty
- Weak pulse
- Cyanosis
- Low blood pressure due to decreased cardiac output
- Reduction of breathing sounds heard in one side of the chest
- Distended neck veins
- Trachea may be pushed to one side of neck (deviated)

If you seal a sucking chest wound with an occlusive dressing and find that the patient declines rapidly, you will have to lift a corner of the seal to let air escape. The patient should respond almost immediately as pressure is released from the heart and uninjured lung. Reseal the wound and monitor the patient. You may have to continue to unseal and reseal the wound.

REMEMBER: Whenever you apply an occlusive dressing to a pneumothorax patient, stay alert for tension pneumothorax.

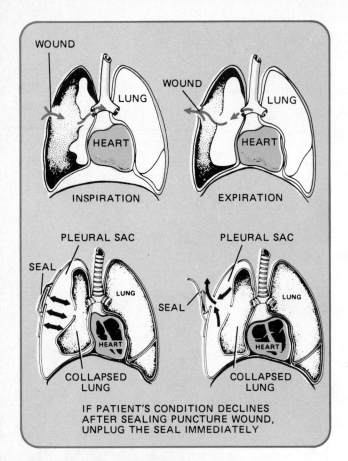

Figure 10-22: Tension pneumothorax.

Impaled Objects. As discussed in Chapter 8, an impaled object should be left in place. The object must be stabilized with bulky dressings, pads, or a doughnut-shaped stabilizer made from cravats. You should use tape to hold all dressings and pads in place. If tape proves to be ineffective due to blood or sweat on the patient's skin, hold the dressings and pads in place with wide cravats. These should be tied on the patient's side. Make certain that nothing touches the impaled object during transport.

Specific Closed Chest Injuries

Closed chest injuries include rib fractures, flail chest, and compression injuries.

Rib fractures usually result from blunt trauma or compression. Often, you will not know for sure if a rib is fractured; however, some ribs are more susceptible to injury than others. The upper four pairs of ribs are rarely fractured because they are protected by the structures of the shoulder girdle. The fifth through tenth pairs of ribs are the ones most commonly fractured. The freedom of movement found in the "floating" ribs often prevents them from being fractured.

A conscious coherent person with fractured ribs usually can point out the exact injury site. Seldom is there any deformity associated with the injury. The symptoms and signs of fractured ribs include:

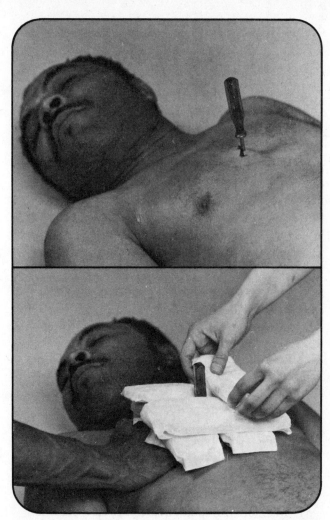

Figure 10-23: Stabilizing and dressing an object impaled in the chest.

- Pain at the site of the fracture, with increased pain upon moving
- Tenderness over the site of the fracture
- Shallow breathing, sometimes with the patient reporting a crackling sensation at or near the site of fracture.
- Characteristic stance, with the patient leaning toward the injured side and holding his hand over the fracture site.

Care of Fractured Ribs Always provide care for possible fractured ribs. You will probably help reduce the patient's pain, and you will provide protection for his lungs and the blood vessels that are located between the ribs (intercostal arteries and veins). Remember, evaluating fractured ribs requires x-ray analysis by a physician. If you suspect rib fracture, provide appropriate care.

Apply at least three cravats around the patient's chest and arm. Position one cravat just below the level of the fracture. The second cravat overlaps the first and should be directly over the injury site. The third cravat overlaps the second and should be above the fracture site. The arm on the injured side

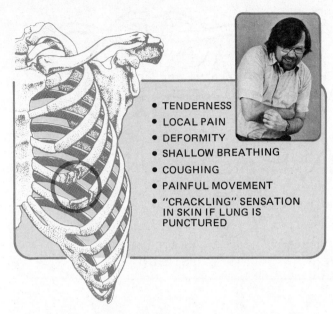

- TENDERNESS
- LOCAL PAIN
- DEFORMITY
- SHALLOW BREATHING
- COUGHING
- PAINFUL MOVEMENT
- "CRACKLING" SENSATION IN SKIN IF LUNG IS PUNCTURED

Figure 10-24: Characteristic stance of a patient with rib fractures.

can be placed across the chest, and a fourth cravat should be applied as a swathe to support the angle of the arm.

Flail chest usually occurs when three or more consecutive ribs on the same side of the chest are fractured, each in at least two places. This produces a section of chest wall that will move independently of the rest of the chest wall. Often, this movement is in the opposite direction to the rest of the chest wall. This is known as paradoxical respiration. The same problem occurs when the sternum is broken away from its cartilage attachments with the ribs. Both of these conditions are called flail chest. EMTs see flail chests most often at motor vehicle accidents, usually caused by the patient being forced against the vehicle's steering wheel. The symptoms and signs of flail chest include:

- The symptoms and signs of fractured ribs
- The failure of a section of the chest wall to move with the rest of the chest when the patient is breathing. Typically, paradoxical respirations are observed.

Care for Flail Chest Do not attempt to bind, strap, or tape the injured section of ribs or the loose sternum. Instead, you must try to hold the flail section in place. To care for a flail chest you should:

1. Carefully locate the edges of the flail section by gently feeling the injury site.
2. Apply a thick pad of dressings over the site. This pad should be several inches thick. A small pillow can be used in place of the pad of dressings. A small sandbag or other such soft, lightweight item can also be used.
3. Use large strips of tape to hold the pad in place. (Place the tape as shown in Fig. 10-27.) The tension on the tape bears down on the pad, which, in turn, depresses the flail section. If tape will not hold, use wide cravats.
4. Administer a high concentration of oxygen. Assisted ventilation may be necessary.
5. Treat for shock.
6. Monitor the patient, taking extra care to look for signs of heart or lung injury.
7. Transport as soon as possible with the patient in a semi-reclined position. If the patient cannot tolerate this position, gently place him on the injured side.

Complications of Chest Injuries

The lungs, heart, and great vessels can be injured in accidents involving the chest. Some of the more serious problems seen are:

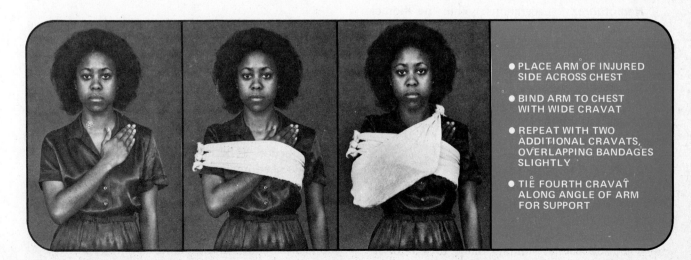

- PLACE ARM OF INJURED SIDE ACROSS CHEST
- BIND ARM TO CHEST WITH WIDE CRAVAT
- REPEAT WITH TWO ADDITIONAL CRAVATS, OVERLAPPING BANDAGES SLIGHTLY
- TIE FOURTH CRAVAT ALONG ANGLE OF ARM FOR SUPPORT

Figure 10-25: Care of fractured ribs utilizes cravats applied to hold the arm against the chest.

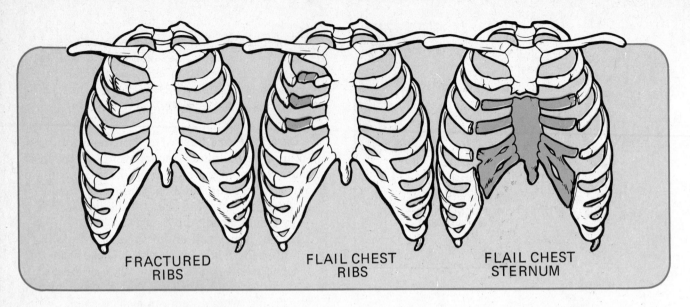

FRACTURED RIBS   FLAIL CHEST RIBS   FLAIL CHEST STERNUM

Figure 10-26: Rib fractures and flail chest.

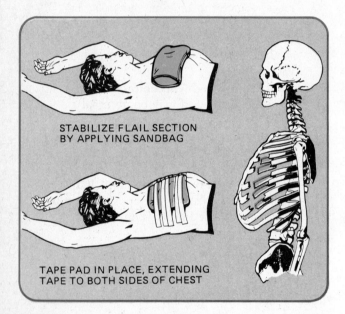

STABILIZE FLAIL SECTION
BY APPLYING SANDBAG

TAPE PAD IN PLACE, EXTENDING
TAPE TO BOTH SIDES OF CHEST

Figure 10-27: Care for flail chest.

Hemothorax   Lacerations within the thoracic cavity can be produced by penetrating objects or fractured ribs. Blood will flow into the pleural space, the lung will collapse, and the heart will be forced against the uninjured lung.

Hemopneumothorax   This is a combination of air and blood, producing the same results—a collapsed lung and pressure on the heart and uninjured lung.

Cardiac Tamponade   This occurs when sharp or blunt injury to the heart causes blood to flow into the surrounding pericardial sac. This unyielding sac fills with blood and compresses the chambers of the heart to a point where they will no longer fill adequately, sending blood back into the veins. The patient's neck veins will bulge, his pulse

will become very weak, and successive blood pressure measurements will show systolic and diastolic readings that approach each other as the patient's condition deteriorates.

The difference in pressure between systolic and diastolic readings is called **pulse pressure**. If a chest injury patient shows a steadily decreasing pulse pressure, this is a reliable sign of serious injury in the thoracic cavity. A pulse pressure below 15 mmHg is critical.

Traumatic Asphyxia   This is not a condition, but a group of symptoms and signs that can be associated with sudden compression of the chest. When this occurs, the sternum exerts severe pressure on the heart, forcing blood out of the right atrium, up into the jugular veins in the neck. THIS IS A TRUE EMERGENCY, requiring immediate transport. Artificial ventilation with oxygen is probably the only way to keep the patient alive during transport.

Tension Pneumothorax   This can arise two ways. We have discussed the problem of air escaping from a punctured lung into the thoracic cavity with no exit for this air due to the application of an occlusive dressing. It is possible for a patient to have a closed chest injury where a lung is punctured (e.g.: by a fractured rib). Air will build up within the closed thoracic cavity, quickly impairing heart and lung function. THIS IS A TRUE EMERGENCY. Such patients need immediate advanced medical care.

The signs of tension pneumothorax include increasing respiratory difficulty, a weak pulse, cyanosis, and low blood pressure noted due to the decrease in cardiac output. The veins of the neck may appear distended and the trachea may be pushed off to one side.

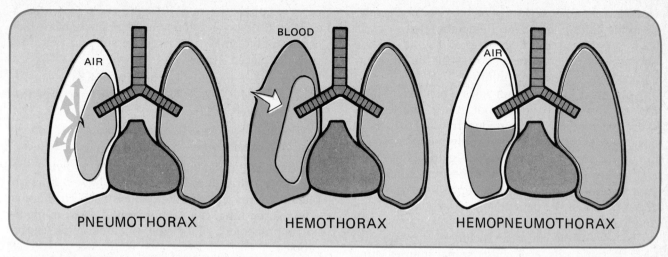

Figure 10-28: Conditions produced by chest injuries.

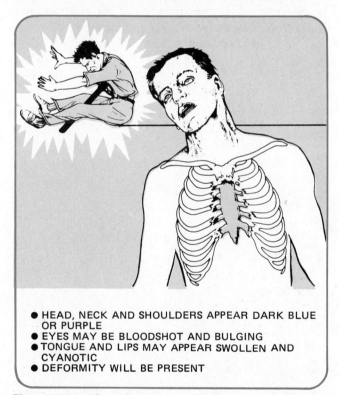

- HEAD, NECK AND SHOULDERS APPEAR DARK BLUE OR PURPLE
- EYES MAY BE BLOODSHOT AND BULGING
- TONGUE AND LIPS MAY APPEAR SWOLLEN AND CYANOTIC
- DEFORMITY WILL BE PRESENT

Figure 10-29: The symptoms and signs of traumatic asphyxia.

NOTE: Except for pneumothorax, and cases of tension pneumothorax caused by an occlusive dressing, there is little the EMT can do for major complications occurring with chest injuries. Immediate transport and continued administering of oxygen may be all that you can do. If basic life support measures are provided, often requiring artificial ventilation with oxygen, you may be able to keep the patient alive until more advanced medical procedures can be delivered.

SUMMARY

The skull is made up of the cranium and the face. The vertebral column is connected to the skull.

That portion of the spine running through the neck is called the cervical spine. The ribs are attached to the thoracic spine. The midback contains the lumbar spine, while the sacral spine and coccyx are lower back structures. The skull, spinal column, sternum, and ribs form the axial skeleton.

The brain is protected by the skull. The spinal column protects the spinal cord. The brain and spinal cord are part of the central nervous system.

Injuries to the skull include open and closed head injuries. If the cranium remains intact, the injury is classified as a closed head injury.

Open head injuries involve fractures of the cranium (skull fractures). There can be direct injury to the brain in open head injuries. Closed head injuries include indirect injuries to the brain, such as concussions and contusions.

Skull fractures may be obvious or difficult to detect. Always look for wounds to the head, deformity of the skull, bruises behind the ear, discolorations around the eyes, sunken eyes, unequal pupils and blood or clear fluid flowing from the ears and/or nose.

Brain injury can occur with head injuries. Look for signs of skull fracture, loss of awareness, confusion, unequal pupils, and paralysis.

When caring for a patient with injuries to the cranium, you should maintain an open airway using the MODIFIED JAW-THRUST technique. Provide resuscitative procedures, if needed. Keep the patient at rest and talk to the patient to try to prevent loss of consciousness. Control bleeding, but avoid pressure over the site of a fracture. Do NOT remove impaled objects, bone fragments, or any other objects from skull wounds.

Facial fractures often cause airway obstruction. You should maintain an open airway using the modified jaw-thrust technique.

Neck and spinal injuries can be very serious. The secondary survey is very important in detecting signs of possible spinal injuries. Always look for weakness, numbness, loss of feeling, pain or paralysis to the limbs of a patient. Remember that you will have to probe or pinch the feet and hands of the unconscious patient. Assume that the unconscious trauma patient has spinal injuries.

You must follow certain rules when caring for a patient who may have neck or spinal injuries. Always consider the unconscious trauma patient to have neck or spinal injuries. Apply manual traction for the head and neck, place an extrication collar, and secure the patient to a long spine board. Do your best to immobilize the patient's head and neck and as much of the patient's body as possible. Continuously monitor the patient.

Injuries to the chest can include soft tissue injuries, fractured ribs, flail chest, spinal injuries, lung injuries and heart injuries.

If pain and tenderness at the site indicate rib fractures, you should place the arm of the patient that is on the same side as the fracture against the chest. Apply three overlapping cravats and a swathe. If rib or breastbone movements indicate flail chest, apply a thick pad over the site and tape this pad into place.

An object impaled in the chest should not be removed. Stabilize the object with pads and tape the pads into place.

Penetrating chest wounds ("sucking" chest wounds) require you to apply a sealed occlusive dressing. If the patient worsens after applying the occlusive dressing, he may have tension pneumothorax. Loosen the occlusive seal. If there is a punctured lung, the patient should show immediate improvement, if tension pneumothorax is the problem.

The complications associated with chest injuries require immediate transport. Basic life support, including ventilation with oxygen, may be the only way you can keep some patients alive.

11 *medical emergencies*

SECTION ONE: COMMON MEDICAL EMERGENCIES

OBJECTIVES By the end of this section, you should be able to:

1. Define "medical emergency." (p. 234-5)

2. List the major diagnostic symptoms and signs associated with medical emergencies. (p. 236)

3. Relate coronary artery disease to specific changes in arterial walls. (p. 237-8)

4. Compare and contrast the symptoms and signs of angina pectoris and acute myocardial infarction. (p. 239-41)

5. List the emergency care procedures for angina pectoris. (p. 240)

6. List the emergency care procedures for possible acute myocardial infarction. (p. 240)

7. Define "congestive heart failure" and explain its symptoms and signs in terms of this definition. (p. 241, 3)

8. Describe the emergency care for possible congestive heart failure. (p. 243)

9. List the symptoms and signs of stroke. (p. 245)

10. Describe the emergency care provided for stroke. (p. 245)

11. Define "dyspnea" and relate this term to respiratory distress. (p. 244)

12. List the symptoms and signs of respiratory distress. (p. 244, 6)

13. Compare and contrast emphysema and chronic bronchitis in terms of symptoms and signs. (p. 247)

14. Describe the emergency care procedures for chronic obstructive pulmonary disease. (p. 246-7)

15. List the symptoms and signs of asthma. (p. 247-8)

16. Describe the emergency care procedures for asthma. (p. 248)

17. Describe the emergency care procedures for hyperventilation. (p. 248)

18. Compare and contrast diabetic coma (diabetic ketoacidosis) and insulin shock (hypoglycemia) in terms of symptoms, signs, and emergency care. (p. 250)

19. Describe what occurs during each phase of a convulsive seizure and relate specific emergency care procedures to each phase. (p. 249-51)

20. List the general symptoms and signs associated with acute abdominal distress. (p. 252-3)

21. Describe the emergency care procedures for acute abdomen. (p. 253)

22. List the general symptoms and signs of an infectious disease. (p. 253)

23. List how communicable diseases may be transmitted. (p. 253)

24. Describe the basic procedures for:

    A. Protecting yourself from communicable diseases. (p. 252-3)

    B. Making the ambulance ready after transporting a patient with a possible communicable disease. (p. 253)

SKILLS As an EMT, you should be able to:

1. Determine if a patient is having a medical emergency.

2. Assess patients for:
   - Disorders of the heart
   - Stroke
   - Respiratory distress, including hyperventilation
   - Chronic obstructive pulmonary disease
   - Diabetic emergencies

- Convulsive seizures
- Acute abdomen
- Possible infectious disease

3. Provide emergency care for possible angina pectoris, acute myocardial infarction, and congestive heart failure.

4. Provide emergency care for possible stroke.

5. Provide emergency care for possible chronic obstructive pulmonary disease, asthma, and hyperventilation.

6. Provide emergency care for diabetic coma and insulin shock.

7. Provide emergency care for all three phases of a convulsive seizure.

8. Provide emergency care for acute abdomen.

9. Provide emergency care for possible infectious diseases.

10. Protect yourself from communicable diseases.

11. Ready an ambulance for the next run after transporting a patient with a possible communicable disease.

12. Promptly and efficiently deliver oxygen to patients having medical emergencies.

TERMS you may be using for the first time:

Chronic—a medical problem that is consistently present over a long period of time.

Episodic—a medical problem that affects the patient at irregular intervals.

Acute—a medical problem with a sudden onset.

Coronary (KOR-o-nar-e) **Artery**—a blood vessel that supplies the muscle of the heart.

Myocardium—heart muscle.

Atherosclerosis (ATH-er-o-skle-RO-sis)—a build-up of fatty deposits and other particles on the inner wall of an artery. This build up is called **plaque.** Calcium may deposit in the plaque, causing the wall to become hard and stiff.

Arteriosclerosis (ar-TE-re-o-skle-RO-sis)—''hardening of the arteries'' caused by calcium deposits.

Occlusion—the blockage of an artery.

Aneurysm (AN-u-riz'm)—the dilation of a weakened section of an arterial wall.

Coronary Artery Disease (CAD)—the narrowing of a coronary artery brought about by atherosclerosis. Occlusion occurs in many cases.

Angina Pectoris (AN-ji-nah PEK-to-ris)—the sudden pain occurring when a portion of the myocardium is not receiving enough oxygenated blood.

Acute Myocardial Infarction (AMI)—occurs when a portion of myocardium dies when deprived of oxygenated blood.

Congestive Heart Failure (CHF)—the failure of the heart to pump efficiently, leading to excessive blood or fluids in the lungs, the body, or both.

Pulmonary Edema—when the pulmonary vessels are engorged with blood and the alveoli contain excess fluids and foam. This may be associated with congestive heart failure.

Dyspnea (disp-NE-ah)—difficult breathing.

Rales—abnormal breathing sounds heard in the lungs. A powdery or gravelly sound can be heard with a stethoscope.

Ascites (a-SI-tez)—the noticeable distention of the abdomen caused by the accumulation of excessive fluids.

Hyperventilation—a temporary condition of rapid, deep breathing that reduces the carbon dioxide level of the blood.

Diabetic Coma—a condition that begins with the build-up of sugar (hyperglycemia) in the blood. Sugar and water are lost in the kidneys, leading to a state of unconsciousness.

Insulin Shock—a condition that occurs to the diabetic when there is a sudden drop in the level of blood sugar (severe hypoglycemia).

Acute Abdomen—inflammation in the abdominal cavity producing intense pain.

Diaphoresis (DI-ah-fo-RE-sis)—profuse perspiration. The patient is said to be diaphoretic (DI-ah-fo-RET-ik).

WHAT ARE MEDICAL EMERGENCIES?

In the basic level EMT course, there is much emphasis placed on injury. However, the EMT also is expected to provide care for medical emergencies.

These are problems that the layperson would call illness or sickness. In emergency care, a medical emergency occurs as a result of one of the following factors:

- A defect in the structure or function of an organ or organ system. This can be present at birth (congenital) or acquired during life. Heart disease is an example.

- A disease caused by an infectious organism such as a bacterium or virus. An example of this would be bacterial meningitis.
- The effect of a harmful substance, such as a poison or a drug.

Medical emergencies do not include any problems caused by trauma, nor do they include problems that are primarily psychological or emotional in nature. The problems related to trauma have been studied in preceding chapters and will be completed in the environmental emergencies chapter. Psychological and emotional emergencies are given a special heading in emergency care. We will cover these in Chapter 14.

Environmental and medical emergencies come together when we start to consider the effect of harmful substances. A patient's severe reaction to a wasp sting would be an example. Poisonings are usually environmentally induced emergencies, yet the medical problems faced are the concern of the EMT in primary care. Drug abuse presents itself as a medical emergency, closely linked to special patient management and psychological emergencies. Therefore, drug abuse and poisoning will be covered in Section 2.

As an EMT, you will have to be familiar with:
- Cardiovascular emergencies—including heart attack and stroke.
- Respiratory emergencies—including respiratory distress, emphysema, and asthma.
- Diabetes—including the problems associated with its management.
- Disorders and diseases of the brain—including convulsive disorders such as epilepsy.
- Abdominal distress—including the abdominal disorders and diseases classified as acute (sudden onset) abdominal distress.
- Communicable diseases—including the major bacteria- and virus-induced illnesses of our society.

Medical problems can be chronic, consistently present over a long period of time. Diabetes and bronchitis are examples of medical problems that are chronic. As an EMT, your care for chronic medical problems will be required in cases that have suddenly turned worse, or where complications have quickly changed the patient's condition. These types of medical emergencies will require you to provide some very basic emergency care measures and to transport the patient. Other medical problems can be episodic, affecting the patient at irregular intervals and leaving him unaffected at other times. The patient expects problems, but the onset may not be predictable. Some patients with epilepsy or asthma have episodes that will require you to respond, provide care, and transport.

The unknown medical problem faces the EMT when the patient has an acute medical problem occurring for the first time. Acute refers to a sudden onset, as when a heart attack occurs without warning, or an abdominal inflammation suddenly produces severe pain. Carefully gathering and evaluating symptoms and signs will be your only way to be certain that you are dealing with a specific acute medical emergency.

Problems of detecting and providing care for medical emergencies may arise at the accident scene. Always remember that a medical emergency requiring immediate EMT-level care can be hidden because of an accident. A patient having a heart attack or stroke, or a patient having trouble managing his diabetes may fall and injure himself. Caring for the injury and letting the medical emergency go undetected can lead to serious, life-threatening problems for the patient. This is another reason why you must conduct a proper patient assessment.

The stress of an accident may set off both known and unknown medical problems. A heart attack, stroke, or seizure may occur at an accident scene. A complete patient assessment and monitoring of vital signs may be the only way you can be prepared for such events.

Detecting Medical Emergencies

Interviews with the patient and other individuals at the medical emergency scene may be the primary way of obtaining information. The patient, his family, neighbors, or fellow workers may be able to alert you to a known medical problem. In some cases, a medical identification device may prove to be the major factor in determining what could be wrong with the patient. For acute cases, what the patient tells you and what you determine from the physical examination will probably be your only sources of information.

The symptoms and signs gathered and evaluated during the patient assessment are critical in determining the nature of the medical emergency. Keep in mind that you have been developing an understanding of illness and disease since childhood. In many cases, you can tell someone is probably ill. You cannot make a diagnosis, but you can draw certain conclusions. You are aware that pain, aches, fever, nausea, vomiting and other such indicators point to illness. Take this knowledge and apply it through the discipline of the patient survey.

The symptoms gathered from the patient, combined with certain signs, may lead you to determine what possible type of medical emergency is causing problems for the patient. You will have to pay strict attention to:

- Pain, anywhere in the body
- Feelings of "temperature" or fever, and chills
- A tight feeling in the chest
- An upset stomach
- Unusual bowel or bladder habits
- Unusual thirst or hunger
- An odd taste in the mouth
- "Burning" sensations
- Dizziness or feelings of faintness
- Numbness or tingling sensations

Diagnostic signs are collected during the patient survey, including:

- Altered states of consciousness
- Pulse rate and character—remember that a pulse rate above 120 or below 50 beats per minute indicates a true emergency for the adult patient.
- Breathing rate and character—a true emergency exists when the adult patient's respirations are over 30 per minute.
- Skin temperature, condition, and color
- Pupil size, equality, and response
- Color of the lips, tongue, and earlobes
- Breath odors
- Abdominal tenderness
- Muscular activity—spasms and paralysis
- Bleeding or discharges from the body

REMEMBER: If anything about the patient's general state of health appears to be unusual, assume there is a medical emergency. If the patient has atypical vital signs, assume there is a medical emergency. Consider valid all patient complaints relating to the way he feels. If the patient says he is not feeling "normal" in any way, assume there is a medical emergency. Transport all possible medical emergencies so that a physician can make a diagnosis and provide needed care. Your role as an EMT is not to diagnose, but to assess the patient and provide the proper initial care appropriate for a certain set of symptoms and signs.

DISORDERS OF THE CARDIOVASCULAR SYSTEM

Cardiovascular diseases are major health problems in the United States. A large percentage of the medical emergencies seen by EMTs deals with such problems as heart attacks, strokes, heart failure, or some other disorder of the cardiovascular system. Before beginning this segment of the chapter, review the basics of the cardiovascular system:

- The heart is a cone-shaped, hollow organ, roughly the size of a man's clenched fist.

- The superior surface of the heart is the *base*, while the inferior point is known as the *apex*.
- The heart is located in the midportion of the thoracic cavity. The base of the heart is directly behind the sternum, at about the level of the third rib. The lower portion of the heart extends from behind the sternum into the lower left chest. The apex terminates between the fifth and sixth ribs.
- The heart is vertically divided down the middle by a septum; thus there is a "right heart" and a "left heart."
- Each side of the heart has two chambers, an upper atrium and a lower ventricle. The right atrium receives blood from the body and the right ventricle sends blood to the lungs. Blood returning from the lungs enters the left atrium, to be sent to the left ventricle and pumped out into systemic (the entire body) circulation.
- One-way valves control the direction of blood flow in the heart. They are located between atria and ventricles, and in the great arteries that leave the ventricles.
- Heart action is controlled by electrical impulses sent from the cardiac control center of the brain. Epinephrine (adrenalin) released into the bloodstream also affects heart action.

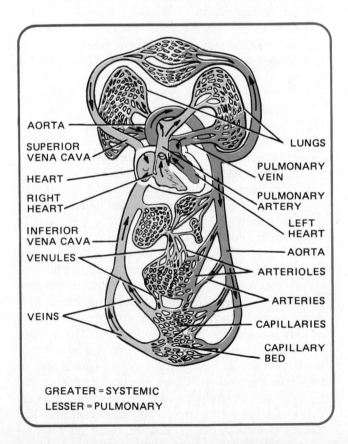

Figure 11-1: Anatomy of the cardiovascular system.

- Blood leaves the heart by way of the arteries. These turn into smaller vessels known as arterioles. The arterioles lead into the capillary beds where exchange between the blood and the tissues takes place. *Venules* take blood from the capillaries to the veins. Blood returns to the heart by way of the veins.

- The circulation of blood between the heart and the lungs is the pulmonary circuit. The circulation of blood pumped from the heart, out to the body, and returned to the heart is the systemic circuit.

To better understand cardiovascular disease, you must know two additional terms. The heart has its own set of blood vessels to supply its tissues with oxygen and food, and to remove carbon dioxide and other wastes. This is the **coronary** (KOR-o-nar-e) **system.** Of chief concern in heart disease are the **coronary arteries.** The muscle of the heart is the **myocardium** (mi-o-KAR-de-um). The health of the myocardium and the amount of oxygenated blood reaching this tissue are of great importance in heart disease.

The Nature of Cardiovascular Diseases

Most of the cardiovascular emergencies covered in this section are caused, directly or indirectly, by changes in the walls of arteries. These arteries can be part of the systemic circulatory system, the pulmonary circulatory system, or the coronary system. Two conditions, **atherosclerosis** (ATH-er-o-skle-RO-sis) and **arteriosclerosis** (ar-TE-re-o-skle-RO-sis), are involved in the changes found in these artery walls.

Atherosclerosis is a build-up of fatty deposits on the inner walls of arteries. This build-up causes a narrowing of the inner vessel diameter, restricting the flow of blood. Fats and other particles combine to form this deposit known as **plaque.** As time passes, calcium can be deposited at the site of the plaque, causing the area to harden. In arteriosclerosis, the artery wall becomes hard and stiff due to calcium deposits. This ''hardening of the arteries'' causes the vessel to lose its elastic nature, changing blood flow and increasing blood pressure.

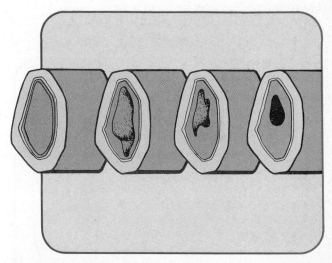

Figure 11-3: Atherosclerosis . . . the process of plaque formation.

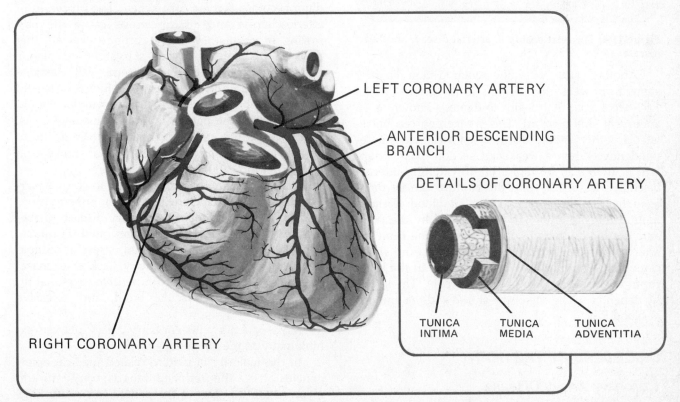

LEFT CORONARY ARTERY

ANTERIOR DESCENDING BRANCH

DETAILS OF CORONARY ARTERY

TUNICA INTIMA   TUNICA MEDIA   TUNICA ADVENTITIA

RIGHT CORONARY ARTERY

Figure 11-2: The coronary artery system.

Throughout the entire process of both athero-sclerosis and arteriosclerosis, the amount of blood passing through the artery is restricted. The rough surface formed in the artery can lead to blood clots being formed, causing increased narrowing of the artery. The clot and debris from the plaque form a **thrombus** (THROM-bus). These thrombi can reach a size where they **occlude** (cut off) blood flow completely, or they may break loose to become **emboli** (EM-bo-li) and move to occlude the flow of blood somewhere in a smaller artery. In cases of partial or complete blockage, the tissues beyond the point of blockage will be starved of oxygen and may die. If this blockage involves a large area of the heart or brain, the results may be quickly fatal.

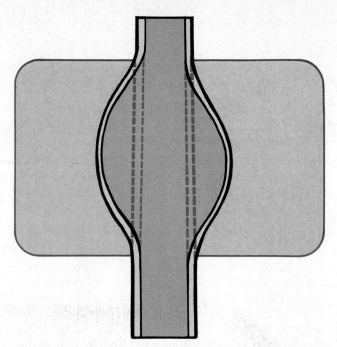

Figure 11-5: Formation and rupture of an aneurysm. A weakened area in the wall of an artery will tend to balloon out, forming a sac-like aneurysm which may eventually burst.

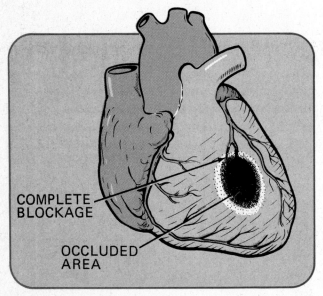

Figure 11-4: The relationship of arterial disease and heart disease.

Another cause of cardiovascular system disorder stems from weakened sections in the arterial walls. Each weak spot that begins to dilate is known as an **aneurysm** (AN-u-riz'm). This weakening can be related to other arterial diseases, or it can exist independently. When a weakened section of an artery bursts, there can be rapid, life-threatening internal bleeding. Tissues beyond the rupture can be damaged by the cut-off of oxygenated blood. Tissues around the site often can be damaged by the pressure exerted on them by the blood pouring from the artery. If a major artery ruptures, death from shock can occur very quickly. When an artery in the brain ruptures, a severe form of stroke occurs. The severity depends on the site of the stroke and the amount of blood loss.

DISORDERS OF THE HEART

Coronary Artery Disease

Physical and emotional stress cause the heart to

work harder. For this to happen, the myocardium must receive more oxygenated blood than usual. This presents no problem when the heart and its coronary vessels are normal. However, when coronary vessels are diseased, their ability to carry blood is reduced. Since the blood supply to the heart is reduced, so is the oxygen supply, and the myocardium becomes starved for oxygen. The processes of arteriosclerosis and atherosclerosis cause the narrowing or **occlusion** of the coronary vessels that leads to this state of oxygen starvation. As plaque and calcium form on the inner arterial wall, elasticity is reduced, limiting the vessel's ability to dilate to increase the blood flow to the heart muscle. Should a vessel burst, the patient is in an immediate crisis. Usually, it is the effect on the myocardium due to partial blockage of a coronary artery that shows itself as the first indication of heart disorder.

Factors identified as contributors to coronary artery disease (CAD) include sex (male), hypertension, smoking, family history of coronary disease, diabetes, race (Caucasian), excessive saturated fat intake, high cholesterol level in the blood, stressful occupation or environment, a sedentary (lack of exercise) existence, an aggressive competitive personality, obesity, heavy or muscular build, and excessive sugar intake.

Most patients with coronary artery disease exhibit many of the above factors.

In the majority of cardiac-related medical emergencies, it is the reduced blood supply to the myocardium that causes the patient to require EMS assistance and care.

Angina Pectoris

Remember, when the heart muscle has to work harder because of physical or emotional stress, healthy coronary arteries dilate to supply the myocardium with more oxygenated blood. When vessels are narrowed by coronary artery disease, the supply of oxygenated blood cannot meet the increased demand, even for a few seconds. In some patients, a severe pain develops as myocardial tissue becomes oxygen-starved. This pain is **angina pectoris** (AN-ji-nah PEK-to-ris) or, literally, a pain in the chest.

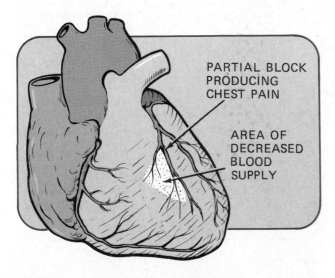

Figure 11-6: Angina pectoris produces pain in the chest that may be similar to that of a heart attack.

The pain of an angina attack generally diminishes and disappears when the physical or emotional stress ends. Seldom does this painful attack last longer than *3 to 5 minutes*. As the heart rate returns to normal, the supply of blood moving through the diseased coronary arteries can meet the decreased demand. This means that rest is indicated for a person experiencing an angina attack.

Nitroglycerine tablets are prescribed for persons subject to angina attacks caused by coronary artery disease. At the onset of an episode, the patient places a tablet under his tongue, allowing the medicine to enter the bloodstream quickly. Nitroglycerine works to dilate the coronary arteries. In turn, blood pressure is reduced as is the myocardial workload. Emergency medical personnel can help angina patients to take their medication, as well as to place them in a restful position and provide emotional support. You should administer oxygen to the angina patient. Transport the patient, even if his pains disappear.

A complete guide to symptoms, signs, and emergency care for angina pectoris is provided in Scansheet 11-1.

Acute Myocardial Infarction

Acute myocardial infarction (AMI) is a condition in which a portion of the myocardium dies as a result of oxygen starvation. This is brought on by the narrowing or occlusion of the coronary artery that supplies the region with blood.

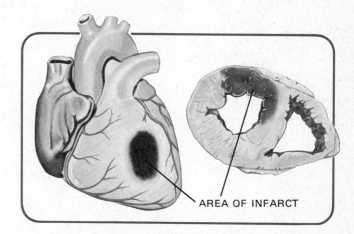

Figure 11-7: Cross-section of a myocardial infarction.

The AHA reports nearly one million cases of AMI in the United States each year. Over 650,000 deaths annually are the result of heart disease. A major factor in heart disease is *sudden death*, cardiac arrest that occurs within two hours of the onset of symptoms. Each year, approximately 350,000 people die suddenly from cardiac arrest away from hospitals. Cardiologists believe that many of these people could be saved if they received prompt and efficient care in the early warning stages, or CPR immediately upon onset of cardiac arrest. Thus it is vital that EMTs be able to recognize a possible AMI and to furnish appropriate care from first contact to transfer at the medical facility.

A variety of factors can cause an AMI. Coronary artery disease in the form of atherosclerosis is usually the underlying reason for the incident. However, for some patients, factors often regarded as harmless may be responsible for setting off the heart attack. These factors include unusual exertion, severe emotional distress, and unrelieved fatigue. These patients may have a pre-existing, undetected disturbance in heart rate and rhythm known as **arrhythmia** (ah-RITH-me-ah), undetected coronary artery disease, or prolonged chronic problems with respiration.

The complications from acute myocardial infarction are both common and dangerous. About 85% to 90% of all AMI victims experience some sort of arrythmia. Some of the arrythmias associated with AMI may be lethal. Arrythmias often associated with AMI include:

• **Asystole** (a-SIS-tol-e)—cardiac standstill

ANGINA PECTORIS

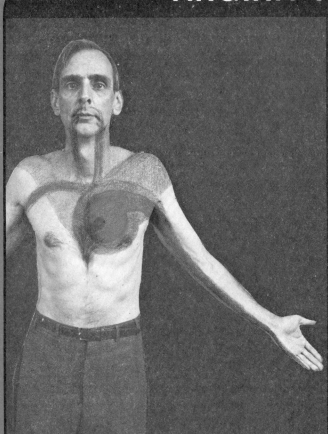

SIGNS AND SYMPTOMS:

- EARLY SYMPTOMS ARE OFTEN MISTAKEN FOR INDIGESTION
- AS AN ATTACK WORSENS, PAIN ORIGINATES BEHIND STERNUM AND RADIATES TO:
  - EITHER OF THE UPPER EXTREMITIES (USUALLY THE LEFT) WITH PAIN RADIATING TO THE SHOULDER, ARM, AND ELBOW. IN SOME CASES THE PAIN MAY EXTEND DOWN THE LIMB TO THE LITTLE FINGER.
  - THE NECK, JAWS, AND TEETH
  - THE UPPER BACK
  - THE SUPERIOR, MEDIAL ABDOMEN
- THE PAIN MAY NOT ORIGINATE UNDER THE STERNUM
- SOME PATIENTS HAVE PAIN ONLY IN THE JAW, OR THE TEETH
- SHORTNESS OF BREATH
- NAUSEA
- PAIN LASTS THROUGHOUT ATTACK AND IS NOT INFLUENCED BY MOVEMENT, BREATHING, OR COUGHING
- PAIN USUALLY LASTS 3 TO 5 MINUTES
- PAIN DIMINISHES WHEN PHYSICAL OR EMOTIONAL STRESS ENDS
- PATIENT USUALLY REMAINS STILL

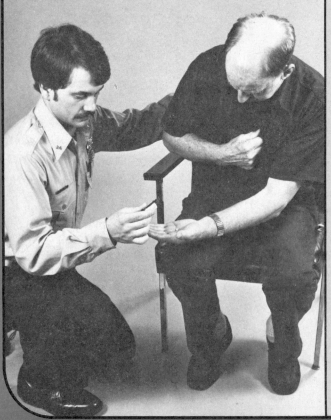

EMERGENCY CARE

- PROVIDE EMOTIONAL SUPPORT

- SUPPLY OXYGEN AT A HIGH FLOW RATE

- PLACE THE PATIENT IN A REST-FUL, COMFORTABLE POSITION

- ASSIST THE PATIENT WITH MEDICATION (NITROGLYCERIN)

SCAN 11.1

- **Ventricular fibrillation** (ven-TRIK-u-lar fi-bre-LAY-shun)—when the ventricles no longer beat with a full, steady, symmetrical pattern.
- **Atrial fibrillation** or **atrial flutter**—a highly irregular, inefficient atrial contraction.
- **Bradycardia** (bra-de-KAR-de-ah)—when the heart rate is below 40 to 50 beats per minute.
- **Tachycardia** (tak-e-KAR-de-ah)—when the heart rate climbs above 120 beats per minute.

Another common complication seen with AMI is **mechanical pump failure,** or the inability of the heart to function normally due to damaged tissues. This can lead to cardiac arrest, cardiogenic shock (11%), fluids "backing up" in the lungs and other body organs (congestive heart failure, 60%), and body cell death due to oxygen starvation. About 4% of all AMI victims develop aneurysms in the ventricles that can lead to mechanical pump failure or lethal arrythmias. Nearly 2% of AMI patients suffer *cardiac rupture* as the dead tissue area of the myocardium bursts open. (Even though resuscitative measures are not usually effective for such patients, you must provide basic life support.)

Scansheet 11-2 presents the symptoms, signs, and care for acute myocardial infarction. Note that on the Scansheet there is a comparison of

angina pectoris and AMI. As an EMT, you should know the major differences between the two as you evaluate a possible heart attack patient. When in doubt, treat as if there is an AMI.

REMEMBER: Transportation of a patient with a heart condition must be carried out in a sane, careful fashion. A high-speed ride with siren wailing only increases the patient's fear and apprehension, placing additional stress upon the heart. Conceivably, the patient's condition could worsen and he could die due to complications brought about by improper methods used in transport.

Congestive Heart Failure

Congestive heart failure (CHF) may be brought on by an AMI, diseased heart valves, hypertension, or some form of obstructive pulmonary disease such as emphysema. This condition is often a complication of acute myocardial infarction, occurring several days after the heart attack.

The problem arises when a damaged or weakened heart cannot pump enough blood to maintain proper circulation throughout the body. The problem typically starts as **left heart failure,** related to damage in the left ventricle. Blood becomes "backed up," first in the pulmonary vessels, and finally in

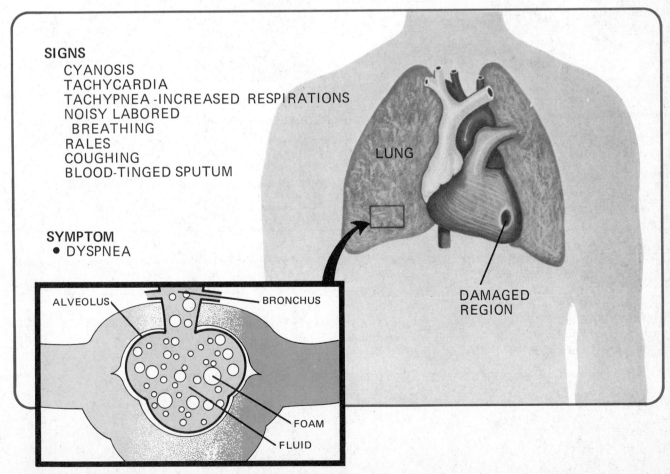

SIGNS
CYANOSIS
TACHYCARDIA
TACHYPNEA -INCREASED RESPIRATIONS
NOISY LABORED
 BREATHING
RALES
COUGHING
BLOOD-TINGED SPUTUM

SYMPTOM
- DYSPNEA

LUNG

DAMAGED REGION

ALVEOLUS   BRONCHUS

FOAM

FLUID

Figure 11-8: Mechanical pump failure is a complication of AMI.

ACUTE MYOCARDIAL INFARCTION (AMI)

RESPIRATORY:
- DYSPNEA — SHALLOW OR DEEP RESPIRATIONS
- COUGH THAT PRODUCES SPUTUM

BEHAVIORAL:
- ANXIETY, IRRITABILITY, INABILITY TO CONCENTRATE
- DEPRESSION
- FEELING OF IMPENDING DOOM
- MILD DELIRIUM, PERSONALITY CHANGES
- FAINTING
- OCCASIONAL THRASHING ABOUT AND CHEST-POUNDING

CIRCULATORY:
- SIGNS OF SHOCK
- INCREASED PULSE RATE, SOMETIMES IRREGULAR
- REDUCED BLOOD PRESSURE

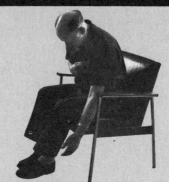

AN AMI CAN LEAD TO:
- MECHANICAL HEART FAILURE
- SHOCK (USUALLY WITHIN 24 HOURS)
- CONGESTIVE HEART FAILURE (IMMEDIATELY, OR UP TO A WEEK OR MORE LATER)

PAIN:
- MARKED DISCOMFORT, CONTINUES WHEN AT REST
- COMPRESSING, CONSTRICTING, OR ACHING PAIN RATHER THAN A SHARP OR THROBBING PAIN
- USUALLY NOT ALLEVIATED BY NITROGLYCERIN
- MAY LAST SEVERAL MINUTES
- ORIGINATES UNDER STERNUM AND MAY RADIATE TO ARMS, NECK, OR JAW

- CARDIAC ARREST (40% DIE BEFORE THEY REACH THE HOSPITAL)

EMERGENCY CARE

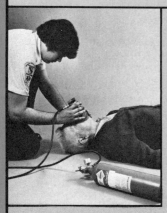

FOR THE UNCONSCIOUS PATIENT
- ESTABLISH AND MAINTAIN AN AIRWAY
- PROVIDE PULMONARY RESUSCITATION OR CPR IF NEEDED
- ADMINISTER HIGH CONCENTRATION OF OXYGEN
- TRANSPORT IMMEDIATELY
- IF PATIENT DEVELOPS RESPIRATORY OR CARDIAC ARREST, DELIVER OXYGEN WITH A BAG-VALVE-MASK UNIT OR A DEMAND VALVE RESUSCITATOR

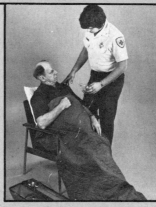

FOR THE CONSCIOUS PATIENT
- KEEP THE PATIENT CALM AND STILL
- TAKE HISTORY AND DETERMINE VITAL SIGNS
- HELP PATIENT WITH MEDICATIONS
- ADMINISTER HIGH CONCENTRATION OF OXYGEN
- CONSERVE BODY HEAT
- TRANSPORT AS SOON AS POSSIBLE IN A SEMI-RECLINED OR SITTING POSITION
- MONITOR VITAL SIGNS DURING TRANSPORT

EMERGENCY CARE MAY BE COMPLICATED BY MANY FACTORS. IF THE PATIENT IS CONSCIOUS, HIS IRRITABILITY, RESTLESSNESS, AND FEELING OF IMPENDING DOOM MAY MAKE HIM UNCOOPERATIVE AND UNWILLING TO SETTLE DOWN, EVEN THOUGH IT IS VITAL THAT HE DO SO. MANY AMI PATIENTS WILL RESIST THE PLACEMENT OF A FACE MASK FOR OXYGEN DELIVERY. IF HE RESISTS AFTER AN EXPLANATION OF THE IMPORTANCE OF OXYGEN, USE A NASAL CANNULA AT 8 LITERS/MINUTE. PROVIDE NEEDED OXYGEN, BUT DO NOT UPSET THE PATIENT.

DISTINGUISHING BETWEEN ANGINA AND AMI

ANGINA PECTORIS
- PAIN FOLLOWS EXERTION OR STRESS
- PAIN RELIEVED BY REST
- PAIN USUALLY RELIEVED BY NITROGLYCERIN
- PAIN LASTS 3 TO 5 MINUTES
- NOT ASSOCIATED WITH ARRHYTHMIAS
- BLOOD PRESSURE USUALLY NOT AFFECTED

AMI
- PAIN OFTEN RELATED TO STRESS OR EXERTION, BUT MAY OCCUR WHEN AT REST
- REST USUALLY DOES NOT RELIEVE PAIN
- NITROGLYCERIN MAY RELIEVE PAIN
- PAIN LASTS ½ HOUR TO SEVERAL HOURS
- OFTEN ASSOCIATED WITH ARRHYTHMIAS
- BLOOD PRESSURE IS OFTEN REDUCED, BUT MANY PATIENTS HAVE "NORMAL" BP

WARNING!

IF THERE IS ANY DOUBT AS TO WHICH CONDITION THE PATIENT IS SUFFERING FROM, TREAT FOR AMI.

SCAN 11-2

the systemic vessels. Increased pressure in these vessels forces fluids from the blood into the body tissue causing a swelling known as **edema** (e-DE-mah). **Pulmonary edema** usually occurs first, with fluids building up in the microscopic alveoli of the lungs. Poor respiratory exchange leads to shortness of breath (**dyspnea**—disp-NE-ah), with noisy and labored respirations. Powdery or gravelly sounds known as **rales** can be heard with the stethoscope. Some patients cough up blood-tinged sputum.

Left heart failure, if left untreated, commonly causes **right heart failure,** as edema of the liver, spleen, and lower extremities develops. The abdomen becomes noticeably distended by fluids, producing a condition known as **ascites** (a-SI-tez).

The symptoms and signs of congestive heart failure can include:

- Tachycardia (rapid pulse, 120 or above)
- Dyspnea (shortness of breath)
- Normal or elevated blood pressure
- Cyanosis
- Pulmonary edema with rales, sometimes coughing up of pink sputum
- Patient may be anxious or confused
- Edema of lower extremities
- Enlarged liver and spleen, with abdominal distention (develop late)
- Engorged pulsating neck veins (develop late)

Note that the patient will probably wish to remain in a seated or semi-reclined position. This should be encouraged since it allows for less labored respiration. Keep the patient calm and conserve body heat. Whereas some AMI patients will fight a face mask, the "oxygen hungry" patients with congestive heart failure often accept oxygen therapy without difficulty.

Give a high concentration of oxygen unless the patient has emphysema, chronic bronchitis, or an unclassified form of obstructive pulmonary disease (COPD). For these patients, 24% oxygen delivered by venturi mask is recommended. If the patient fears the mask, a nasal cannula can be used for short transport. It is best to call the emergency department physician for recommendations as to the flow rate of the oxygen. Some patients can only tolerate several liters per minute. (See Chapter 6 for more information on oxygen delivery to COPD patients.)

Cardiac Pacemakers

Many people wear cardiac pacemakers that keep the heart beating at a steady, efficient rate. These devices replace the heart's own natural pacemaker when it becomes defective or damaged.

On occasion, you may find a patient with a cardiac pacemaker having the symptoms and signs of an AMI, angina pectoris, or congestive heart failure. The pacemaker will not prevent someone from hav-

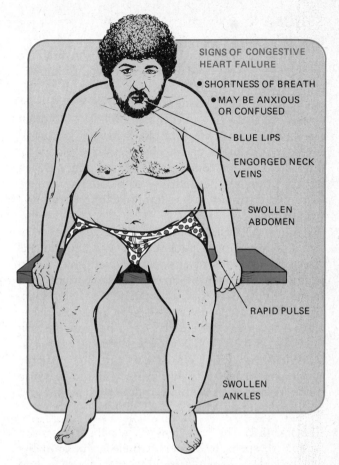

SIGNS OF CONGESTIVE HEART FAILURE
- SHORTNESS OF BREATH
- MAY BE ANXIOUS OR CONFUSED
- BLUE LIPS
- ENGORGED NECK VEINS
- SWOLLEN ABDOMEN
- RAPID PULSE
- SWOLLEN ANKLES

Figure 11-9: The signs of congestive heart failure.

ing any of these problems. Care will be the same as for any patient with these problems. Transport all angina pectoris patients having a pacemaker. Remember, as an EMT, you do not have the training or equipment necessary to evaluate the pacemaker in terms of efficiency and proper function.

Even though it would be rare, you may respond to find a patient suffering a medical emergency due to a pacemaker malfunction. This is a serious emergency and requires IMMEDIATE TRANSPORT. You cannot evaluate or repair the device. Indications of pacemaker problems include a very slow pulse rate (below 50, possibly going as low as 35 beats per minute), often fixed, but at times irregular. The patient almost certainly will be faint, dizzy, or very weak.

Coronary Artery Bypass Patients

The coronary artery bypass has become a relatively common procedure in cardiac surgery. Should you find a patient who has had this surgery, or an unconscious patient with a midline surgical scar on the chest, provide care as you would for any patient with the same symptoms and signs. Treat the AMI patient with a bypass as you would any patient with an AMI. If cardiac arrest occurs, provide CPR in the same prompt, efficient manner.

STROKE

Often thought of as a disorder of the brain, a stroke or **cerebrovascular accident** (CVA) is initially a problem of the cardiovascular system. It is the result of damage (accident) to one of the arteries (-vascular) supplying oxygenated blood to the brain (cerebro-). The pathway of blood may be occluded by a clot (thrombus or embolism), a large plaque of fatty deposits, or compression of the artery by an adjacent tumor. The pathway of blood also can be disrupted by an artery bursting, resulting in cerebral hemorrhaging.

Age and physical condition influence the type of stroke suffered by a patient. This and the various sizes and locations of arteries involved give varied symptoms and signs. Sometimes the patient may have nothing more than a headache when first evaluated. This can be enough reason to transport, especially if the patient is elderly, has a previous history of stroke, or has chronic heart or pulmonary disease.

When providing emergency care for possible stroke patients, do all you can to calm and reassure them. Transport carefully, avoiding high speed and the use of sirens.

REMEMBER: The conscious CVA patient may not be able to speak to you; nonetheless, he probably will be able to hear everything that you say and understand what is going on around him. He will undoubtedly be frightened, in need of thoughtful and compassionate care.

See Scansheet 11-3 for the symptoms, signs, and emergency care of stroke patients.

RESPIRATORY SYSTEM DISORDERS

Dyspnea and Respiratory Disorders

The term **dyspnea** (disp-NE-ah) means labored or difficult breathing. It is not a primary illness, but a condition brought about by a number of medical, traumatic, and environmental causes. This problem can be related to lung diseases, heart conditions, allergic reactions, pneumothorax, and carbon monoxide poisoning, just to name a few. In most cases, dyspnea occurs when a disease has caused some kind of direct interference with either the flow of air into and out of the lungs, or with the exchange of oxygen and carbon dioxide within the lungs. In the typical dyspnea patient, the problem causing the interference originates in the lungs, as in the case of asthma.

Dyspnea is just one of a series of stages seen in **respiratory distress.** As something occurs to limit air flow or exchange, the patient will begin to increase

the rate and depth of his respirations. This is followed by dyspnea, in the form of shortness of breath. Hypoxia follows, resulting from the decreased supply of oxygen. The patient may be gasping for air, cyanotic, and possibly suffering problems with vision. At the same time blood oxygen levels are too low and carbon dioxide levels are on the increase. The respiratory control center is at first stimulated, causing the patient to breathe rapidly. With time, this center is depressed and the breathing rate slows. Unless this condition is corrected, the patient will have a temporary cessation of breathing **(apnea)**, becoming unconscious. He will exhibit dilated pupils. Respirations will cease and the patient will go into cardiac arrest. Basically, the patient will have suffocated **(asphyxia).**

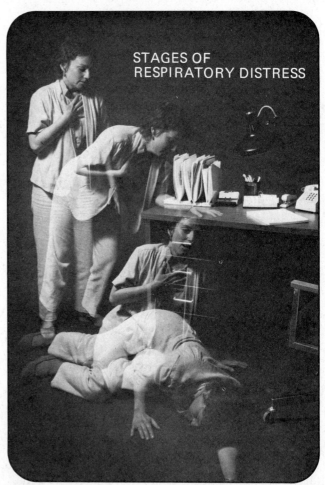

Figure 11-10: The stages of respiratory distress. A. Slight distress, B. Dyspnea, C. Apnea, D. Asphyxia.

Emergency Care for Dyspnea

It is fairly obvious when a person is suffering from dyspnea. The symptoms and signs are shown in Figure 11-11. When the distress is not due to trauma, it is often difficult to determine the exact medical or environmental problem. An efficient patient interview is very important. Question the patient, family members, fellow workers, and by-

STROKE – CEREBROVASCULAR ACCIDENT

CAUSES OF CEREBROVASCULAR ACCIDENTS – STROKE

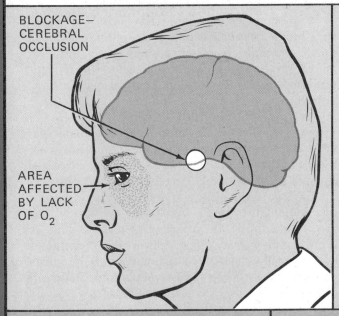

BLOCKAGE–
CEREBRAL
OCCLUSION

AREA
AFFECTED
BY LACK
OF O_2

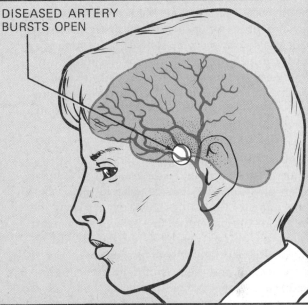

DISEASED ARTERY
BURSTS OPEN

CEREBRAL THROMBOSIS BLOCK–
AGE IN ARTERIES SUPPLYING
OXYGENATED BLOOD WILL RE-
SULT IN DAMAGE TO AFFECTED
PARTS OF THE BRAIN.

CEREBRAL HEMORRHAGE AN ANEURYSM OR OTHER WEAKENED
AREA OF AN ARTERY BURSTS. THIS HAS TWO EFFECTS:
- AN AREA OF THE BRAIN IS DEPRIVED OF OXYGENATED BLOOD.
- POOLING BLOOD PUTS INCREASED PRESSURE ON THE BRAIN,
  DISPLACING TISSUE AND INTERFERING WITH FUNCTION.

CEREBRAL HEMORRHAGE IS OFTEN ASSOCIATED WITH ARTERIO-
SCLEROSIS AND HYPERTENSION.

SYMPTOMS AND SIGNS OF STROKE

- HEADACHE
- CONFUSION AND/OR DIZZINESS
- LOSS OF FUNCTION OF EXTREMITIES
  (Usually on one side of the body)
- COLLAPSE
- FACIAL FLACCIDITY AND LOSS OF
  EXPRESSION
- IMPAIRED SPEECH
- UNEQUAL PUPIL SIZE
- RAPID, FULL PULSE
- DIFFICULT RESPIRATION
- NAUSEA
- CONVULSIONS
- COMA

EMERGENCY CARE OF STROKE PATIENT

CONSCIOUS PATIENT
- ASSURE AN OPEN AIRWAY
- KEEP PATIENT CALM
- ADMINISTER OXYGEN
  AS REQUIRED
- MONITOR VITAL SIGNS
- TRANSPORT IN SEMI RE-
  CLINING POSITION
- GIVE NOTHING BY MOUTH

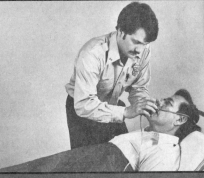

UNCONCIOUS PATIENT
- MAINTAIN OPEN AIRWAY
- PROVIDE OXYGEN AS REQUIRED
- MONITOR VITAL SIGNS
- TRANSPORT IN LATERAL RECUMBENT POSITION
- KEEP AFFECTED LIMBS UNDERNEATH PATIENT
- USE PROTECTIVE PADDING

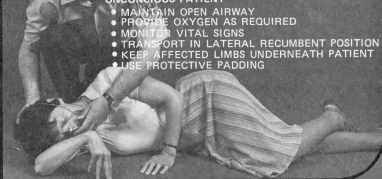

SCAN 11.3

standers. Do not accept responses using medical terms. Someone may tell you the patient has asthma when he really has chronic bronchitis or emphysema. The information gained from an interview should be weighed with the signs determined during the physical examination. Medical identification devices and prescription medicines being taken by the patient also can serve as sources of information. Do not try to determine what the medications indicate, but relay the names of the drugs to the emergency department physician. This must be done immediately if the patient has taken the medications and is still in distress.

Once the medical problem is known, a specific course of action can be taken. If the reason for the respiratory distress cannot be determined, you must assure an open airway, treat for shock, and transport the patient. Providing 100% oxygen may be dangerous for the patient. Many EMS Systems start the patient on 24% oxygen by venturi mask and radio the emergency department physician to ask if the concentration and method of delivery should be changed. Some patients fight the mask, believing it

will interfere with their breathing. Explain to them that they will receive more oxygen if they wear the mask. If they still refuse, try using a nasal cannula.

Chronic Obstructive Pulmonary Disease

Chronic obstructive pulmonary disease includes *chronic bronchitis, emphysema*, and many undetermined respiratory illnesess that cause the patient problems like those seen in emphysema. Chronic bronchitis can be seen in children and teenagers; however, chronic obstructive pulmonary disease is mainly a problem of the middle-aged or older patients. This may be due to the long-term reactions of tissues in the respiratory tract to smoking, allergens, chemicals, air pollutants, or repeated infections.

Chronic bronchitis and emphysema are compared in Figure 11-12. In chronic bronchitis, the bronchiole lining is inflamed. Excess mucus is formed and released. The cells in the bronchioles that normally clear away accumulations of mucus are not able to do so. The sweeping apparatus on these cells, the cilia, have become paralyzed.

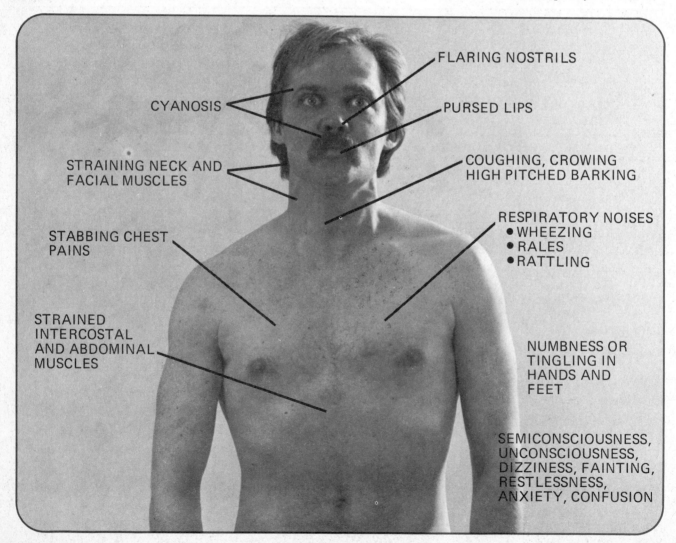

Figure 11-11: The symptoms and signs of respiratory distress.

The symptoms and signs of chronic bronchitis include:

- Patient is usually an older person
- Patient is usually a current or past heavy smoker
- Persistent cough
- Shortness of breath, with the tendency to tire easily
- Tightness in chest
- Periods of dizziness in some cases
- Cyanosis, edema of the lower extremities, and patient wanting to sit upright at all times occur in advanced cases.

In emphysema, the walls of the alveoli and bronchioles break down, greatly reducing the surface area for respiratory exchange. The lungs begin to lose elasticity and the alveoli and bronchioles secrete excess mucus. These factors combine to trap stale air in the lungs, reducing the effectiveness of normal breathing efforts.

The symptoms and signs of emphysema can include:

- Patient is usually an older person
- Patient is a current or past heavy smoker, or has been exposed to industrial smoke and gases
- Patient often has past history of respiratory problems or respiratory allergies
- Signs that are the same as chronic bronchitis
- Advanced cases have:

  Rapid pulse, occasionally irregular

  Breathing in puffs through pursed lips

  Blood pressure usually normal

  Barrel-chest appearance

  Wheezing

The emergency care is essentially the same for both bronchitis and emphysema:

1. Assure an open airway.
2. Monitor vital signs.
3. Allow the patient to assume the most comfortable position.
4. Loosen any restrictive garments.
5. Keep the patient warm, but not overheated.
6. Do all you can to reduce stress.
7. Administer oxygen at 24% by venturi mask. Follow local guidelines . . . usually 100% oxygen at 2 to 5 liters per minute to deliver 24%.
8. Transport as soon as possible

Take great care in administering oxygen to the chronic obstructive pulmonary disease patient. A high flow rate of oxygen will increase the blood concentration of oxygen, but it will not lower the carbon dioxide levels. This could cause the patient to reduce his breathing efforts too soon and develop respiratory arrest (see Chapter 6).

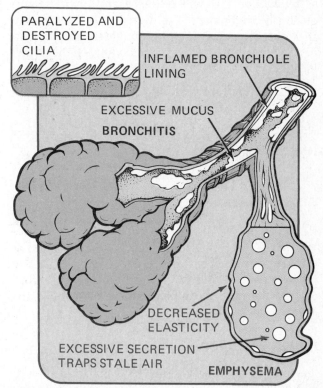

Figure 11-12: Chronic bronchitis and emphysema are chronic obstructive pulmonary diseases.

Asthma

Seen in young and old patients alike, asthma is an episodic disease. This is far different from chronic bronchitis and emphysema, both of which *continually* afflict the patient. Between episodes, the asthmatic patient can lead an essentially normal life. When an asthma attack occurs it may be triggered by an allergic reaction to something inhaled, swallowed, or injected into the body. Attacks can be precipitated by insect stings, air pollutants, infection, strenuous exercise, or emotional stress.

When an asthma attack occurs, the small bronchioles that lead to the airsacs of the lungs become narrowed because of contractions of the smooth muscles that make up the airway. To complicate matters, there is an overproduction of thick mucus. Between the contractions and the mucus, the small passages practically close down, severely restricting airflow. The airflow is mainly restricted in one direction. When the patient inhales, the expanding lungs exert an outward force, increasing the diameter of the airway, allowing air to flow into the lungs. During exhalation, the opposite occurs and the stale air becomes trapped in the lungs. This requires the patient to forcefully exhale the air, producing the characteristic wheezing sounds associated with asthma.

The patient having an asthmatic attack will not usually have chest pains or an increased pulse rate. The rhythm of the pulse will be normal. There will be no doubt that he is having difficulty with his expirations. Wheezing sounds can be heard without a stethoscope. He will be tense and anxious, and obviously frightened. The veins in the neck may stick out. He may hunch his shoulders and pull up his chest wall in an attempt to breathe. Other signs include cyanosis and coughing.

To provide care, you should:
1. Try to reassure and calm the patient.
2. Assist the patient in taking any prescribed asthma medications.
3. Help the patient position himself so he feels most comfortable.
4. Provide oxygen.
5. Transport—oxygen may only provide temporary relief.

WARNING: Anaphylactic shock is a complication of asthma. This must be considered as a possibility any time you are caring for an asthma patient. Bronchiospasms may occur before the patient develops anaphylactic shock.

Hyperventilation

A **hyperventilating** patient breathes too rapidly and too deeply. Often fear or stress will set off the attack. Some patients will have chest pains or other symptoms of an impending heart attack. Some patients report a tingling sensation in the upper extremity and may display a cramping of the fingers. The patient may tell you that he has attacks of hyperventilation. Even with this information, you should stay alert for changes in vital signs. The patient's problem in the past *may* have been hyperventilation, but this time it could be something more serious. Remember, hyperventilation may indicate a medical problem.

In most cases, the hyperventilating patient will not be cyanotic. This is a reliable clue that allows you to rule out severe respiratory distress.

The carbon dioxide level in the blood of a hyperventilating patient is too low. Having the patient breathe into a paper bag (not plastic) increases the carbon dioxide level in the blood, bringing it closer to normal. This usually controls the attack. If you are unable to control hyperventilation by this method, there may very well be a more serious medical problem. Transport the patient, monitoring vital signs. Do not provide oxygen unless there are signs of oxygen deficiency or you are ordered to do so by a physician.

NOTE: Hyperventilation is not only a condition, it can also be a sign. When occurring by itself, hyper-

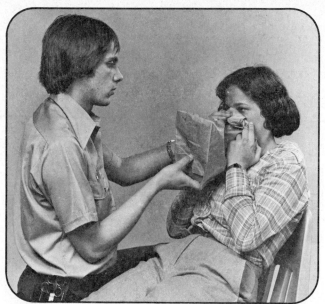

Figure 11-13: Have the hyperventilating patient rebreathe into a paper bag.

ventilation is seldom a problem for the EMT. However, patients with respiratory distress or AMI's also may show hyperventilation. You must assess all hyperventilating patients. Remember that cyanosis usually indicates a problem more serious than the condition of hyperventilation.

DIABETES MELLITUS

The cells of the body need glucose as a source of energy. More complex sugars are converted into this simple sugar, which is then absorbed into the bloodstream. This blood sugar cannot simply pass from the bloodstream into the body's cells. In order to enter the cells, **insulin** must be present. Without insulin, the cells can be surrounded by glucose and still starve for this sugar. When sugar intake and insulin are balanced, the body can effectively use sugar as an energy source. If, for some reason, insulin production decreases, the glucose cannot be utilized by the cells. This glucose remains in circulation, increasing in concentration as more sugars are digested by the person, who is now experiencing feelings of great hunger. The level of blood sugar climbs, eventually to be spilled over into the urine. The urine output of the body increases in an effort to rid the body of excess sugar in the blood.

The condition brought about by decreased insulin production is known as **diabetes mellitus** or sugar diabetes. The person suffering from this condition is a diabetic. The problem may begin as a child with *juvenile diabetes,* or it may develop as the person ages, called *maturity onset* diabetes. Diabetes is seen more often in older people. There are at least 5 million diabetics in the United States. The danger of undetected and untreated diabetes is severe. As the condition develops, the diabetic can become weak and show a loss of weight even though he has increased his sugar and fat intake. He will take in large quantities of water to offset the loss of fluids through extensive urination. Acids and ketones (compounds like fingernail polish remover) begin to concentrate in the blood. This can cause coma and lead to death.

There is no cure for diabetes; it can only be controlled. Some patients can do this by strictly following medically supervised diets. About 30% must take daily doses of insulin. Therefore, there are two possible sources of problems for the diabetic who is taking insulin: an overuse, or an underuse of insulin. Either can prove to be life-threatening.

Diabetic Coma and Insulin Shock

Diabetic coma results from a decreased insulin supply. Enough insulin is not being produced by the body or the person is not taking effective dosages of insulin. The body attempts to overcome the lack of sugar in the cells by using other foodstuffs for energy, notably stored fats. However, fats are not an efficient alternative to glucose and the waste products of their utilization greatly increase the acidity of the blood **(acidosis).** If allowed to go untreated, acidosis and the loss of fluids brought on by the high level of glucose in the blood eventually lead to diabetic coma.

Insulin shock occurs when there is too much insulin in the blood. Typically, this is caused when a diabetic:

- Takes too much insulin
- Has reduced his sugar intake by not eating, giving him an excess of insulin in the blood
- Has overexercised or overexerted himself, thus using sugars faster than normal

In any case, sugar rapidly leaves the blood supply and enters the cells. Not enough sugar remains for the brain, leading to unconsciousness. Permanent brain damage can occur quickly if the sugar is not replenished.

The terms "diabetic coma" and "insulin shock" are most commonly used in EMT-level emergency care. Diabetic coma is the end result of severe **hyperglycemia** (HI-per-gli-SE-me-ah), or too much sugar in the blood. Physicians consider diabetic coma to be a part of *diabetic ketoacidosis* (KE-to-as-i-DO-sis), occurring when the body breaks down too many fats trying to obtain fuel compounds. The diabetic patient with severe hyperglycemia has not developed diabetic coma until he is unconscious. However, since this is a complex diagnosis and utilizes many medical terms, most EMS Systems have their EMTs use the term diabetic coma.

Insulin shock is part of a severe case of **hypoglycemia** (HI-po-gli-SE-me-ah), or too little sugar in the blood. If any of the symptoms and signs described in Scansheet 11-4 are detected for a diabetic patient, you are to consider him to have developed insulin shock.

Care for Diabetic Emergencies

Many students find that they confuse diabetic coma and insulin shock. For this reason, the signs, symptoms, and procedures for care are presented side by side on Scansheet 11-4. Note that diabetic coma has a slow onset, while insulin shock comes on suddenly. This is because some sugar still reaches the brain in hyperglycemic states. When insulin shock occurs, the hypoglycemia is so severe that it is possible that no sugar is reaching the brain. Diabetic coma patients have dry, warm skin and a rapid, weak pulse. Insulin shock patients have moist skin, often cold and "clammy." Their pulse beat is full and rapid. The diabetic coma patient has acetone breath while the insulin shock patient usually does not. Continue to make the comparison for yourself.

As you consider evaluating the patient, keep in mind that many diabetic coma patients and some insulin shock patients will appear to be intoxicated. Always suspect a diabetic problem in cases that seem to involve no more than intoxication. Also keep in mind that the patient intoxicated on alcohol may also be a diabetic, with the alcohol smell covering over the acetone smell characteristic of diabetic coma. The alcoholic diabetic is a good candidate for emergency care because he tends to neglect taking insulin during periods of prolonged drinking.

Whenever you are in doubt as to whether a CONSCIOUS patient is suffering from diabetic coma or insulin shock, GIVE THE PATIENT SUGAR. The "sugar for everyone" policy is correct for conscious patients since diabetic coma patients will not be hurt by what you do provided they are transported. Insulin shock patients need sugar as soon as possible. Giving anything by mouth to an unconscious patient is a dangerous policy, since it may lead to aspiration. A "sprinkle" of granulated sugar under the tongue is acceptable in some EMS Systems, but no one advocates administering liquids by mouth to the unconscious patient.

CONVULSIVE DISORDERS (INCLUDING EPILEPSY)

In a conscious, healthy individual, muscular movements are usually smooth and coordinated. However, if the normal functions of the brain are upset by injury, infection, or disease, the electrical

DIABETIC EMERGENCIES

DIABETIC COMA	INSULIN SHOCK
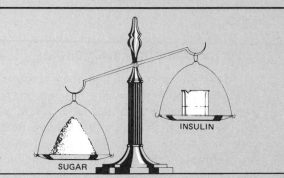	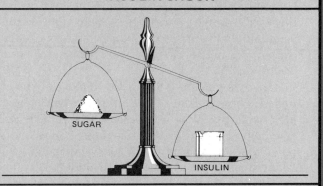

DIABETIC COMA

CAUSES:
- THE DIABETIC'S CONDITION HAS NOT BEEN DIAGNOSED AND/OR TREATED.
- THE DIABETIC HAS NOT TAKEN HIS INSULIN.
- THE DIABETIC HAS OVEREATEN, FLOODING THE BODY WITH A SUDDEN EXCESS OF CARBOHYDRATES.
- THE DIABETIC SUFFERS AN INFECTION WHICH DISRUPTS HIS GLUCOSE / INSULIN BALANCE.

EMERGENCY CARE:
- IMMEDIATELY TRANSPORT TO A MEDICAL FACILITY

SYMPTOMS AND SIGNS:
- GRADUAL ONSET OF SYMPTOMS AND SIGNS, OVER A PERIOD OF DAYS.
- PATIENT COMPLAINS OF DRY MOUTH AND INTENSE THRIST.
- ABDOMINAL PAIN AND VOMITING COMMON.
- GRADUALLY INCREASING RESTLESS, CONFUSION, FOLLOWED BY STUPOR.
- COMA, WITH THESE SIGNS:
  - SIGNS OF AIR HUNGER — DEEP, SIGHING RESPIRATIONS.
  - WEAK, RAPID PULSE.
  - DRY, RED, WARM SKIN.
  - EYES THAT APPEAR SHRUNKEN.
  - NORMAL OR SLIGHTLY LOW BLOOD PRESSURE.
  - BREATH SMELLS OF ACETONE — SICKLY SWEET, LIKE NAIL POLISH REMOVER.

INSULIN SHOCK

CAUSES:
- THE DIABETIC HAS TAKEN TOO MUCH INSULIN.
- THE DIABETIC HAS NOT EATEN ENOUGH TO PROVIDE HIS NORMAL SUGAR INTAKE.
- THE DIABETIC HAS OVEREXERCISED, OR OVEREXERTED HIMSELF, THUS REDUCING HIS BLOOD GLUCOSE LEVEL.
- THE DIABETIC HAS VOMITED A MEAL.

EMERGENCY CARE:
- CONSCIOUS PATIENT — ADMINISTER SUGAR. GRANULAR SUGAR, HONEY, LIFESAVER OR OTHER CANDY PLACED UNDER THE TONGUE.
- AVOID GIVING LIQUIDS TO THE UNCONSCIOUS PATIENT. PROVIDE "SPRINKLE" OF GRANULATED SUGAR UNDER TONGUE . . .
- TURN HEAD TO SIDE.
- TRANSPORT TO THE MEDICAL FACILITY.

SYMPTOMS AND SIGNS:
- RAPID ONSET OF SYMPTOMS AND SIGNS, OVER A PERIOD OF MINUTES.
- DIZZINESS AND HEADACHE.
- ABNORMAL, HOSTILE, OR AGGRESSIVE BEHAVIOR, WHICH MAY BE DIAGNOSED AS ACUTE ALCOHOLIC INTOXICATION.
- FAINTING, CONVULSIONS, AND OCCASIONALLY COMA.
- NORMAL BLOOD PRESSURE.
- FULL RAPID PULSE.
- PATIENT INTENSELY HUNGRY.
- SKIN PALE, COLD, AND CLAMMY; PERSPIRATION MAY BE PROFUSE.
- COPIOUS SALIVA, DROOLING.

SPECIAL NOTES: DIABETIC COMA AND INSULIN SHOCK

WHEN FACED WITH A PATIENT WHO MAY BE SUFFERING FROM ONE OF THESE CONDITIONS:
- DETERMINE IF THE PATIENT IS DIABETIC. LOOK FOR MEDICAL ALERT MEDALIONS OR INFORMATION CARDS; INTERVIEW PATIENT AND FAMILY MEMBERS.
- IF THE PATIENT IS A KNOWN OR SUSPECTED DIABETIC, AND INSULIN SHOCK CANNOT BE RULED OUT, ASSUME THAT IT IS INSULIN SHOCK AND ADMINISTER SUGAR.

OFTEN A PATIENT SUFFERING FROM EITHER OF THESE CONDITIONS MAY SIMPLY APPEAR DRUNK. ALWAYS CHECK FOR OTHER UNDERLYING CONDITIONS—SUCH AS DIABETIC COMPLICATIONS—WHEN TREATING SOMEONE WHO APPEARS INTOXICATED.

activity of the brain can become irregular. This irregularity can bring about uncontrolled muscular contractions (a seizure). Unconsciousness is common to convulsive seizures.

Convulsive seizures are seen with:

- Epilepsy (grand mal or major seizure)
- CVA (stroke)
- Brain injury
- High fever
- Infection
- Severe gastrointestinal distress
- Measles, mumps, and other childhood diseases
- Eclampsia (see Chapter 12)
- Undetected reasons

A convulsive seizure has three distinct phases:

1. Tonic Phase—the body becomes rigid, stiffening for no more than 30 seconds. Breathing may stop, the patient may bite his tongue (rare), and bowel and bladder control could be lost.
2. Clonic Phase—the body jerks about violently, usually for no more than one or two minutes (some can last five minutes). The patient may foam at the mouth and drool. His face and lips often become cyanotic.
3. Postictal Phase—this begins when convulsions stop. The patient may regain consciousness immediately and enter a state of drowsiness and confusion, or he may remain unconscious for several hours. Headache is not uncommon.

Epilepsy

Epilepsy is an **episodic** disorder, that is, chronic. It may result from the effects of scar tissue in the brain following head injury or surgery, a reduced flow of blood to the brain, or a brain tumor. More often than not, the cause of a person's epilepsy remains a mystery.

Epilepsy may cause two forms of seizure: a **grand mal**, or major seizure characterized by convulsions; or a **petit mal**, or minor seizure that does not produce convulsions. A petit mal seizure may go unnoticed by everyone except the patient and knowledgeable members of his family. A conscientious use of special medications usually allows most epileptics to live normal lives without convulsions of any type.

When a person develops a grand mal seizure, he often experiences sudden brain cell activity known as an ''aura.'' He may see bright light or a sudden burst of colors. He may also experience the sensation of certain smells. Whatever the sensation, he knows that a seizure is coming. Usually the person

will let family members or associates know of the coming attack, and will then lie down. Emergency care is the same for epilepsy as for the other types of convulsive seizures.

Emergency Care for Convulsive Disorders

The basic emergency care for seizure patients is to:

1. Place the patient on the floor or ground.
2. Loosen restrictive clothing.
3. Protect the patient from injury, but do NOT try to hold the patient still during convulsions.
4. After convulsions have ended, keep the patient at rest positioned for drainage from the mouth.
5. Take vital signs.
6. Protect the patient from embarrassment by having onlookers give the patient privacy.
7. If this is the patient's first attack, or he has had others but is not under the care of a physician, transport him to a medical facility, monitoring vital signs. If the patient has had other attacks, ask if you may call his physician. The doctor may wish to see the patient, have the patient transported to a hospital, or change the patient's medications.

NOTE: Never place anything in the mouth of a convulsing patient. Many objects can be broken and obstruct the patient's airway. In the past ''bite sticks'' were used to try to keep patients from biting their tongues. These were made from tape-padded tongue depressors. Many groups studying the care of epileptic patients no longer recommend the use of ''bite sticks.'' Most patients do not bite their tongue during a seizure.

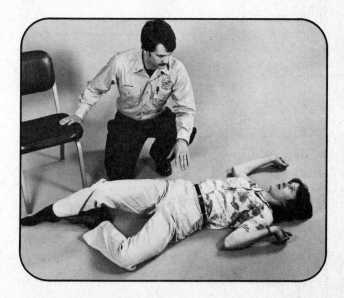

Figure 11-14: Protect the patient from injury.

ACUTE ABDOMINAL DISTRESS (ACUTE ABDOMEN)

Many abdominal problems start out as simple "indigestion" in the mind of the patient as he waits for it to "go away." However, when pain does not go away, or it becomes so severe that it frightens the patient and his family, emergency medical services may have to respond. Sometimes, after arrival at the hospital, it is determined that the cause of the pain is nothing more than indigestion. Other times it may prove to be such problems as:

- Appendicitis
- Intestinal obstruction
- Strangulated hernia (see Chapter 8)
- Inflammation of the gallbladder
- Perforated ulcer
- Kidney stones
- Ectopic pregnancy (see Chapter 12)
- Inflammation of the pancreas
- Inflammation of the abdominal cavity membranes (peritonitis)

The general symptoms and signs of acute abdomen can include:

- Pain—localized (confined to a small area) or diffuse (generalized, widespread)
- Nausea and vomiting
- Diarrhea or constipation
- Rapid pulse
- Low blood pressure (sometimes elevated when patient is in severe pain)
- Rapid shallow breathing (usually a response to pain)
- Fever
- Distention of the abdomen (may be pronounced)
- Tenderness (local or diffuse)
- Soft or rigid abdomen

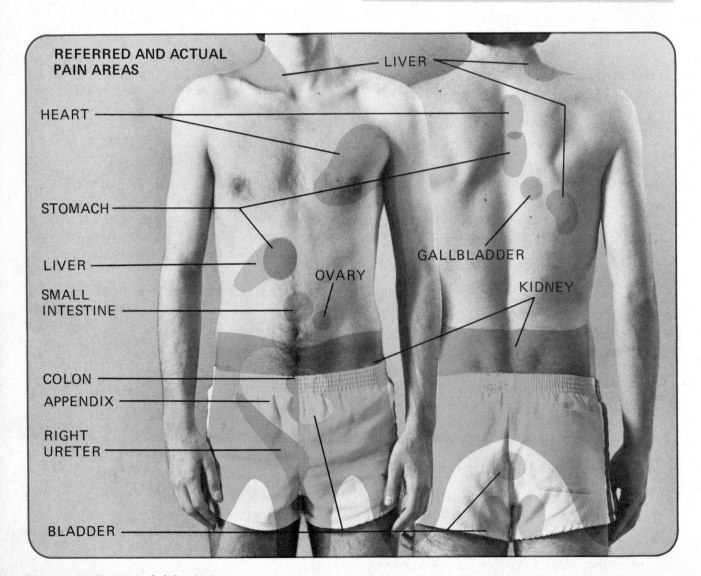

REFERRED AND ACTUAL PAIN AREAS

LIVER

HEART

STOMACH

LIVER

SMALL INTESTINE

OVARY

GALLBLADDER

KIDNEY

COLON

APPENDIX

RIGHT URETER

BLADDER

Figure 11-15: Patterns of abdominal pain.

- Abdominal wall muscle spasms
- An obvious protrusion
- Bleeding from the rectum, blood in the urine, nonmenstrual bleeding from the vagina
- Fear

As you look for these indicators, consider the patient's overall appearance. Does he appear ill? Is he restless? Does he try to lie perfectly still in an effort to alleviate the pain? Does he try to draw his knees up against his abdomen (**guarded abdomen**)? All of these point to acute abdominal distress.

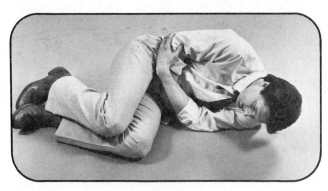

Figure 11-16: Guarded abdomen.

Emergency Care for Acute Abdominal Distress

The symptoms and signs of acute abdominal distress should not be taken lightly. What you do and do not do can be critical for the patient. Do not try to guess the nature of the distress. . . TRANSPORT THE PATIENT. You should also:

1. Maintain an open airway and be on the alert for vomiting.
2. Treat for shock.
3. Position the patient on his back with knees flexed but stay on the alert for vomiting.
4. Reassure the patient. . .do not try to diagnose.
5. Administer oxygen if there is shallow breathing or other indications of respiratory difficulties.
6. Do not give anything to the patient by mouth.
7. Attempt to collect information as to the time of onset, if it was gradual or sudden, the nature of the pain (stabbing, gnawing, sharp), any chills or fever, any unusual bowel movements, any bleeding.

NOTE: Anti-shock garments may be ordered for some patients who are in acute abdominal distress (see Appendix 4A).

COMMUNICABLE DISEASES

As an EMT, you may have to care for and transport a patient who has an infectious disease. This may be noticeable because the patient shows:

- Fever
- Profuse sweating (diaphoresis)
- Vomiting or diarrhea
- A rash or other lesions on the skin
- Headache, stiff neck, chest pain, abdominal pain
- Coughing or sneezing

Your role will be to transport, maintain an open airway, treat for shock, keep the patient warm, and give nothing by mouth. However, your duties go beyond this. If the disease is communicable, you must protect yourself and make certain that no one else using the ambulance or its supplies will contract the disease.

The typical patient requiring your services because he is "ill" will not cause you to take any unusual steps to protect yourself. You should avoid touching any discharges from the body (when necessary, wear surgical gloves). You should avoid touching stools or contaminated articles of clothing and bed linens. Do not touch your face in case you have

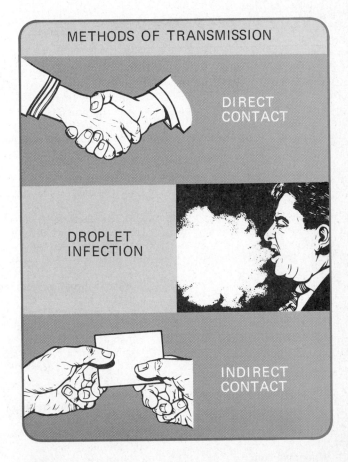

Figure 11-17: How communicable diseases may be transmitted.

touched something contaminated. Wash your hands and face. Ask the emergency department physician if you need to do anything else or if you need special immunization or antibiotic treatment. Ask to be informed if the patient is diagnosed as having a communicable disease. It means you will need to be examined also.

When in quarters, unload and properly dispose of any contaminated bedding, properly discard all disposable items used by the patient, and clean any nondisposable items used in patient care. This includes disinfecting respiratory equipment and the ambulance cot. Unless directed otherwise, air the ambulance and scrub its patient compartment.

NOTE: Some systems have disposal of contaminated items done at the hospital.

Remember to care for yourself. Remove and plastic bag your clothing. This clothing should be laundered separately, as soon as possible, using a disinfecting laundry product. Shower thoroughly with a disinfecting soap, and make sure you clean your fingernails.

If the emergency department physician believes that the patient's disease requires special proce-

dures, he will tell you. You are to follow his directions. Make certain that he contacts your organization's medical officer so that there will be proper supervision for the special cleaning of equipment and caring for personnel.

SUMMARY

For specific care procedures, review the scansheets and lists provided in this chapter.

A chronic illness is one that is constantly present over a long period of time. Some medical problems are episodic, only affecting the patient at irregular intervals. When a medical problem has a sudden onset, it is said to be acute.

Detecting medical problems depends on a proper patient assessment, including patient and bystander interviews, looking for medical identification devices, taking vital signs, and conducting a physical examination. You must gather symptoms and signs and relate these to possible medical problems.

Most cardiovascular emergencies can be related to changes in arterial walls. Atherosclerosis is the build-up of fatty deposits to form plaque on the in-

Table 11.1: Communicable Diseases

Disease	Mode of Transmission	Incubation Period
Chickenpox (varicella)	Direct contact. . .moist crusts are infectious	14 to 16 days
Diphtheria	Person to person by respiratory droplets, or indirectly from contaminated objects	2 to 5 days
German measles (rubella)	Air-borne droplets	14 to 21 days
Infectious hepatitis	Contact with objects contaminated by person's feces (including their hands)	25 to 30 days
Measles (rubeola)	Air-borne droplets and secretions from the mouth, nose, and eyes	10 to 12 days
Meningitis (bacterial)	Oral and nasal secretions	2 to 10 days
Mumps	Droplets of saliva or objects contaminated by saliva	14 to 21 days
Pneumonia (bacterial and viral)	Droplets and secretions from mouth and nose	several days
Scarlet fever (scarlatina)	Nose and throat secretions; pus from ears	several days
Staphylococcal skin infections (staph)	Direct contact with sore, its discharge, or contaminated objects	several days
Syphilis	Venereal contact: saliva, semen, vaginal discharge, and blood can carry the organism into open cuts	10 days to several months
Tuberculosis (TB)	Respiratory secretions, contaminated objects, organisms on patient's hands	4 to 6 weeks
Typhoid fever	Feces, urine, and contaminated objects	7 to 21 days
Whooping cough (pertussis)	Respiratory secretions and air-borne droplets	5 to 21 days

ner wall of an artery. When calcium deposits form, arteriosclerosis has occurred. Both can occlude an artery. This can take place in a coronary artery, leading to coronary artery disease. This disease is associated with smoking, hypertension, poor diet, stressful living, and lack of exercise.

Angina pectoris is a condition where the patient suffers chest pains during emotional or physical stress. This pain indicates that all areas of the myocardium are not receiving an adequate supply of oxygenated blood. The pain usually lasts from 3 to 5 minutes and is relieved by rest and nitroglycerine. Administer oxygen and transport the patient.

Acute myocardial infarction occurs when an area of the myocardium dies because it has not received enough oxygenated blood. The patient will usually have chest pains that do not go away after rest. The pain may last several minutes or longer. He will have difficult breathing, increased pulse rate, and reduced blood pressure in some cases. The patient will be anxious, depressed, and have feelings of impending doom. Maintain an open airway, keep the patient calm, administer oxygen, help him take medications, treat for shock, and transport as soon as possible.

Avoid the use of siren and excessive speed during transport.

Congestive heart failure is related to a damaged or weakened heart that can no longer maintain proper circulation. Blood is "backed up" into pulmonary, then systemic vessels. Fluids are forced from the blood into the tissues. In left heart failure, pulmonary edema brings about dyspnea (difficult, labored breathing). Rales can sometimes be heard. Right heart failure produces edema of the liver, spleen, and lower extremities. Ascites, or an abdomen distended by fluids, may develop.

Allow the congestive heart failure patient to assume a comfortable position, keep him calm, and conserve body heat. Unless the patient suffers from COPD, administer a high concentration of oxygen. If he has COPD, deliver no higher than 24% oxygen by venturi. Transport as soon as possible.

A patient with a cardiac pacemaker can still suffer angina pectoris, AMI, or congestive heart failure. Do not try to evaluate the efficiency of the pacemaker. Treat as you would any patient having the same problem and transport. The same holds true for a patient who has had a coronary artery bypass.

A stroke or cerebrovascular accident (CVA), is caused by occlusion or bursting of an artery supplying the brain. The conscious patient will usually be confused and have a headache, loss of extremity function (often to one side only), facial flaccidity, impaired speech, unequal pupils, and a rapid full pulse. Often the patient will have nausea, and may develop coma.

If the stroke patient is conscious, maintain an open airway, keep him calm, administer oxygen if needed, and transport in a semi-reclined position. Do the same for the unconscious patient, but transport in a lateral recumbent position, with affected limbs padded and placed under the body.

Administer a high concentration of oxygen to a patient with dyspnea, unless he has chronic bronchitis, emphysema, or other form of COPD. The COPD patient should receive 24% oxygen by venturi. Reassure and calm the asthma patient, assisting him with medications. Transport all asthmatic patients. . .oxygen may provide only temporary relief.

Hyperventilation, as a condition and not a sign of more serious problems, can be cared for by having the patient breathe into a paper bag.

Diabetes mellitus can usually be controlled by diet, or diet and insulin. When the diabetic patient does not take enough insulin or he takes too much sugar, he becomes hyperglycemic and may develop diabetic coma. This has a slow onset, with the patient complaining of thirst. He may become restless, then confused, possibly going into a state of stupor followed by unconsciousness. The pulse will be rapid and weak, respirations will be deep, and the skin will be warm and dry. The patient will have acetone breath. Transport immediately, and provide sugar to the conscious patient if you cannot tell if he is developing diabetic coma or insulin shock.

Insulin shock develops from severe hypoglycemia when the patient takes too much insulin or too little sugar. It has a rapid onset, with the patient complaining of hunger. Often the patient has a headache and dizziness. The pulse is rapid and full, the skin is cold and clammy, and there is no acetone breath. Provide sugar, but do not give liquids to the unconscious patient (sprinkle granulated sugar under the tongue). Transport as soon as possible.

Convulsive seizures, including epilepsy, require you to protect the patient from physical harm and embarrassment. Transport of the patient is the best policy.

Acute abdomen has many different symptoms and signs, including pain, nausea, vomiting, rapid pulse, and rapid shallow breathing. Do not try to diagnose the source of the problem. Maintain an open airway, treat for shock, provide oxygen as needed, and transport. Place the patient on his back with the knees flexed. Stay alert for vomiting.

A patient may have a communicable disease if he has fever, diaphoresis (profuse sweating), vomiting or diarrhea, a rash or lesions, headache, coughing, or sneezing. Nontrauma-related neck, chest, or abdominal pain may also indicate an infectious disease. Transport the patient, treating for shock. Protect yourself from contamination during care and transport. Consult with the emergency department physician and follow his directions for personal care and the disposal, cleaning, and sterilization of equipment and supplies.

SECTION TWO: POISONING AND DRUG ABUSE

OBJECTIVES By the end of this section, you should be able to:

1. Define "poison" and state the four ways in which a poison can enter the body. (p. 257)

2. Define "poison control center" and describe the role of such centers when you are providing emergency care for a poisoning patient. (p. 259)

3. List the symptoms and signs of ingested poisoning and describe the emergency care for patients who have ingested a poison, plus any exceptions to these procedures. (p. 259-60)

4. List the symptoms and signs of inhaled poisoning and describe the emergency care for patients who have inhaled a poison. (p. 260-1)

5. List the symptoms and signs of absorbed poisoning and describe the emergency care for patients who have absorbed a poison. (p. 261)

6. List the symptoms and signs of an injected poisoning and describe the emergency care for pa-

tients who have been injected with a poison. (p. 261-2)

7. List the symptoms and signs of snakebite and describe the emergency care for patients who have been bitten by a snake. (p. 262-3)

8. Describe the special problems faced when dealing with a patient under the influence of alcohol. (p. 263-4)

9. Describe the symptoms and signs of alcohol abuse and alcohol withdrawal. (p. 263-4)

10. Summarize the emergency care provided for the alcohol abuse patient. (p. 264)

11. Define "uppers," "downers," "hallucinogens," "narcotics," and "volatile chemicals." (p. 264-5)

12. Describe in general a patient under the influence of each of the above substances. Include a description of drug withdrawal. (p. 264-5)

13. Summarize the emergency care provided for drug abuse patients. (p. 265-6)

SKILLS As an EMT, you should be able to:

1. Detect obvious cases of ingested, inhaled, absorbed, and injected poisons.

2. Contact your local poison control center and provide them with the patient information they require.

3. Receive and carry out instructions given by a poison control center.

4. Provide the proper care for a patient who is a

poisoning victim, including the correct use of Syrup of Ipecac and activated charcoal.

5. Detect when a patient is the victim of snakebite and provide prompt efficient emergency care.

6. Determine if a patient is having a medical emergency, or if he has abused alcohol or drugs.

7. Provide emergency care for patients under the influence of alcohol or drugs, and for patients suffering alcohol or drug withdrawal.

TERMS you may be using for the first time:

Poison—any solid, liquid, or gaseous chemical that can harm the body by altering cell structure or processes.

Venom—a poison produced by living organisms such as certain snakes, spiders, and marine life forms.

Syrup of Ipecac—a compound used to induce vomiting in appropriate cases involving conscious poison victims.

Withdrawal—referring to alcohol or drug withdrawal, where the patient's body reacts severely when deprived of the abused substance.

Delerium Tremens (DT's)—a severe reaction that can be part of alcohol withdrawal. The patient's hands tremble, hallucinations may occur, the patient displays atypical behavior, and convulsions may take place. Severe alcohol withdrawal with the DT's can lead to death.

Uppers—stimulants such as amphetamines that affect the central nervous system to excite the user.

Downers—depressants such as barbiturates that affect the central nervous system to relax the user.

Narcotics—a class of drugs that affect the nervous system and change many normal body activities. An intense state of relaxation is associated with their use.

Hallucinogens—mind-affecting or -altering drugs that act on the central nervous system to produce excitement and distortion of stimuli from the environment.

Volatile Chemicals—vaporizing compounds, such as cleaning fluid, that are breathed in by the abuser to produce a "high."

POISONING

A **poison** is any chemical that can harm the body. Associated with this damage are symptoms and signs that indicate the patient is having a medical emergency. In the United States, there are more than one million cases of poisoning annually. While some of these cases are the results of murder or suicide attempts, most are accidental. These accidents usually involve common substances such as medications, petroleum products, cosmetics, and pesticides. In fact, a surprisingly large percentage of chemicals in everyday use contain substances that are poisonous if misused.

We usually think of poisons as being some kind of liquid or solid chemical that has been ingested by the poisoning victim. This often is the case, but keep in mind that many living organisms are capable of poisoning people. Certain snakes, lizards, spiders, scorpions, insects, and some fish and marine life forms produce poisons called **venoms.** Usually, these venoms are injected into victims by a bite or sting. Poisonous plants such as poison ivy contain substances that cause reactions when they come into contact with the skin. There are also mushrooms and other common plants that can be poisonous if eaten. These include some varieties of house plants, like the rubber plant and poinsettia. Bacterial contaminants in food may produce **toxins** (poisons), some of which can be deadly (e.g., botulism or food poisoning).

Poisons can be taken into the body by way of ingestion, inhalation, absorption (through the skin) and injection (through tissues and the bloodstream). A great number of substances can be considered to be poisons, with different people reacting differently to various poisons. As odd as it may seem, what may be a dangerous poison for one person may have little effect on another. For most poisonous sub-

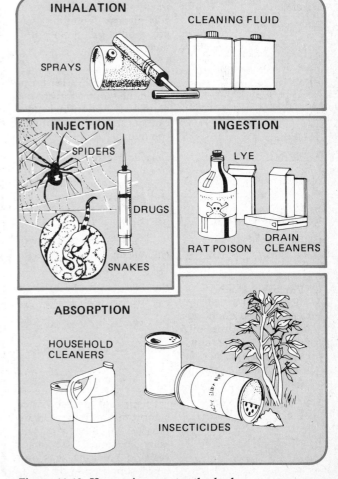

Figure 11-18: How poisons enter the body.

stances, the reaction is far more serious in children than in adults.

Once in the body, poisons can do damage in a variety of ways. A poison may act as a corrosive or irritant, destroying skin and other body tissues. A poisonous gas can act as a suffocating agent, displacing oxygen in the air. Some poisons are systemic poisons, causing harm to the entire body or to an entire body system. These poisons can critically depress or overstimulate the central nervous system, cause vomiting and diarrhea, prevent red blood cells from carrying oxygen, or interfere with the normal biochemical processes in the body. The actual effect and extent of damage rendered by a poison depends on the nature of the poison, its concentration, and sometimes on how it enters the body.

TYPES OF POISONS

Ingested poisons can include many common household and industrial chemicals, medications, improperly prepared foods, plant toxins, petroleum products, and agricultural products made specifically to control rodents, weeds, insects, and crop diseases.

Inhaled poisons take the form of gases, vapors, and sprays. Again, many of these substances are

Table 11.2: Common Poisons

POISON	HELPFUL SYMPTOMS AND SIGNS
ACIDS	Burns on or around the lips. Burning in mouth, throat, and stomach, often followed by heavy vomiting.
ALKALIS (ammonia, bleaches, detergents, lye, washing soda, certain fertilizers)	Check to see if mouth membranes appear white and swollen. There may be a "soapy" appearance in the mouth. Abdominal pain usually present. Vomiting may occur, often full of blood and mucus.
ARSENIC (rat poisons)	"Garlic breath," with burning in the mouth, throat, and stomach. Abdominal pain can be severe. Vomiting is common.
ASPIRIN	Delayed reactions, including ringing in the ears, rapid and deep breathing, dry skin, and restlessness.
CARBON MONOXIDE	Cherry red skin
CHLOROFORM	Slow, shallow breathing with chloroform odor on breath. Pupils are dilated and fixed.
CORROSIVE AGENTS (disinfectants, drain cleaners, household acids, iodine, pine oil, turpentine, toilet bowl cleaners, styptic pencil, water softeners, strong acids)	(SEE ACIDS)
FOOD POISONING	Difficult to detect since symptoms and signs vary greatly. Usually, you will note: abdominal pain, nausea and vomiting, gas and bowel sounds, and diarrhea.

POISON	HELPFUL SYMPTOMS AND SIGNS
IODINE	Upset stomach and vomiting. If a starchy meal has been eaten, the vomitus may appear blue.
METALS (copper, lead, mercury, zinc)	Metallic taste in mouth, with nausea and abdominal pains. Vomiting may occur. Stools may be bloody or dark.
PETROLEUM PRODUCTS (some deodorizers, heating fuel, diesel fuels, gasoline, kerosene, lighter fluid, lubricating oil, naphtha, rust remover, transmission fluid)	Note characteristic odors on patient's breath, on clothing, or in vomitus.
PHOSPHORUS	Abdominal pain and vomiting. Vomitus may be phosphorescent.
PLANTS (poison ivy, poison oak, poison sumac)	Swollen, itchy areas on the skin, with quickly forming "blister-like" lesions.
PLANTS—Ingested (azalea, castor bean, elderberry, foxglove, lily of the valley, mountain laurel, mushrooms and toadstools, nightshade, oleander, poinsettia, rhododendron, rhubarb, rubber plant, some wild cherries)	Difficult to detect, ranging from nausea to coma. Always question in cases of apparent child poisoning.
STRYCHNINE	The face, jaw, and neck will stiffen. Strong convulsions occur quickly after ingesting.

commonly used in the home, industry, and agriculture. Such poisons include carbon monoxide (from car exhaust and wood burning stoves), ammonia, chlorine, the gases produced from volatile liquid chemicals (including many industrial solvents), and insect sprays.

Absorbed (through the skin) **poisons** may or may not damage the skin. However, most are corrosives or irritants that will injure the skin and then be slowly absorbed into body tissues and the bloodstream. Included in this group of poisons are many of the insecticides and agricultural chemicals in common use. Corrosive activity usually does not stop with the skin. It will continue destroying tissues and then be absorbed by the body, possibly causing widespread damage. Contact with a variety of plant materials and certain forms of marine life can harm the skin and possibly be absorbed into tissues under the skin.

Injected poisons come from a number of sources. Insects, spiders, snakes, and certain marine forms are able to inject venoms into the body. The poison may be a drug or caustic chemical self-induced by way of a hypodermic needle. Unusual industrial accidents also can be a source of poisons being injected into the body. Caustics, acids, and industrial solvents may be forced into the body in cases of open wounds.

POISON CONTROL CENTERS

Emergency care of patients in poisoning cases presents special problems for the EMT. Symptoms and signs can vary greatly. Some poisons produce a characteristic set of symptoms and signs very quickly, while others are slow to appear. Those poisons that act almost immediately usually produce obvious signs of poisoning, and the particular poison or its container is often still at hand. Slow-acting poisons can produce effects that mimic an infectious disease or some other medical emergency.

There will be times when you will not know the substances that caused the poisoning. In some of these cases, an expert may be able to tell, based on the combination of certain symptoms and signs. Even when you know the source of the poison, correct emergency care procedures may still be in question. Many times, this is because the ideas about proper care keep changing as more research is done on poisoning. This constant change makes it impossible to print guides and charts for poison control and care that will be up-to-date when you use them. Even the information printed on labels of chemical containers may no longer be accurate at the time of the poisoning. All these factors mean proper emergency care techniques are best selected when based on expert opinion.

To overcome these problems, a network of **poison control centers** has been established throughout the country. In most localities, a poison control center can be reached 24 hours a day. The staff can tell you what should be done for most cases. You should know the telephone number for the center serving your area. Carry this number with you at all times.

So that you can best help the poison control center, note and report any containers at the scene of the poisoning. Let them know if the patient has vomited and describe the vomitus. When possible, gather information from the victim or from bystanders before you call the center. An accurate description of symptoms and signs may be needed before the poison control center can tell you what to do for the patient.

Many people have the impression that the poison control center should be called only for cases of ingested poison. The staff of the center can provide you with valuable information for *all* types of poisoning.

Regional Problems

Learning how to detect the effects of some poisons takes experience. Many can be learned through careful study. Keep in mind that your community may have special poisoning problems. Not every community is exposed to rattlesnakes, jellyfish, or powerful agricultural chemicals. Many EMS Systems have compiled lists of special poisoning problems for their areas. Check if this has been done for the area in which you will be an EMT.

EMERGENCY CARE FOR POISONING

Ingested Poisons

You must gather information quickly in cases of possible ingested poisoning. If at all possible, do so while you are making a primary survey. Note any *containers* that may contain poisonous substances. See if there is any *vomitus*. Check if there are any substances on the patient's clothes or if the patient's clothing indicates the nature of his work (farmer, miner, etc.). Can the *scene* be associated with certain types of poisonings? Question the patient and any bystanders.

The symptoms and signs for ingested poisons can include any or all of the following:

- Burns or stains around the patient's mouth
- Unusual breath odors, body odors, or odors on the patient's clothing or at the scene
- Abnormal breathing
- Abnormal pulse rate and character

- Sweating
- Dilated or constricted pupils
- Excessive saliva formation or foaming at the mouth
- Pains in the mouth or throat, or painful swallowing
- Stomach or abdominal pain
- Abdominal tenderness, sometimes with distention
- Upset stomach or nausea
- Retching, vomiting
- Diarrhea
- Convulsions
- Altered state of consciousness

To provide the proper emergency care, call the poison control center. Follow the directions given to you by the center's staff. In most cases of ingested poisoning, emergency care will consist of diluting the poison in the patient's stomach with one or two glasses of water or milk, and then inducing the patient to vomit. Never attempt to dilute the poison or induce vomiting if the patient is unconscious.

For *conscious* patients, typical procedures for care include:

1. Maintain an open airway.
2. CALL THE POISON CONTROL CENTER. If directed to do so. . .
3. Dilute the poison by having the patient drink one or two glasses of water or milk. Do NOT give anything by mouth if the patient is having convulsions, unless otherwise directed by a physician or poison control center.
4. If supplies are available, induce vomiting by giving the patient two tablespoons of Syrup of Ipecac followed by no less than 8 ounces of water (one full glass). If the patient is a child under the age of 10, use only one tablespoon of Syrup of Ipecac.
5. Position the patient so that he will not aspirate any vomitus and transport IMMEDIATELY. Place patient in a semi-reclined position and monitor closely for vomiting. If he becomes unconscious, place him in a lateral recumbent position to help prevent aspiration of vomitus.
6. If transport is delayed, wait 15 to 20 minutes for the patient to vomit. If the patient does not vomit after this time, give another dose of ipecac and water.
7. Save all vomitus.
8. Instead of inducing vomiting, you may be directed to give the patient two tablespoons of activated charcoal mixed vigorously in 8 ounces of water. If you are directed to induce vomiting and then give charcoal, give

the patient ipecac and water, followed by charcoal and water after the patient has vomited.

WARNING: Do NOT induce vomiting if the patient is not fully conscious, has been convulsing, or if the source of the poison is a strong acid, alkali, or petroleum product. Vomiting of such substances can cause severe tissue damage and usually will cause the patient to aspirate the vomitus. Examples of these substances are oven cleaners, drain cleaners, toilet bowl cleaners, lye, ammonia, bleaches, kerosene, and gasoline. Always check for burns around the patient's mouth and the odor of petroleum products on his breath.

When practical, transport the poisoned patient as soon as possible, calling the poison control center en route. Actions to dilute the poison and to induce vomiting are carried out during transport. Transport without delay is *critical* if the poisoned patient is unconscious.

Inhaled Poisons

WARNING: If you suspect inhaled poisons, approach the scene with care. If the source of the poison is an industrial compound, chlorine, or ammonia, use protective clothing and breathing apparatus. Make certain that your entire body is protected. Move the patient from the scene as quickly as possible.

Gather information from the patient and bystanders without delay. Note if there are any indications of inhaled poisons, including broken or breached containers, distinctive odors, signs of fire or smoke, and poor ventilation. Possible sources of the poison can be automobile exhaust, stoves, charcoal grills, industrial solvents, and spray cans.

The symptoms and signs of inhaled poisons vary depending upon the source of the poison. They include:

- Unconsciousness or altered states of behavior (depression or euphoria)
- Shortness of breath
- Coughing
- Rapid or slow pulse rate
- Eyes may appear to be irritated, or the patient may complain of burning eyes.
- The patient may complain of burning sensations in his mouth, nose, throat, or chest.
- Burning or itching (often complaints are made about the underarms, groin, and moist areas of the body).
- Severe headache
- Nausea and vomiting
- Carbon monoxide poisoning can cause the

lips and skin of white patients to turn cherry red.
• Spray paint or other substances may be found on the patient's face.

Emergency care consists of removing the patient from the source of the inhaled poison, maintaining an open airway, providing needed life support measures, and administering oxygen. It may be necessary to remove contaminated clothing from the patient. Avoid touching this clothing since it may cause skin burns. Since some poisonous gases condense into liquids, you may have to care for the patient's chemical burns (see page 302). Transport the patient as soon as possible. If the patient is unconscious, place him in a lateral recumbent position in case of vomiting.

REMEMBER: Unless you are trained to enter a scene involving poisonous gases and have the proper equipment, do NOT try to provide care for a patient in a poisonous atmosphere.

Absorbed Poisons

Absorbed poisons usually irritate or damage the skin. A poison can be absorbed with little or no damage to the skin, but such cases are very rare. The patient, bystanders, and what you observe at the scene will help you to determine if you are dealing with a case of absorbed poisoning. In the vast majority of cases, absorbed poisoning will be detected because of skin reactions to chemicals or plants at the scene.

The symptoms and signs of absorbed poisoning include any or all of the following:

• Skin reactions (from mild irritations to chemical burns)
• Itching
• Irritation of the eyes
• Headache
• Increased relative skin temperature
• Anaphylactic shock (rare)

Emergency care for absorbed poisoning includes moving the patient from the source of the poison and using water to immediately flood all the areas of the patient's body that have been exposed to the poison. After the initial water wash, remove all contaminated clothing (including shoes, jewelry, and watches) and wash the affected areas of the patient's skin with soap and water. When no soap is available, continue to flood the exposed areas of the patient's skin. Dry chemicals should be brushed from the skin before flushing. More specific directions for chemical burns will be covered in Chapter 13. Be on the alert for anaphylactic shock. Remember, this is a true emergency requiring immediate transport.

NOTE: You are responsible for any clothing or jewelry removed from the patient.

Injected Poisons

Insect stings, spider bites, and snakebites are typical sources of injected poisons. Commonly seen are reactions to wasp, hornet, bee, ant, and scorpion stings. The bite of the black widow and brown recluse spiders also can produce a medical emergency. Insect stings and bites are rarely dangerous; however, 5% of the population *will* have an allergic reaction to the venom and a few people may develop shock.

As an EMT, you are not expected to be able to classify insects and spiders as to genus and species. Proper identification of these organisms is best left to experts. If the problem has been caused by a creature that is known locally and is not normally dangerous (such as bees, wasps, and puss caterpillars), the major concern will be anaphylactic shock. If this does not appear to be a problem, care is usually simple. However, if the cause of the bite or sting is unknown, or the organism is unknown, the patient should be seen by a physician. Do not to try to classify spiders and scorpions. Call the emergency department, or take the patient to a medical facility and let experts decide on the proper treatment. If the dead organism is at the scene, be sure it is dead, but do not touch it with your hands. Transport the dead organism along with the patient.

Poisons also can be injected into the body by way of a hypodermic needle. Drug overdose and drug contamination, which can produce serious medical emergencies, will be covered later in this section.

Gather information from the patient, bystanders, and the scene. The symptoms and signs of injected poisoning can include:

• Noticeable stings or bites on the skin
• Puncture marks (especially note forearms and legs)
• Localized pain or itching
• Burning sensations at the site followed by pain spreading throughout the limb
• Swelling or blistering at the site
• Weakness or collapse
• Difficult breathing and unusual pulse rate
• Headache and dizziness
• Nausea and vomiting
• Muscle cramps, chest tightening, joint pains
• Excessive saliva formation, profuse sweating
• Anaphylactic shock

Emergency care for injected poisons includes:

1. Treating for shock, even if the patient does not present any signs of shock.

2. Scraping away bee and wasp stingers and venom sacs. Do NOT pull out stingers, always scrape them from the patient's skin. Carefully scrape the site using a blade or a card.
3. Placing a covered ice bag or cold pack over the bitten or stung area.

Some patients sensitive to stings or bites carry medication to help prevent anaphylactic shock. Help all such patients to take their medications. Your EMT course may include training in how to administer injectable medications for cases when the patient cannot do this himself. This is a serious legal medicine question. Make certain you follow local policies. **REMEMBER:** Be certain to look for medical identification devices.

Snakebites

Snakebites require special care. Over 8,000 people in the United States are bitten by poisonous snakes each year. The symptoms and signs of poisoning may take several hours to develop. Very few people die from snakebite. If death does result, it is usually not a rapidly occurring event unless anaphylactic shock develops. Most victims who will die live for one to two days.

The bite from a diamondback rattler or coral snake is considered very serious. Since each person reacts differently to snakebites, you should consider the bite from *any* known poisonous snake to be a serious emergency. Staying calm and keeping the patient calm is critical. There *is* time to treat the bite and to transport the patient.

Unless you are dealing with a known local species that is not considered poisonous, consider *all* snakebites to be from poisonous snakes. The patient or bystanders may say that the snake was not poi-

sonous, but they could be wrong. If the dead or captured snake is at the scene, your role as an EMT is not to identify the snake, but to provide care and to transport the dead snake along with the patient. Arrange for the *separate* transport of a live specimen. Do not attempt to transport a live snake in the ambulance.

Should you see the live, uncaptured snake, take great care or you may be its next victim. When possible, note its size and colorations. Unless you are an expert, do not try to catch the snake.

The symptoms and signs of snakebite may include:

- A noticeable bite on the skin—This may appear as nothing more than a discoloration.
- Pain and swelling in the area of the bite—This may be slow to develop, from 30 minutes to several hours.
- Rapid pulse and labored breathing
- Progressive general weakness
- Vision problems (dim or blurred)
- Nausea and vomiting
- Convulsions
- Drowsiness or unconsciousness

The emergency care for snakebite includes:

1. Keep the patient calm.
2. Treat for shock, conserve body heat.
3. Contact the poison control center.
4. Locate the fang marks and clean this site with soap and water.
5. Remove any rings, bracelets, or other constricting items on the bitten extremity.
6. Keep any bitten extremities immobilized—the application of a splint will help. Try to keep the bite at the level of the heart; or, when this is not possible, below the level of the heart.

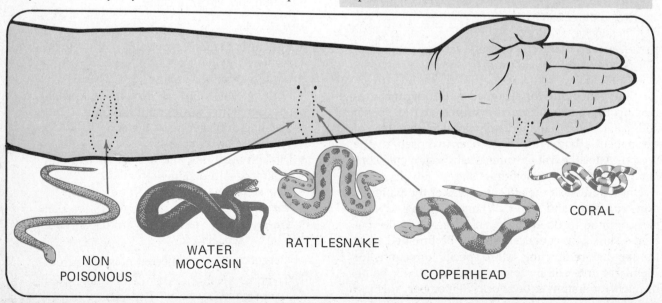

NON POISONOUS   WATER MOCCASIN   RATTLESNAKE   COPPERHEAD   CORAL

Figure 11-19: Venomous snakes and their bites.

7. Apply a light constricting band above and below the wound. This is to restrict the flow of lymph, not the flow of blood.

8. Transport the patient, carefully monitoring vital signs.

Apply a constricting band above and below the fang marks. Each band should be about 2 inches from the wound, but NEVER place one band on each side of a joint, such as above and below the knee. If the bite is to a finger, one band can be applied to the wrist of the affected extremity. The constricting bands should be from a snakebite kit or made of ³/₄ to 1¹/₂ inch wide soft rubber. If only one band is available, place it above the wound (between the wound and the heart). If no bands are available, use a handkerchief.

The constricting bands should be placed so that you can slide your finger underneath them. Do not place them so they cut off arterial flow. Monitor for a pulse at the wrist or ankle, depending upon the extremity involved. Check to be certain that tissue swelling has not caused the constricting bands to become too tight.

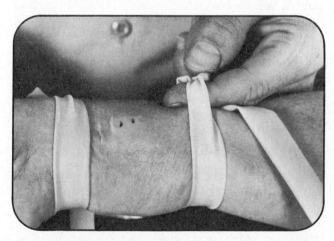

Figure 11-20: Care for snakebite.

Do not place an ice bag or cold pack on the bite unless you are directed to do so by a physician. Do not cut into the bite and suction or squeeze unless you are directed to do so by a physician. NEVER suck the venom from the wound using your mouth.

ALCOHOL AND DRUG ABUSE

ALCOHOL ABUSE

Even though alcohol is socially acceptable when used in moderation, it is still a drug. As with any other drug, abuse can lead to illness, poisoning of the body, antisocial behavior, and even death. As an EMT, you must take a professional approach when caring for a patient under the influence of alcohol. Remember, the patient needs your care and concern.

The intoxicated patient is not a joke. There can be serious medical problems or injuries that require your care. Take special precautions when working with the intoxicated patient. He may attempt to injure himself, bystanders, or even those trying to care for him.

The EMS System believes that EMTs should provide care for the patient suffering from alcohol abuse the same as for any other patient. An alcohol problem is not looked upon as a crime, but as a disease. To provide proper care, you must determine quickly that the patient's difficulties are caused by alcohol and that it is the *only* problem. Remember, diabetes, epilepsy, head injuries, high fevers, and other *medical* problems may make the patient appear to be drunk. If allowed to do so, conduct a primary and secondary survey and an interview. In some cases, the interview will have to depend on bystanders for meaningful results.

When needed, call the police for assistance so that you can conduct the patient assessment, provide care, and transport the patient. Protect yourself by staying alert for violent behavior.

The signs of alcohol abuse in an intoxicated patient include:

- The odor of alcohol on the patient's breath or clothing. By itself, this is not enough to conclude alcohol abuse. Be certain that this odor is not "acetone breath" as experienced by the diabetic.
- Swaying and unsteadiness of movement.
- Slurred speech and the inability to carry on a normal conversation. Do not be fooled into thinking the situation is not serious because the patient jokes or acts humorously.
- A flushed appearance to the face, often with the patient sweating and complaining of being warm.
- Nausea and vomiting or the desire to vomit.

The alcoholic patient may not be under the influence of alcohol, but suffering from **alcohol withdrawal.** This can be a severe reaction occurring when the patient cannot obtain alcohol, or when he is too sick to drink alcohol. The alcohol withdrawal patient may experience hallucinations and **delirium tremens (DT's).** In some cases, the DT's can be fatal. The patient with the DT's may show:

- Confusion and restlessness
- Atypical behavior, to the point of seeming "mad" or demonstrating "insane" behavior
- Some DT patients will have hallucinations
- Gross tremor (obvious shaking) of the hands
- Profuse sweating
- Convulsions (common, can be very serious)

- The symptoms and signs of shock due to fluid loss (rare)

Note that some of the signs seen in alcohol abuse are similar to those found in medical emergencies. Be CERTAIN that the only problem is alcohol abuse. There may be other signs, such as depressed vital signs, due to the patient mixing alcohol and drugs. When interviewing the intoxicated patient or one suffering from alcohol withdrawal, NEVER ask the patient if he is 'taking drugs'. He may react to these questions as if you are gathering evidence of a crime. Ask him if he has been taking any medication while drinking.

The basic care for the intoxicated patient and the patient suffering alcohol withdrawal consists of:

1. A proper survey and interview to detect any medical emergencies or injuries. Look carefully for fractures and indications of other injuries.
2. Monitoring vital signs, staying alert for respiratory problems.
3. Talking to the patient to keep him as alert as possible.
4. Helping the patient when he vomits so that he will not aspirate the vomitus.
5. Protecting the patient from hurting himself, without the illegal use of restraint.
6. Treating for shock
7. Staying alert for convulsions
8. Transporting the patient in a position to allow for drainage should the patient vomit.

NOTE: In some systems, patients under the influence of alcohol who are not suffering from a medical emergency or apparent injury are not transported. They are given over to the police. This may not be wise since the EMT might have missed a medical problem or injury. ALL PATIENTS WITH THE DT's SHOULD BE TRANSPORTED TO A MEDICAL FACILITY.

DRUG ABUSE

Drugs may be simply classified as uppers (stimulants), downers (depressants), narcotics, hallucinogens (mind-affecting drugs), and volatile chemicals. **Uppers** are stimulants affecting the nervous system to excite the user. An example would be amphetamines. **Downers** are depressants such as barbiturates, meant to affect the central nervous system to relax the user. **Narcotics** affect the nervous system and change many of the normal activities of the body. Often they produce an intense state of relaxation and feelings of well-being. Heroin is a commonly abused narcotic. **Hallucinogens,** such as LSD, are mind-affecting drugs that act on the nervous system to produce an intense state of excitement or a distortion of the user's surroundings. **Vol-**

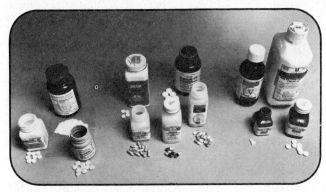

Figure 11-21: Abused substances.

atile chemicals are depressants sniffed or inhaled by the user. These compounds act upon the central nervous system. Cleaning fluid is a commonly abused volatile chemical.

As an EMT, you will not need to know the names of very many abused drugs or their specific reactions. It is far more important for you to be able to detect possible drug abuse at the overdose level and to relate certain signs to certain types of drugs and drug withdrawal. Your care for the drug abuse patient will be basically the same for all drugs and will not change unless ordered by a poison control center or emergency department physician. Table 11.3 provides some of the names of commonly abused drugs. Do no worry about memorizing this chart. Read it through so that you can place some of the more familiar drugs into categories in terms of drug type.

Signs of Drug Abuse

The symptoms and signs of drug abuse and drug overdose can vary from patient to patient, even for the same drug. Often, you will have to carefully combine the information gained from symptoms, signs, the scene, bystanders, and the patient in order to be certain that you are dealing with drug abuse. In many cases, you will not be able to determine or discover the substance involved. When questioning the patient and bystanders, you will get better results asking if the patient has been taking any medications rather than using the word ''drugs.''

Some significant symptoms and signs related to specific drugs include:

- Uppers—Excitement, increased pulse and breathing rates, rapid speech, dry mouth, dilated pupils, sweating and the complaint of having gone without sleep for long periods.
- Downers—Sluggish, sleepy patient lacking typical coordination of body and speech. Pulse and breathing rates are low, often to the point of a true emergency.
- Hallucinogens (mind-affecting drugs)—Fast

Table 11.3: Commonly Abused Substances

UPPERS	DOWNERS	NARCOTICS	MIND-AFFECTING DRUGS	VOLATILE CHEMICALS
AMPHETAMINE (Benzedrine, bennies, pep pills, ups, uppers, cartwheels)	AMOBARBITAL (blue devils, downers, barbs, Amytal)	CODEINE (often in cough syrup)	DMT	CLEANING FLUID (carbon tetrachloride)
BIPHETAMINE (bam)	BARBITURATES (downers, dolls, barbs, rainbows)	DEMEROL	LSD (acid, sunshine)	FURNITURE POLISH
COCAINE (coke, snow)		DILAUDID	MESCALINE (peyote, mesc)	GASOLINE
DESOXYN (black beauties)	CHLORAL HYDRATE (knockout drops)	HEROIN ("H," horse, junk, smack, stuff)	MORNING GLORY SEEDS	GLUE
DEXTROAMPHETAMINE (dexies, Dexedrine)	GLUTETHIMIDE (doriden, goofers)	METHADONE (dolly)	PCP (angel dust, hog, peace pills)	HAIR SPRAY
METHAMPHETAMINE (speed, meth, crystal, diet pills, Methedrine)	METHAQUALONE (Quaalude, ludes, Sopor, sopors)	MORPHINE	PSILOCYBIN (magic mushrooms)	NAIL POLISH REMOVER
METHYLPHEMIDATE	NON-BARBITURATE SEDATIVES (various tranquilizers and sleeping pills: Valium, Miltown, Equanil, meprobamate, Thorazine, Compazine, Librium, reserpine)	OPIUM (Op, poppy)	STP (serenity, tranquility, peace)	PAINT THINNER
PRELUDIN	PARALDEHYDE	PENTAZOCINE (Talwin)		
	PENTOBARBITAL (yellow jackets, barbs)			
	PHENOBARBITAL (goofballs, phennies, barbs)			
	SECOBARBITAL (red devils, barbs, Seconal)			

pulse rate, dilated pupils and a flushed face. The patient often "sees" things, has little concept of real time and may not be aware of the true environment. Often, what he says makes no sense to the listener.

- Narcotics—Reduced rate of pulse and breathing, often with a lowering of skin temperature. Pupils are constricted, muscles are relaxed and sweating is profuse. The patient is very sleepy and does not wish to do anything. In overdoses, coma is a common event.

- Volatile chemicals—Dazed or showing temporary loss of contact with reality. The patient may develop coma. The inside of the nose and mouth may show swollen membranes. The patient may complain of a "funny numb feeling" or "tingling" inside the head.

When reading the above list, you should have noticed that many of the indications of drug abuse are similar to those for quite a few medical emergencies. As an EMT, you must NEVER assume drug abuse, or drug abuse occurring by itself. You must be on the alert for medical emergencies, injuries, and combinations of drug abuse problems and other emergencies.

In addition to seeing the effects of long-term drug use and overdose, you will have to deal with cases of severe drug withdrawal. As with reactions to drugs, withdrawal varies from patient to patient and from drug to drug. In most cases of drug withdrawal, you will see:

- Shaking
- Anxiety
- Nausea
- Confusion and irritability
- Profuse sweating
- Increased pulse and breathing rates

Care for Drug Abuse Patients

When providing care for drug abuse patients, you should:

1. Provide life-support measures if required.
2. Call the poison control center or the emergency department in accordance with local policies.
3. Monitor vital signs and be alert for respiratory arrest.
4. Talk to the patient to gain confidence and to help maintain his level of consciousness.

5. Protect the patient from hurting himself, without using illegal restraint.
6. Treat for shock.
7. Look closely for signs of fractures and internal injuries.
8. Check carefully for head injuries.
9. Look for gross tissue damage on the extremities resulting from the injection of drugs. Dress and bandage all such sites.
10. Transport the patient as soon as possible, monitoring vital signs, staying alert for convulsions, and watching for vomiting that could obstruct the airway.
11. Continue to reassure the patient throughout all phases of care.

NOTE: Some sources still recommend that EMTs induce vomiting if an overdose was taken within 30 minutes of their arrival at the scene. The time of overdose is very difficult to determine, or to obtain from bystanders. *It is best not to induce vomiting unless directed by a physician.* In most cases, vomiting is induced in the same way as in cases of ingested poisons.

CAUTION: Many drug abusers may appear calm at first and then become violent as time passes. Always be alert and ready to protect yourself. If the patient creates an unsafe scene and you are not a trained law enforcement officer, GET OUT and find a safe place until the police arrive. Be extra cautious if you know the patient has been using PCP.

SUMMARY

If you are dealing with a possible poisoning, always look for evidence at the scene that may indicate poisoning and the nature of the poison. Learn to make use of your local poison control center.

There is a wide variety of symptoms and signs associated with ingested poisons. Always look for burns or stains around the patient's mouth. Expect unusual breathing, pulse rate, and sweating. Abdominal pain, nausea, and vomiting are common. Be sure to save all vomitus.

Inhaled poisons can cause shortness of breath or coughing. Often, the patient will have irritated eyes, rapid or slow pulse rate, and changes in skin color. It is possible to relate cherry colored skin to carbon monoxide poisoning.

Absorbed poisons usually irritate or damage the skin. Look for irritated eyes.

Injected poisons sometimes cause pain and swelling at the site. Difficult breathing and unusual pulse rate are often seen.

In all cases of poisoning, contact your local poison control center. For conscious patients, you will usually be directed to dilute ingested poisons with water or milk. The next step will probably be to induce vomiting with ipecac and water or as directed by the poison control center. Transport the patient as soon as possible, and position to reduce the chances of aspiration of vomitus. Charcoal and water may be given when vomiting is not called for or after vomiting has occurred.

WARNING: Do NOT induce vomiting if the poison is a strong acid, alkali, or petroleum product.

In cases of inhaled poisons, remove the patient from the source. Provide life support measures as needed. It may be necessary to remove contaminated clothing.

Remove the patient from the source of an absorbed poison and flood with water all body areas that have come into contact with the poison. Remove contaminated clothing and jewelry. Continue to flood the exposed areas of the patient's skin, or wash with soap and water.

When treating injected poisons other than snakebite, treat for shock, scrape away stingers and venom sacs, and place a covered ice bag or cold pack over the stung area. For snakebite, you should keep the patient calm, clean the site and keep any bitten extremities immobilized. Treat for shock. Apply a constricting band above and below the wound site.

Patients suffering from alcohol abuse are to receive the same level of professional care as any other patient. Be certain the problem is due to alcohol or alcohol withdrawal. There may be a medical problem or injuries. Try to detect the odor of alcohol, slurred speech, swaying and unsteadiness of movement. Find out if the patient is nauseated. Be alert for vomiting. In cases of alcohol withdrawal, look for hand tremors that may indicate the DT's. In all cases of alcohol abuse, monitor vital signs and be alert for respiratory arrest.

Drug abuse can show itself in many ways, depending on the drug, the patient, and whether you are dealing with withdrawal or overdose. Withdrawal from most drugs will produce shaking, anxiety, nausea, confusion and irritability, sweating, and increased pulse and breathing rates.

Uppers usually speed up activity, speech, pulse, breathing and tend to excite the user. Downers do just the opposite. Hallucinogens (mind-affecting drugs) increase pulse rate, dilate the pupils, and cause the patient to see things and to lose touch with reality. Narcotics reduce pulse and breathing rates. Pupils of narcotic patients usually will be constricted. The patient may appear sleepy and may not wish to do anything. Volatile chemicals act as depressants, causing the patient to be dazed.

In cases of drug abuse or withdrawal, provide life-support measures as needed. Monitor vital signs and be alert for respiratory arrest. Treat for shock. Provide emotional support to the patient.

12 childbirth and pediatrics

SECTION ONE: CHILDBIRTH

OBJECTIVES By the end of this section, you should be able to:

1. Name the components of the sterile emergency obstetric pack and describe the uses for each item. (p. 268-9)

2. Name and locate the anatomical structures of pregnancy. (p. 269)

3. List and describe the THREE stages of labor. (p. 269-70)

4. Describe how to evaluate the mother before delivery. (p. 270-1)

5. Describe how to prepare the mother, the delivery scene, and personnel prior to delivery. (p. 271-2)

6. Describe, step by step, what the EMT should do during each of the three stages of labor. (p. 270-6)

7. Describe the care given to both mother and infant after delivery, including airway and umbilical cord care. (p. 273-7)

8. List the typical complications of delivery and state what you should do in each situation. (p 277-83)

9. Describe the courses of action taken by the EMT in cases of multiple births, premature births, abortions (miscarriages), and stillbirths. (p. 279-83)

10. List all those emergencies involving birth that require immediate transport. (p. 277-83)

11. Describe what the EMT can do to comfort parents during normal and abnormal deliveries. (p. 270, 271, 272, 276, 277, 279, 283)

SKILLS As an EMT, you should be able to:

1. Evaluate a woman in labor and assist her in the delivery of her child.

2. Provide postdelivery care for the newborn, including proper airway and umbilical cord care.

3. Provide resuscitative measures for newborns in respiratory and cardiac arrest.

4. Assist in delivery of the placenta.

5. Provide postdelivery care for the mother, including emotional support and care of the afterbirth.

6. Provide emergency care and needed basic life support procedures for abnormal deliveries, including breech and premature birth.

7. Properly provide oxygen for the newborn when required.

TERMS   you may be using for the first time:

Fetus (FE-tus)—the baby as it develops in the womb.

Uterus (U-ter-us)—the womb where the fetus develops.

Cervix (SUR-viks)—the neck of the uterus that enters the birth canal.

Vagina (vah-JI-nah)—the birth canal.

Amniotic (am-ne-OT-ic) **Sac**—the "bag of waters" that surrounds the developing fetus.

Placenta (plah-SEN-tah)—the organ of pregnancy where exchange of oxygen, foods, and wastes occurs between mother and fetus.

Umbilical (um-BIL-i-cal) **Cord**—the fetal structure containing the blood vessels that travel to and from the placenta.

Labor—the three stages of delivery that begin with the contractions of the uterus and end with the expulsion of the placenta.

Afterbirth—the placenta, membranes of the amniotic sac, umbilical cord, and some tissues from the lining of the uterus that are delivered after the birth of the baby.

Crowning—when part of the baby is visible through the dilated cervix.

Vulva (VUL-vah)—the female external genitalia.

Cephalic (se-FAL-ik) **Presentation**—when the baby appears head first during birth. This is the normal presentation.

Breech Presentation—when the baby appears buttocks first during birth.

Eclampsia (ek-LAM-se-ah)—a complication of pregnancy that can lead to convulsions and coma.

Ectopic (ek-TOP-ik) **Pregnancy**—when implantation of the fertilized egg is not in the body of the uterus, but in the the oviduct (fallopian tube), cervix, or abdominopelvic cavity.

Abortion—spontaneous (miscarriage) or induced termination of pregnancy.

Premature Infant—newborn weighing less than 5.5 pounds, or delivered before the seventh month of pregnancy.

CHILDBIRTH

THE ROLE OF THE EMT

Participating in the delivery of a baby is usually a wonderful and exciting event for the EMT. In most cases, you will be dealing with a natural event, not an emergency. Seldom is childbirth outside of a medical facility an emergency, except perhaps to an untrained attendant! Our society presently believes that birth is meant to occur in a hospital delivery room. Hospital care of mother and newborn does reduce the chance of problems and can correct most immediate complications. However, the vast majority of babies ever born were not delivered in any type of medical facility. This holds true today, for the majority of the world's women do not have access to modern medical facilities for the purpose of giving birth.

Birth is a natural process. The anatomy of the human female and that of the baby allow the process to occur with few immediate problems. Nonetheless, EMTs need to know the procedures that can help mother and baby before, during, and after delivery, as well as the techniques that can be employed when complications arise.

REMEMBER: EMTs do not deliver babies . . . mothers do! Your primary role will be to *help* the mother as she delivers her child.

Equipment and Supplies

Assisting the mother and providing care is much easier if a few basic items are kept as part of the ambulance supplies. You will need a sterile obstetrical kit that contains the items required for preparation of the mother, delivery, and initial care of the newborn. This kit should include:

- Several pairs of sterile surgical gloves
- 5 towels or sheets for draping the mother
- 1 dozen 4 × 4 gauze pads (sponges)
- 1 small rubber-bulb syringe
- 3 cord clamps or hemostats
- Umbilical cord tape
- 1 pair of surgical scissors
- 1 baby blanket
- Several individually wrapped sanitary napkins

In addition, you will find use for a stainless steel basin, two large plastic bags, and disposable masks, paper gowns, and caps.

Occasionally, emergency service personnel have to assist in the delivery of a baby without a sterile delivery pack. Again, keep in mind that most babies have been born without such packs being on hand.

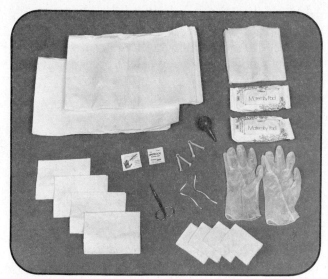

Figure 12-1: Contents of a disposable OB kit.

A few simple supplies will aid you in assisting the mother:

- Clean sheets and towels to drape the mother and wrap the newborn

- Heavy flat twine or new shoelaces to tie the cord (do NOT use thread, wire, or light string since these may cut through the cord)

- A towel or plastic bag to wrap the placenta after its delivery

- Clean, unused rubber gloves. If none is available, carefully wash your hands, if possible.

ANATOMY OF PREGNANCY AND DELIVERY

The developing baby is called a **fetus** (FE-tus). During pregnancy, the fetus grows in its mother's **uterus** (U-ter-us), a muscular organ often called the womb. When the mother is in labor, the muscles of the uterus contract at ever-shortening intervals and push the baby through the neck of the uterus known as the **cervix** (SUR-viks). The cervix must dilate some 4 inches during labor to allow the baby's head to pass into the **vagina** (vah-JI-nah) or birth canal so that delivery can take place.

More than just the fetus develops within the uterus during pregnancy. Attached to the wall of the uterus is a special organ called the **placenta** (plah-SEN-tah). Composed of both maternal and fetal tissues, the placenta serves as an exchange area between mother and fetus. Oxygen and foods from the mother's bloodstream are carried across the placenta to the fetus. Carbon dioxide and certain other wastes cross from fetal circulation to maternal circulation. Since the placenta is an *organ of pregnancy*, it is expelled after the baby is born.

The mother's blood does *not* flow through the body of the fetus. The fetus has its own circulatory system. Blood from the fetus must be sent through the placenta and return to its body. This is done by way of the blood vessels contained in the **umbilical** (um-BIL-i-kal) **cord.** The umbilical cord is fully expelled with the birth of the baby and the delivery of the placenta.

While developing in the uterus, the fetus is enclosed and protected within a thin, membranous ''bag of waters'' known as the **amniotic** (am-ne-OT-ik) **sac.** This sac contains one pint to one quart of liquid called amniotic fluid, which allows the fetus to float during development. In the vast majority of cases, the amniotic sac breaks during labor and the fluid gushes from the birth canal. This is a normal condition of childbirth.

Crowning is when the ''**presenting**'' part of the baby first bulges from the vaginal opening. The presenting part of the baby usually is the head. The normal headfirst birth is called a **cephalic** (se-FAL-ik) **delivery.** If the buttocks, or both feet of the baby deliver first, the birth is called a **breech birth.**

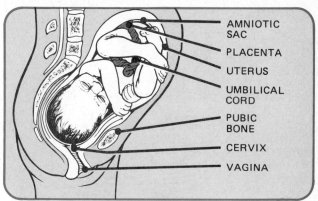

Figure 12-2: The structures of pregnancy.

THE STAGES OF LABOR

There are three stages of labor:

1. *First Stage*—starts with contractions and ends when the baby enters the birth canal.
2. *Second Stage*—the time from when the baby is in the birth canal until it is born.
3. *Third Stage*—begins when the baby is born and continues until the afterbirth (placenta, umbilical cord, and tissues from the amniotic sac and the lining of the uterus) is delivered.

The contractions of the uterus that occur during the first stage of labor move the baby downward and *dilate* the cervix. The cycle of contractions starts far apart and becomes shorter as birth approaches. Typically, these contractions range from every 30 minutes down to three minutes apart or less. Labor pains accompany the contractions.

As the fetus moves and the cervix dilates, the amniotic sac usually breaks. The beginning of cervical dilation signals the end of the first stage of labor. Most women giving birth for the first time will re-

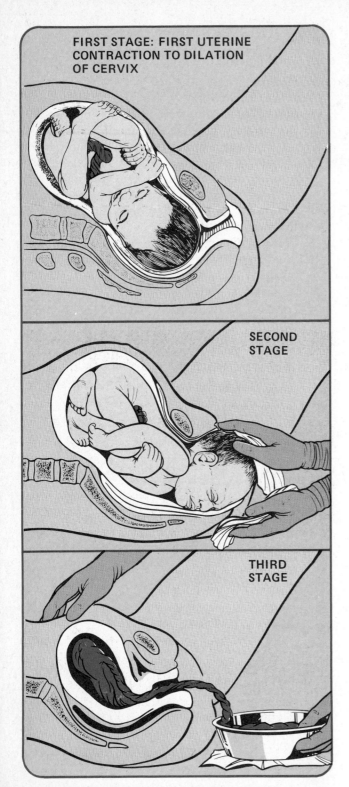

FIRST STAGE: FIRST UTERINE CONTRACTION TO DILATION OF CERVIX

SECOND STAGE

THIRD STAGE

Figure 12-3: The three stages of labor.

main in this stage for an average of 12 hours. Some women may remain in this stage for no more than four hours.

The second stage of labor includes the full dilation of the cervix and increasingly frequent contractions. Labor pains become more severe. In the second stage of labor, the cramping and abdominal pains associated with the first stage of labor still may be present, but most women report a major new discomfort, that of feeling they have to move their bowels. The moment of birth is nearing and the EMT will have to decide whether to transport, or to keep the mother where she is and prepare to assist with delivery.

THE NORMAL DELIVERY

Evaluating the Mother

A simple series of questions and an examination for crowning will allow you to make the decision for transport. However, do not let the ''urgency'' of this decision upset the mother. Your patient needs emotional support at this time. Your calm, professional actions will help her feel more at ease and assure her that the required care will be provided for both her and the unborn child.

Begin to evaluate the mother:

1. Ask her name and age.

2. Ask if this is her *first* pregnancy. The average time of labor for a women having her first baby usually lasts about 16 to 17 hours. The time in labor is considerably shorter for each subsequent birth.

3. Ask her how long she has been having labor pains, how often she is having pains, and if her ''bag of waters'' has broken. At this point, with a woman having her first delivery, you may feel that you can make a decision about transport. You should continue with the evaluation procedure. Also, you should begin to time the frequency and length of the contractions.

4. Ask her if she is straining or if she feels as though she needs to move her bowels. If she says yes, this means that the baby has probably moved into the birth canal and is pressing the vaginal wall against the rectum. Birth will probably occur very soon. The mother may tell you that she can feel the baby trying to move out through her vaginal opening. In such cases, birth is probably very near.

5. Examine the mother for **crowning.** This is a visual inspection to see if there is bulging at the vaginal opening, or if the presenting part of the baby is visible. Crowning means birth is imminent.

Examining for crowning may be very embarrassing to the mother, the father, and any bystanders. For this reason, it is very important that you fully explain what you are doing and why. Be certain that you protect the mother from the stares of bystanders. In a polite, but firm manner, ask everyone who does not belong at the scene to leave. Carefully help the patient remove enough clothing to allow

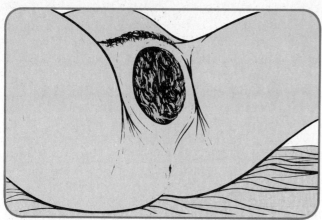

Figure 12-4: Crowning of the infant's head occurs in the second stage of labor.

you an unobstructed view of the **vulva** (VUL-vah), or external genitalia.

REMEMBER: A professional appearance coupled with a professional approach to a problem instills confidence in patients and bystanders alike.

If this is the woman's first delivery, she is not straining, and there is no crowning, there is little reason why she cannot be transported to a medical facility for delivery. On the other hand, if this is not her first delivery, and she is straining, crying out, and complaining about having to go to the bathroom, birth may occur too soon for transport. If the mother is having contractions about 2 minutes apart, birth is very near. Crowning certainly means that it is too late to transport the mother.

You may find a patient who is afraid of transport because she believes that birth will occur along the way. Assure her that you think there is enough time before delivery. Let her know that you are trained to assist with the delivery and that the ambulance is well-equipped to handle her needs and care for the newborn should she deliver en route.

If your evaluation of the patient leads you to believe that birth is too near at hand for transport, prepare the mother for delivery. Remember, as part of the preparation, the patient will need emotional support.

REMEMBER: Do not allow the mother to go to the bathroom, even though she says that she has to move her bowels. Do not attempt to hold the mother's legs together or use any other "folk" method to attempt to delay the delivery.

Preparing the Expectant Mother

When your evaluation leads you to believe birth is imminent, you must immediately prepare the mother for delivery. To do so, you should:

1. Control the scene so that the mother has privacy. If you are not in a private home and transfer to the ambulance is impractical (crowning is present), ask any bystanders to leave.

2. Place the mother on a bed, sturdy table, or the ambulance stretcher. You will need about 2 feet of work space below the woman's legs on which to place and initially care for the newborn. Space is limited on the ambulance stretcher, but having the patient positioned there may speed transport if complications arise.

NOTE: Do NOT delay positioning the mother. If time permits, and the mother is to be placed on a table or other hard surface, lay down a folded blanket, towels, or even newspapers with a sheet over them to make a cushion. If delivery is to be on a bed, firm up the mattress with plywood, table leaves, or other such rigid materials that can be placed between the mattress and the springs. Such firmness will tend to keep blood and other fluids pooled in the work area. A rubber sheet, plastic bag, or newspapers placed under the sheet will help prevent the mattress from becoming soaked. Do NOT leave the patient to find all these materials.

3. Have the mother lie down on her back with her thighs spread, her knees flexed, and her feet flat. Use one or two pillows to elevate her head and shoulders. A folded blanket should be used to lift her buttocks approximately 2 inches above the supporting surface.

4. Position your partner, the father, or someone the mother agrees to have assist you at the mother's head, opposite from the side where you will be working (work on the mother's right if you are right-handed, or on her left if you are left-handed). This person should stay alert to help turn the mother's head should she vomit. As well, this person should provide emotional support to the mother, soothing and encouraging her.

5. Position the OB pack on a table or chair on the same side where you will be working. All items must be within easy reach.

6. If time allows, put on any protective items such as a mask or gown.

7. Remove any clothing or underclothing that obstructs your view of the vaginal opening. Put on sterile gloves from the OB kit. Use sterile sheets or sterile towels to cover the mother as shown in Figure 12-5. Clean sheets, clean cloths, towels, or material such as tablecloths can be used if you do not have an OB kit.

NOTE: If delivery is to take place in an automobile, position the mother flat on the seat. Arrange her legs so that she has one foot resting on the seat and the other foot resting on the floor.

Delivering the Baby

Position yourself to the mother's side in such a way that you have a constant view of the vaginal

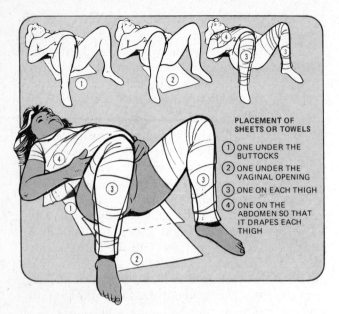

Figure 12-5: Preparing the mother for delivery.

opening. Be prepared for the baby to come at any moment. Look to see if there is crowning, or if part of the baby's head becomes visible with each contraction. Do NOT assume that birth is not about to happen soon if the baby is not visible or if the area of the baby seen is "less than the size of a fifty-cent piece."

Be prepared for the patient to experience pain. Delivering a child may be a natural process, but it is always accompanied by severe pain. Your patient may also have intense feelings of nausea. If this is her first child, she may be very frightened. All these factors may cause your patient to be uncooperative at times. You must remember that the patient is in pain, and probably feels ill. She will need emotional support.

During delivery, talk to the mother. Ask her to relax between contractions. Continue to time each contraction from the beginning of the contraction to the beginning of the next contraction. Encourage her not to strain unless she feels she must. Remind her that her feeling of a pending bowel movement is just pressure caused by the baby moving into her birth canal. Ask her to breathe deeply through her mouth. She may feel better if she pants, though she should be discouraged from breathing rapidly and deeply enough to bring on hyperventilation. If her "bag of waters" breaks, remind her that this is normal.

NOTE: Until there are signs of complications, consider the delivery to be normal if there is a cephalic presentation.

The steps for assisting the mother with a normal delivery are:

1. Continue to keep someone at the mother's head in case she vomits. If no one is on hand to help, be alert for vomiting.

2. Position your hands at the mother's vaginal opening when the baby's head starts to appear. Do NOT touch her skin.

3. Place one hand below the baby's head as it is delivered. Spread your fingers evenly around the baby's head (see Scansheet 12-1), remembering that its skull contains "soft spots" or **fontanelles**. Support the baby's head, but avoid pressure to these soft areas of the skull. Use your other hand to help cradle the baby's head. This slight pressure may help prevent an explosive delivery. DO NOT PULL ON THE BABY!

4. If the umbilical cord is wrapped around the baby's neck, *gently* loosen the cord. If you are too rough with the cord, it will tear. Try to place two fingers under the cord at the back of the baby's neck. Bring the cord forward, over the baby's upper shoulder and head. If you cannot loosen and reposition the cord, the baby cannot be delivered. Immediately clamp the cord in two places using the clamps provided in the OB kit. Be very careful not to injury the baby. With extreme care, cut the cord between the two clamps. Gently unwrap the ends of the cord from around the baby's neck.

5. If the amniotic sac does not break, use your finger to puncture the membrane. Pull the membranes away from the baby's mouth and nose.

6. Most babies are born face down and then rotate to the right or left. Be ready to support the baby's head so that it does not touch the mother's anal area. When the entire head of the baby is visible, continue to support the head with one hand and reach for the rubber bulb syringe. Compress the syringe BEFORE placing it in the baby's mouth. Carefully insert the tip of the syringe about 1 to 1.5 inches into the baby's mouth and release the bulb to allow fluids to be drawn into the syringe. Withdraw the tip and discharge the syringe's contents onto a towel. Repeat this procedure two or three times in the baby's mouth and once or twice in each nostril. The tip of the syringe should not be inserted more than 1/2 inch into the baby's nostril.

7. The upper shoulder (usually with some delay) will deliver next, followed quickly by the lower shoulder. You must support the baby throughout this entire process. Gently guide the baby's head downward, to assist the mother in delivering the baby's upper shoulder. If the lower shoulder is slow to deliver, assist the mother by gently guiding the baby's head upward.

8. Support the baby throughout the entire birth process. Once the feet are born, lay the baby on its side with its head slightly lower than its body. This is done to allow blood, fluids, and mucus to drain from the mouth and nose. Note the time of birth.

CAUTION: Babies being born are slippery! Make certain that you offer proper support. Some deliveries are explosive. Do not squeeze the baby, but do provide adequate support. You can prevent an explosive delivery by using one hand to maintain slight pressure on the baby's head.

Caring for the Newborn

Even with a normal delivery, each step in the care of the baby is essential for its survival. To care for the newborn, you should first place the baby on the bed or padded table surface, keeping the baby as close to the level of the vagina as possible. Remember, the infant is still connected to the placenta. Too high or too low a position may cause circulation problems. This is not the time to place the baby on the mother's abdomen!

CAUTION: Keep the baby on its side, with the head positioned slightly lower than its body. This will help provide proper drainage.

The initial care for the newborn includes:

1. *Clear the baby's airway*—Use a sterile gauze pad to clear mucus and blood from around the baby's nose and mouth.

2. *Keep the baby on its side*—With the head slightly lower than the body, again suction the mouth and nose with a rubber bulb syringe. If necessary, you can cradle the baby in your arms. However, it is best to keep the baby on the cot or table surface.

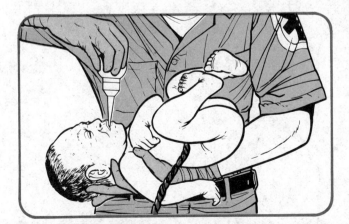

Figure 12-6: Suctioning the mouth of the newborn is accomplished by squeezing the bulb, then inserting it into the infant's mouth. The bulb is released to suction, then the tip is removed from the mouth and the bulb is squeezed to remove its contents.

3. *Establish that the baby is breathing*—Usually the baby will be breathing on its own by the time you clear the airway. A newborn infant should begin breathing *within 30 seconds*. If it is not, then you must "encourage" the baby to breathe. Snap one of your index fingers against the soles of the baby's feet. Do NOT hold the baby up by its feet and slap its bottom! Care of a nonbreathing infant will be covered later in this chapter.

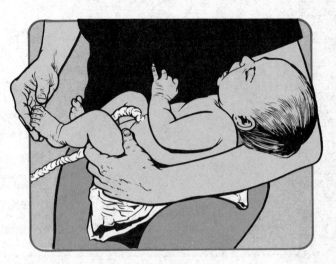

Figure 12-7: It may be necessary to encourage the newborn to breathe.

Do not become alarmed if the hands and feet of a breathing newborn appear slightly blue. It is not uncommon for this blue color to remain for some time.

4. *Keep the infant warm*—If the environment is too cool, you may have to wrap the baby in a baby blanket, clean towel, or sheet prior to clamping and cutting the cord.

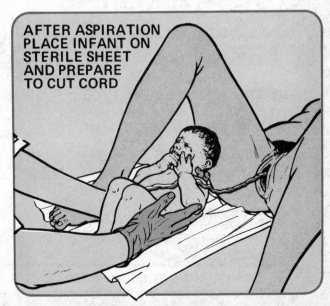

AFTER ASPIRATION PLACE INFANT ON STERILE SHEET AND PREPARE TO CUT CORD

Figure 12-8: Placing the infant before clamping the umbilical cord.

NORMAL DELIVERY

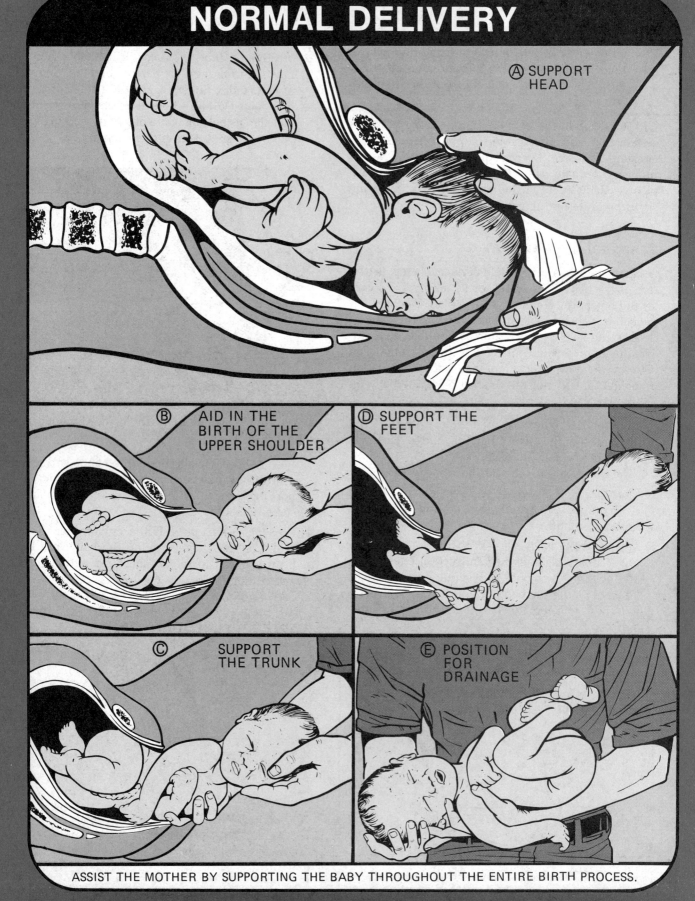

Ⓐ SUPPORT HEAD

Ⓑ AID IN THE BIRTH OF THE UPPER SHOULDER

Ⓓ SUPPORT THE FEET

Ⓒ SUPPORT THE TRUNK

Ⓔ POSITION FOR DRAINAGE

ASSIST THE MOTHER BY SUPPORTING THE BABY THROUGHOUT THE ENTIRE BIRTH PROCESS.

SCAN 12-1

5. *Prepare to clamp and cut the umbilical cord.*

Do not wash the infant. Sometimes the mother may request you do so, but this is best done at the medical facility.

Cutting the Umbilical Cord

In a normal birth, the infant must be breathing on his own before you clamp and cut the cord. The general procedure for umbilical cord care is as follows:

1. Use the sterile clamps or umbilical tape found in the OB kit. If you do not have a kit, then use clean shoelaces. Use extreme care with any tying done to the cord, forming the knot slowly to avoid cutting the cord. Ties should be made using a square knot. Wait until strong pulsations of the cord have stopped before tying or clamping it.
2. Apply one clamp or tie to the cord about 10 inches from the baby. This allows for IV lines to be used at the hospital, if they are needed.
3. Place a second clamp or tie about three inches closer to the baby.
4. Cut the cord between the clamps or knots using sterile surgical scissors. NEVER untie or unclamp a cord once it is cut. Do NOT attempt to adjust a clamp or retie a knot. Should bleeding continue, apply another tie or clamp as close to the original one as possible.
5. Be careful when moving the baby so that no trauma is brought to the clamped cord. If the cord does not remain closed off completely, the baby may bleed to death. In most cases, the cord vessels will collapse and seal themselves.

CAUTION: Do not tie, clamp, or cut the cord of a baby who is not breathing on its own, unless you have to perform CPR on the infant.

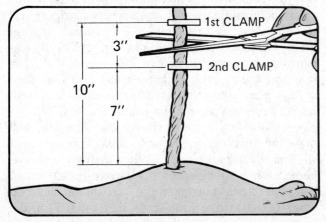

Figure 12-9: A newborn is separated from its mother by cutting the umbilical cord.

NOTE: Some EMS Systems recommend that umbilical tape be used to tie the baby's clamped cord once it is cut. Tying is done with the OB kit's umbilical tape placed about one inch from the infant's body. The cord is slowly compressed with the tape and a square knot is tied. Both the tape and the clamp are left in place. Your instructor will tell you if this is the policy for your area.

If you are assisting at a birth when off duty, you will probably be able to find all the items you need to tie and cut the cord. It is best to tie and cut the cord as soon as possible. If no clamps or tying devices are on hand, you may delay clamping and tying the cord if the infant will receive this care within 30 minutes. If you tie the cord and believe it will be some time before transport and transfer, you can soak scissors in alcohol for several minutes and use them to cut the cord. If the baby is still attached to the placenta when the organ is delivered, wrap the placenta in a towel and transport infant and placenta as a unit. The placenta should be placed at the same level as the baby, or slightly higher. Careful monitoring of the baby must be maintained.

Recording the Birth

If adhesive tape is available, double face it and write the mother's last name and the time of delivery on a piece of tape and loosely secure this tape around the baby's wrist. Do not allow the adhesive to come into contact wth the baby's skin. Your partner should record the exact time of birth in accordance with local policy. Usually, this is done on a record of live birth.

Wrap the newborn warmly in a baby blanket and let the mother hold him on her abdomen. During the delivery of the placenta, have your partner hold the baby, unless the mother insists otherwise.

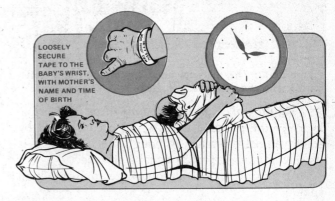

LOOSELY SECURE TAPE TO THE BABY'S WRIST, WITH MOTHER'S NAME AND TIME OF BIRTH

Figure 12-10: Wrap the baby and place it on the mother's abdomen.

Caring for the Mother

Care for the mother includes helping her deliver the placenta, controlling vaginal bleeding, and making her as comfortable as possible.

Delivering the Placenta   The third stage of labor is the delivery of the placenta with its umbilical cord section, membranes of the amniotic sac, and some of the lining tissues of the uterus. Placental delivery begins with a brief return of the labor pains that stopped when the baby was born. In most cases, the placenta will be expelled within a few minutes after the baby is born, although the process may take 30 minutes or longer. If mother and baby are doing well and there are no respiratory problems or significant uncontrolled bleeding, transportation to the hospital can be delayed up to 20 minutes while awaiting delivery of the placenta.

Save all afterbirth tissues. The attending physician will want to examine the placenta and other tissues for completeness since any afterbirth tissues remaining in the uterus pose a serious threat to the mother. Try to catch the afterbirth in a container. Place the container in a plastic bag, or wrap it in a towel, paper, or plastic. If no container is available, catch the afterbirth in a towel, paper, or a plastic bag. Label this material "placenta" and include the name of the mother and the time the tissues were expelled.

REMEMBER: If the placenta does not deliver within 20 minutes of the baby's birth, transport the mother and baby to a medical facility without delay.

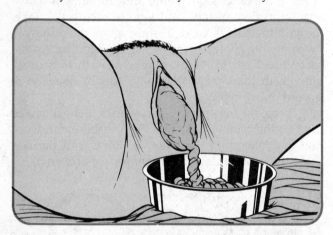

Figure 12-11: The placenta must be collected and transported with the mother and baby.

Control of Vaginal Bleeding After Birth   Delivery of the placenta is ALWAYS accompanied by some vaginal bleeding. Although the blood loss is usually around ½ pint, it may be profuse.

To control vaginal bleeding after delivery, you should:

1. Place a sanitary napkin, over the mother's vaginal opening. Do NOT place anything in the vagina.
2. Have the mother lower her legs and keep them together. Tell her that she does not have to "squeeze" them together. Elevate her feet.

3. Massage the mother's lower abdomen to help contract her uterus, which will help control bleeding. Feel the mother's abdomen until you note a "grapefruit-size" object. This is her uterus. Rub this area lightly with a circular motion. It should contract and become firm, and bleeding should diminish.
4. If the mother so desires, have her nurse the baby. This also will aid in the contraction of the uterus.

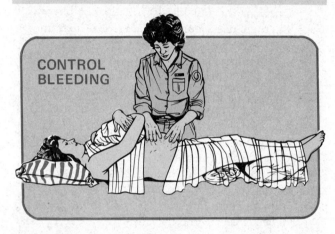

CONTROL BLEEDING

Figure 12-12: After delivery of the placenta, you will have to control vaginal bleeding.

The skin between the vulva and the anus is known as the **perineum** (per-i-NE-um). A slight tearing of tissue can occur at the vaginal opening during the birth process. The mother may feel discomfort from this torn tissue, with the discomfort extending from the vaginal opening through the perineum. Let her know that this is normal and that the problem will be cared for quickly at the medical facility.

Providing Comfort to the Mother   Keep contact with the mother throughout the entire birth process and after she has delivered. Your care for the mother does not end when you have completed your duties with the placenta and vaginal bleeding. Be aware that she has just undergone a tremendous emotional experience and small acts of kindness will be appreciated and remembered. Childbirth is a rigorous task, and a woman may be physically exhausted at the conclusion of delivery. Wiping her face and hands with a damp washcloth and then drying them with a towel will do wonders to refresh her and prepare her for the trip to the hospital. Replacing of blood-soaked sheets and blankets will make the trip more comfortable. Make sure that both she and the baby are warm. When delivery occurs at home, ask a member of the family or a trusted neighbor to help you clean up. You should clean up whatever disorder EMS care has caused in the house; however, you should not delay transport in order to do this. It may be necessary for you to return to the house after transport. If so, you will have to be accompanied by a member of the family.

REMEMBER: Birth is an exciting and joyous event. Talking to the mother and paying attention to her new baby are part of total patient care. Treat your patient as you would wish a member of your family to be treated.

COMPLICATIONS OF DELIVERY

While most babies are born without difficulty, complications may occur during and after delivery. We have already considered three such complications: the cord around the neck; an unbroken amniotic sac; and infants who need encouragement to breathe. These problems can be corrected by simple procedures. However, there are other complications that can threaten the life of both mother and newborn.

Conditions of High-Risk

Risk of complications during and immediately following the birth increases when the expectant mother:

- Is over age 35
- Has hypotension or hypertension
- Has diabetes
- Has predelivery bleeding
- Has an infection
- Is drug-dependent (heroin, methadone, alcohol)
- Is taking certain medications (lithium carbonate, magnesium, reserpine)

A proper patient interview may be your only way of obtaining any of this information.

The Nonbreathing Baby

Remember that a newborn should begin breathing *within 30 seconds* after delivery. This is about the time it should take you to place the infant on his side in a head-low position and suction his mouth and nose. If breathing does not begin, the stimulus of snapping your fingers against the soles of the baby's feet must be your next approach. If this fails, establish an open airway. If the infant does not start to breathe on his own, provide four gentle breaths (puffs from the cheeks). Determine if the baby is breathing and if he has a brachial pulse. Begin pulmonary resuscitation *immediately* if there's a pulse but no breathing.

Rescue breathing efforts may initiate spontaneous breathing, but the infant will struggle to breathe. When this happens, you should provide a gentle breath each time the infant attempts to breathe in.

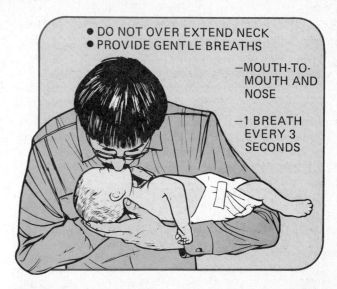

Figure 12-13: Pulmonary resuscitation of the newborn. Do NOT overextend the neck. Provide gentle breaths mouth-to-mouth and nose once every 3 seconds.

If you do not detect a brachial pulse for the nonbreathing newborn, begin CPR immediately in accordance with AHA guidelines. Current recommendations call for the cord to be clamped and cut when a newborn requires CPR.

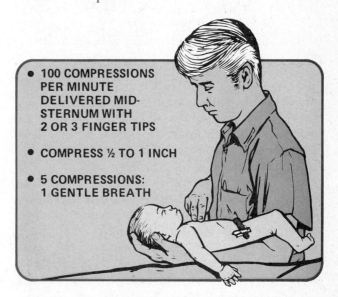

Figure 12-14: CPR for the infant: 100 compressions/minute delivered at midsternum with 2 or 3 fingers. Compress 1/2 to 1 inch. Deliver 5 compressions:1 breath.

Transport the mother and baby to the hospital, while you continue resuscitation efforts until spontaneous heart and lung action begin, or until care is transferred to the staff of the emergency department. Extreme care must be taken when moving the mother and baby. Remember, the mother has yet to deliver the placenta and she still carries a portion of the clamped umbilical cord.

The infant may begin spontaneous normal breathing. Should this happen, you can give oxygen. There is a danger of giving too much oxygen to a newborn, but if the time from birth to transfer at the medical facility is short (around 20 minutes), the benefits outweigh the dangers. Do NOT blow a stream of oxygen directly into the baby's face. Make a tent of aluminum foil above the infant's head and let the oxygen enter this tent. When possible, use a humidified source of oxygen.

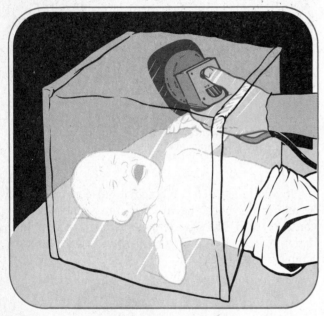

Figure 12-15: Providing oxygen to the infant.

Do not give up hope! Newborn babies have been saved without brain damage even after 20 minutes of continued resuscitation. Be aware, however, that some babies are **stillborn** (born dead), having died several hours prior to birth. They sometimes have a strong disagreeable smell and large blisters on the skin. In addition, their heads may be very soft. Under no circumstances should you attempt to resuscitate the infant. Turn your full attention to the mother. She will need care that shows concern for her loss. Discourage her from viewing the dead baby.

NOTE: Mechanical resuscitation devices should *not* be used on infants. There is a technique for bag-valve-mask ventilation, but this is considered *advanced* life support by the AHA and most systems. Do not use such techniques unless they are part of local guidelines and you have received formal training in the procedures.

Prolonged Delivery

Contractions every 2 or 3 minutes are a highly reliable sign that birth is imminent. If the baby is not delivered after 20 minutes of contractions that are 2 to 3 minutes apart, a prolonged delivery is indicated. Explain this to the mother and transport to a medical facility without delay.

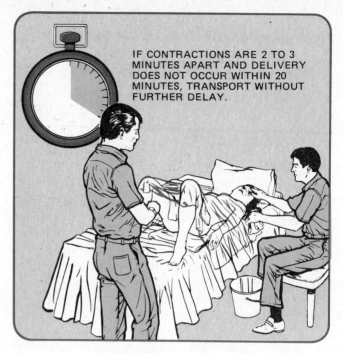

IF CONTRACTIONS ARE 2 TO 3 MINUTES APART AND DELIVERY DOES NOT OCCUR WITHIN 20 MINUTES, TRANSPORT WITHOUT FURTHER DELAY.

Figure 12-16: Indications of prolonged delivery.

PRE-DELIVERY EMERGENCIES

Excessive Pre-birth Bleeding

If a woman in labor begins to bleed excessively from the vagina, you should:

1. Place the patient in a supine position and begin to treat for shock. Do NOT hold the patient's legs together.
2. Place a sanitary napkin over the vaginal opening. DO NOT PLACE ANYTHING IN THE VAGINA.
3. Administer a high concentration of oxygen.
4. Transport as soon as possible.
5. Replace pads as they become soaked, but save all pads to evaluate blood loss.
6. Save all tissue that is passed.

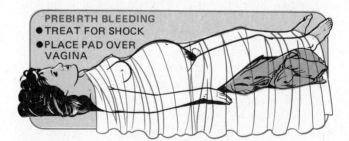

PREBIRTH BLEEDING
● TREAT FOR SHOCK
● PLACE PAD OVER VAGINA

Figure 12-17: Attempt to control excessive pre-birth bleeding. Immediate transport is required.

A pregnant woman does not have to be in labor to have excessive bleeding from the vagina. Bleeding in early pregnancy may be due to a miscarriage. If the bleeding occurs late in pregnancy, there may be problems involving the placenta. **Placenta previa** (plah-SEN-tah PRE-vi-ah) is a condition where the placenta is formed in an abnormal location that will not allow for a normal carry of the fetus. **Abruptio placentae** (ab-RUP-she-o plah-SEN-ti) is a condition where the placenta separates from the uterine wall. Care for patients with these problems is the same as for any excessive pre-birth bleeding.

Eclampsia

Eclampsia (ek-LAM-se-ah) is unique to pregnancy. It is the advanced stage of **toxemia** (poisoning of the blood) **of pregnancy.** This is seen most often in young women having their first child. In the early stages, extreme swelling of the face, hands, and feet is characteristic. Usually, the patient will have an elevated blood pressure. When the condition is severe, the patient will complain of headache, visual difficulties, and pain in the upper abdomen. Apprehension and shakiness are common. At its worst, eclampsia can cause potentially fatal seizures.

All patients with eclampsia require transport. If the patient is *convulsive*, you should:

1. Treat as you would any seizure patient, protecting her from harming herself.
2. Position the unconscious eclampsia patient on her side to allow drainage and keep the tongue from blocking the airway.
3. When conscious, reposition the patient on her back and elevate the head and shoulders.
4. Administer a high concentration of oxygen.

Ectopic Pregnancy

In normal pregnancy, the fertilized egg will begin to divide in the **oviduct** (fallopian tube) and eventually implant in the wall of the uterus. In an **ectopic** (ek-TOP-ik) **pregnancy,** implantation may take place in an oviduct, the cervix of the uterus, or in the abdominopelvic cavity. Women with this type of pregnancy may have acute abdominal pain, a rapid weak pulse, and will go into shock. There may be slight vaginal bleeding. This is a TRUE EMERGENCY, requiring immediate transport, positioning and treating for shock. Oxygen should be provided. Do NOT give the woman anything by mouth.

Accidents

If a pregnant woman is injured in an accident, such as a motor vehicle collision or a fall, treat her injuries as you would any other patient's. Remember that maintenance of respiration and circulation, and the control of bleeding are vital not only to the mother, but to the fetus. A developing fetus is critically dependent on the uninterrupted oxygenated blood supply that enters the placenta. Since the patient may have undetected internal bleeding, transport all pregnant women involved in accidents as soon as possible.

Question the alert, conscious patient to determine if she received any blows to the abdomen, pelvis, or back. Examine the unconscious patient for abdominal injuries. When in doubt, examine the patient, but be certain to provide privacy.

A pregnant woman who is an accident victim naturally will worry about her unborn child. Provide emotional support and remind her that the developing baby is well protected in the uterus. Reassure her she is being transported to a medical facility that can take care of her needs and the needs of the unborn child.

Miscarriage and Abortion

Miscarriage is the common term given to a **spontaneous abortion.** For a number of reasons, the fetus and placenta may deliver before the 28th week of pregnancy, before the baby can live on its own. Excessive bleeding can occur, requiring you to treat the mother as you would a patient with excessive pre-birth bleeding. Remember to save all tissues that are passed and all blood-soaked pads. Emotional support is very important. NEVER refer to the miscarriage as a "spontaneous abortion." Not all patients will associate the word "abortion" with the term "miscarriage."

An **induced abortion** is one that is the result of actions taken to stop the pregnancy. Some women take excessive dosages of certain drugs, poisons, and other chemicals. Such patients will require care for the overdose or the poisoning. In some cases, women insert objects into the vagina to try to mechanically disrupt the pregnancy. There can be excessive internal and external bleeding.

Women having a miscarriage that requires them to seek emergency care generally have cramping abdominal pains not unlike those associated with the first stage of labor. Bleeding can range from moderate to severe. There may be a noticeable discharge of tissue particles and blood from the vagina.

Women undergoing self-induced or nonmedical abortions can show the same clinical picture as those having spontaneous abortions. However, the pain involved is usually much greater and bleeding will be more severe.

Care is basically the same for both types of abortion:

1. Help stem vaginal bleeding by treating for shock and placing a sanitary napkin over the vaginal opening. Do NOT pack the vagina.
2. Transport as soon as possible, positioning the patient for shock.

3. Provide oxygen.
4. Replace and save all blood-soaked pads.
5. Save all tissues that are expelled. Do NOT replace or pull out any tissues that are being expelled through the vagina.

Ruptured Uterus

The uterus may *rupture* during labor. This is a rare occurrence, but when it does happen, it is a TRUE EMERGENCY requiring transport without delay. Be alert for this problem if the mother has had a cesarean section or any other surgery performed on her uterus. If the patient has had a number of full-term pregnancies, she may also be a candidate for a ruptured uterus. The previous pregnancies may have weakened the wall of the uterus.

A patient may have a ruptured uterus if she reports a tearing sensation in her abdomen and constant pain. Labor typically appears as if it is going to be extended. Contractions may start out being very forceful, then stop completely. There may not be any major vaginal bleeding. Transport the patient without delay, provide oxygen, and treat for shock. You may have to provide resuscitative measures for the mother.

ABNORMAL DELIVERIES

Anytime a patient has a breech or limb presentation, or a prolapsed umbilical cord, provide oxygen in high concentrations.

Breech Presentation

Breech presentation is the most common abnormal delivery. It involves a buttocks-first delivery. Through prompt and efficient emergency care, you can assist in the delivery of the baby. Should delivery not be possible, the care you provide can save the infant's life. Even though care at a breech birth is an EMT-level skill, keep in mind that this *is* an emergency. Many hospitals have recently increased the number of cesarean sections in deliveries involving breech presentations. This is a warning that more problems have been associated with breech births than was once believed.

If you evaluate a woman in labor and find the buttocks rather than the head presenting, prepare the mother for delivery and:

1. Allow the buttocks and trunk to deliver spontaneously. Provide support as they emerge.
2. Support the baby by allowing the body to rest on the palm of your hand and letting the legs dangle astride your arm.
3. The head will deliver of its own accord, but if the head does not deliver WITHIN 3 MINUTES, special care procedures must be initiated immediately.

When the head does not deliver in 3 minutes, two things are happening that require special care. First of all, the umbilical cord is squeezed against the vaginal wall by the baby's head, reducing blood flow through the cord. Reduced circulation means reduced oxygen supply to the baby. The second problem occurs when the baby attempts spontaneous breathing. Its face will be pressed against the wall of the birth canal, obstructing the nose and mouth. Since oxygen flow through the cord is obstructed, spontaneous breathing is essential.

In a breech presentation where the head does not deliver within 3 minutes, quickly explain to the mother what you are going to do and:

1. Carefully place your gloved hand in the vagina, keeping your palm toward the baby's face. Usually, the baby will be in a face-down position.

2. Form a "V" with your fingers, placing the index finger on one side of the baby's nose and the middle finger on the other side. Push the vaginal wall away from the baby's face.
3. Assure an open path to the infant's mouth by inserting the tip of your finger into the infant's mouth.
4. Maintain the airway until the head is delivered.
5. If the head delivers, support the head and apply enough support along the baby's body to prevent an explosive delivery. After delivery, care of the baby, cord, mother, and placenta is the same as in a cephalic delivery.

If the head is not delivered **within 3 minutes** of the established airway, maintain the airway and transport mother and child as a unit. Administer oxygen to the mother.

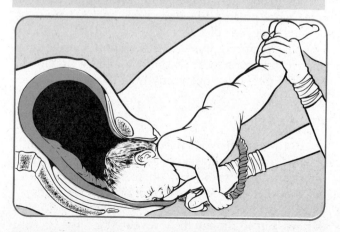

Figure 12-18: Procedures in a breech birth.

Take extreme care to maintain the airway being provided for the infant. You may be able to keep the mother on her back, or it may be necessary to place her in a knee-chest position (follow local guidelines).

REMEMBER: Do NOT attempt to deliver the baby by pulling on its legs.

Prolapsed Umbilical Cord

This is a TRUE EMERGENCY, usually seen early in labor. During delivery, the umbilical cord presents first. The cord is squeezed between the vaginal canal walls and the head of the baby. The cord is pinched and oxygen supply to the baby may be totally interrupted. Such an emergency requires IMMEDIATE TRANSPORT to a medical facility, keeping the mother in an exaggerated shock position with a pillow or blanket under her hips. Be certain to provide her with oxygen to increase the concentra-

tion carried over to the infant. Wrap the exposed cord, using a sterile towel from the OB kit. The best results are obtained if this towel is kept moist with *sterile saline*.

It will be necessary for you to insert several fingers of a gloved hand into the mother's vagina so that you can push up on the baby's head to keep pressure off the cord. You will be pushing up through the cervix. This may be the only chance that the baby has for survival, so continue to push up on the baby until you are relieved by a physician.

Limb Presentation

If, on evaluation of the mother, you find an upper or lower limb presenting, transport the mother immediately to a medical facility. Keep her in the delivery position (follow local guidelines). This also applies if there is a compound presentation of an arm and a leg, or a shoulder and an arm. Administer oxygen to the mother.

There is often a prolapsed cord with the compound presentation. Follow the same procedures as you would for any delivery involving a prolapsed cord. Remember, you have to keep pushing up on the baby until relieved by a physician. The baby must be kept off the cord if it is to survive.

On rare occasions, a baby will have shoulders too large to fit through the pelvic bones (symphysis pubis) and the hollow of the sacrum. The head will deliver, but the shoulders become wedged. Suction the baby's mouth and nose and carefully transport without delay. Provide oxygen to the mother.

REMEMBER: In the case of a limb presentation, do not try to pull on the limb or replace the limb into the vagina. Do NOT place your hand into the vagina, unless there is a prolapsed cord.

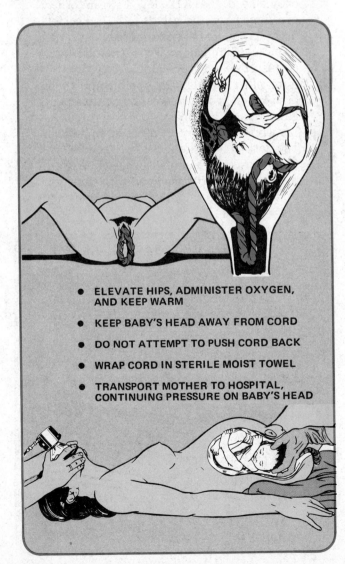

- ELEVATE HIPS, ADMINISTER OXYGEN, AND KEEP WARM
- KEEP BABY'S HEAD AWAY FROM CORD
- DO NOT ATTEMPT TO PUSH CORD BACK
- WRAP CORD IN STERILE MOIST TOWEL
- TRANSPORT MOTHER TO HOSPITAL, CONTINUING PRESSURE ON BABY'S HEAD

Figure 12-19: Prolapsed umbilical cord.

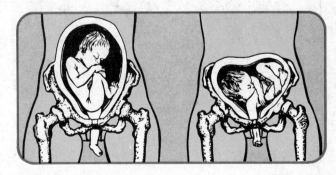

Figure 12-20: Limb presentations.

Multiple Birth

Multiple birth, usually in the form of twins, is not considered to be a complication, provided that the deliveries are normal. Twins generally are delivered in the same manner as a single delivery, one birth following the other. If the mother is under a doctor's care, she will probably be aware that she is carrying twins. Without this information, you should consider a multiple birth to be a possibility if the mother's abdomen appears unusually large before delivery, or it remains very large after delivery of the baby. If the birth is multiple, labor contractions will continue and the second baby will be delivered shortly after the first. Usually, this is within minutes of the first birth. The placenta or placentas are delivered normally.

When assisting in the delivery of twins, clamp or tie the cord of the first baby to prevent bleeding from the second baby via the cord. Assist the mother with the delivery of the second baby, then provide care for the babies, umbilical cords, placentas, and the mother as you would in a single baby delivery. The babies will probably be smaller than in a single birth, so care should be taken to keep them warm during transport.

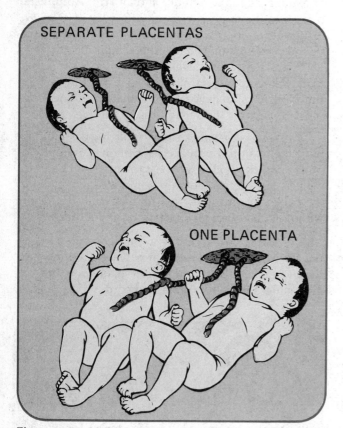

Figure 12-21: Multiple birth.

Premature Birth

By definition, a **premature baby** is one that weighs less than 5.5 pounds at birth, or one that is born before the seventh month of pregnancy. Since you will probably not be able to weigh the baby accurately, you will have to make a determination based on the mother's information and the baby's appearance. By comparison with a normal full-term baby, the head of a premature infant is much larger in proportion to the small, thin, red body.

Premature babies need special care from the moment of birth. The smaller the baby, the more important the initial care. You should take the following steps when providing care for the premature infant:

1. Keep the baby warm. Once breathing, the baby should be wrapped snugly in a warm blanket. Additional protection can be provided by an outer wrap of aluminum foil. Premature babies lack fat deposits that would normally help keep them warm.
2. Keep the airway clear. Continue to suction fluids from the nose and mouth using a rubber bulb syringe. Keep checking to see if additional suctioning is required.
3. Watch the umbilical cord for bleeding. Examine the cut end of the cord carefully. If there is any sign of bleeding, even the slightest, apply another clamp or tie closer to the baby's body.
4. Provide oxygen. Deliver the oxygen into the top of an aluminum foil tent placed over the baby's head. Do NOT blow a stream of oxygen directly on the baby's face. If available, use a humidified oxygen source.
5. Avoid contamination. The premature infant is susceptible to infection. Keep it away from other people. Do not breathe on its face. When available, wear disposable paper gowns, caps, and masks.
6. Transport the infant in a warm ambulance. The desired temperature is between 90° and 100°F. Use the ambulance heater to warm the patient compartment prior to transport. In the summer months, all compartment

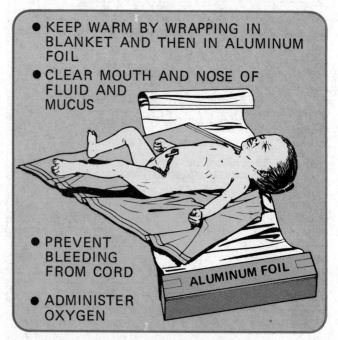

- KEEP WARM BY WRAPPING IN BLANKET AND THEN IN ALUMINUM FOIL
- CLEAR MOUTH AND NOSE OF FLUID AND MUCUS
- PREVENT BLEEDING FROM CORD
- ADMINISTER OXYGEN

ALUMINUM FOIL

Figure 12-22: Premature infants need special care.

windows should be closed and the air conditioning should be turned off.

7. Call ahead and alert the medical facility.

When a premature infant carrier is available, make certain that you are completely familiar with its use. In some areas, a mobile intensive care unit may be able to respond and transport the baby.

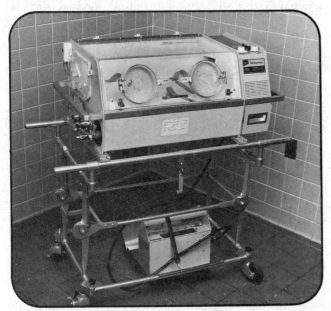

Figure 12-23: A premature infant carrier.

The Stillborn Infant

As noted earlier, some babies die up to several hours before birth. These babies are not to receive resuscitation. Any other babies who are born in pulmonary or cardiac arrest are to receive basic life support measures. When death appears to be imminent, you should prepare to provide life support.

Nothing is quite so sad as a baby born dead or one that dies shortly after birth. It is a tragic moment for both the parents and the emergency care personnel. Your thoughtfulness may provide the distraught parents with spiritual comfort. Christian parents may ask you to baptize the baby should it be stillborn or if death appears likely. This is acceptable practice for emergency personnel. Regardless of your own religious belief, you should comply with the parents' request. Ask the parents if they know the exact words of baptism for their denomination. Say exactly what they tell you. If they are not sure, simply sprinkle drops of water on the baby's head and say: "I baptize thee in the name of the Father, and of the Son, and of the Holy Spirit." In some cases, the parents may request that you modify the above by saying, ". . .and of the Holy Ghost."

Needless to say, resuscitative efforts should be continued during and after the baptism and continued until transfer at the hospital.

SUMMARY

The fetus developing in the uterus is surrounded by the amniotic sac. While developing, the fetus receives nourishment and oxygen through the placenta. It is connected to the placenta by way of the umbilical cord.

The first stage of labor starts with contractions and ends when the baby enters the vagina. The second stage of labor ends with birth. The third stage ends with the delivery of the placenta.

Evaluate the mother to see if she is about to deliver. Consider if this is her first baby, how far apart the contractions are, if she feels pressure or feels as if she may have a bowel movement, if her "bag of waters" has broken, or if she feels the baby moving into her vagina.

If you believe that birth will occur shortly, provide the mother with as much privacy as possible, position her on her back, with her knees bent, feet flat, and legs spread apart. Remove any clothing obstructing your view of the vaginal opening. See if any part of the baby is visible or visible upon contractions. This is crowning. If the head appears first, this is a cephalic presentation.

Assist the mother as she delivers her baby. Carefully support the head of the infant as it is born. Provide support for its entire body and head as birth proceeds.

If you notice the umbilical cord around a baby's neck, gently loosen the cord with your fingers. When the cord will not loosen, you will have to clamp it in two locations and cut between the clamps.

If the amniotic sac does not break, puncture it and pull it away from the baby's mouth and nose.

In caring for the newborn, clear the baby's airway and make certain that the baby is breathing. If it is not breathing, "encourage" it by snapping your index finger on the soles of its feet. (Never lift and spank the baby.) For nonbreathing babies with a brachial pulse, provide mouth-to-mouth and nose resuscitation. If there is no pulse, provide CPR. If CPR is necessary, you will have to clamp and cut the cord.

If the environment is cold, you may have to partially wrap the newborn before cutting the cord. Do not tie, clamp, or cut a cord until the baby is breathing on its own, unless you must provide CPR for the infant.

Always wrap the newborn in a blanket to keep it warm.

Assist the mother as she delivers the placenta and save all tissues for transport. Help control vaginal bleeding with clean pads over the vaginal opening and massage the abdomen over the site of the uterus. Remove all wet towels and sheets. Wipe clean the mother's face and hands.

REMEMBER: Throughout the entire birth process, provide emotional support to the mother.

Be ready for complications during a delivery. Provide an airway with your fingers in cases of breech birth. Maintain this airway until the baby is born or until you hand the mother over to trained professionals at a medical facility. Transport mothers with pre-birth bleeding, prolapsed umbilical cords, or limb presentations to a medical facility as soon as possible. Administer oxygen. If there is a prolapsed cord, you will have to insert several fingers into the vagina to push the baby off the cord.

If there is severe bleeding before delivery, pad the vaginal opening, treat for shock, administer oxygen, and transport as soon as possible.

Expect a multiple birth if contractions continue after a baby is born. Tie or clamp the umbilical cord of the first child before the next delivers.

Keep premature babies warm, maintain a clear airway, monitor the cord for bleeding, provide oxygen to a tent over the baby's head, and protect from contamination.

In cases of miscarriage and abortion, be certain to provide emotional support to the mother. Pad her vaginal opening if there is bleeding. Save all blood-soaked pads and any passed tissues. Treat for shock.

In cases of stillborns, remain professional and provide emotional support to the mother, father, and other family members.

SECTION TWO: PEDIATRIC EMERGENCIES

OBJECTIVES By the end of this section, you should be able to:

1. State the age limits for infant and child. (p. 286)
2. Describe how to conduct a primary survey on the infant and the child patient. (p. 286-90)
3. State, step by step, the basic life support procedures for both infant and child patients. (p. 287)
4. Describe the changes in the interview method used when the patient is a child. (p. 286, 8)
5. List the normal vital signs for the infant and the child patient. (p. 289)
6. List in general what special problems are searched for during the secondary survey when the patient is an infant and when the patient is a child. (p. 288-90)
7. State the appropriate basic EMT-level care for pediatric emergencies involving:
   - Fever (p. 293)
   - Convulsions (p. 294)
   - Acute abdomen (p. 294)
8. Define sudden infant death syndrome (SIDS) and state the EMT's role in a possible SIDS-related infant death. (p. 294-5)
9. Describe EMT care procedures for impaled fishhooks and rings stuck on fingers. (follow local guidelines). (p. 290-1)
10. Describe the symptoms and signs associated with bike fork compression injury and state the emergency care for such an injury. (p. 291)
11. State the common burn injuries received by infants and children. (p. 290)
12. Define child abuse in terms of the battered child syndrome and sexual assault. (p. 291-2, 5)
13. List the typical injuries associated with the battered child. (p. 292)
14. State the EMT's role in cases of possible child abuse, including care for possible sexual assault. (p. 292-3)

SKILLS As an EMT, you should be able to:

1. Determine if a patient is a child or an infant.
2. Conduct a proper primary survey on infants and children.
3. Control your emotions and remain professional during a pediatric emergency.
4. Provide appropriate basic life support for both infants and children.
5. Properly conduct an interview of a child patient.
6. Conduct a secondary survey physical examination on infants and children, detecting atypical vital signs, possible injuries, and indications of possible medical emergencies.
7. Provide prompt and efficient care in cases of injury when the patient is an infant or child.
8. Evaluate infants and children for possible medical emergencies.
9. Provide emotional support to parents in cases of possible sudden infant death syndrome.
10. Act as a professional in cases of possible child abuse.

TERMS   you may be using for the first time:

Bike Fork Compression Injury—an injury sustained when the victim's heel is caught in the spokes of a bicycle or tricycle. The foot is driven into the fork of the front wheel, producing crushing injuries to the tissues behind and around the ankle.

Sudden Infant Death Syndrome (SIDS)—the unexplained sudden death of an apparently healthy infant while asleep. Death can usually be related to respiratory arrest.

Child Abuse—assault of an infant or child that produces physical and emotional injuries. Sexual assault is included as a form of child abuse.

INFANTS AND CHILDREN— SPECIAL PATIENTS

By definition, an infant is anyone under one year of age. A child is anyone from one to eight years of age. In the past, any patient over eight years of age was to be treated using adult techniques. Even though this may be true in terms of pulmonary resuscitation and CPR, such a statement cannot be made for all aspects of care. Even when exact age guidelines are established, there must be some variations in care based on the size of the patient.

The maturity of the patient can be significant. One hardly expects a nine-year-old child to be able to deal with an emergency in the same fashion as a 14-year-old adolescent. The procedures of the interview and the amount of emotional support required certainly would be different for the two age groups. Add to this the fact that many children and individuals in their early adolescence have been observed to react to crises in a regressive manner. This means that a patient who is usually a mature 10-year-old may act more like a six-year-old in an emergency. Care for the patient must be applied as needed by the individual in the particular situation.

The concept of adolescent medicine is fairly new. The lower limits of systolic blood pressure used to indicate the onset of shock cannot be the same for a 12-year-old and a 17-year-old patient. One cannot apply children's blood volumes to the 14-year-old. In most cases, adult blood volumes cannot be applied to the 14-year-old patient either. Such factors require you to judge the individual in terms of body size and apparent emotional and physical maturity.

Your own reactions to a pediatric emergency make infants and children special patients. A broken bone is a broken bone and a bleeding wound is a bleeding wound. The principles of emergency care are essentially the same, regardless of the age of the injured patient. Yet we all react more intensely to the cries of children. We immediately want to stop the suffering and correct all problems. Those in emergency medicine must control their emotions so as not to be overwhelmed by cries of pain, expressions of fear, and the unnerving silence of children who *should* be crying. There is no doubt that you

should be strongly motivated to care for the infant or child patient, and that you should want him to "feel better." However, unless you control your emotions so that you are objective and efficient, what is really needed to help the child may not be provided. If you let your emotions control your actions, the emotional support and comfort needed by child, family, and bystanders will not be part of the care you provide. Unless you are calm and professional, the emotional reactions of the patient and others at the scene may become more intense.

Always keep in mind that parents, family, friends, and bystanders at the scene need your support. In fact, unless each individual believes that you are concerned and wish to help, you may not be allowed to provide care, or you may be prevented from providing effective care. There is usually little time for long conversations. Identify yourself and show through your interactions with the child that you are concerned. The *way* you provide care shows that you are a well-trained professional.

THE PRIMARY SURVEY AND BASIC LIFE SUPPORT

Details for the procedures used in the primary survey and basic life support for infants and children were presented in Chapters 3 through 5. The next page is provided to remind you of what to do to establish and maintain an open airway, provide pulmonary resuscitation and CPR, control profuse bleeding, and treat for shock.

THE SECONDARY SURVEY

The Patient Interview

Obviously, you will not be able to interview an infant. Young children can be interviewed if you take your time and keep your language as simple as possible. If the parents or guardians are at the scene and are not injured or ill, talk with them, but do not exclude the child. Talking with the parents will help gain the child's confidence. However, if you do not follow this by talking *directly* to the child, you may find the child unwilling to accept your help, and the parents losing confidence in your ability to help their child.

PRIMARY SURVEY AND BASIC LIFE SUPPORT: PEDIATRIC EMERGENCIES

INFANTS (birth to 1 year)

Establishing Unresponsiveness: Infant should move or cry when gently tapped or shaken.
Airway: Use head-tilt, neck-lift method, but provide only a *slight* tilt. Do NOT close the airway by using too great a tilt.
Evaluating Breathing: Use the LOOK, LISTEN, and FEEL approach. If infant is struggling to breathe, but not cyanotic, immediate transport is recommended.

CLEARING THE AIRWAY:
- Use mouth-to-mouth and nose technique.
- Provide 4 gentle breaths in rapid succession.
If there is evidence of airway obstruction:
- Make certain you have not overextended the neck.
- Straddle infant over your arm with the head lower than the trunk. Strike directly between the shoulder blades.
- Support head by placing your hand around the jaw and chest. Add support by placing your forearm on your thigh.
- Rapidly deliver 4 back blows with heel of your free hand. Strike directly between the shoulder blades.
- Place your free hand on infant's back, sandwiching him between your two hands. Turn infant over and place his back on your thigh.
- Rapidly deliver 4 chest thrusts as if providing external chest compressions for CPR.
- If airway remains obstructed, but patient is conscious, continue back blows and chest thrusts.
- If airway remains obstructed, but patient is unconscious, place your thumb in patient's mouth, over the tongue. Wrap your other fingers around lower jaw and look for an obstruction. Do NOT attempt blind finger sweeps. When performing finger sweeps, use your little finger.
- If patient is unconscious and obstruction has not been dislodged, provide 4 breaths and repeat back blows, chest thrusts, looking for and removing visible obstructions.

RESCUE BREATHING:
- Open airway without overextending the neck
- Use mouth-to-mouth and nose technique
- Provide gentle breaths, noting the chest rise
- Deliver 4 breaths in rapid succession
- If airway is clear and patient still not breathing, determine a pulse but no breathing, provide rescue breathing.
- Deliver 1 gentle breath every THREE SECONDS. Check for pulse every few minutes.

CPR:
- If patient unresponsive and not breathing:
  Open airway
  Provide 4 gentle breaths in rapid succession
  Look, listen, and feel for breathing. If no indication of obstruction, but patient still unconscious and not breathing . . .
- Determine BRACHIAL PULSE. If no pulse and no breathing, provide CPR.
- Compress breastbone, between the nipples, using the tips of 2 or 3 fingers.
- Depress the sternum ½ to 1 inch.
- Compress at a rate of 100 per minute.
- Interposed ventilation as a gentle breath, mouth-to-mouth and nose, 1 EVERY 5 COMPRESSIONS ("1, 2, 3, 4, 5, breathe").
- Check brachial pulse every few minutes.

BLEEDING:
- Use direct pressure as a primary method
- When necessary, use elevation, pressure points, or a blood pressure cuff. Tourniquet is a *last* resort.
- Consider blood loss of 25 ml or more to be very serious.

SHOCK:
- Consider infant in shock if blood loss is 25 ml or more.
- Consider infant in severe shock if systolic blood pressure is under 50 mmHg.
- Consider shock more severe if evidence of dehydration (vomiting, diarrhea, exposure to high temperatures, overheating, high skin temperature).
- Assure adequate breathing and circulation, and control serious bleeding
- Administer oxygen per local guidelines
- Elevate lower extremities, but avoid placing pressure on cervical spine and head
- Splint fractures
- Avoid rough handling
- Prevent loss of body heat
- Give nothing by mouth
- Transport as soon as possible, monitoring vital signs

CHILDREN

Establishing Unresponsiveness: Child should move or cry when gently tapped or shaken.
Airway: Use head-tilt, neck-lift method, but provide only a *slight* tilt for the small child. For larger children, provide an adequate head-tilt, but do NOT close the airway by tilting the head too far.
Evaluating Breathing: Use the LOOK, LISTEN, and FEEL approach. If child is struggling to breathe, but not cyanotic, immediate transport is recommended. Should child be in respiratory arrest, or cyanotic and cannot breathe, make certain airway is open and unobstructed so you can begin rescue breathing efforts.

CLEARING THE AIRWAY:
- Make certain you have the proper head-tilt.
- Use the mouth-to-mouth and nose technique for small children and the mouth-to-mouth technique for large children.
- Provide 4 gentle breaths in rapid succession.
If there is evidence of airway obstruction:
- Treat the small child as you would an infant.
- If child too large to straddle your forearm, kneel and "drape" patient across between your arms for turning, kneel and "drape" patient across your thigh. Keep the patient's head lower than the trunk.
- Rapidly deliver 4 back blows with heel of your free hand. Provide blows directly between the shoulder blades.
- Place the child on his back, on a hard surface. Provide support for his head and back as you move him from your thigh.
- Rapidly deliver 4 chest thrusts as if providing external chest compressions for CPR.
- If airway remains obstructed, but patient is conscious, continue back blows and chest thrusts.
- If airway remains obstructed, but patient is unconscious, place your thumb in patient's mouth, over the tongue. Wrap your other fingers around lower jaw and look for an obstruction. Do NOT attempt blind finger sweeps.

- If patient is unconscious and obstruction has not been dislodged, transport as soon as possible, providing 4 breaths and repeating back blows, chest thrusts, looking for and removing visible obstructions.

RESCUE BREATHING:
- Open airway without overextending the neck
- Use mouth-to-mouth and nose technique for small children and mouth-to-mouth for larger children.
- Provide gentle breaths, noting the chest rise
- Deliver 4 breaths in rapid succession
- If airway is clear and patient still not breathing, determine a pulse.
- If no pulse, provide CPR. Should there be a pulse, but no breathing, provide rescue breathing.
- Deliver 1 gentle breath every FOUR SECONDS. Check for pulse every few minutes.

CPR:
- If patient unresponsive and not breathing:
  Open airway
  Provide 4 gentle breaths in rapid succession
  Look, listen, and feel for breathing. If no indication of obstruction, but patient still unconscious and not breathing . . .
- Determine a CAROTID PULSE. If no pulse and no breathing, provide CPR.
- Apply compressions to breastbone, between the nipples, using the tips of three fingers for small child. Larger children, use the heel of one hand.
- Depress the sternum 1 to 1½ inches.
- Compress at a rate of 80 per minute.
- Interposed ventilation as a gentle breath, mouth-to-mouth and nose or mouth-to-mouth, 1 EVERY 5 COMPRESSIONS ("1 and 2 and 3 and 4 and 5 and breathe").
- Check for carotid pulse every few minutes.

BLEEDING:
- Use direct pressure as a primary method
- When necessary, use elevation, pressure points, or a blood pressure cuff. Tourniquet is a *last* resort.
- Consider blood loss of 500 ml (½ liter or about 1 pint) or more to be very serious.

SHOCK:
- Consider child in shock if blood loss is 500 ml or more.
- Consider child in shock if systolic blood pressure is under:
  50 mmHg in pre-school children
  60 mmHg in children up to age 12
  70 mmHg in teenagers
- Consider shock to be more severe if evidence of dehydration (vomiting, diarrhea, exposure to high temperatures, overheating, high skin temperature)
- Assure adequate breathing and circulation, and control serious bleeding
- Administer oxygen per local guidelines
- Elevate lower extremities, but avoid placing pressure on cervical spine and head
- Splint fractures
- Avoid rough handling
- Prevent loss of body heat
- Give nothing by mouth
- Transport as soon as possible, monitoring vital signs

All patients have some degree of fear at the emergency scene. Infants and children usually are more fearful than adults because they lack the experience to understand illness and injury. In addition, the infant or child is easily frightened by the unknown. Since so many things are unknowns to a child, it is easy to see why emergencies can be so scary for children. The infant is unclear as to what comprises the world immediately around him. The elements associated with the emergency (pain, noise, bright lights, cold, etc.) often set off a reaction of pure panic on the part of the infant.

Keep in mind that any problems faced by the child will be intensified if his parents are not at the scene. Children find security by interacting with their parents as they face new problems and emergencies. Asking for his parents may be the child's first priority, even above that of having you help him or relieve his pain.

When you are dealing with a child patient, you should:

- Identify yourself to the child. Keep this very simple. For example, "Hi. My name is Mark. What's yours?"

- Let him know that someone will call his parents.

- If the child has a toy on the scene and wants it, let him have the toy.

- Sit or kneel with the child so as not to tower over him.

- SMILE at the child. This is one sign from an adult that carries a lot of weight with most children.

- Touch the child on the forehead and hold his hand. If the child does not wish to be touched, he will let you know. Do not force the issue; simply smile and provide comfort to the child by way of conversation.

- Do not let the child see scissors, clamps, or other tools and equipment.

- Let the child see your face and speak directly to him. Speak clearly and slowly, making certain that the child can hear you.

- Stop occasionally to find out if the child understands what you have said or asked. Even if you communicate easily with children, never assume that a child has understood you. Find out if you have been understood by questioning the child periodically.

- Determine as quickly as you can if there are any life-threatening problems and care for them. If there are no problems of this nature, continue with patient survey and interview at a relaxed pace. Fearful children cannot take the pressure of a rapidly paced examination and a lot of "meaningless" questions all being controlled by a stranger.

- Always tell the child what you are going to do as you take vital signs and do a physical examination. Do not try to explain the entire procedure at once. Explain one step, do the procedure, then explain the next step.

- NEVER LIE TO THE CHILD. Tell him when he may feel pain during the physical examination. If he asks if he is sick or hurt, tell him so, but be certain to add that you are there to help and you will not leave. Let the child know that other people also will be helping him.

The Physical Examination

Vital Signs   You will need to determine vital signs for the infant or child patient. Do not tell the child that you are going to "take" his pulse or his blood pressure. Some children will think that you are literally going to take something away from them. Try to obtain pulse, respirations, and relative skin temperature as you talk to the child patient. This will give you time to gain the child's confidence before trying to measure blood pressure. Be certain to show the child the blood pressure cuff. Let him see the surface of the cuff that will be placed against his arm. This will help dispel fear that the cuff contains needles or objects that may hurt. Wrap the cuff around an area of your wrist or arm that will accept the small size of the pediatric cuff. Pump the bulb to show that the procedure will not hurt. Tell him that it will feel "tight" for a little while.

Remember that a child is naturally curious, even when he is in pain. If he expresses an interest in your stethoscope, let him listen. Should he want to operate your pen light, let him do so. Such activities build a rapport with the child that will reduce his fears and make the child more receptive to your care.

Table 12-1 lists the vital signs for infants and children. Keep in mind that a child will have even less understanding than an adult as to why you are doing certain things. Most children will remain confident in what you are doing if you continue to talk with them and keep direct eye contact whenever possible.

Head-to-Toe Survey   A head-to-toe survey of infants and children is done in much the same manner as for adult patients. If the parents are at the scene, explain what you are going to do and the importance of the physical examination. Unless there are possible neck or spinal injuries, the child should be held in the mother's or father's lap. Kneel

Table 12.1: Vital Signs: Infants and Children

	INFANT	CHILD
Pulse Rate	140 to 150 (birth) 110 (6 months)	Range: 80 to 150 100 (avg. 1 year old) 95 (2 to 4 years) 90 (5 to 10 years) 85 (10 to 15 years) 75 to 80 (15 years +)
Breathing Rate	40 (birth) 30 (6 months)	Range: 16 to 44 28 (avg. 1 year old) 25 (2 to 4 years) 24 (5 to 10 years) 20 (10 to 15 years) 16 to 18 (15 years +)
Systolic Blood Pressure	60 to 80 (birth 90 (6 months)	Range: 90 to 150 90 (avg. 1 year old) 100 (2 to 4 years) 100 to 110 (5 to 10 years) 110 (10 to 15 years) 110 to 120 (15 years +)
Diastolic Blood Pressure	Very serious if below 50 or above 75 mmHg	Very serious if below 50 or above 75 mmHg for child 1 to 5 years. Very serious if below 60 or above 85 for ages 5 to 12. Very serious if below 60 or above 105 from age 12 to adult.

tioned during an objective examination. Nonetheless, you should protect the child from the stares of onlookers. Many children around the age of eight go through a stage of intense modesty. You may have to keep explaining why you must remove certain articles of clothing. Take your time so as not to rush the child into accepting all that is happening to him.

The young adolescent is often worried about the changes occurring to his body. Keep in mind that this is a new experience for the patient and he may be uncertain if these changes are "normal." Handling the clothing of a teen-age girl can be a little awkward for the male EMT. In most cases, a simple description of the survey will set the patient at ease. However, you should make sure that the parents understand what you are going to do and why it must be done. Whenever possible, conduct the examination in the presence of a female EMT. Do NOT delay patient evaluation and care because you or the patient may be embarrassed. As a professional, you must put such feelings aside and act in a manner that will allow the patient to relax and understand that there is no need for embarrassment.

The head-to-toe survey is done to look for the same signs of injury and illness as in the case of the adult patient. However, you should take special care with the following:

- Head—Remember that an infant has "soft spots" (fontanelles) on the skull. Make certain you do not apply pressure to these spots. Keep in mind that many accidents involving infants and children produce head injuries.
- Nose and ears—Blood and clear fluids are often missed during the survey. Look carefully and relate these findings to skull fractures.
- Neck—Cervical spine injuries can occur more easily with pediatric patients since the head is large compared to the rest of the body. In medical emergencies, the neck may be sore, stiff, or swollen.
- Chest—Listen closely for even air entry and the sounds of breathing. Be alert for rales and wheezes.
- Abdomen—Note any tender areas.
- Pelvis—Be on the alert for rectal bleeding.
- Extremities—You MUST do a neurological assessment for both infants and children.

and try to stay at the child's eye level. Explain to the child that you are going to ask questions from time to time as you check from the "top" of his head to the "tips" of his toes. Tell the child what you are going to do *before* you do it, and warn him of any possible pain. Simply tell the child that what you do may hurt a little, but the pain will go away quickly. Let him know that you must do what you are doing so that you can help him. Always tell the child that you need his help.

Many EMT squads carry a doll or a stuffed animal to give to the child during the physical examination. If a toy is carried on the ambulance, it must be made of materials that allow for proper sanitizing. Such a toy serves to provide comfort to the child and allows you to explain the survey to the child. You can point to an area on the toy and tell the child this is where you must touch him during the survey. You also can use the toy to explain what you need to do when providing emergency care. This type of one-to-one communication not only helps you and the child, it also helps to build parent and bystander confidence, letting them know that a professional compassionate emergency medical technician is caring for the child.

Young children usually suffer no embarrassment when articles of clothing are removed or reposi-

The neurological evaluation often produces special problems. Infants have to be watched carefully to see their responses to your touching, squeezing, and pushing. It is often necessary to treat all infants as if they were unconscious patients, and test them for reaction to painful stimuli. Always note if the conscious infant or child patient's eyes look in the direction of your hand or your face as you touch him. Children should follow your movements with

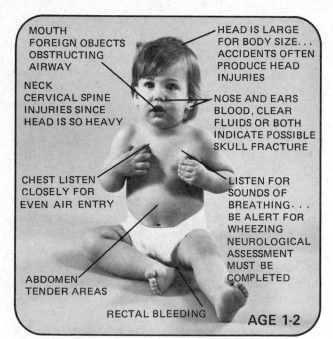

MOUTH
FOREIGN OBJECTS
OBSTRUCTING
AIRWAY

HEAD IS LARGE
FOR BODY SIZE. . .
ACCIDENTS OFTEN
PRODUCE HEAD
INJURIES

NECK
CERVICAL SPINE
INJURIES SINCE
HEAD IS SO HEAVY

NOSE AND EARS
BLOOD, CLEAR
FLUIDS OR BOTH
INDICATE POSSIBLE
SKULL FRACTURE

CHEST LISTEN
CLOSELY FOR
EVEN AIR ENTRY

LISTEN FOR
SOUNDS OF
BREATHING. . .
BE ALERT FOR
WHEEZING
NEUROLOGICAL
ASSESSMENT
MUST BE
COMPLETED

ABDOMEN
TENDER AREAS

RECTAL BLEEDING   AGE 1-2

Figure 12-24: Special survey considerations.

their eyes. Notice if the patient stays alert, responds only when you call his name or speak loudly, or if he lapses quickly into a sleepy state. See if the patient will squeeze your fingers, or a ball or other toy. If you reach a point in the evaluation where you do not think spinal injuries are likely, continue to test the young child's neurological reactions by simple childhood games such as "peek-a-boo." Holding your hand up to the young child's hand will often lead the patient to compare the size of his hand with yours. In doing so, the child will move his fingers and will press against your hand. If the child does not respond, see if he wants to play "pattycake," or to hold an object that requires him to use both hands and eyes in coordination. The stethoscope is ideal for this purpose, provided the child shows no fear of the instrument.

INJURIES COMMON TO CHILDREN

When providing emergency care for the child patient, always tell him what you are going to do before you do it. Try to make him feel special. Tell the child that he is very brave and has been a big help to you. Carry a brightly colored adhesive bandage and apply this to suitable dressings. Make a fuss over using this tape only for him, calling it a "battle ribbon" or some other special name.

Head Injuries

Again, remember that head injuries are common in accidents involving infants and children. Take special care in noting any signs of injury. If the injury appears to be minor and the parents do not want you to transport the child, warn them to watch

the child closely for at least 48 hours. Tell them what you are looking for when you conduct the patient assessment and tell them to do the same over the next few days. They should awaken the child every couple hours the night of the head injury and check for any indications of problems. If the child is difficult to awaken, has headaches, or clear fluids or blood in the ears or nose, ask them to call a physician or take the child IMMEDIATELY to a medical facility. Stress that, once any of the signs of head problems appear, care *cannot* be delayed.

In addition to noting obvious scalp, cranial, and facial injuries, you should look for:

- Vomiting, typically seen in cases of head injury.
- Clear fluids, or clear fluids and blood coming from the nose, ears, or ears and nose.
- Drowsiness or lapsing into a sleepy state.
- Problems with speech, including the inability to talk.
- Headache, though this is often delayed.
- Unequal pupils
- Cases where the child says he is seeing double.
- Any convulsion associated with a head injury.
- A stiff or sore neck occurring several days after a head injury (possible meningitis . . .transport!).

Burns

You should look carefully for burns when caring for young children. They are often the victims of first and second degree burns to the hands and face resulting from contact with hot water, steam, cooking utensils, and hot radiators. If you note that the burn is on both hands, or if you note that the child shows evidence of past burns, transport the child, no matter how minor the burn. The emergency department staff may wish to examine the child to determine if the child is being abused, or if the child is retarded and has not had the benefit of proper medical evaluation.

Rings Stuck on Fingers

Parents' lack of knowledge of dealing with minor childhood problems often leads to the EMS System being called to a nonemergency situation. This is the case for rings stuck on fingers. Sometimes the parents do not call but bring the child to the rescue squad's station. In either case, by the time you see the child, a good bit of tugging on the ring has taken place and the child's finger is swollen. Many squads have a ring cutter, ring saw, jeweler's saw, or fine hacksaw blade for these "emergencies." However, the ring is often valuable, requiring removal of the ring without destroying it.

The first course of action is to hold the child's finger under warm water for a short period of time. Often, the ring will expand and can be removed with a few gentle tugs. If this fails, try to slide the ring off after lubricating the finger with grease, butter, cooking oil, or petroleum jelly. Do not use petroleum lubricating oil, heating oil, or motor vehicle oil. These can burn or irritate the child's skin.

Your next course of action is the opposite of the first. Immerse the finger in ice water for several minutes to reduce the swelling. Try to move the ring to a place on the finger where it will be loose and massage the finger from tip to hand. After several minutes of massaging, lubricate the finger and try to slip the ring off.

Before resorting to cutting the ring, try to slide three or four inches of thin string under the ring toward the hand. Then wrap the string tightly around the finger below the ring for about three-quarters of an inch. While holding the wrapping snugly in place with one hand, grasp the upper end of the string with your other hand and pull downward over the ring. This starts an unwrapping process. If the finger is not too badly swollen, the ring may slide over the string that is still wrapped around the finger and continue to move as you continue to unwrap the string. It may be necessary to repeat this procedure several times.

When all else fails, you will have to CAREFULLY cut the ring off the child's fnger. Before doing so, make sure that the child understands you will cut only the ring and not his finger.

Bike Fork Compression Injury

Children often ride on the cross bars of bicycles. When the passenger is not careful, the heel of one foot may catch in the spokes of the front wheel. The foot is quickly carried into the fork of the front wheel, where it jams. Bent spokes are usually your first clue of a bike fork compression injury.

Expose the injured foot and look for areas of pale or white skin behind the ankle. The tissue has probably been crushed. Considerable pain usually accompanies this injury. Examine the patient for other possible injuries, looking carefully for fractures to the leg. If there are no apparent leg fractures or dislocations, immobilize the ankle as you would for a fractured ankle, using a folded pillow. Transport the patient to a medical facility.

Trapped Extremities

Children often put their head, legs, arms, feet, hands, or fingers into places where they become trapped. In some localities, specially trained personnel from the rescue squad or fire service are called to handle these situations. If you must act in such emergencies, begin by having the child relax. Once this is done, he may be able to slowly free himself, or free himself with you helping to guide the part from the point of entrapment. Lubricating substances can be used to help slide the child free. If nothing else works, you may have to cut away the material holding the child. Explain what you are going to do, step by step, then proceed with great caution and make sure that the trapped part is well protected by padding and that the rest of the child's body is safe. Delay working if the child becomes upset. It is important that he does not move around or struggle to free himself. Do not chop or tear away obstructions. Careful sawing is usually the best approach. Once the child is freed, conduct a proper patient assessment and care for all injuries. Usually, minor abrasions and lacerations are all that result. The parents should be told to call or see a physician since tetanus shots may be required.

Impaled Fishhook

Too often, people start pulling on an impaled fishhook to remove it from the skin. But the barb on a fishhook usually grabs and the hook cannot be pulled free. Next people try to push the point through the skin and cut off the barb. The hook then can be worked back through the wound. This type of action is very painful in some cases and can be dangerous. It can only be done safely in cases where the hook is superficially impaled. The best course of action is to transport the child to a medical facility. It is true that the same procedure may be used at the hospital, but it will be done by a trained physician who knows where nerves, blood vessels, muscles, and tendons are. A local anesthetic can make the procedure painless. In some cases, the doctor may have to make an incision to remove the hook. The wound can be properly cleaned and the child can receive a tetanus shot or booster, as required. Do not take this type of wound any less seriously than any other impaled object.

THE BATTERED CHILD SYNDROME

At one time, people thought child abuse was a rare phenomenon. It now appears that this problem has always been part of our culture and is on the increase. For example, the Commonwealth of Virginia recently has reported between 30,000 and 35,000 cases of child abuse annually. But the problem is thought to be even more serious than the statistics would have you believe. For every battered child seen by an emergency department or family physician, there are apparently many more *unreported* cases that never receive such care.

Many surveys have tried to find the number of children classified as "battered." These are the children beaten with fists, hair brushes, straps, pool cues, razor strops, bottles, broom handles, baseball bats, pots and pans, and almost any object that can serve as a weapon. Included in this group are children intentionally burned by hot water, steam, open flames, cigarettes, and other thermal sources. Battered children include those thrown down steps, pushed out of windows and over railings, and even pushed from moving cars.

The horror grows as we find children who are shot, stabbed, electrocuted, and suffocated. The Bureau of Community Health Services reports 1,000 to 4,000 deaths a year from child abuse and neglect. At least 300 of these victims are infants. Emergency department physicians indicate on various surveys that 10% of ALL children under 5 years of age are battered children.

Child abusers are mothers, fathers, sisters, brothers, grandparents, babysitters, white-collar workers, blue-collar workers, unemployed persons, the rich, the poor. There is no distinction as to race, creed, sex, or ethnic background. In other words, ANYONE can be a child abuser.

Indications of Child Abuse

Child abuse can take several different forms, often occurring in combination. These forms include:

- Psychological abuse
- Neglect
- Physical assault
- Sexual assault

A child's psychological problems and pathologic behavior are difficult to trace back to specific abuse. This is typically not a direct problem in the realm of the EMT. What constitutes neglect is a serious legal question. As a child goes without proper food, shelter, clothing, supervision, and love, the effects surely will be seen, but seldom is this the major part of an emergency response. Sexual assault and molestation are problems seen by EMTs. This will be covered later in this section. For now, let us consider only the physically battered child.

The best way to describe the types of injuries that can be inflicted in child abuse cases is to say, "if it can happen to the body, it has been done by a child abuser." In child abuse cases, you will find:

- Bruises, abrasions, lacerations, and incisions of all sizes and forms. These include welts, swollen limbs, split lips, black eyes, and loose or broken teeth.
- Broken bones, with all types of fractures. Many battered children have multiple fractures, often in various stages of healing or have fracture-associated complications.
- Head injuries, with concussions and skull fractures.
- Abdominal injuries include ruptured spleens, livers and lungs lacerated by broken ribs, internal bleeding from blunt trauma, and lacerated and avulsed genitalia.

There are times when you will treat an injured child and never think he has been abused. The child relates well with his parents and there appears to be a strong bond between them. However, there are certain indications that abuse may be occurring in or outside the home. Be on the alert for the following:

- Repeated responses to provide care for the same child or children in a family.
- Indications of past injuries. This is why you must do a physical examination and why you must remove articles of clothing. Pay special attention to the back and buttocks.
- Poorly healing wounds or improperly healed fractures. It is rare for a child to receive a fracture, be given proper orthopedic care and then show angulations and large "bumps" and "knots" of bone at the "healed" injury site.
- Indications of past burns, or fresh bilateral burns. Children seldom put both hands on a hot object or touch the same hot object again (true, some do. . .this is only an indication, not proof).
- Many different types of injuries to both sides of the front and back of the body. This gains even more importance if adults on the scene insist that the child "falls a lot."
- Fear on the part of the child to tell you how he was injured. Combine this with the adults on the scene indicating they do not wish to leave you alone with the child.

Pay attention to the adults as you treat the child. Do they have trouble controlling anger? Do you feel that at any moment there may be an emotional outburst? Do any of the adults appear to be in a deep state of depression? Are there indications of alcohol or drug abuse? Do any of the adults speak of suicide or seeking mercy for their unhappy children?

The Role of the EMT

Remember that you are an EMT charged with providing emergency care for an injured child. You are not a physician trained to detect abuse, a police officer, court investigator, judge, or one-person jury. Provide prompt and efficient care, controlling your emotions and holding back any accusations. Do NOT give any indications to the parents or other adults at the scene that you suspect them of child abuse. Do NOT ask the child if he has been abused. To do so when others are around could produce too great a stress for the injured child to handle. Properly assess the patient and provide appropriate care. If you are suspicious about the mechanism of injury, transport the child even though the severity of injury may not warrant such action.

ALWAYS report your suspicions to the emergency department staff in accordance with local policies. Almost every medical facility staff will take action to see if your fears are well founded. If for some reason you do not believe that the medical staff at an institution has taken you seriously, or you believe they do not wish to become involved (this would probably never happen), then you MUST report your suspicions to the juvenile authorities of the local police department. This may not be a legal requirement in your state, but it is a professional one.

Maintain patient and family confidentiality. Do not tell your family or friends that you saw a possible case of child abuse. Do not name the child or his family. Report the problem to your superior officer at the squad or service where you work. This will allow for past responses to be checked and future responses to be noted in case a pattern in a family develops to indicate possible abuse. Even when talking to your partner, the hospital staff, and your squad leaders, use the terms "suspicious" and "possible." Do not call someone a child abuser. If you break confidentiality, you could be sued. Keep in mind that the courts can deal harshly with those who provide patient care and then violate the confidentiality of the patient, the family, and the home. Also keep in mind that rumors about abuse may, in the long run, cause mental or physical harm to your child patient.

Sexual Assault

It is not certain how many children are victims of sexual molestation and abuse. The problem ranges from adults exposing themselves to children, to adults touching children's genitals or having children touch their genitals, to sexual intercourse, oral sex and sexual torture. Many of the cases reported are for adults exposing themselves. The other extreme, where there is physical injury to the child, also is usually reported. The cases in between, especially those causing emotional injury or minor physical injury, are usually not reported, and therefore are difficult to estimate. However, it is believed that 10% of all boys and 20% of all girls are in some way molested or abused sexually before they reach the age of 18. At least 5% of all abuse victims are also sexually abused.

In some cases, you may find a child who obviously has been sexually assaulted or has unexplained genital injury. In rare cases, the child himself may tell you that he was sexually assaulted. When any of these things occur, remain professional and control your emotions. Do not allow the child to become embarrassed. Do not say anything that may make the child believe that *he* is to blame for the sexual assault (many believe that they are). Tell the child that the people at the hospital will help him and that he should not be embarrassed.

Provide care as needed. Do not examine the genitalia unless there is obvious injury. Discourage the child from going to the bathroom (for both defecation and urination). Do not let the child wash or change clothes. It is very important that you do not give the patient anything by mouth. Transport the child and report your suspicions to the medical staff, making certain they understand that you are talking about possible sexual assault. As with all cases of child abuse, maintain patient and family confidentiality.

MEDICAL PROBLEMS COMMON TO CHILDREN

Like adults, children can suffer a variety of medical problems from "belly-ache" to heart attack. While emergency care measures for medical problems are the same for children as for adults, there are a few problems common to childhood that deserve attention.

Fever

Above-normal body temperature is one of the most important signs of an existing or impending acute illness. Fever usually accompanies such childhood diseases as measles, mumps, chicken pox, mononucleosis, pneumonia, and Reye's syndrome. The fever also may be due to heatstroke or some other noninfectious disease problem. NEVER regard a fever as unimportant. Do not try to diagnose or accept what the parents believe may be the problem. As an EMT, you cannot tell specifically what is wrong with the child, or what is likely to happen over the next few hours.

Many EMS Systems use relative skin temperature as a sign. If the infant or child feels too warm, or if he feels hot, then prepare the patient and transport. If you work with a squad that takes temperature by thermometer, be aware that a mild fever can quickly turn into a life-threatening one. Any child one to five years old with an oral temperature above 103°F MUST be transported. Any child from five to twelve with a temperature above 102°F MUST be transported.

High temperature can cause convulsions, coma, permanent damage to the central nervous system, or even death. Should you find an infant or child with a high fever:

1. Remove the child's clothing, but do not allow him to be exposed to conditions that may bring on sudden chills.
2. Cover the child with a towel that has been saturated in tepid water.
3. Transport as soon as possible, protecting the patient from temperature extremes.

Do NOT: use rubbing alcohol to cool the patient; submerge the child in a tub of cold water; or cover the child with a towel saturated with ice water. It is not the duty of an EMT to administer aspirin or other such fever-reducing compounds. In fact, it is probably illegal for you to do so in your locality.

Convulsions

High fever, epilepsy, meningitis, diabetic states, and many other medical problems can bring on convulsions. Usually, you will arrive after the convulsion has passed. You should assure an open airway, staying on the alert for vomiting. Interview the patient and any family members and bystanders who saw the convulsion. Ask how long it lasted and what part of the body was twitching. Assess the child for symptoms and signs, and note any injuries sustained during the convulsion. Transport all infants and children who have undergone a convulsive seizure. If the patient has another seizure in your presence, care for the patient the same as you would an adult. Keep in mind that the child will be in great need of emotional support.

Acute Abdomen

Infants and children can develop abdominal pain for a variety of reasons—appendicitis, intestinal influenza, gas pains, indigestion, bacterial infection of the bowels, and intussusception (in-tus-sus-SEP-shun)—the telescoping of one section of intestine into the adjoining one. You will not be able to tell one problem from another, nor would the basic EMT-level emergency care rendered be different if you could. Consider any abdominal pain or cramp to be serious in the child patient. Intermittent cramps may be just as serious a problem as steady cramps or pain. Fever, vomiting, blood in the stools, and lumps in the abdomen all indicate a potentially serious problem. Treat the child as you would an adult with acute abdomen. Remember, you will have to provide much more emotional support. Transport the child to a medical facility as soon as possible. If the parents cannot decide if they want their child to be transported, lead them away from the child and explain why it is important for the child to be seen by a physician.

Poisoning

Children are often the victims of accidental poisoning. The procedures described in Chapter 11, Section Two apply to infant, child, and adult. There are *some* special types of poisonings not often associated with adult patients, however. These special cases include:

- Aspirin Poisoning—Look for hyperventilation, vomiting, and sweating. In severe cases, convulsions, coma, or shock.
- Lead Poisoning—This usually comes from ingesting pieces of lead-base paints. Look for nausea with abdominal pain and vomiting. Muscle cramps, headache, muscle weakness, and irritability are often present.
- Iron Poisoning—Iron compounds such as ferrous sulfate are found in some vitamin tablets. As little as one gram of ferrous sulfate can be lethal to a child. Within 30 minutes to several hours, the child will show nausea and vomiting, often accompanied by bloody diarrhea. Typically, the child will go into shock; however, this may be delayed up to 24 hours as the child at first appears to be getting better.
- Petroleum Product Poisoning—The patient will usually be vomiting, with coughing or choking. In most cases, you will smell the distinctive odor of a petroleum distillate (gasoline, kerosene, heating fuel, etc.). Aspiration pneumonia is a serious problem for victims of petroleum poisoning.

REMEMBER: Care for poisonings as directed by your local poison control center.

Sudden Infant Death Syndrome

In the United States, **sudden infant death syndrome** (SIDS) strikes between 6,500 and 7,500 apparently healthy babies each year. These babies receive proper care, and frequently pass physical examinations within days of their sudden death. Some relationships have been drawn to family history of respiratory problems, but there is still no accepted reason for why these babies die.

The cause of SIDS can usually be related to respiratory failure. As an EMT, provide basic life support measures for the possible SIDS patient. Be certain the parents receive emotional support and that they know everything is being done for the child at the scene and in transport.

Parents who lose a child to SIDS often suffer intense guilt. If parents express such feelings, remind them that SIDS occurs to apparently healthy babies who are receiving the best parental care. In cases of SIDS, do not be embarrassed to express your sorrow for their loss, but do so only after a

Table 12.2: How to Distinguish Between SIDS and Child Abuse and Neglect*

Sudden Infant Death Syndrome	Child Abuse and Neglect
Incidence: Deaths: 6,500 - 7,500/year Highest: 2 to 4 months of age When: Winter Months	*Incidence:* Deaths: 1,000 to 4,000/year Deaths in Infants: 300/year When: No seasonal difference
Physical Appearance: • Exhibits no external signs of injury. • Exhibits ''natural'' appearance of dead baby: 　—Lividity—settling of blood; frothy drainage from nose/mouth 　—Small marks, e.g., diaper rash looks more severe 　—Cooling/rigor mortis-takes place quickly in infants (about 3 hours) • Appears to be well-developed baby, though may be small for age. • Other siblings appear normal and healthy.	*Physical Appearance:* • Distinguishable and visible signs of injury. 　—Broken bone(s) 　—Bruises 　—Burns 　—Cuts 　—Head trauma, e.g., black eye 　—Scars 　—Welts 　—Wounds • May be obviously wasted away (malnutrition). • Other siblings may show patterns of injuries commonly seen in child abuse and neglect.
May Initially Suspect SIDS • All of the above characteristics 　　PLUS • Parents say that infant was well and healthy when put to sleep (last time seen alive).	*May Initially Suspect Child Abuse/Neglect* • All of the above characteristics 　　PLUS • Parents' story does not ''sound right'' or cannot account for all injuries on infant.

NOTE: The determination of whether the child is or is not a SIDS victim is the responsibility of the medical examiner or medical coroner. **It is NOT the responsibility of the Emergency Medical Technician.**

*Bureau of Community Health Services (HSA/PHS): Training Emergency Responders: Sudden Infant Death Syndrome. An Instructor's Manual. 1979, p. C-3

physician has officially informed them of the child's death.

REMEMBER: Speaking with a suspicious tone or asking inappropriate questions may only increase the parents' sorrow.

SUMMARY

An infant is anyone under one year of age. Traditionally, a child is anyone from one to eight years of age; however, this does not mean that all factors applying to the care of adults can be used for individuals from 8 to 18 years of age.

Remember that you are a professional. Learn to control your emotions so that you can provide prompt and efficient care. You will need to provide emotional support to the patient, parents, and bystanders in cases of pediatric emergencies.

When conducting a primary survey, establish responsiveness by shaking or gently tapping the infant or child. Take care in establishing an airway. Too great a head-tilt may close the infant's or small child's airway. Deliver rescue breathing and interposed ventilations by the mouth-to-mouth and nose technique for infants and small children. The mouth-to-mouth method may be used for larger children. Clear the airway by providing four gentle breaths in rapid succession, four back blows, four chest thrusts (as you would in CPR), and finger probes (only when you can see the object and use your little finger for probing).

Rescue breathing is provided to the infant at the rate of one gentle breath (puff) every three seconds. For the child patient, the rate is one gentle breath every four seconds.

Establish an infant's pulse by feeling for the brachial pulse. Use the carotid pulse for children. For infants in cardiac arrest, compress the infant's sternum along the midline, directly between the nipples. Use the tips of two or three fingers to compress ¹/₂ to 1 inch. Provide 100 compressions per minute with 1 interposed ventilation every 5 compressions.

For the child in cardiac arrest, compress the sternum along the midline, directly between the nipples. Use the tips of two or three fingers for the young child and the heel of one hand for older children. Compress the sternum 1 to 1¹/₂ inches. Provide 80 compressions per minute with 1 interposed ventilation every 5 compressions.

An infant is considered to be in shock if he has lost 25 milliliters or more of blood, or his systolic blood pressure falls below 50 mmHg. A child is considered in shock if he has lost 500 milliliters or more of blood, or if his systolic blood pressure falls below 50 mmHg (preschooler), 60 mmHg (to age 12), or 70 mmHg (teenager).

Take your time with the interview when the patient is a child. Talk to the parents, but also direct questions to the child. Show the child, the parents, and bystanders that you are a concerned professional. Tell the child what you are going to do before you do it. Do not lie to the child. Tell the child when he may experience pain. Apply the correct values for vital signs to infant and child (see Table 12-1). Do not use adult vital sign figures for infants and children.

When conducting a physical examination of an infant or child patient, use the head-to-toe approach. Take special care to look for head injuries, signs of skull fracture, cervical spine injuries, unusual breathing sounds, abdominal tenderness, and rectal bleeding. ALWAYS conduct a neurological assessment. You may have to treat the infant as if he were an unconscious patient and depend upon response to painful stimuli.

In cases of head injury, note drowsiness, speech problems, vomiting, headache, unequal pupils, double vision, clear fluids or clear fluids and blood in the nose or ears, convulsions, and a stiff or sore neck (within days of the injury). Be certain parents are aware of what to look for if they do not allow you to transport the child.

Treat a bike fork compression injury as you would a broken ankle. Immobilize with a pillow splint and transport. Attempt to slide stuck rings off of fingers by using a lubricant. The same type of lubricant can be used to help free trapped extremities. Do not push the barb of a fishing hook through the patient's skin. Transport the patient and have a physician perform the procedure.

Always be alert to possible child abuse. Look for indications of injuries and behavior that may lead you to suspect physical or sexual abuse. Report all suspicions to the emergency department staff. Do a complete head-to-toe survey so that you will detect all obvious injuries and indications of past abuse. Remember to maintain patient and family confidentiality.

Do not underestimate the significance of fever, convulsions, and abdominal pain in infants and children. Any of these require you to transport the patient. Remember that many children are accidental poisoning victims, often by aspirin, lead, iron, and petroleum products. Follow the instructions of your local poison control center.

Sudden infant death syndrome victims should receive resuscitative measures. The parents will need strong emotional support. If they express feelings of guilt, tell them that SIDS occurs to thousands of apparently healthy babies each year. Even with the very best of care, these babies still die. Do not be embarrassed to express your own sorrow.

13 environmental emergencies

SECTION ONE: ENVIRONMENTAL EMERGENCIES

OBJECTIVES By the end of this section, you should be able to:

1. Define first, second, and third degree burns. (p. 299)

2. State the factors used in determining the severity of burns. (p. 299-300)

3. Define "rule of nines" and fill out a body chart for both adult and child patients. (p. 300)

4. List the factors used to distinguish between critical, moderate, and minor burns. (p. 300-1)

5. Describe the proper emergency care for thermal, chemical, and electrical burns. (p. 301-3)

6. Describe the proper emergency care for thermal and chemical burns to the eyes. (p. 303-4)

7. Describe the emergency care provided for smoke inhalation victims. (p. 304-5)

8. Use symptoms and signs to distinguish between heat cramps, heat exhaustion, and heatstroke. (p. 305-6, 7)

9. List the steps in caring for heat cramps, heat exhaustion, and heatstroke. (p. 307)

10. State how to distinguish between incipient, superficial, and deep frostbite. (p. 306, 8)

11. Describe the emergency care for incipient, superficial, and deep frostbite. (p. 308-9)

12. State how to detect and treat hypothermia. (p. 309-10)

13. Describe basic care procedures for the victim of an electrical accident. (p. 312)

14. Describe the EMT's role in hazardous materials accidents. (p. 312)

15. Describe emergency care procedures for radiation accidents. (pp. 316-7)

SKILLS As an EMT, you should be able to:

1. Classify burns as first, second, or third degree.

2. Use the rule of nines to determine the severity of a burn.

3. Provide care for thermal, chemical, electrical, and radiation burns.

4. Provide care for patients suffering from smoke inhalation.

5. Detect and care for heat cramps, heat exhaustion, and heatstroke.

6. Classify problems due to exposure to cold in terms of:
   - hypothermia
   - incipient frostbite (frostnip)
   - superficial frostbite (frostbite)
   - deep frostbite (freezing)

7. Provide care for patients with problems due to exposure to cold.

8. Provide care for special emergencies, including: electrical accidents, hazardous materials accidents, and radiation accidents.

TERMS you may be using for the first time:

First Degree Burn—a burn involving only the epidermis

Second Degree Burn—a burn involving the epidermis and the dermis, but not penetrating the dermis

Third Degree Burn—a full thickness burn with damage extending through the dermis

Alkali—a substance that is chemically basic, as opposed to being neutral or acid

Hyperthermia (HI-per-THURM-i-ah)—heat-related injury including heat cramps, heat exhaustion, and heatstroke

Heat Cramps—a condition brought about by loss of body fluids and salts due to profuse perspiration.

Heat Exhaustion—heat prostration. A mild form of shock caused when blood pools in the blood vessels of the skin in an attempt to rid the body of excess heat.

Heatstroke—commonly called "sunstroke." A true emergency where the patient stops sweating in response to the high temperatures around him.

Hypothermia (HI-po-THURM-i-ah)—a generalized cooling that may reduce the body temperature to a point where the body can no longer generate enough heat to support life

Incipient Frostbite—frostnip

Superficial Frostbite—commonly called "frostbite," where exposure to cold damages the skin and subcutaneous layers

Deep Frostbite—freezing of body tissue

Ionizing Radiation—the product of atomic decay, including alpha particles, beta particles, and gamma rays

Overpressure—an increase in pressure above normal atmospheric pressure limits

Dynamic Pressure—energy released as an airborne shock wave.

ENVIRONMENTAL FACTORS

Nearly any element or combination of elements in our daily lives can cause injury. From a practical point of view, environmental emergencies are those related to:

- Excessive heat
- Excessive cold
- Water and ice
- Electricity
- Hazardous materials
- Radiation

Often, it is the combination of two or more of the above that causes serious injury and complicates emergency care efforts. Excessive heat can cause shifts in the regulatory mechanisms of the body, leading to a true emergency. This can be combined with burns received from fires. Water is not only a danger in terms of drowning, but its temperature may bring about injury due to excessive cold. Electricity not only will burn the skin, but also will change vital chemical activities within the body.

Our skin is the first line of defense against the environment. For this reason, many environmental injuries involve the skin. The eyes sustain injuries usually avoided by other organs. Thus, the eyes also are involved in many environmental emergencies. Our airway opens the respiratory system to the outside, making the lining of the airway susceptible to damage from many environmental factors. Respiratory injury can extend from the nasal membranes to the level of microscopic structures of the lungs.

Body organs and their chemical activities can be altered because of environmental factors. Radiation can affect the cells deep within the body. Electricity can disrupt nerve, muscle, and heart actions. Many hazardous materials can destroy or alter cells that make up the body's tissues. Sometimes this action is rapid and dramatic; at other times it is slow and subtle.

As an EMT, you must be prepared to provide care for a variety of environmental emergencies. Keep in mind that such emergencies can occur anywhere, at any time.

EMS System Responsibilities

EMTs assess and provide care for patients who receive injuries due to environmental factors. However, EMTs are not usually trained to combat *all* the sources of injury, or to control *all* scenes involving environmental factors. Keep this in mind and remember that *your* safety must be the first consideration.

Typically, EMTs are trained to control the fire scene, but not to fight fires. They are capable of handling certain electrical emergencies, but are limited in rescue procedures. Water rescue, hazardous materials rescue, and radiation accident rescue all require specialized training. Even when other branches of emergency and rescue services attend victims, special training is required to guarantee the safety of the emergency care provider in such hazardous accidents.

REMEMBER: Do only what you have been trained to do. "Heroic" efforts can place you and your fellow rescuers in danger and may even delay proper care for the patient.

BURNS

Many EMS System responses involve burns. You must be able to classify, evaluate, and care for burn injuries.

For most cases involving burns, we tend to think only of injury to the skin. Since the skin is the part of the body constantly in direct contact with the environment, such an assumption is valid, but burns can do much more than injure the skin. Injuries from burns often involve structures below the skin, including muscles, bones, nerves, and blood vessels. The eyes can be injured beyond repair when burned. Respiratory system structures can be damaged, with possible airway obstruction, respiratory failure, and respiratory arrest. In addition to the physical damage caused by burns, patients also may suffer emotional and psychological problems that begin at the emergency scene and could last a lifetime.

Classifying Burns

Burns can be classified according to the agent causing the burn. The source of the burn also can be used to make the classification more specific. For example, the source of the burn can be heat. This can be reported as "thermal burns from contact with a radiator." You should report the *agent* causing the burn and, when practical, the *source* of the agent. The agent of burn can be:

- Thermal—including flame, radiation or excessive heat from fire, steam, and hot liquids and hot objects.
- Chemicals—including various acids, bases, and caustics
- Electricity—including AC current, DC current, and lightning
- Light—typically involving the eyes, with burns caused by intense light sources or ultraviolet light (includes sunlight).
- Radiation—Usually from nuclear sources. Ultraviolet light also is considered to be a source of radiation burn.

Never assume the source of the burn. What may appear to be a thermal burn could be from radiation. You may find minor thermal burns on the patient's face and forget to consider light burns to his eyes. Always gather information from your observations of the scene, bystanders' reports, and the patient interview.

Burns involving the skin can be classified as partial thickness and full thickness burns. **Partial thickness burns** can involve the epidermis, or the epidermis and the upper dermis, but they do not include burns that pass through the dermis to damage underlying tissues (see Chapter 8). A **full thickness burn** will pass through the epidermis and dermis, causing injury to subcutaneous layers. Both partial and full thickness burns are described by an evaluation system using the term "degree," with burns involving the skin classified as first, second, or third degree. The least serious burn is the first degree burn.

- *First Degree Burn*—A superficial injury that involves only the epidermis. It is characterized by pain, reddening of the skin, and perhaps some swelling. The burn will heal of its own accord without scarring. Since the skin is not burned through, this type of burn is evaluated as a *mild partial thickness burn.*
- *Second Degree Burn*—The first layer of skin is burned through and the second layer is damaged, but the burn does not pass through to underlying tissues. There will be deep intense pain, intense reddening, blisters, and a mottled (spotted) appearance to the skin. Burns of this type have swelling and blistering for 48 hours after the injury as plasma and tissue fluids are released and rise to the top layer of skin. A second degree burn is called a *partial thickness burn.* When treated with reasonable care, second degree burns will heal themselves and produce very little scarring.
- *Third Degree Burn*—This is a *full thickness burn,* with all the layers of the skin damaged. Some third degree burns are difficult to tell from second degree burns; however, there usually are areas charred black or areas that are dry and white. The patient may complain of severe pain, or, if enough nerves have been damaged, he may feel no pain at all (except at the periphery of the burn where adjoining second degree burns may be causing pain). This type of burn may require skin grafting. As third degree burns heal, dense scars form.

Determining the Severity of Burns

Whenever you must determine the severity of a burn, consider the following factors:
- Source of the burn
- Body regions burned
- Degree of burn
- Extent of burned areas
- Age of patient
- Other patient illnesses and injuries

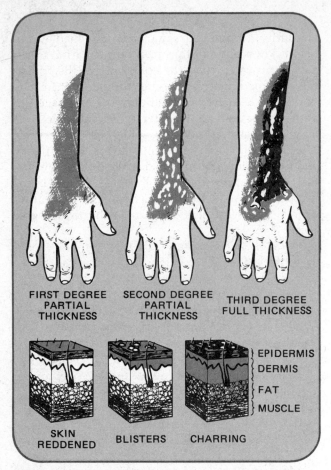

FIRST DEGREE
PARTIAL
THICKNESS

SECOND DEGREE
PARTIAL
THICKNESS

THIRD DEGREE
FULL THICKNESS

EPIDERMIS
DERMIS
FAT
MUSCLE

SKIN
REDDENED

BLISTERS

CHARRING

Figure 13-1: Severity of burns.

The source of the burn can be significant in terms of patient assessment. A minor burn caused by nuclear radiation is of more concern than one caused by thermal sources. Chemical burns are of special concern since the chemical may remain on the skin and continue to burn for hours, or even days, eventually entering the bloodstream. This sometimes happens with certain alkaline chemicals.

Any burn of the face is of special concern, since it may involve injury to the airway or injury to the eyes. The hands and feet also are areas of special concern because scarring may cause some loss of movement of fingers or toes. Special care is required to prevent aggravation to the injury by patient movement, and to prevent the damaged tissues from sticking together prior to transfer at the hospital. Circumferential burns (burns to major joints) can be very serious. Burns of this type may interrupt circulation to the tissues distal to the burn site. When the groin, buttocks, or medial thighs are burned, the chances for bacterial contamination present unusual problems that can be far more serious than the damaged tissues themselves.

The degree of burn is important. In second and third degree burns, the outer layer of the skin is penetrated. This can lead to contamination of exposed tissues and invasion of the circulatory system.

It is important that you be able to estimate the extent of the burn area. The amount of skin surface involved can be calculated quickly by using the

"**Rule of Nines.**" Each of the following areas represents 9% of the body surface: the head and neck, each upper limb, the chest, the abdomen, the upper back, the lower back and buttocks, the front of each lower limb, and the back of each lower limb. These make up 99% of the body's surface. The remaining 1% is assigned to the genital region.

These figures apply only to adults. The system for infants and children is far more complex, as shown in Figure 13-2. At the emergency scene, it is more practical to consider the infant's head and neck as 18%, each upper limb 9%, the chest and abdomen 18%, the entire back 18%, each lower limb 14%, and the genital region 1%. True, this adds up to 101%, but it is only used to give a rough determination. Note that the head of the infant receives an 18% value. The head of a child is much larger in proportion to the rest of the body than in the adult.

Age is a major factor in burn cases. Infants, children under age 5, and adults over 60 have more severe body reactions to burns and different healing patterns than do other age groups. Burn intensity and body area involvement that would be classified as minor to moderate for a young adult may be fatal for an infant or the aged.

Obviously, patients with respiratory illnesses will be placed in greater jeopardy when exposed to heated air or chemical vapors. Likewise, the stress of an environmental emergency leading to a burn will undoubtedly be of concern to patients with heart disease. Patients with respiratory ailments, heart disease, kidney disease, or diabetes will react more severely to burn damage. What may be a minor burn for a healthy adult could be of major significance to these types of patients.

Injuries other than burns may compromise the individual's health. When the *stress* of a burn is added, the seriousness of a patient's emergency may lead to shock or some other life-threatening problem. Treat all burns as more serious if accompanied by other injuries.

Classifying the Severity of Burns

Burns must be classified as to severity. Once the factors affecting severity have been noted, the following classification can be used:

Critical Burns
- ALL burns complicated by injuries of the respiratory tract, soft tissues, and bones.
- Third degree burns involving the face, hands, feet, groin, or major joints.
- Third degree burns involving more than 10% of the body surface.
- Second degree burns involving more than 30% of the body surface.

Moderate Burns
- Third degree burns that involve less than

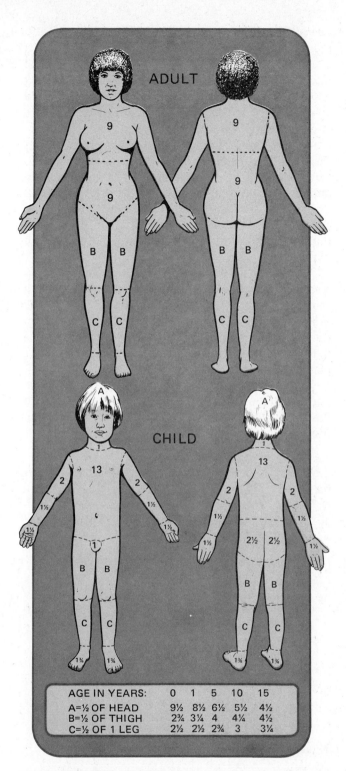

Figure 13-2: The Rule of Nines.

AGE IN YEARS:	0	1	5	10	15
A=½ OF HEAD	9½	8½	6½	5½	4½
B=½ OF THIGH	2¾	3¼	4	4¼	4½
C=½ OF 1 LEG	2½	2½	2¾	3	3¼

10% of the body surface, excluding face, hands, feet, groin, or major joints.
- Second degree burns that involve 15 to 30% of the body surface.
- First degree burns that involve 50 to 75% of the body surface.
  Minor Burns
- Third degree burns involving less than 2% of the body surface, excluding face, hands, feet, groin, or major joints.

- Second degree burns that involve less than 15% of the body surface.
- First degree burns that involve less than 20% of the body surface.

EMERGENCY CARE FOR BURNS

Other emergencies receive care before burns. Airway obstruction, severe breathing difficulties, respiratory arrest, cardiac arrest, severe bleeding, shock, spinal injuries, severe head injuries, open chest wounds, and open abdominal wounds take priority over burns. This holds true for the individual patient with any of these emergencies as well as burns, or when deciding the order of treatment and transport at the multiple-patient scene.

Certain *medical* problems are cared for before burns. These include heart attack, stroke, heatstroke, poisoning, and abnormal childbirth. Again, this applies to both the single-patient and the multiple-patient scene.

Burns involving the respiratory tract are considered *high-priority emergencies.* This is the only burn that most EMS Systems rate as highly as the injuries and medical problems listed previously. Immediate transport is called for if the patient has burns that can be classified as critical. Since age can be a factor, immediate transport is usually recommended for any child or elderly patient with deep or extensive second or third degree burns. Likewise, a patient with known chronic respiratory disease, heart disease, past history of stroke, or diabetes will usually be considered for immediate transport.

If more than one patient is injured, transport is generally done in the order of estimated severity, but some consideration is given to the benefits of awaiting care. Patients with respiratory tract injury, or complications involving respiration or heart action, are typically given first transport. Some systems next transport those patients with severe burns covering 60 to 80% of the body surface. They justify waiting on patients with severe burns over 80% or more of the body on the grounds that death is likely and the other patients have a higher chance of survival if transported as soon as possible. Pain is also a consideration for order of transport. Remember that third degree burn patients with the most serious burns will often have little or no pain due to the damage of nerve endings. It may seem cruel to let a second degree burn patient in pain wait, but if the third degree burn patient has more serious injuries, he is to be transported first.

NOTE: The order of patient care and transport varies according to locality. The above is only one example. Follow your local guidelines. More will be said about the triage of patients in Chapter 14.

REMEMBER: If in doubt when evaluating a burn,

overclassify. If you are uncertain whether a burn is first degree or second degree, consider the burn to be second degree. If you are uncertain as to whether a burn is second or third degree, consider it third degree.

Treating Thermal Burns

CAUTION: Do NOT attempt to rescue people trapped by fire unless you are trained to do so, and have the equipment and personnel required. The simple act of opening a door could cost you your life. In some fires, opening a door or window can greatly intensify the fire or even cause an explosion. Problems at the fire scene will be covered in Chapter 16.

As an EMT, you will have to care for thermal burns caused by scalding liquids, steam, contact with hot objects, flames, and flaming liquids and gases. On rare occasions, you may be called to care for sunburn. Seldom is this a problem requiring transport, except for severe cases involving infants and young children. These patients usually have other heat-related injuries that are the primary reason for transport.

The basic care for thermal burns is set forth in the next Scansheet. Local protocols may vary somewhat depending upon the procedures used at the local burn center or medical facility. Third degree burns are to be wrapped with dry sterile dressing or a burn sheet. Some burn centers recommend moist dressings for partial thickness burns to 9% or less of the body and dry dressings for more severe cases. EMTs do not treat burns, they provide *supportive care* for burns until the patient can be transferred to the staff of a medical facility. NEVER apply ointments, sprays, or butter to the burn site. To do so would delay needed treatment while the emergency department staff removes these substances.

Treating Chemical Burns

CAUTION: Some scenes where chemical burns have occurred can be very hazardous. Always evaluate the scene. There may be large pools of dangerous chemicals around the patient. Acids could be spurting from broken containers. There may be toxic fumes present. If the scene will place you in danger, do NOT attempt a rescue unless you are trained for such a situation and have the needed equipment and personnel at the scene.

Chemical burns require *immediate* care. Hopefully, people at the scene will begin this care before you arrive. At many industrial sites, workers and First Responders are trained to provide initial care for accidents involving the chemicals in use. Most major industries have emergency deluge-type safety showers to wash dangerous chemicals from the body. This will not always be the case. Be prepared for situations where nothing has been done and there is no running water near the scene.

Immediate action is called for with chemical burns. The primary procedure of care is to WASH AWAY the chemical by using flowing water. Simply wetting the burn site is not enough. Continuous flooding of the affected area is required, using a copious, but gentle flow of water. Avoid hard sprays that may damage badly burned tissues. Continue to wash the area for several minutes, removing contaminated clothing, shoes, socks, and jewelry from the patient AS YOU APPLY THE WASH. If the chemical burns prove to be mild, wash again with mild soap and water. Do NOT apply soap to major burns.

Once you have washed the burned areas, apply a sterile dressing or burn sheet, treat for shock, and transport the patient. When possible, find out the exact chemical or mixture of chemicals involved in the accident. Be on the alert for delayed reactions that may cause renewed pain, or interfere with the patient's ability to breathe.

Should the patient complain of increased burning or irritation, wash the burned areas again with flowing water for several minutes. Avoid removing dressings once they are in place.

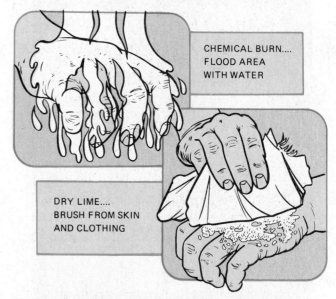

CHEMICAL BURN....
FLOOD AREA
WITH WATER

DRY LIME....
BRUSH FROM SKIN
AND CLOTHING

Figure 13-3: Emergency care for chemical burns.

Many of the chemicals used in industrial processes are mixed acids. Their combined action can be immediate and severe. The pain produced from the initial chemical burn may mask any pain being caused by renewed burning due to small concentrations left on the skin. When the chemical is a strong acid (e.g., hydrochloric or sulfuric acid), a combination of acids, or an unknown, play it safe and continue washing even after the patient claims he is no longer in pain.

There are some special situations:
• If dry lime is the burn agent, do NOT wash

CARE FOR THERMAL BURNS

TYPE OF BURN	TISSUE BURNED		TISSUES BELOW SKIN	COLOR CHANGES	PAIN	BLISTERS
	OUTER LAYER OF SKIN	2nd LAYER OF SKIN				
1st DEGREE	+	−	−	RED	+	−
2nd DEGREE	+	+	−	DEEP RED	+	+
3rd DEGREE	+	+	+	CHARRED BLACK OR WHITE	+/−	+ /−

FIRST AND SECOND DEGREE

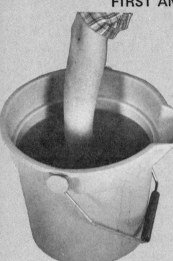

- IMMERSE IN COLD WATER 2-5 MINUTES
- COVER ENTIRE BURN WITH DRY STERILE DRESSING
- TRANSPORT, AND CONTINUE COLD WATER APPLICATION

FOR EXTENSIVE FIRST, SECOND & THIRD DEGREE BURNS

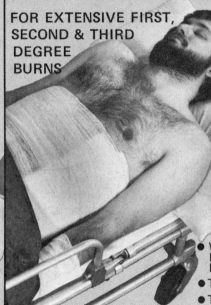

- WRAP AREA WITH DRY STERILE DRESSING
- TREAT FOR SHOCK
- TRANSPORT

IF HANDS OR TOES ARE BURNED

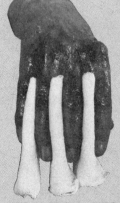
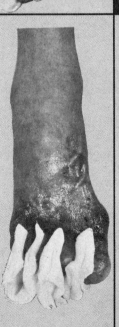

- SEPARATE DIGITS WITH STERILE GAUZE PADS
- MOISTEN PADS WITH STERILE WATER

BURNS TO THE EYES

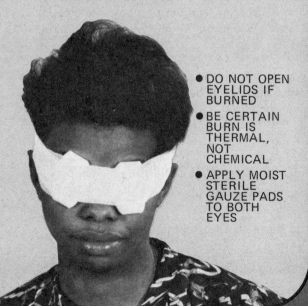

- DO NOT OPEN EYELIDS IF BURNED
- BE CERTAIN BURN IS THERMAL, NOT CHEMICAL
- APPLY MOIST STERILE GAUZE PADS TO BOTH EYES

SCAN 13-1

the burn site with water. To do so will create a corrosive liquid. *Brush* the dry lime from the patient's skin, hair, and clothing. Make certain you do not contaminate his eyes or airway. Use water *only* if the lime has been brushed from the body, contaminated clothing and jewelry has been removed, and the process of washing can be done quickly and continuously with running water.

● Carbolic acid (phenol) does not mix with water. When available, use *alcohol* for the initial wash, followed by a long steady wash with water.

● Concentrated sulfuric acid produces heat when water is added. An initial wash with mild soapy water can be used if the burns are not severe when you begin to provide care.

● Hydrofluoric acid is used for etching glass and in many other manufacturing processes. Since burns may be delayed, treat *all* patients who may have come into contact with the chemical. First apply a bicarbonate of soda solution and then flood with water. If burning sensations are severe when you arrive, immediately begin the water wash. Do NOT delay care and transport to find any neutralizing agents.

Anytime a patient is exposed to a caustic chemical and may have inhaled the vapors, provide humidified oxygen and transport as soon as possible. This is very important when the chemical is an acid known to vaporize at standard environmental temperatures (e.g., hydrochloric or sulfuric acid).

Chemical Burns to the Eyes   A corrosive chemical can burn the globe of a person's eye before he can react and close the eyelid. Even with the lid shut, chemicals can seep through onto the globe. To care for chemical burns to the eye, you should:

1. IMMEDIATELY flood the eyes with water.
2. Keep running water from a faucet, low pressure hose, bucket, cup, bottle, rubber bulb syringe, or other such source flowing into the burned eye. The flow should be from the medial (nasal) corner of the eye to the lateral corner. Since the patient's natural reaction will be to keep his eyes tightly shut, you may have to hold the eyelids open.
3. Continue washing the eye for the following time periods:

Acid Burns—At least 5 minutes

Alkali Burns—At least 15 minutes

Unknown Caustic—At least 20 minutes

4. After washing, cover both eyes with moistened pads, and transport as soon as possible. You may find it to the patient's advantage to wash during transport.

5. Wash the patient's eyes for 5 more minutes if he begins to complain about renewed burning sensations or irritation.

WARNING! Do NOT use neutralizers such as vinegar or baking soda in a patient's eyes.

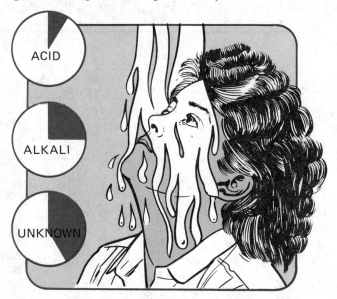

Figure 13-4: Care of chemical burns to the eyes.

Smoke Inhalation

Smoke inhalation is a serious problem associated with the scenes of thermal and chemical burns. The smoke from any fire source contains poisonous substances. Modern building materials and furnishings often contain plastics and other synthetics that release toxic fumes when they burn or are overheated. It is possible for the substances found in smoke to burn the skin, irritate the eyes, injure the airway, cause respiratory arrest and, in some cases, to cause cardiac arrest.

As an EMT, you will most likely see irritation of the eyes and injury of the airway associated with smoke. Irritation to the skin and eyes may be treated by simple flooding with water. Your first priority will be the patient's airway. The patient usually will have difficulty breathing, often accompanied by coughing. Note if his breath has a "smoky" smell or the odor of chemicals involved at the scene. In cases of smoke or toxic gas inhalation, you should:

1. Move the patient to a safe area.
2. Do a primary survey and supply life support measures as needed.
3. Administer oxygen in high concentration and continue this throughout transport. When possible, the oxygen should be humidified.
4. Care for possible spinal injuries and any other injury or illness requiring care at the scene.
5. Treat for shock. Most conscious patients are

able to breathe more easily when kept in a semi-seated position.

6. Transport as soon as possible, providing oxygen and monitoring the patient's vital signs.

NOTE: The body's reaction to toxic gases and foreign matter in the airway often can be delayed. It is a good procedure to have all smoke inhalation patients seen by a physician.

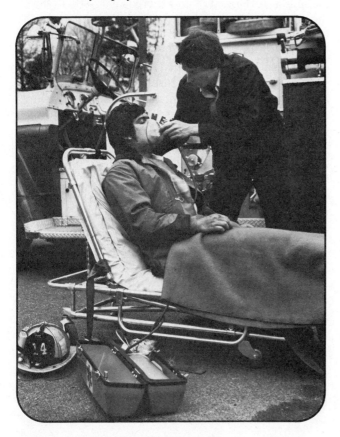

Figure 13-5: Care for smoke inhalation.

EMERGENCIES DUE TO EXCESSIVE HEAT

Heat is generated as a result of constant chemical processes within the body. A certain amount of this heat is required to maintain normal body temperature. The excess heat is given off by the body through three major avenues:

- *Respiration*—the air we exhale is warm. As the body overheats, respirations become more rapid.
- *Radiation*—heat is released at the surface of the skin. When there is an excess of heat in the body, blood flow to the skin increases, sometimes pooling in the vessels of the skin. This allows for more heat to be lost through the skin.
- *Evaporative Heat Loss*—perspiration is given off from glands in the dermis of the skin. As this

perspiration evaporates, the skin is cooled and heat is lost in the process.

Consider what can happen to the body when it is placed in a hot environment. Air being inhaled is warm, possibly warmer than the air being exhaled. The skin may actually absorb more heat than it radiates. Add to this high humidity, slowing down the evaporation of perspiration. To make things even more difficult, consider all this in an environment that lacks circulating air or a breeze which would speed up radiation and evaporation heat loss. What exists now is the environment often associated with emergencies due to excessive heat, or **hyperthermia.** This is why a "heat wave" greatly increases EMS responses for heat-related emergencies.

Since evaporative heat loss is reduced, moist heat can produce dramatic body changes in a short period of time. However, moist heat usually tires individuals very quickly, frequently stopping them from overexerting and harming themselves. Yet some people continue to push, running the risk of placing their bodies in a state of emergency.

Dry heat often deceives individuals. They continue to work in or remain exposed to excess heat far beyond the point that their bodies can tolerate. This is the reason why you may see problems caused by dry heat exposure that are worse than those seen in moist heat exposure.

The same rules of care apply to heat-related emergencies as to any emergency. You will still have to perform patient surveys and interviews. Do NOT overlook other possible problems. Collapse due to heat exposure may result in a fall that can fracture bones. A history of high blood pressure, heart disease, or lung problems may have quickened the effects of heat exposure. What appears to be a problem related to heat exposure could be a heart attack. Age, diseases, and existing injuries all must be considered when evaluating the patient. Always consider the problem to be greater if the patient is very young, elderly, injured, or has a chronic disease.

There are three common emergencies brought about by exposure to excessive heat:

- HEAT CRAMPS—brought about by long exposure to heat. The emergency scene temperature does not have to be much greater than what would be considered to be a "normal" environmental temperature. The individual perspires heavily, often drinking large quantities of water. As the sweating continues, salts are lost by the body, bringing on painful muscle cramps. Researchers are trying to determine if the loss of water alone is enough to cause heat cramps. Most medical authorities still believe it is a combination of water and salt loss that brings on the condition.
- HEAT EXHAUSTION—the typical heat ex-

haustion patient is a healthy individual who has been exposed to excessive heat while working or exercising. This is a mild form of shock caused by blood pooling in the skin as the body attempts to rid itself of excess heat. This problem is often seen with firefighters, construction workers, dock workers and those employed in poorly ventilated warehouses. Heat exhaustion is more of a problem during the summer and reaches a peak during prolonged heat waves.

- HEATSTROKE—this is a TRUE EMERGENCY, brought about when a person fails to sweat in response to the increase in temperature around him. Athletes, laborers, and others who exercise or work in hot environments are common victims. More cases of heatstroke are reported on hot, humid days. However, many cases occur from exposure to dry heat. Even though heatstroke is commonly called ''sunstroke,'' it can be caused by excessive heat other than from the sun. ALL cases of heatstroke are serious and require sending the patient to a medical facility as soon as possible.

The symptoms and signs of heat cramps, heat exhaustion, and heatstroke are compared in the next Scansheet. Care procedures also are listed.

EMERGENCIES DUE TO EXCESSIVE COLD

As noted in the section on heat-related emergencies, the human body generates heat, trying to keep a temperature of 98.6°F (37°C). This involves a balance of the heat being generated, the heat lost, and the heat absorbed from the environment. If the environment is too cold, body heat can be lost faster than it can be generated. The body attempts to adjust by reducing respirations, perspiration, and circulation to the skin. Muscular activity will increase in the form of shivering to generate more heat. The rate at which fuel foods are burned within the body increases to produce more heat. At a certain point, enough heat will not be available to all parts of the body, leading to damage of exposed tissues, a general reduction of body functions, or the cessation of a vital body function. An EMT's actions can prevent long rehabilitation due to cold-related injuries, keep body parts from becoming nonfunctional, and may even save the patient's life.

Cold-related emergencies can be the result of local cooling or general cooling. **Local cooling** injuries are those affecting particular parts of the body. They are grouped under the heading of *frostbite*. **General cooling** affects the entire body. This problem is known as **hypothermia** (hi-po-THURM-i-ah).

The body can lose heat by **conduction**. This is a direct transfer of heat from the warm body into the cold environment. Heat also can be lost by **convection** as cool air passes over the body surface and carries away body heat. If a person's body or clothing becomes wet, **waterchill** becomes a problem. Water conducts heat away from the body 240 times faster than still air. The effects of a cold environment also can be made worse by **windchill**. The more wind, the more heat loss by the body. Wind increases the effects of cold temperatures. For example, if it is 10°F outside and there is a 20 MPH wind, the amount of heat lost by the body is the same as if it were -25°F.

When evaluating the effects of cold temperatures on a patient, you must consider temperature, windchill, waterchill, exposed areas of the body, clothing, length of exposure, health of the patient, existing injuries, age, and how active the patient was during exposure. Patients with injuries or chronic illnesses will show the effects of cold much sooner than healthy people. The elderly will be more quickly affected. The unconscious patient lying on the cold ground will tend to have greater cold-related problems than one who is conscious and able to walk about.

Local Cooling

Local cooling is **frostbite**. Most commonly affected are the ears, nose, hands, and feet. When a part of the body is exposed to intensely cold air or liquid, blood flow to that particular part is limited by the constriction of blood vessels. When this happens, tissues do not receive enough warmth to prevent freezing. In the most severe cases, gangrene can set in and ultimately lead to the loss of tissues.

There are three degrees of frostbite:

- FROSTNIP—this is incipient frostbite, brought about by direct contact with a cold object or exposure of a body part to cold air. Windchill and waterchill can be major factors. This condition is not serious. Tissue damage is minor and the response to care is good. The tip of the nose, the tips of the ears, the upper cheeks, and the fingers (all areas generally exposed) are most susceptible to frostnip.

- SUPERFICIAL FROSTBITE—commonly called ''frostbite.'' The skin and subcutaneous layers become involved. If frostnip goes untreated, it becomes superficial frostbite.

- FREEZING—this is deep frostbite where the skin, the subcutaneous layers, and the deeper structures of the body are affected. Muscles, bones, deep blood vessels, and organ membranes can become frozen.

NOTE: As an EMT, do not listen to bystanders' myths and folktales about care of frostbite. NEVER

HEAT RELATED EMERGENCIES

CONDITION	MUSCLE CRAMPS	BREATHING	PULSE	WEAKNESS	SKIN	PERSPIRATION	LOSS OF CONSCIOUSNESS
HEAT CRAMPS	+	VARIES	VARIES	+	MOIST-WARM-NO CHANGE	HEAVY	SELDOM
HEAT EXHAUSTION	–	RAPID SHALLOW	WEAK	+	COLD CLAMMY	HEAVY	SOMETIMES
HEAT-STROKE	–	DEEP THEN SHALLOW	FULL RAPID	+	DRY–HOT	LITTLE OR NONE	OFTEN

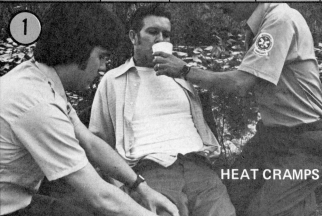

HEAT CRAMPS

SIGNS AND SYMPTOMS: SEVERE MUSCLE CRAMPS (USUALLY IN THE LEGS AND ABDOMEN) EXHAUSTION, SOMETIMES DIZZINESS OR FAINTNESS

EMERGENCY CARE PROCEDURES:
- MOVE PATIENT TO A NEARBY COOL PLACE
- GIVE PATIENT SALTED WATER TO DRINK, OR COMMERCIAL ELECTROLYTE FLUIDS
- HELP EASE CRAMPS BY MUSCLE MASSAGE. MASSAGE WITH PRESSURE IS MORE EFFECTIVE THAN LIGHT RUBBING ACTION
- APPLY WARM, MOIST TOWELS TO THE FOREHEAD AND OVER CRAMPED MUSCLES FOR ADDED RELIEF
- IF CRAMPS PERSIST, OR IF MORE SERIOUS SIGNS AND SYMPTOMS DEVELOP, READY THE PATIENT AND TRANSPORT

SIGNS AND SYMPTOMS: RAPID SHALLOW BREATHING, WEAK PULSE, COLD CLAMMY SKIN, HEAVY PERSPIRATION, TOTAL BODY WEAKNESS, AND DIZZINESS LEADING TO UNCONSCIOUSNESS

EMERGENCY CARE PROCEDURES:
- MOVE THE PATIENT TO A NEARBY COOL PLACE
- KEEP THE PATIENT AT REST
- REMOVE ENOUGH CLOTHING TO COOL THE PATIENT WITHOUT CHILLING HIM
- GIVE PATIENT SALTED WATER TO DRINK, OR COMMERCIAL ELECTROLYTE FLUIDS. DO NOT ADMINISTER FLUIDS TO UNCONSCIOUS PATIENT
- TREAT FOR SHOCK, BUT DO NOT COVER TO THE POINT OF OVERHEATING PATIENT
- IF UNCONSCIOUS, FAILS TO RECOVER RAPIDLY, HAS INJURIES OR MEDICAL HISTORY, TRANSPORT AS SOON AS POSSIBLE

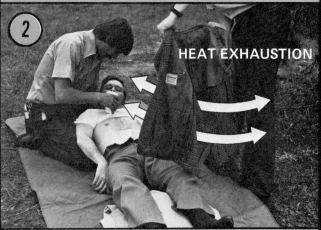

HEAT EXHAUSTION

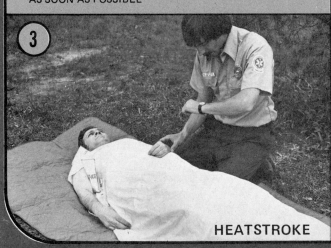

HEATSTROKE

SIGNS AND SYMPTOMS: DEEP BREATHS, THEN SHALLOW BREATHING, RAPID, STRONG PULSE, THEN RAPID WEAK PULSE; DRY, HOT SKIN, DILATED PUPILS; LOSS OF CONSCIOUSNESS (POSSIBLE COMA) CONVULSIONS OR MUSCULAR TWITCHING

EMERGENCY CARE PROCEDURES:
- COOL PT.–IN ANY MANNER, RAPIDLY. MOVE PT. OUT OF SUN, OR AWAY FROM HEAT SOURCE. REMOVE CLOTHING–WRAP IN WET TOWELS OR SHEETS. POUR COLD WATER OVER WRAPPINGS. BODY HEAT MUST LOWER RAPIDLY OR BRAIN CELLS DIE!
- WRAP COLD PACKS OR ICE BAGS, IF AVAILABLE & PLACE ONE UNDER EACH ARMPIT, EACH WRIST, EACH ANKLE, AND EACH SIDE OF PATIENT'S NECK
- TRANSPORT AS SOON AS POSSIBLE
- IF TRANSPORT DELAYED, FIND TUB OR CONTAINER–IMMERSE PT. UP TO FACE IN COOLED WATER. MONITOR IN ORDER TO PREVENT DROWNING
- MONITOR VITAL SIGNS THROUGHOUT PROCESS

SCAN 13-2

rub a frostbitten or frozen area. NEVER rub snow on a frostbitten or frozen area. To do so can cause serious damage to the already injured tissues.

As an EMT, you will need to know the symptoms, signs, and care procedures for all three degrees of frostbite. Notice how the symptoms and signs of frostbite are progressive. First, the exposed skin reddens. Then, as exposure continues, the skin takes on a gray or white blotchy appearance. Exposed skin surfaces become numb, due to reduced circulation. If the freezing process is allowed to continue, all sensation is lost and the skin becomes dead white.

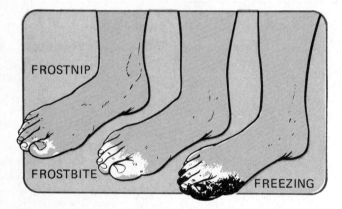

Figure 13-6: The three degrees of frostbite.

Table 13.1: Exposure to Excessive Cold

CONDITION	SKIN SURFACE	TISSUE UNDER SKIN	SKIN COLOR
Frostnip	Soft	Soft	Initially Red, then White
Frostbite	Hard	Soft	White and Waxy
Freezing	Hard	Hard	Blotchy, White to Yellow-Gray to Blue-Gray

Frostnip/Incipient Frostbite

The symptoms and signs of frostnip include:

- Slow onset—frostnip usually takes some time to develop.
- Patient unawareness—most people with frostnip are not aware of the problem until someone indicates that there is something unusual about their skin color.
- Skin color changes—the area of the skin affected will at first redden, then it blanches (becomes white). Once blanching begins, the color change can take place very quickly.
- Loss of sensation—the affected area will feel numb to the patient.

Emergency care for frostnip is simple. . .warm the affected area. Usually, the patient can apply warmth from his own bare hands, blow warm air on the site or, if the fingers are involved, hold them in the armpits. During recovery from frostnip, the patient may complain about "tingling" or burning sensations, which is normal. If the condition does not respond to this simple care, begin to treat for frostbite.

Superficial and Deep Frostbite

The symptoms and signs of superficial frostbite are:

- The affected area of the skin appears white and waxy.
- The affected area will feel frozen, but only on the surface. The tissue below the surface MUST still be soft and have its normal "bounce."

The symptoms and signs of freezing include:

- The skin will turn mottled or blotchy. The color will turn to white, then grayish yellow and finally a grayish blue.
- The tissues feel frozen to the touch, without the underlying resilience characteristc of superficial frostbite.

Initial care for superficial frostbite and for deep frostbite is the same:

When the patient can be transported to a medical facility without delay, protect the frostbitten area by covering the site of injury and handling the affected part as gently as possible.

Where practical, transport should be as soon as possible, but if transport must be delayed, get the patient indoors and keep him warm. Do not allow the patient to smoke. Smoking causes blood vessels to constrict, increasing any circulation problems in the damaged tissues. Rewarm the frozen part. To do so, you will need a container to heat water and a container to immerse the entire site of injury WITHOUT the limb touching the sides or bottom. If you cannot find a suitable container, fashion one from a plastic bag supported by a cardboard box or wooden crate. Proceed as follows:

1. Heat some water to a temperature between 100°F and 105°F. You should be able to put your finger into the water without experiencing discomfort.
2. Fill the container with the water and prepare the injured part by removing any clothing, bands, or straps.
3. Fully immerse the injured part of the body. Do NOT allow the frostbitten area to touch the sides or bottom of the container. When the water cools below 100°F, remove the limb and add more warm water. The patient may complain of pain as the affected area rewarms.

4. If you complete rewarming the part (it no longer feels frozen and is turning red or blue in color), gently dry the affected area and apply a sterile dressing. Place pads of dressing material between fingers and toes before dressing hands and feet. Next, cover the site with blankets or whatever is available to keep the affected area warm. Do NOT allow these coverings to come in direct contact with the injured area. Best results are obtained if you first build some sort of framework on which the coverings can rest.

5. Make certain you keep the entire patient as warm as possible without overheating. Continue to monitor the patient.

6. Assist circulation by rhythmically and carefully raising and lowering the affected limb.

7. Transport as soon as possible with the affected limb slightly elevated. Keep the entire patient warm.

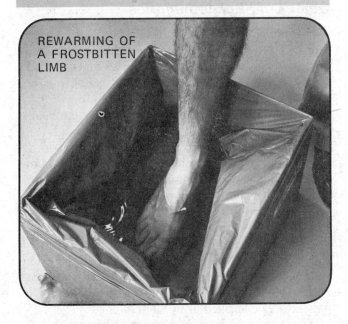

REWARMING OF A FROSTBITTEN LIMB

Figure 13-7: Rewarming the frozen part.

General Cooling/Hypothermia

The generalized cooling of the human body is known as **systemic hypothermia** (HI-po-THURM-i-ah). Exposure to cold reduces body heat. With time, the body is unable to maintain its proper internal temperature. If allowed to continue, hypothermia leads to death. Be aware that hypothermia can develop in temperatures *above* freezing.

Hypothermia is often a serious problem for the aged. During the winter months, many older people attempt to live in rooms that are kept too cool. Failing body systems, chronic illness, poor diet, and a lack of exercise combine with a cold environment to bring about hypothermia.

The symptoms and signs of hypothermia include:

- Shivering (early stages when body core temperature is above 88°F)
- Feelings of numbness
- Drowsiness, and unwilling to do even the simplest of activities, plus decreased level of consciousness.
- Slow breathing and pulse rates (seen in cases of prolonged hypothermia)
- Failing eyesight (seen in cases of prolonged hypothermia)
- Coordination difficulties (the patient may stagger)
- Unconsciousness, usually the patient has a "glassy stare" (seen in extreme cases).
- Freezing of body parts (seen in the most extreme cases). Action must be taken immediately as the patient may be near death.

Table 13.2: The Stages of Systemic Hypothermia

Body Temperature	Symptoms
99°F to 96°F	Intense, uncontrollable shivering.
95°F to 91°F	Violent shivering persists. If victim is conscious, he has difficulty speaking.
90°F to 86°F	Shivering decreases, is replaced by strong muscular rigidity. Muscle coordination is affected. Erratic or jerky movements are produced. Thinking is less clear. General comprehension is dulled. There may be total amnesia. The victim is generally still able to maintain the appearance of psychological contact with his surroundings.
85°F to 81°F	Victim becomes irrational, loses contact with his environment, and drifts into a stuporous state. Muscular rigidity continues. Pulse and respirations are slowed.
80°F to 78°F	Victim becomes unconscious. He does not respond to the spoken word. Most reflexes cease to function. Heartbeat becomes erratic.
Below 78°F	Cardiac and respiratory centers of the brain fail. Ventricular fibrillation occurs; probable edema and hemorrhage in the lungs; death.

The care of mild hypothermia requires you to:

1. Do patient surveys and interviews to determine the extent of the problem.

2. Keep the patient dry. Remove any wet

clothing and replace with dry items, or wrap the patient in blankets. Be sure to wrap the patient's head, leaving the face exposed.
3. Use heat to raise the patient's body temperature. This can be done during transport. If transport is delayed, move the patient to a warm environment if at all possible. Gently apply heat to the patient's body in the form of heat packs, hot water bottles, electric heating pads, hot air, radiated heat, and your own body heat and that of bystanders. DO NOT WARM THE PATIENT TOO QUICKLY. Rapid warming will release pooled blood, possibly causing serious heart problems (ventricular fibrillation).

If transport must be delayed, a warm bath is very helpful, but you must keep the patient alert enough so that he does not drown. *Constant* monitoring is necessary for unconscious patients. Again, do not warm the patient too quickly.
4. Provide oxygen. Do NOT use oxygen from a cold cylinder.
5. If the patient is alert, give him warm liquids.
6. Except in the mildest of cases (shivering), transport the patient, with his head lower than his feet. PROVIDE OXYGEN and monitor vital signs.
7. NEVER allow a patient to remain in, or return to, a cold environment. Hypothermia will probably recur.

NOTE: You will not be providing very much help to patients with mild to moderate hypothermia if you simply wrap them in blankets. Their bodies can no longer generate enough heat to make such care useful. Provide external heat sources, but rewarm the patient *slowly*. Handle the patient with great care.

In very serious cases of hypothermia, the patient's body core temperature usually falls below 80°F. The patient will have problems with breathing and a slowed pulse rate. Cardiac arrest is possible. Parts of the patient's body may be frozen. Consider serious any case of hypothermia in which the patient is unconscious, even if the core temperature is above 80°F.

DO NOT TRY TO REWARM THE SEVERE HYPOTHERMIA PATIENT. Even if you rewarm the patient slowly, you may cause the patient to develop lethal ventricular fibrillation. For the severe hypothermia patient, you should:

1. Handle the patient as gently as possible. Rough handling may cause ventricular fibrillation.
2. Place the patient in a head-down position.

Make certain he has an open airway.
3. Provide oxygen. Do NOT use oxygen from a cold cylinder.
4. Wrap the patient in blankets. If available, use insulating blankets.

In extreme cases of hypothermia, you will find the patient unconscious, with no discernable vital signs. The patient will feel very cold to your touch (the core temperature of the body may be below 80°F), but it is possible that the patient is still alive! Begin resuscitative measures. The patient may not reach biological death for over 30 minutes. The staff at the emergency department will not pronounce a patient biologically dead until after he is rewarmed as resuscitative measures are being applied. This means that you cannot assume a severe hypothermia patient is dead on the basis of body temperature and lack of vital signs.

Other Cold-Related Injuries

Chilblains   These are lesions that occur from repeated prolonged exposures of bare skin to temperatures of 60°F or lower. The lesions are red, swollen areas that the patient reports as hot, tender, and itchy. Chilblains are chronic, that is, they linger. There is no emergency care procedure for chilblains other than to protect the injured area and try to prevent recurrence. Keep in mind that the role of the EMT does not include diagnosis. Therefore, recommend that the patient see a physician to make certain that chilblains are the problem.

Trench Foot   Sometimes called immersion foot, **trench foot** is a condition that develops when the lower extremities remain in water that is just above freezing for a prolonged period. The affected part becomes swollen and appears waxy and mottled. It feels cold to touch and to the patient. The patient may complain of numbness.

To provide care, remove wet shoes and stockings. Do not open any blisters that may have developed. Gently rewarm the extremity and wrap it lightly with sterile dressing. The extremity may become red and hot. Dress the affected limb, placing strips of dressing between the toes. Keep the limb slightly elevated. Severe disability can occur with trench foot. Make certain that you transport the patient to a medical facility.

Protecting The Accident Victim From Cold

The injured patient is more susceptible to the effects of cold. As an EMT, you should begin to protect the accident victim before extrication and throughout care and transport. The major course of action is to prevent additional body heat loss. Although it may be neither practical nor possible to replace wet clothing, you can at least create a barrier to the cold with blankets, a salvage cover, an aluminized blanket, a survival blanket, or even articles of clothing. A plastic trash bag can serve as protection from wind and water, and it will help prevent heat loss. Keep in mind that the greatest area of heat loss may be the head. Provide some sort of head covering for the patient.

When the patient's injuries allow, place a blanket between his body and the cold ground. If the patient will remain trapped in wreckage for a period of time, plug holes in the wreckage with blankets or salvage covers. If available, use a 500-watt incandescent lamp to generate heat within the wreckage.

When administering oxygen to patients exposed to cold, do not use a cold cylinder. When possible, keep the cylinder inside the warm ambulance. If extrication procedures take a long time, make certain that you are not delivering cold oxygen to the patient.

INJURIES DUE TO ELECTRICITY

WARNING: The scenes of injuries due to electricity are often very hazardous. If the source of electricity is still active, do NOT attempt a rescue unless you have been trained to do so and have the necessary equipment and personnel. Gaining access to the patient at an electrical accident is covered in Chapter 16.

Electric current and lightning can cause severe damage to the body. The skin is burned where the energy enters the body, and where it leaves into a ground. Along the path of this flow tissues are damaged, significant chemical changes take place in the nerves, heart, and muscles, and the body processes are disrupted or completely shut down. The victim of an electrical accident may have any or all of the following symptoms and signs:

- Burns where the energy enters and exits the body
- Disrupted nerve pathways, displayed as paralysis
- Muscle tenderness, with or without muscular twitching
- Respiratory difficulties or arrest (the tongue may swell and obstruct the airway)
- Irregular heart beat or cardiac arrest
- Elevated blood pressure
- Restlessness or irritability if conscious, or loss of consciousness
- Visual difficulties
- Fractured bones and dislocations from severe muscle twitching or from falling. This can include the spinal column.
- Convulsions (severe cases)

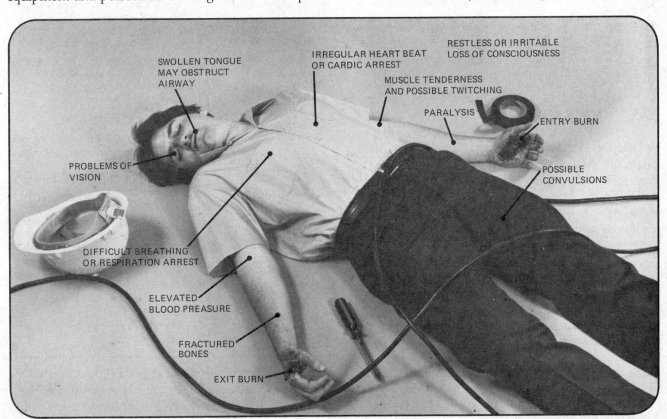

Figure 13-8: Injury due to electrical shock.

As with all patients, establishing and maintaining an open airway will be your primary responsibility, followed by assurance of circulation. As you provide care, remember to look for dislocations and fractures, and the signs of spinal damage.

Patients who are victims of electrical accidents may require care for electrical burns. To care for such burns, you should:

1. Make certain you and the patient are in a SAFE ZONE (see Chapter 15).
2. Provide airway care (remember that electrical shock may cause severe swelling along the airway).
3. Provide basic life support as required.
4. Care for spinal injuries, head injuries, and severe fractures.
5. Evaluate the burn, looking for at least two burn sites: contact with the energy source and contact with a ground.
6. Apply dry sterile dressings to the burn sites.
7. Treat for shock and administer oxygen.
8. Transport as soon as possible. Some problems have a slow onset, requiring you to transport even what you would consider to be a case of "mild" electrical shock. If there are burns, there may also be more serious hidden problems. In any case of electrical shock, problems with the heart may develop.

REMEMBER: The major problem caused by electrical shock is usually *not* the burn. Respiratory and cardiac arrest are real possibilities. Be prepared to provide basic life support measures.

HAZARDOUS MATERIALS

WARNING: Do NOT attempt a rescue when an accident involves hazardous materials unless you have been trained to do so, have the needed equipment, and have the personnel necessary to assure a safe scene. As an EMT, you would do well to take a hazardous materials course as part of your continuing education.

One of the undesirable aspects of our modern world is the growing number of hazardous materials. They are needed to manufacture essential and beneficial products. Hazardous materials also can be the waste products of manufacturing. Even though safety procedures have been set down, and followed for the most part, accidents involving hazardous materials do occur. They take place at factories, along railroads, and on local, state, and federal highways.

You must understand that as an EMT, you will be highly skilled in emergency care. However, without specialized training, you are still a layperson when it comes to hazardous materials. Special training is required to understand hazardous materials, work at the scene of accidents involving these materials, and render the scene safe. You CANNOT judge the state of a container or the probability of explosion without the benefit of specialized training. Do NOT think that you can use safety equipment unless you have been trained in the care, field testing, and actual use of the equipment. With hazardous material accidents, you may be able to do nothing more than stay a safe distance away from the scene and wait for expert help to arrive.

Table 13.3: Hazardous Materials (a partial list)

Material	Possible Hazard
Benzene (benzol)	Toxic vapors; can be absorbed through the skin. Destroys bone marrow.
Benzoyl peroxide	Fire and explosion.
Carbon tetrachloride	Damages internal organs.
Cyclohexane	Explosive. Eye and throat irritant.
Diethyl ether	Flammable. Can be explosive. Irritant to eyes and respiratory tract. Can cause drowsiness or unconsciousness.
Ethyl acetate	Irritates eyes and respiratory tract.
Ethylene dichloride	Strong irritant.
Heptane	Respiratory irritant.
Hydrochloric acid	Respiratory irritant; exposure to high concentration of vapors can produce pulmonary edema. Can damage skin and eyes.
Hydrofluoric acid	Vapors can cause pulmonary edema and severe eye burns. Vapors and liquid can burn skin. Vapors can be lethal.
Hydrogen cyanide	Highly flammable. Very toxic through inhalation or absorption.
Methyl isobutyl ketone (hexose)	Strong irritant of eyes and mucous membranes.
Methylene chloride	Eye damage.
Nitric acid	Produces a toxic gas (nitrogen dioxide). Skin irritant. Can cause self-ignition of cellulose products (e.g.: sawdust).
Organochloride (Chlordane, DDT, Dieldrin, Lindane, Methoxychlor)	Eye and skin irritant. Toxic fumes and smoke.
Perchloroethylene	Toxic if inhaled or swallowed.
Silicon tetrachloride	Water-reactive to form toxic hydrogen chloride fumes.
Tetrahydrofuram (THF)	Damages eyes and mucous membranes.
Toluol (toluene)	Toxic vapors. Can cause organ damage.
Vinyl chloride	Flammable and explosive. Listed as a carcinogen.

Regardless of your training, should you arrive at the scene of a hazardous materials accident, ESTABLISH A SAFE ZONE. Keep unauthorized people out of this zone and try to convince people to leave the immediate area. Stay upwind from the site and

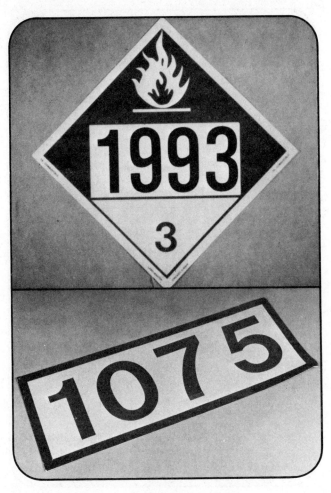

Figure 13-9: Hazardous materials placards.

avoid being downhill in case there are flowing liquids that are burning or otherwise unsafe. Make sure that you do not set up your position in a low-lying area in case fumes are escaping and hanging close to the ground. Likewise, avoid placing yourself higher than the accident scene so that you will not be in the path of escaping gases or heated air.

CALL FOR THE HELP YOU WILL NEED. The support services required at the scene of a hazardous materials accident may include fire services, special rescue personnel, local or state hazardous materials experts, and law enforcement personnel for crowd control. If the accident has taken place at an industrial site or along a railway, the company experts in hazardous materials need to be notified. Much of this can be done by a single call to your dispatcher.

Local back-up support will want to know certain facts, including:

- Type of hazardous material—gas, liquid chemical, cooled chemical, dry chemical, radioactive liquid, radioactive gases, or solid radioactive materials.

- Specific name of the material, or its identification number.

- How much material is at the scene.

- Current state of the material—escaping as a gas, leaking as a liquid, being blown into the air, in flames, or apparently still contained.

- How long you estimate that the scene has been dangerous.

- Other hazardous materials near the scene.

- Estimated number of possible patients in the danger zone.

You *do* have sources of information. Vehicle drivers, plant or railroad personnel, and perhaps even bystanders may be able to tell you the name of the hazardous material. In many cases, there will be a colored placard on the vehicle, tank, or railroad car. This placard will have a four-digit identification number. Older placards are usually orange and have an identification number preceded by the letters "UN" or "UA." Your dispatcher may have access to the name of the material through this identification number. There also may be an invoice, shipping manifest (trains), or bill of lading (trucks) that can confirm the identity of the substance.

The Chemical Transportation Emergency Center (CHEMTREC) has been established in Washington, D.C., by the Chemical Manufacturers Association. They can provide you with information about the hazardous material. They have a 24-hour, toll-free telephone number for the continental United States: 800-424-9300. In the Washington, D.C. area, the number is 202-483-7616. CHEMTREC will accept collect calls. When you call, keep the line open so that changes in the scene can be reported to CHEMTREC, and the center can confirm that they have contacted the shipper or manufacturer. CHEMTREC will be able to direct you as to your initial course of action. If there is no identification number and no one knows what is being carried, you may have no other choice than to wait for experts to arrive at the scene.

Initial actions at the scene can be directed according to information sent to you by your dispatcher, hazardous materials expert, or CHEMTREC. Often, this initial action is based on the procedures presented in *Hazardous Materials, The Emergency Response Handbook* (DOT P 5800.2), published by the Department of Transportation. When you call your dispatcher or CHEMTREC:

1. Give your name and call back number.
2. Explain the nature and location of the problem.
3. Report the identification number if there is a safe way for you to obtain this information.
4. When possible, supply the name of the shipper or manufacturer.
5. Describe the type of container.

6. Report if the container is on railcar, truck, open storage, or housed storage.
7. Give the carrier's name and the name of the consignee.
8. Report local conditions.
9. Keep the line of communication open at all times.

During the entire process, keep in a safe area. Do NOT step in any spilled materials. Do NOT think that the scene is safe simply because the substance has no apparent odor. Do what you can to keep people away from the scene.

As soon as possible, decide who will take charge of the scene. If this has not been decided in planning sessions prior to the incident, you or another professional at the scene should become the 'incident commander' (IC) until experts arrive to take over responsibility.

Providing Emergency Care

After a safety zone is created, you may do the following, if trained to do so:

1. Put on 100% full body protective clothing and self-contained positive pressure breathing apparatus (you must know how to check out and properly wear such equipment).
2. Isolate the accident area and keep the safe zone clear of unauthorized and unprotected personnel.
3. Evaluate the scene in terms of possible fire or explosion (this takes *special* training).
4. Move any patients as soon as possible. If the scene offers no immediate danger (expert judgment is required to determine this), begin life support measures within the danger zone.
5. Provide basic life support. For pulmonary resuscitation and CPR, use oxygen with a demand valve so you do not have to take off your own protective gear.
6. Administer oxygen to any patient having difficulty breathing.
7. IMMEDIATELY flush with water the skin, clothing, and eyes of anyone coming into contact with the hazardous material. Continue the wash for no less than 15 minutes.
8. Remove contaminated clothing, shoes, and jewelry from all patients and personnel. Flush the person's skin with water.
9. Transport the patient(s) as soon as possible, treating for shock, administering oxygen, and taking all steps necessary to maintain normal body temperature. (Remove your protective gear as recommended by local guidelines.)

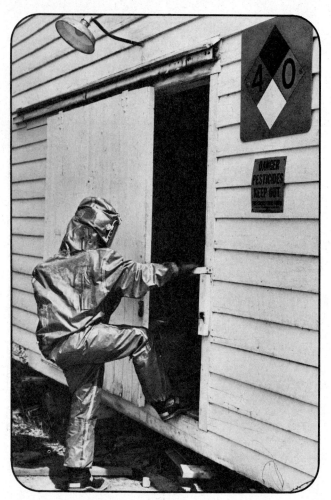

Figure 13-10: The use of proper equipment is required at a hazardous materials accident.

NOTE: After reading this section, you may well ask, "What can I do besides wait for experts to arrive?" Some materials will allow you to act. This is why you need to provide your dispatcher with all the information available. There are materials that will require experts to respond before you can gain access and provide care. Remember, you are an EMT, not an expert in hazardous materials.

RADIATION ACCIDENTS

WARNING: An EMT is not expected to be an expert in radiation accidents. Do ONLY what you have been trained to do. Every state has a procedure for emergency services to follow when radioactive substances are involved in an accident. It behooves all emergency care personnel to learn and understand those procedures, especially if duties are performed in heavily traveled transportation corridors.

"Radiation" is a general term that applies to the transmission of energy. This can include nuclear energy, ultraviolet and visible light, heat, sound, and X rays. When we speak of radiation accidents, we are referring to **ionizing** radiation. This radiation is from an atomic source, and is used to generate electricity, provide isotopes for medicine and industry, and to make nuclear weapons. Whenever atomic materials are made or used, there is a certain amount of waste and contaminated material produced. The sources of radiation seen in accidents include not only the radioactive materials in use, but also radioactive waste materials.

In most radiation accidents, industrial experts will be promptly available to provide you with instructions for your safety and the care of the patient(s). Away from the industrial site, local rescue experts, or state/federal officials may direct your activities. When in doubt, call your dispatcher to secure directions, or obtain an Interagency Radiological Assistance Plan (IRAP) by calling the nearest IRAP Regional Coordinating Office.

Types of Radiation

The three major types of ionizing radiation include **alpha particles**, **beta particles**, and **gamma rays**. Neutron radiation also exists but is rarely encountered, being found primarily in association with nuclear reactor fuels. Neutrons can penetrate deep within the tissues and cause serious tissue damage and death.

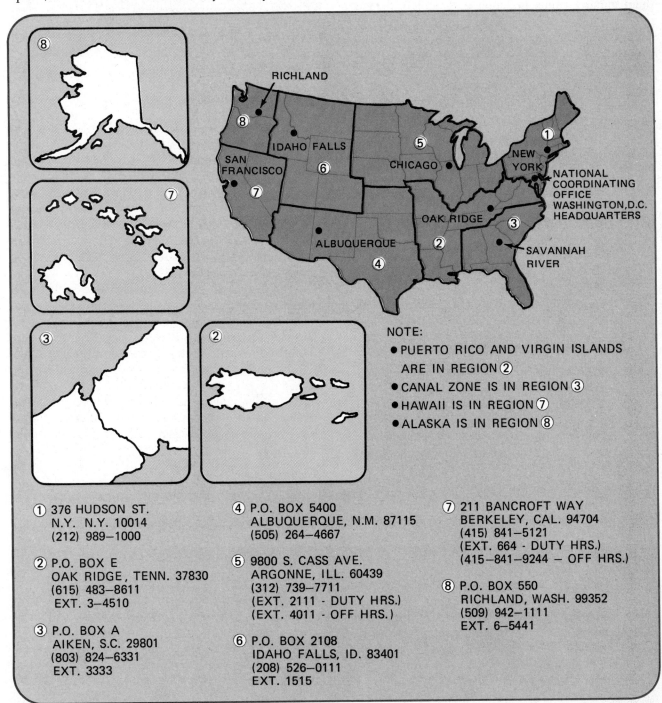

① 376 HUDSON ST.
N.Y. N.Y. 10014
(212) 989–1000

② P.O. BOX E
OAK RIDGE, TENN. 37830
(615) 483–8611
EXT. 3–4510

③ P.O. BOX A
AIKEN, S.C. 29801
(803) 824–6331
EXT. 3333

④ P.O. BOX 5400
ALBUQUERQUE, N.M. 87115
(505) 264–4667

⑤ 9800 S. CASS AVE.
ARGONNE, ILL. 60439
(312) 739–7711
(EXT. 2111 - DUTY HRS.)
(EXT. 4011 - OFF HRS.)

⑥ P.O. BOX 2108
IDAHO FALLS, ID. 83401
(208) 526–0111
EXT. 1515

⑦ 211 BANCROFT WAY
BERKELEY, CAL. 94704
(415) 841–5121
(EXT. 664 - DUTY HRS.)
(415–841–9244 – OFF HRS.)

⑧ P.O. BOX 550
RICHLAND, WASH. 99352
(509) 942–1111
EXT. 6–5441

Figure 13-11: IRAP Regional Coordinating Offices.

Alpha particles do little damage since they can be absorbed by a layer of clothing, a few inches of air, paper, or the outer layer of skin. This is a low-energy source of radiation. Beta particles are higher in energy level, but can be stopped by heavy clothing. This is not to say that the danger of exposure to alpha and beta radiation can be taken lightly. Irradiated dust particles and smoke can be inhaled, particles can contaminate open wounds, and irradiated foodstuffs can be ingested. Once inside the body, they continue to cause cell damage until they are removed, or until they decay.

Gamma rays and X rays can be considered the same thing. Gamma radiation is extremely dangerous, carrying high levels of energy able to penetrate thick shielding. The rays easily pass through clothing and the entire body, inflicting extensive cell damage.

Since ionizing radiation cannot be seen, felt, or heard, some sort of detection instrument is needed to measure the radiation given off by a radiation source. The most commonly used device is the Geiger counter. The rate of radiation is measured in *roentgens per hour* (r/hr) or milliroentgens per hour (mr/hr, 1000 mr = 1 r).

The Effects of Radiation on the Body

Simply stated, ionizing radiation causes changes in the body cells. Depending on the dosage received, the changes can be in cell division, cell structure, and cell chemical activities. If enough radiation is absorbed, leukemia and other cancers may result. At a certain dosage level, death is a certainty.

Determining exposure, absorption, and damage done by radiaton requires highly specialized training. Look at the problem in a practical manner. If you are working for one hour in an area where the Geiger counter reading is 100 r/hr, you will probably tolerate the dose with no ill effects. Should your exposure be 200 r/hr, you may become ill. Increase this to 300 r/hr and you will become very ill. At 400 r/hr, you will probably die in a short time.

How much radiation a person receives depends on the source of radiation, the length of time exposed, the distance from the source, and the shielding between the person and the source. The amount of radiation at the patient's initial location may be 300 r/hr. If you are only exposed for 20 minutes, this is the same radiation equivalent as working one hour at a 100 r/hr scene. The amount of radiation may drop off quickly as the patient is decontaminated and as you move the patient away from his initial position. If you wear protective gear, the amount of radiation absorbed will be considerably less than the Geiger counter reading.

Keep in mind that if care requires 60 minutes at a scene of 300 r/hr, three EMTs can take turns pro-

viding the care. Each will be exposed for only 20 minutes, so that the exposure per person does not exceed the equivalent of working for 1 hour at 100 r/hr.

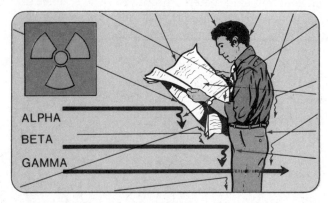

Figure 13-12: Factors determining radiation received.

Types of Radiation Accidents

As an EMT, you may respond to two types of radiation accidents: clean or dirty.

In the **clean accident,** the patient is exposed to radiation, but is not contaminated by the radioactive substance, particles of radioactive dust, or radioactive liquids, gases, or smoke. If the patient is properly decontaminated before you arrive, there is little danger to you, provided that the source of radiation is no longer exposed at the scene. The body itself does not become radioactive.

The **dirty accident,** often associated with fire at the scene of a radiation accident, exposes the patient to radiation and contaminates him with radioactive particles or liquids. The scene may be highly contaminated, even though the primary source of radiation is shielded when you arrive. If you are the first to arrive, you may have to wait for technical assistance unless you have radiation detection instruments and know how to use them. Otherwise, what you consider to be a clean accident may be a dirty one.

Rescue and Care Procedures

Your duties at the scene should include:

1. Protecting yourself from exposure.
2. Noting any hazard labels that indicate there may be a radiation hazard.
3. Alerting your dispatcher so you can obtain expert assistance.
4. Carrying out those rescue procedures you are trained to do when appropriate equipment is at the scene.
5. Providing emergency care for the *decontaminated* patient.
6. Helping prevent the spread of radiation through the control of contaminated articles.

When arriving at the scene, look for RADIA-TION HAZARD LABELS. These labels have a purple "propeller" symbol on a yellow background. Notify your dispatcher immediately to inform proper authorities and send technical assistance to the scene. If your dispatcher tells you to leave the scene, or if a radiation expert tells you to leave, do so promptly and safely. Otherwise, park upwind, as far from the scene as practical, behind any shielding of considerable mass. Thick metal or concrete walls, earth banks, and even heavy vehicles and construction equipment offer some additional shielding.

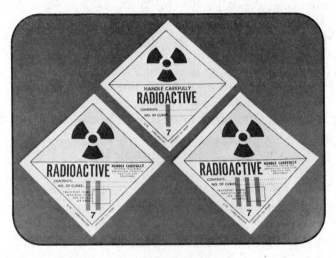

Figure 13-13: Radiation hazard labels.

You will have to wait for technical assistance unless you are trained to measure the radiation level and have the proper protective clothing and breathing equipment to allow a rescue. If you are trained in such rescue, remember to approach from upwind, avoiding when possible any dust clouds or smoke. If radiation levels are high, extricate the patient as quickly as possible, even when this means no survey, no immediate basic life support, and no splinting "where he lies." The rule is to *"get in and out quickly."*

Before care can be given, the patient must be decontaminated. Move the patient to the edge of the ACCIDENT ZONE (this is determined by local standards). Quickly remove the patient's clothing, shoes, and jewelry. If available, plastic bag these articles and place the bag in a metal container that has a tightly fitting lid. After removing the patient's clothing, remove your own protective garments and breathing apparatus. Bag these articles and place them in the container and close the lid. Some breathing apparatus may be too large to fit in this container. If this is the case, leave the apparatus next to the container. Make certain someone guards this container so that it can be removed properly.

Care can now be rendered, provided the level of radiation on the patient's skin does not exceed locally set limitations. Place yourself and the patient in a shielded area.

There are four types of radiation accident patients that may require your care:

- *Clean/patient received an external dose of radiation*—the patient is no danger to the EMT.
- *Dirty/patient received an internal dose of radiation*—after external cleansing there is no danger to the EMT. Should rescue breathing be required before decontamination, use oxygen and a demand valve or a bag-valve-mask unit.
- *Dirty/patient externally contaminated*—there is danger to the EMT. Avoid contact until patient decontamination is possible. Unless radiation levels are high, basic life support and care for life-threatening problems is possible. Use oxygen with a demand valve or a bag-valve-mask unit for rescue breathing.
- *Dirty/external surface contamination and wounds*—Take care not to contaminate yourself during care. Use oxygen with a demand valve or a bag-valve-mask unit if rescue breathing is required. The wounds should be cleaned separately from the adjacent skin. Dress the wounds.

Anytime you suspect that a patient has received internal contamination, save all vomitus and body wastes for transport. Keep them in a sealed, properly labeled metal container. Swab the anterior portions of the patient's nostrils and place the swabs in a sealed metal container. Label the container. Take nothing from the scene unless directed to do so by the radiation officer in charge.

Transport and Decontamination

Before you can transport the patient, he should be washed. Ask for a safe area to do this that will be guarded in case of contaminated water run-off. Before transport, cover the ambulance stretcher mattress with a blanket. Wrap the patient in the blanket and fashion a head covering from a towel. Only the patient's face should show when he is ready for transport. Transport the patient to the medical facility in accordance with your local radiation accident plan. You should radio ahead to alert the staff to the situation and to give your estimated time of arrival.

Decontamination or disposal of the equipment and clothing left at the scene will be done by those in charge of the radiation accident. Your ambulance, clothing, and supplies will be decontaminated by radiation experts. This is one reason why keeping an accurate ambulance equipment and supply inventory is so important. The experts must know what you used at the scene. You may be asked to help in the process, but you do not have the training to assure a proper job.

This leaves the most important decontamination procedure—your own personal decontamination. Shower with copious quantities of water, carefully washing your entire body. Pay particular attention to your hair, orifices, and parts of the body that usually rub together (medial arm and lateral chest, etc.). Allow the shower to run for some time after you complete washing to flush contaminants deep into the sanitary system. Have yourself checked by radiation experts and a physician.

NOTE: There is always some degree of risk when providing care at the radiation accident scene and when trying to provide care for the contaminated patient. Be *certain* to follow all local guidelines to the letter.

EXPLOSIONS

Fire and hazardous materials often lead to explosions. An explosion is defined as the rapid release of energy. The magnitude of an explosion depends on several factors, including the type of explosive agent, the space in which the agent is detonated, and the degree of confinement of the explosion.

The damage done is a result of the shock wave that is generated during the release of energy. As the wave extends outward in all directions, two types of pressure are generated. **Overpressure** is the pressure increase over the normal atmospheric pressure. Overpressure surrounds an object as the shock wave hits it and tends to crush the object inward. **Dynamic pressure** may be compared to a strong wind, striking each object in its path as the shock wave moves outward. Objects are pushed over or torn apart, and debris is picked up and propelled outward.

Injury is usually related to the distance from the point of detonation. The closer the victim, the more injuries. Typical injuries can include ruptured ear drums, ruptured internal organs, internal bleeding, contusions of the lungs (due to rapid pressure changes), burns, lacerations, impaled objects, fractures, and crushing injuries.

Explosions often produce superheated air that can cause severe respiratory system damage and thermal burns. When providing care at the scene of an explosion, be alert for these problems.

Basic life support is the first priority of care. A complete patient assessment is the only way you can detect most major injuries. Transport is required, even for what may appear to be only minor injuries. This is justified because there can be a delay in certain injuries appearing as obvious signs. When you transport, always assume there are internal injuries.

SUMMARY

Burns can be caused by heat (thermal), chemicals, electricity, light, and radiation.

As an EMT, you must be able to classify burns in terms of first, second, and third degree. See Scansheet 13-1 for the factors involved in this classification.

Care for all burns, keeping in mind that burns are more serious for children, the elderly, injured patients, and those with a chronic illness. Always monitor vital signs, since the respiratory system may be involved and also the circulatory system.

Any burn to the hands, feet, groin, or face is to be considered a serious burn (exception: simple sunburn). If a whole area of the body is involved, such as the chest, you are to consider this to be a serious burn. Second and third degree burns that involve a major joint must also be considered serious. Learn to use the rule of nines in evaluating burns. Consider critical:

- Any burn that is complicated by injuries to the respiratory tract, soft tissues, and bones.
- Third degree burns to the face, groin, hands, feet, or major joint.
- Third degree burns that involve more than 10% body surface.
- Second degree burns that involve more than 30% body surface.

When in doubt, overclassify. . .consider a questionable first degree burn to be second degree and a questionable second degree burn to be third degree.

Treat minor burns with cold water and a sterile or clean dressing. Do not soak major burns in cold water. Wrap the affected areas in sterile or clean dressings. Treat for shock and transport.

If the patient's eyes or eyelids are burned, cover the eyelids with sterile or clean pads. Moisten with sterile water. Use sterile or clean pads to separate burned fingers and toes before dressing.

The care for chemical burns involves flooding with water, except when cause of the burn is dry lime. Instead, brush away the chemical from the patient's skin and clothing. After washing or brushing, apply dressings, treat for shock, and transport.

When the eyes are involved in cases of chemical burns, take immediate action and flood with water. Use running water for 5 minutes in acid burns, 15 minutes in alkali burns, and 20 minutes in cases of unknown agents.

In the care for patients with electrical burns, your primary concern should be with breathing and pulse. For the actual care of the burn, remember to look for at least two burn sites, one where the electricity entered the patient's body and the other where it exited. Apply sterile or clean dressings, treat for shock, and transport.

Smoke contains many poisonous substances. Move the patient to a safe atmosphere and aid in breathing by administering oxygen. Have the patient see a physician.

Exposure to excessive heat can bring about heat cramps, heat exhaustion, or heatstroke. Heat cramps are seldom a serious problem. Some cases of heat exhaustion can turn serious. All cases of heatstroke are serious. Heatstroke is a true emergency. See Scansheet 13-2 for the symptoms and signs of all three conditions. You must be able to tell one condition from the others.

Care for heat cramps includes cooling the patient, giving salted water or commercial electrolyte fluids, and massaging cramped muscles. In cases of heat exhaustion, you must cool the patient, give salted water or commercial electrolyte fluids, and treat for shock. If the patient does not improve, transport as soon as possible.

Heatstroke requires you to cool the patient as rapidly as possible. Use ice bags, cold packs or cool running water. Transport immediately. This is a true emergency.

Exposure to cold can cause frostnip (incipient frostbite), frostbite (superficial frostbite), or freezing (deep frostbite). The signs for each of these conditions are given in Table 13.1.

Often, the patient can use his own body heat to warm frostnipped areas of the body. Frostbite requires gentle handling of the affected part, keeping the patient warm, dressing the site, and transporting to a medical facility. If transport is delayed, the affected area will have to be rewarmed by immersing it in warm water (100°F to 105°F). Keep the water warm, but still comfortable to your touch. The same basic care also applies to freezing.

Excessive cold can bring about hypothermia. Shivering, feelings of numbness, and drowsiness are most frequently seen in hypothermia. Care for mild to moderate hypothermia involves using external heat sources to slowly raise the patient's body temperature. Hypothermia can be very serious. If the patient becomes unconscious, has problems with breathing, has a slowed pulse rate, has frozen body parts, or is in cardiac arrest, provide needed basic life support, wrap him in an insulated blanket, and transport as soon as possible.

Hazardous materials should be handled by experts. Learn to look for hazardous materials placards. Provide care only when safe to do so. Establish a safe zone and call for the help you will need. When you can provide care, direct your attentions to basic life support and decontamination of the patient.

Radiation accidents require expert assistance. Learn to look for radiation hazard labels. Alert your dispatcher and request the help you will need. Park in a shielded area, wear protective clothing, and use a protective breathing apparatus. Get in and out quickly. Remove the patient's clothing and your contaminated gear. Provide care and decontaminate the patient. Make certain that you shower to decontaminate yourself.

Explosions can cause serious multiple injuries. Basic life support is the priority in care. A complete patient assessment is essential to provide proper care.

SECTION TWO: WATER- AND ICE-RELATED ACCIDENTS

OBJECTIVES By the end of this section, you should be able to:

1. List the common types of injuries associated with swimming and diving accidents. (p. 321-2, 4)

2. List, in correct order, the methods to use when attempting to reach a patient in the water. (p. 322-3)

3. State the basic order of care procedures for patients who are near-drowning victims. (p. 323-4)

4. Describe the techniques of resuscitation applied to the near-drowning victim. (p. 324)

5. Describe, step by step, how to turn a patient in the water, and place him on a long spine board. (p. 324-5)

6. State the basic care procedures for diving accident victims with neck or spinal injury. (p. 324)

7. Describe two special types of problems faced when dealing with scuba diving accident victims and tell what should be done for each type of problem. (p. 324, 6)

8. Describe basic ice rescue procedures. (p. 326-7)

SKILLS As an EMT, you should be able to:

1. Evaluate a patient who is the victim of a swimming or diving accident.

2. Solve the basic problems faced in reaching the patient in water- and ice-related accidents.

3. Apply resuscitation skills and other basic life support measures to the near-drowning patient, and to the diving accident victim.

4. Work as a member of a team to turn a patient in the water and to place him on a long spine board.

TERMS you may be using for the first time:

Asphyxia (as-FIX-si-ah)—to suffocate from lack of air.

Laryngospasm (lah-RING-go-spaz'm)—contraction of the larynx set off when water passes the epiglottis.

Mammalian Diving Reflex—a reaction to cold water that shuts off major blood flow except to the brain, heart, and lungs.

Air Embolism—air bubbles in the bloodstream.

Decompression Sickness—the "bends"; nitrogen is trapped in the body's tissues, possibly finding its way into the bloodstream.

ACCIDENTS INVOLVING THE WATER

WARNING: Do NOT attempt a water rescue unless you have been trained to do so and are a very good swimmer. Except for shallow pools and open, shallow waters with uniform bottoms, the problems faced in water rescue are too great and too dangerous for the poor swimmer and untrained person to attempt. If this bothers you, having to stand by not being able to help, then take a course in water safety and rescue. Otherwise, if you attempt a rescue, you will probably become a victim yourself rather than the person who rescues and provides care.

DROWNING AND NEAR-DROWNING

Drowning is immediately brought to mind when one hears of water-related accidents. This is a valid association, since drowning must be the number one consideration in terms of water-related accidents. Even if the first problem faced by a person in the water may be an injury or a medical emergency, the danger of drowning becomes the first concern.

The process of drowning begins as a person struggles to keep afloat in the water. He gulps in large breaths of air as he thrashes about. When he can no longer keep afloat and starts to submerge, he tries to take and hold one more deep breath. As he does, water may enter his airway. There is a series of coughing and swallowing actions, and the victim involuntarily inhales and swallows water. As water flows past the epiglottis, it contracts the larynx and triggers a reflex spasm. This **laryngospasm** (lah-RING-go-spaz'm) seals the airway so effectively that no more than a small amount of water ever reaches the lungs. Unconsciousness soon results from hypoxia.

About 10% of the people who drown die from true asphyxia, or simply suffocation from the lack of air. In the remaining victims, the laryngospasms subside with the onset of unconsciousness and water freely enters the lungs. What happens next depends on whether the victim is in fresh water or salt water.

In fresh water, water passes through the capillary walls into the bloodstream. Red blood cells swell and burst, the pulmonary membrane is damaged, and the heart may develop ventricular fibrillation. This heart action is lethal and is probably the cause of death in most fresh-water drownings.

In salt-water drownings, water is taken from the bloodstream and pulmonary edema develops. As much as one-quarter of the total blood volume is lost as fluids move into the lungs. Hypoxia becomes a major problem. Death is often the result of the shock that occurs with circulatory collapse.

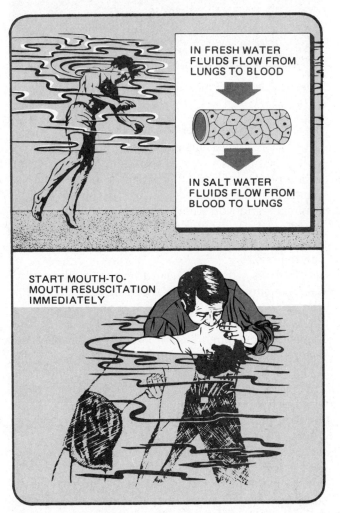

Figure 13-14: Salt water and fresh water have different effects on the body. The care procedures are the same. Begin pulmonary resuscitation as soon as possible.

Keep in mind that the care procedures will be

the same, regardless of the type of water causing the accident. As an EMT, you must start using the term "near-drowning." Obviously, if the patient is breathing and coughing up water, he has not drowned but nearly drowned. This is only part of what we mean as near-drowning. If a victim has "drowned" in layperson's terms, he is not necessarily biologically dead. Resuscitative measures may be able to keep the patient biologically alive long enough for more advanced life support measures to be used to save the patient's life. Only when sufficient time has passed to render resuscitation useless is the victim truly drowned.

The phrase "sufficient time" has a different meaning today when applied to clinically dead patients. The concept of four to six minutes is no longer valid. We now know that patients in cold water can be resuscitated after 45 to 60 minutes in cardiac arrest. Once the water temperature falls below 70°F, biological death may be delayed. The colder the water, the better the patient's chances are for survival. More will be said about this later in the chapter.

Water-Related Injuries

Many different types of injuries occur on, in, or near the water. Boating, waterskiing, diving board accidents, and scuba diving accidents can produce broken bones, bleeding, soft tissue injuries, and airway obstruction. Automobiles may come to rest in the water, with victims showing the same types of injuries normally associated with such accidents, made more complex by the presence of water, and, in some cases additional cold.

A medical emergency may take place while someone is in the water or on a boat. Knowing how the accident occurred may give clues to help detect a medical emergency. As with all patients, the patient survey and interview may be critical in deciding the procedures followed when providing care.

An EMT must consider how accidents can occur. Learn to associate the problems of drowning to scenes other than the pool and the beach. Remember, bathtub drownings do occur. Only a few inches of water are needed for an adult to drown. Even less is required for an infant.

As an EMT, remember to look for the following when your patient is the victim of a water-related accident:

- Airway obstruction—This may be from water in the lungs, foreign matter in the airway or swollen airway tissues (common if the neck is injured in a dive). Spasms along the airway are present in cases of near-drowning.
- Cardiac arrest—Often related to respiratory arrest, or occurring before the near-drowning.
- Signs of heart attack—Through overexertion,

the patient may have greater problems than obvious near-drowning. Some untrained rescuers are fooled into thinking that chest pains are due to muscle cramps produced during swimming.

- Injuries to the head and neck—These can be expected in boating, waterskiing, and diving accidents, but they are also very common in swimming accidents.

- Internal injuries—While doing the patient survey, stay on the alert for fractured bones, soft tissue injuries, and internal bleeding, which is often missed during the first stages of care.

- Hypothermia—The water does not have to be very cold and the length of time in the water does not have to be very long for hypothermia to occur (in some cases of near-drowning, the patient may have a better chance for survival in cold water).

Reaching the Patient

Unless you are a very good swimmer and trained in water rescue, do NOT go into the water to save someone. Such training is available from the American Red Cross and the YMCA in the form of water safety and rescue courses.

The basic order of procedures for a water rescue is to REACH AND PULL, THROW, TOW, and, as a last resort, GO into the water.

When the patient is responsive and close to shore or poolside, begin the rescue by holding out an object for him to grab; then PULL him from the water. When doing this, you must be positioned securely to avoid being pulled into the water. Of all the items that could be used for such a rescue, line (rope) is considered the best choice. If no line is available, use a branch, fishing pole, oar, stick, or other such object. Keep in mind that a towel, blanket, or even an article of your own clothing can work quite well. When no object is near at hand, or conditions are such that you may have only one opportunity to grab the person (strong currents), position yourself flat on your stomach and extend your hand or leg to the patient (not recommended for the non-swimmer). Again, make certain that you are working from a secure position.

Should the person be alert, but too far away for you to reach and pull from the water, THROW an object that will float. A personal flotation device (PFD or lifejacket), or ring buoy (life preserver) is best, if available. The primary course of action is to throw anything that will float and to do so as soon as possible. Buoyant objects that may be at a typical water-related accident scene include foam cushions, plastic jugs, logs, plastic picnic containers, surfboards, flat boards, large beach balls, and plastic toys. Two empty capped plastic milk jugs can keep an adult afloat for hours. Remember that the ambu-

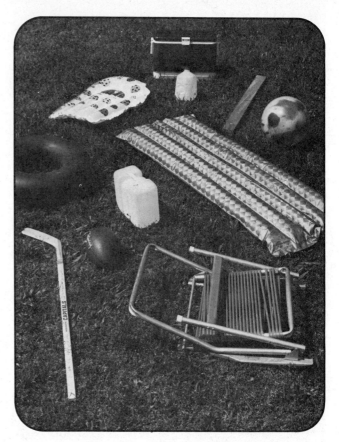

Figure 13-15: Throw the patient any object that will float.

lance has a spare wheel that will float.

Once the conscious patient has an object to hold on to, try to find a way to TOW him to shore. From a safe position, throw the patient a line or another flotation device attached to a line. If you are a good swimmer and you know how to judge the water, wade out to no deeper than your waist should you find it necessary to cut down the distance for throwing the line.

In cases where the near-drowning victim is too far from shore to allow for throwing and towing, or the patient is unresponsive, you may be able to ROW a boat to the patient. Do NOT row to the patient if you cannot swim. Even if you are a good swimmer, wearing a personal flotation device while in the boat is REQUIRED. In cases where the patient is conscious, tell him to grab an oar or the stern (rear end) of the boat. You must exercise great care when helping the patient into the boat. This is even more tricky when in a canoe. Should the canoe tip over, stay with the canoe and hold onto its bottom and side. Most canoes will stay afloat.

If you row to the patient and find that he is unresponsive, you can conduct a quick primary survey from your position in the boat and look for obvious signs of neck or spinal injury before trying to pull him from the water. Of course, this is a judgment call. Should conditions be such that you may lose the chance to grab the patient, then these emergency care procedures must be delayed until after you have the patient safely in the boat.

When reaching and pulling, throwing, and towing fail and a boat is not at the scene, you can GO in the water and swim to the patient. YOU MUST BE A GOOD SWIMMER, trained in water rescue and lifesaving.

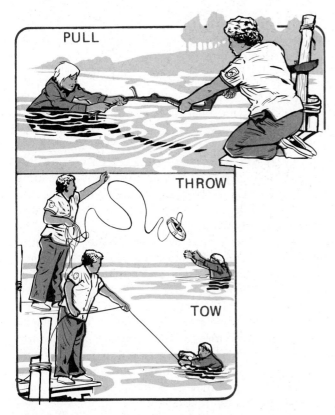

Figure 13-16: If you can, REACH AND PULL the patient from the water. If this fails, THROW him anything that will float and try to TOW him from the water.

Care for the Patient

You will have to provide care for patients who are out of the water when you arrive, in the water when you arrive but rescued by others, or in the water when you initiate care. When needed, begin PULMONARY RESUSCITATION without delay. Do not be surprised to find resistance to the breaths you attempt to provide to the near-drowning patient. You will probably have to apply more force than you would for other patients. Be sure that no foreign objects are in the patient's airway. Remember, you must provide air to the patient's lungs as soon as possible.

A patient having water in the lungs usually will have water in the stomach. If there is enough water in the stomach, there will be added resistance to your efforts to provide rescue breathing or the interposed ventilations of CPR. Since the patient may have spasms along the airway, or swollen tissues in the larynx or trachea, you may find that some of the air you provide will go into the patient's stomach.

Remember, the same problem will occur if you do not properly open the airway, or you are too forceful in providing ventilations. Current AHA guidelines do not call for you to attempt to relieve water or air from the patient's stomach unless the distention interferes with sufficient air exchange.

There is no recommendation to use abdominal thrusts. The trapped air may be relieved by turning the patient on his side and using the palm of the hand to apply pressure to the patient's upper abdomen. The patient's mouth must be cleared before breaths are provided. Forcing trapped air or water out of a patient's stomach should not be done unless suction equipment is ready for immediate use.

Human beings have something in common with many other mammals, a process called the **mammalian diving reflex.** When a person dives into cold water, the body reacts with a series of complex functions that shut off major blood flow to most parts of the body except the heart, lungs, and brain. Whatever oxygen remains in the blood supply is made available to the brain. The colder the water, the more oxygen we tend to divert to the brain. Therefore, for this reason, do not feel that a near-drowning victim should not receive resuscitative care if he has not been breathing for 10 minutes or more. Many such patients have been resuscitated. Recent studies have shown that some freshwater near-drowning patients have been resuscitated, without brain damage, after 45 to 60 minutes. The colder the water, the better the patient's chances.

The Patient Rescued By Others

In all cases of water-related accidents, assume that the unconscious patient has neck and spinal injuries. When the patient is rescued by others while you wait, or is out of the water when you arrive, you should:

1. DO A PRIMARY SURVEY.

2. Provide mouth-to-mouth resuscitation, if needed, as soon as possible. Do not forget to check for airway obstruction.

3. Provide CPR, if needed, as you would for any patient in cardiac arrest.

4. If the patient has an open airway, adequate breathing, and a pulse, look for and control all profuse bleeding.

5. When resuscitative measures are needed, begin them immediately and continue through transport. The near-drowning patient receiving pulmonary resuscitation or CPR should be transported as soon as possible. For all other patients. . .

6. Cover the patient to conserve body heat and complete a SECONDARY SURVEY. Uncover only those areas of the patient's body involved with

the stage of the survey. Care for any problems or injuries detected during the survey, in the order of their priority.

7. Treat for shock, administer oxygen, and transport the patient as soon as possible. When transport is delayed and you believe that the patient can be moved to a warmer place, do so without aggravating any existing injuries. Do NOT allow the near-drowning patient to walk.

The Patient with Possible Spinal Injuries

Injuries to the cervical spine are seen with many water-related accidents. Most often, these injuries are received during a dive or when the patient is struck by a boat, water skier, or ski. Even though *cervical* spine injuries are the most common spinal injuries in water-related accidents, there can be injury anywhere along the spine.

When a patient is unconscious, you may not be able to detect spinal injuries. In water-related accidents, *assume* that the unconscious patient has neck and spinal injuries. Should the patient have head injuries, assume there are neck and spinal injuries also. Keep in mind that a patient found in respiratory arrest or cardiac arrest will need resuscitation started before you can immobilize the neck and spine. Also, you will not be able to carry out a complete survey for spinal injuries while the patient is in the water. Take care to avoid aggravating spinal injuries, but do not delay basic life support. Also, do not delay removing the patient from the water if the scene presents an immediate danger. When possible, keep the patient's neck rigid in a straight line with the body midline. Use the modified jaw-thrust for rescue breathing.

If the patient with possible spinal injuries is still in the water and you are a good swimmer, able to aid in the rescue, secure the patient to a long spine board before removing him from the water. Steps for this procedure are shown on the next Scansheet. This type of rescue requires *special training* in the use of the spine board while in the water. A spine board is a rigid device that can "pop up" very easily from below the water surface. Make certain you know how to control the board and how to work in the water.

Pulmonary resuscitation can begin while the patient is in the water. CPR requires that the patient be out of the water, in a boat, or on land. There is some debate over the value of beginning CPR in the water when the patient is on a long spine board. There is no evidence to prove this will be effective, and the procedure will probably slow down the rescue and increase the risk to the rescuers.

Be realistic when dealing with near-drowning patients. Many of these patients cannot be resuscitated and will have already drowned. Some patients may be resuscitated, but die within 48 hours due to pneumonia, lung damage or brain damage. Even when you provide the best of care, some patients will die. However, you must try to resuscitate the patient. There is no way you will be able to decide if the patient can or cannot be resuscitated successfully. Do your best, to the level of your training.

DIVING ACCIDENTS

Diving Board Accidents

Water-related accidents often involve injuries that occur when people attempt dives or enter the water from diving boards. In the majority of these accidents, the patient is a teenager. Basically the same types of injuries are seen in dives taken from diving boards, poolsides, docks, boats, and the shore. The injury may be due to the diver striking the board or some object on or under the water. If an improper dive is made, injury may result from impact with the water.

Most diving accidents involve the head and neck, but you also will find injuries to the spine, hands, feet, and ribs occurring in many cases. Keep in mind that any part of the body can be injured because of the odd positions the diver may be in when he strikes the water or an object. This means that you must perform *both* the primary and secondary surveys on all diving accident patients unless you are providing life support measures. Do not overlook the fact that a medical emergency may have led to the diving accident.

Care for diving accident patients is the same as for any accident victim, if they are out of the water. Care provided in the water and in removing the patient from the water is the same as for any patient who may have neck and spine injuries. Remember, assume *any* unconscious or unresponsive patient has neck and spinal injuries. There can be delayed reactions in patients with spinal injuries. Compression along the spine may cause a patient with no apparent injuries to suddenly exhibit indications of nerve impairment. Often this begins as a numbness or tingling sensation in the legs.

Scuba Diving Accidents

Scuba (self-contained underwater breathing apparatus) diving accidents have increased as the sport becomes more popular, especially since many untrained and inexperienced people are attempting dives. Today, there are over 1,000,000 people who scuba dive for sport or as part of their job. Add to this a large number who decide to "try it one time," without lessons or supervision.

Scuba diving accidents include all types of body injuries and near-drownings. In many cases, the scuba diving accident was brought about by medical

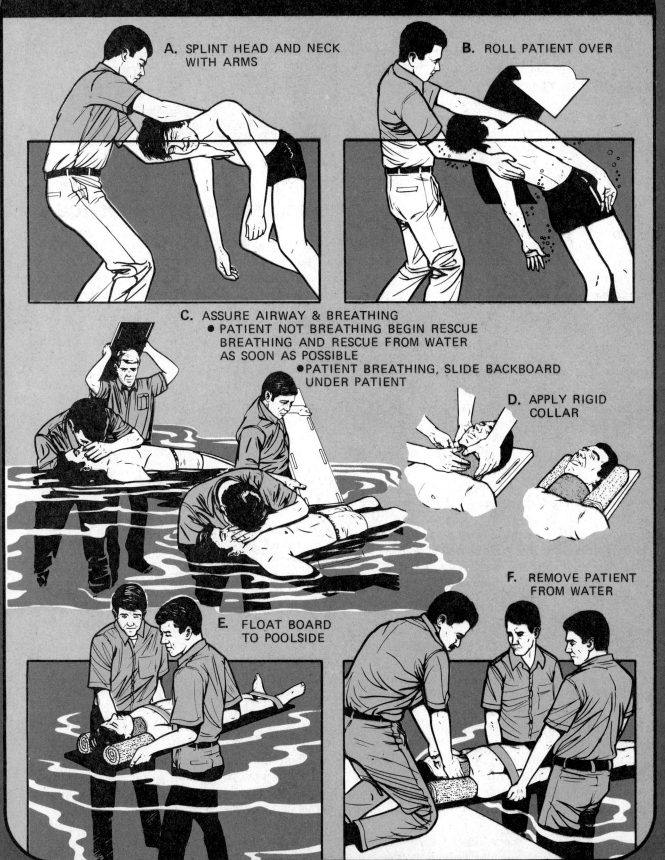

SCAN 13-3

problems that existed prior to the dive. There are two special problems seen in scuba diving accidents: air emboli in the diver's blood and the "bends."

Air emboli (air bubbles in the blood), are most often found in divers who hold their breath during an equipment failure, underwater emergency, or when trying to conserve air during a dive. However, a diver may develop an air embolism in very shallow waters. The onset is rapid, with signs of personality changes. The senses become distorted, often giving the impression that the patient is intoxicated on alcohol. The patient may have convulsions and can rapidly lapse into unconsciousness. Sounds may be heard in the chest, indicating air is trapped outside the lungs in the thoracic cavity.

An automobile accident victim trapped below water takes gulps of air from any air bubbles held inside the vehicle. When freed, the patient may develop air emboli the same as the scuba diver.

The "bends" are really part of what is called **decompression sickness,** usually caused when the diver comes up too quickly from a deep, prolonged dive. The quick ascent causes nitrogen gas to be trapped in the body tissues. It is common for this trapped nitrogen to find its way into the patient's bloodstream. The onset of the "bends" is usually slow for scuba divers, taking from 1 to 48 hours to appear. Because of this delay, carefully consider *all* information gathered from the patient interview and reports from the patient's family and friends. This information may provide the only clues that relate the patient's problems to a scuba dive.

Another way to detect decompression sickness can be gained during the interview stage of patient assessment. Divers increase the risk of decompression sickness if they fly within 12 hours of a dive.

The symptoms and signs of decompression sickness include deep pain to the muscles and joints (the "bends"), choking, coughing, labored breathing, chest pains and blotches on the skin (mottling). In some cases, skin rashes that keep changing in appearance can be found.

Transport all patients with possible air emboli or decompression sickness. Positioning of the patient is critical, to avoid damage to the brain by air bubbles in the blood. Place the patient on the left side in a head-down position. (This should *not* be done if there are any signs of neck or spinal injuries.) Make certain that the patient's head is placed downward by slanting the entire body rather than simply lifting the legs. Continue to monitor the patient and treat for shock. You may have to reposition the patient to assure an open airway.

NOTE: The well-trained scuba diver wears a pre-planned dive chart. This chart may provide you with useful information concerning the nature and duration of the dive.

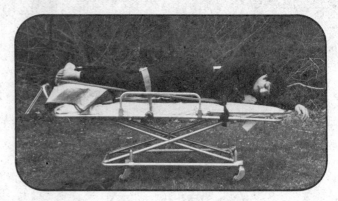

Figure 13-17: Positioning the patient after a scuba diving accident.

ACCIDENTS INVOLVING ICE

Every winter, newspapers report the deaths of numerous persons who fall through ice while skating or attempting to cross an ice-covered body of water. Often, the ice-related accident scene becomes a multiple-rescue problem as people try to reach the victim and also fall through the ice.

There are several ways in which you can reach a patient who has fallen through ice:

- Flotation devices can be thrown to the victim.

- A rope in which a loop has been formed can be tossed to the victim. He can put the loop around his body so that he can be pulled onto the ice and away from the danger area.

- A spine board can be used to spread the rescuer's weight over a larger area to allow crawling out on the ice to reach the patient.

- A small aluminum boat is probably the best device for an ice rescue. It can be pushed stern first by other rescuers and pulled to safety by a rope secured to the bow (front end). The primary rescuer will remain dry and safe should the ice break. The patient can be pulled from the water, or can grasp the side of the boat.

- A ladder is an effective tool often used in ice rescue. It can be laid flat and pushed to the victim, then pulled back by an attached rope. The ladder also can serve as a surface on which a rescuer can spread his weight if he must go on the ice to reach the victim.

When attempting to rescue the victim, remember that he may not be able to do much to help in the process. The effects of cold water may slow his mental and physical capabilities.

You should never enter the water through a hole in the ice in order to find a victim. Whenever possible, never work alone when trying to perform an ice rescue. If you *must* work alone, do not walk out onto the ice, but throw a rope, or push a ladder to the victim. Never go onto ice which is rapidly breaking. Your best course of action will be to work with others, from safe ice surface or the shore. When there is no other choice, you and your fellow rescuers can elect to form a human chain to reach the victim. However, this is not the safest method to employ, even when all the rescuers are wearing PFD's.

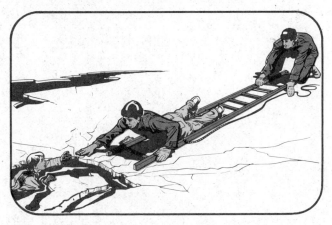

Figure 13-18: The safest way to perform an ice rescue is to work with others.

Expect to find injuries with most patients who have fallen through the ice. Fractures to the bones of the lower extremities are common. Hypothermia may be a problem. Remember that blanket wraps are of little help to patients with mild to moderate hypothermia. They require the slow application of an external source of heat. Transport *all* patients who have fallen through ice. The severe hypothermia patient should not be rewarmed in the field.

There may be injuries that are difficult to detect and problems due to the cold that may be delayed. Keep ice-related accident patients as warm as possible without overheating. Treat them for shock.

SUMMARY

WARNING: DO NOT ATTEMPT A WATER OR ICE RESCUE UNLESS YOU CAN SWIM. DO NOT GO INTO THE WATER UNLESS YOU ARE A GOOD SWIMMER AND HAVE BEEN TRAINED IN WATER RESCUE.

Near-drowning is the number one problem faced in all water- and ice-related accidents. However, injuries of all types do occur and medical problems may have caused the accident.

Often associated with water and ice accidents are airway obstruction, cardiac arrest, heart attacks, head and neck injuries, internal injuries, and hypothermia.

If the victim is in the water, try to REACH and PULL him out, THROW him something that will float, TOW him from the water, or ROW out to him. If you use a boat to reach the person in the water,

you should be wearing a personal flotation device. GO in the water and swim to the patient only if you are trained to do so.

Consider any unconscious patient to have neck and spinal injuries. Care for any patient already out of the water based on primary and secondary surveys and your interviews. Take special care to protect possible neck and spinal injuries.

When providing mouth-to-mouth resuscitation, use the modified jaw-thrust to protect possible neck and spinal injuries.

If you are a *good* swimmer and have been *trained* in water rescue, you may be able to start artificial respirations while the patient is in the water. Starting CPR while the patient is in the water will probably be ineffective. If you are alone and must row a cardiac arrest victim to shore, delay CPR and reach shore as quickly as possible in order to provide uninterrupted, effective CPR.

Many patients in cardiac arrest can be resuscitated even after 10 minutes in arrest. If the water is cold enough, they may last 45 to 60 minutes before reaching biological death.

When patients in water are found unconscious, work to apply an extrication collar and to place the patient on a spine board for floating and lifting from the water. Begin pulmonary resuscitation as soon as possible. Effective CPR is very difficult to perform while the patient is still in the water.

Whenever possible try to support the patient's back and keep the neck rigid and in line with the midline of the back.

All patients in water- or ice-related accidents should be treated for shock. Keep them as warm as possible without overheating. Do NOT allow the near-drowning victim to walk.

Diving accidents usually produce head, neck, and spinal injuries. The hands, feet, and ribs also are frequently injured.

Scuba diving accidents may involve air emboli or decompression sickness. In cases of possible air bubbles in the blood, look for unusual behavior, distorted senses, convulsions, sudden loss of consciousness, and signs of air trapped in the chest cavity. For decompression sickness, expect a delayed reaction, difficult breathing, coughing, choking, chest pains, and changes in the appearance of the skin (blotches or changing rashes). Deep pains in the muscles and joints (the "bends") are typical symptoms in decompression sickness.

In cases of scuba diving accidents, if the possibility of air emboli exists, or if the patient is having the "bends," place the patient on the left side, with the body slanted to keep the head in a sight downward position.

If you must perform an ice rescue, have others help you. Try to throw a line to the victim, or extend a pole to the victim. With the help of others, you may be able to reach the victim by crawling along a ladder or by forming a human chain out to the victim. When caring for the patient, be on guard for problems caused by hypothermia.

14 special patients and situations

SECTION ONE: MANAGEMENT OF SPECIAL PATIENTS

OBJECTIVES By the end of this section you should be able to:

1. Define "special patient" in terms that apply to emergency care. (p. 330)

2. Define "personal interaction." (p. 330)

3. Define crisis from a patient's point of view. (p. 330)

4. List FIVE things an EMT should do when trying to initiate crisis management procedures. (p. 330-1)

5. State the questions EMTs should ask themselves in order to control emotional involvement. (p. 331)

6. Describe the modifications in the approach to care that are made when dealing with elderly patients. (p. 331-2)

7. State how the EMT can establish communication with a deaf patient. (p. 332-3)

8. Describe how an EMT should modify care procedures when the patient is blind. (p. 333)

9. Describe what the EMT can do to establish communication with a non-English speaking patient. (p. 333-4)

10. Define stress reaction, psychiatric emergency, and emotional emergency. (p. 334, 6)

11. Make a list of the terms you can use to describe what you consider to be unusual behavior. (p. 334, 6)

12. Describe how personal interaction relates to caring for patients in emotional emergencies. (p. 336)

13. List at least FIVE injuries or medical problems that may produce behaviors similar to those usually seen in an psychiatric emergency. (p. 337)

14. Describe the actions to be taken by the EMT if the patient is aggressive (p. 337)

15. Describe the actions to be taken by the EMT when caring for a patient attempting suicide. (p. 337-8)

16. State the role of the EMT at the crime scene in relation to patient care and the chain of evidence. (p. 338)

17. Describe what special factors must be considered when providing care for the rape victim. (p. 338)

SKILLS As an EMT, you should be able to:

1. Use personal interaction for patients experiencing a crisis and for patients having an emotional emergency.

2. Initiate crisis management when appropriate.

3. Conduct an efficient interview with elderly patients.

4. Establish effective communication with deaf patients.

5. Provide care and comfort for the blind patient.

6. Establish some form of communication with the non-English speaking patient.

7. Determine if a patient is possibly having an emotional emergency.

8. Provide proper care for the aggressive patient and the patient about to attempt suicide, when your own safety is assured.

9. Provide care at the controlled crime scene, helping to preserve the chain of evidence.

10. Provide care for rape victims that considers their emotional needs, privacy, comfort, and dignity.

TERMS you may be using for the first time:

Crisis—any event seen as a crucial moment or turning point in a patient's life.
Personal Interaction—acting in a calm, professional manner to talk with the patient and listen to what he
is saying so that emotional support can be provided and accepted.
Emotional Emergency—a situation where a patient behaves in a manner that is not considered usual for the occasion. The patient's behavior is often not considered to be socially acceptable.

SPECIAL PATIENTS AND SITUATIONS

Every patient cared for by an EMS System is considered to be special. A patient is a *unique individual*, with his own specific problems and his own ways of attempting to deal with those problems. In emergency care, *"special patients"* are those who require care procedures that are modifications of what is usually done for most patients, or care procedures that are specifically designed to deal with a particular problem. We have already discussed some of these special patients. Caring for a child patient requires modified interview and physical examination procedures. The same is often the case if you are dealing with a patient who has abused drugs or alcohol. Care procedures change once a patient is thought to have a neck or spinal injury. This trauma patient becomes special, requiring the EMT to use procedures of evaluation and care specifically designed for the problem of spinal injury.

Most special patients require you to apply special communications skills and to provide emotional support. How you speak to a patient, what you say, how you express concern, how you listen, and how you indicate that you are listening are very important in special patient emergency care. Collectively, this is **personal interaction,** a skill that takes time to develop and is dependent on experience with many different types of patients.

The process of personal interaction is of great importance when dealing with children, the elderly, deaf patients, blind patients, drug and alcohol abuse patients, patients with emotional emergencies, victims of crime and sexual abuse, and patients who have been injured by friends or members of their own families. Each of these patients may feel that the emergency they are in is a crisis and that they are unable to control any aspect of the situation. Efficient personal interaction may be the key to providing effective total patient care.

The Concept of Crisis

When you are called to the scene of an accident or an illness, you consider the situation to be an emergency. To the patient, the situation may be a **crisis,** considered to be a crucial moment or a turning point in his life. Bystanders may consider the

emergency to be a crisis because they believe that what is happening is beyond their control and their ability to help.

Whenever a crisis exists, real or imagined, it must be managed. As an EMT, you will find yourself having to initiate the first steps in crisis management, or to work with the patient, or his family and friends to begin to deal with the crisis. Your *professional* attitude, your skills at personal interaction, and the emergency care you provide will help the patient begin to deal with his crisis.

Simply put, a person in a crisis is upset. Emotional stress is a part of every injury and illness. For the conscious and alert patient, this emotional stress can be a significant factor, steadily deteriorating the patient's physical and mental stability. If you provide emotional support, you can lessen the emotional stress. By doing so, you not only help the patient begin to cope with a problem, but you also improve his mental and physical well-being. This could keep an emotional emergency from growing worse, or it may be the primary reason why a trauma patient relaxes and avoids developing shock.

Any emergency may require you to practice the skills of crisis management, so remember:

1. Look and act like a *professional* provider of emergency care.
2. Act in a calm *professional* manner. Be careful not to react to what may be meaningless insults or to overreact to what the patient may do or say. Remember, the patient in need of your care is not at his best.
3. Talk *with* the patient and *listen* to what he is saying. Let him know that you are there to help. This tells the patient you are concerned, he is important, and you recognize that he truly has a problem.
4. Avoid improper conversation. You should never offer a simple solution to the patient's problem or tell him that everything is going to be fine. You should avoid comparing yourself to the patient, or telling the patient your own problems. You should not confront the patient and tell him that he is

wrong, or he is not making sense.
5. DO something for the patient. The idea that "actions speak louder than words" is very true in emergency care. Asking if the patient is in pain, controlling minor bleeding, or dressing a minor wound helps a patient deal with the emergency, even if he sees it as a crisis.

Be realistic in caring for patients. You do not have the time to sit down with the patient and go through every phase of crisis intervention, step by step. The sooner you can calmly transport the patient to a medical facility, the sooner he will receive medical care and crisis management help from trained and experienced professionals. Your role with the patient is not a problem-solving role, but one of providing some emotional support and taking the patient to a facility where the patient care team can assess his needs and problems. Never think for a moment that because you are good at working with people, or good at solving your own problems, you can assess patients' abilities to handle crises and determine what they must do to solve problems.

Even though the time you have with a patient is limited, the emotional support you can provide is of great importance. Let the patient know that you are concerned and that you care. To the best of your abilities and training, answer questions asked by the patient. Do not lie to the patient, but try to be positive about his situation.

It is important for the patient to believe that you are concerned about him because he is a person, not just an emergency care problem for you to solve. When possible, do not just talk to the patient, but have a conversation with him. Avoid spending most of your time talking with your partner. Some EMTs develop the habit of stopping conversation with the patient after the initial interview. They provide physical care, reserving conversation for other members of the EMS System. Emotional support cannot be provided unless you develop personal interaction with the patient.

Anyone wishing to become an EMT should be warned about becoming emotionally involved with what is happening at the emergency scene. We discussed this earlier in regard to illness and injury, but we did not mention how this can be a major problem when dealing with patients who are under severe emotional distress. Unless you remain professional, you can become emotionally involved. This may prevent you from providing prompt and efficient care. Your emotional involvement also may harm your emotional stability. Too many EMTs needlessly experience "burn out" in the profession because of this.

When you arrive at the scene of injury, illness, or emotional crisis, make certain that you know why you are there and what you can do. Ask yourself, "Why am I here?" Odds are you were not at the scene when the problem occurred or began, but rather that you were called to the scene. "Why was I called to the scene?" The call was made because someone was in need of emergency care. "What does the patient need?" The patient may need many things, ranging from love and understanding to a solution for a family problem. However, the patient also needs professional-level emergency care. "What am I trained to do as a professional? You are trained to provide emergency care, including emotional support. Once people recognize that there is a problem and they start to do something, then crisis management begins.

There may be one more question you find yourself wondering about: "Did I make a difference?" Almost certainly, you did. The reaction by the patient may not have been what you hoped for and there may not have been any "miracle" turnaround in terms of emotional stress, but you probably helped the patient at the scene and during transport. Your help was not only in terms of illnesses and injuries, but also in coping with emotional stress. The very fact that you transported the patient to a facility where he could receive total patient care must be considered as a major help. In addition to this, the emotional support you provided before transfer probably helped the patient deal with the emergency and made him more receptive to the support offered by other members of the patient care team.

PROBLEMS WITH COMMUNICATION

Difficulties in talking with people can be part of any patient-EMT interaction. However, EMTs report that they have experienced special problems when interviewing children, older patients, deaf patients, blind patients, and patients who speak no English. Interviewing children was covered Chapter 12, Section Two.

The Elderly Patient

Never stereotype patients. Too often, we have a preconceived notion of how someone will act, think, and react. In many cases, a determining factor of how we believe someone will behave is based on age. As with any age group, late adulthood is made of up of individuals of all types and personalities. A person is the total of all his experiences. Someone in late adulthood probably has experienced more than someone in early or middle adulthood. This means that you will find more variations with older patients. Realize that you will probably find that older patients approach things differently than you do.

You should provide care for the older patient as you would for any adult. Make certain that you properly identify yourself as an Emergency Medical Technician, trained to help them. Where you may think that "all old people are alike," the older patient may think that all young people are alike . . . too inexperienced to help. Ask the patient to tell you his name and use it frequently. Never resort to "old timer," "pops," "grandma," or other phrases. REMEMBER, you are talking to an adult, one who has faced other emergencies in his life.

As people age, hearing becomes a problem. A hearing problem may prove to be the reason why an older patient is unresponsive to your questions. Stay alert for the possibility of this problem, but do not assume that an older person cannot hear what you are saying. Avoid shouting whenever possible. Maintain eye contact, speaking directly to the patient. Begin by speaking in your normal voice. When in doubt, ask if he can hear you. If need be, speak directly into his ear.

Words become more important to people as they grow older. People in late adulthood spend more time thinking about what you say and what they are going to say in response. Younger people feel that the conversation is going more slowly than it does with members of their own age group. Consequently, the younger person may assume that the older individual is *thinking* more slowly, or that something must go wrong with the mental processes as people age. This slowness in conversation has been shown to have nothing to do with the mind's slowing down. Older people, through experience, know that words can have many different meanings during a conversation and even more meanings after a conversation is over. They simply spend more time in conversation because they place a high value on what is said. Do not rush the conversation.

You will find that many older people are out of practice in the art of face-to-face communication. In today's society, it is easy for an older person to become isolated, with little opportunity for conversation. This changes the patient's speech patterns. You may find an older patient changing topics or seeming to drift slowly away from the topic of your question. In some cases, this may be due to changes in the circulation to the brain (arteriosclerosis, hardening of the arteries). However, more often than not, this is simply because the older patient is out of practice in the art of conversation.

As an EMT, you must remember that the older patient is an adult who has gone through other emergencies in his life. *Older people know what works for them.* After you are certain that there are no life-threatening problems, allow the older patient to have some control of the pace of the survey and interview.

If the patient's spouse or close friend is at the scene, think of yourself as having more than one patient. You may be caring for a patient while his wife of thirty years watches in total fear, believing that death will take him away. Provide emotional support to *both* individuals. Be watchful of partners and friends, for the stress of the situation could set off a heart attack, convulsion, respiratory problem, or some other medical emergency.

The Deaf Patient

It is unfortunate, but most of us have little experience in communicating with the deaf and almost no skills to help us talk to them. This is true even though there are several million totally deaf people in our country, and many more who have some serious degree of hearing loss.

Seldom will you find a deaf person embarrassed about being deaf. Usually, it is the person with normal hearing who has this problem. Even experienced EMTs find themselves embarrassed trying to interview a deaf patient. The embarrassment usually comes from being asked to do something new or to do something one cannot do well. However, sometimes the uneasy feelings are due to guilt, as if the EMT has done something to cause the person's deafness. Remember, the deaf individual does not blame you for his deafness.

Always keep in mind that any patient might not be able to hear you. He may be able to speak clearly, but still not be able to hear. In most cases, a deaf person will tell you he is deaf or point to his ear and shake his head to indicate, "No, I cannot hear." Some patients may try to speak to you in sign language, using their hands and fingers to make communicating gestures. When in doubt, write, "Are you deaf?" on a card or piece of paper.

Once you are aware of the patient's deafness, see if the patient can read lips. Either write this out or ask him, "Can you read lips?" When speaking to the lip-reading deaf patient, make certain your face is in bright light (use a flashlight if you have to) and you speak slowly, but without distorting how you would normally form words. When you ask a question, point to your mouth to alert the person to the fact that he will have to read your lips. Never turn away from the deaf person while you speak.

Many deaf people cannot read lips, or find the process to be very difficult in an emergency. Your best methods of communication will be through writing and using gestures. If you point to an area on your body and make a face as if you are in pain and point back to the individual, he will usually understand your question. If you are examining the patient, point to your own body before you attempt to do something to his.

Throughout the entire care of a deaf patient, try to keep face-to-face contact, and direct physical contact (touching). Hold his hand, keeping one of your hands free to gesture or to gain his attention by a gentle tap on the shoulder. Point out the arrival of additional help, or other events that may have gone unnoticed.

Some deaf people can speak clearly, some can speak in a voice that may take a little time to understand, and others may not be able to speak at all. If the patient cannot speak, use written communication. Should the deaf patient be able to speak, listen very carefully to what he is saying. If you cannot understand something he has said, do not pretend to understand. This could be a serious mistake in gaining information and patient confidence. Always indicate you do not understand by shaking your head in an obvious "no" gesture.

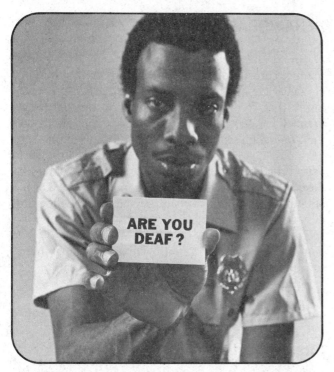

Figure 14-1: A simple prepared card helps to identify the deaf patient.

The Blind Patient

Blind people are seldom embarrassed by their blindness. Again, it is the sighted person trying to communicate with the blind who usually becomes embarrassed. Think for a moment. Why should it be difficult to converse with a blind person? After all, he can hear what you are saying and he is usually very aware of the world around him. Many EMTs claim that the survey and interview of blind patients are really not much different from those of sighted patients. If you remember to tell the blind patient what you are going to do before you do it, if you keep voice and touch contact throughout the period of care, and if you keep the blind person informed of

what is happening around him (the source of strange noises, the arrival of additional help, etc.), you will find little extra difficulty in caring for the blind patient.

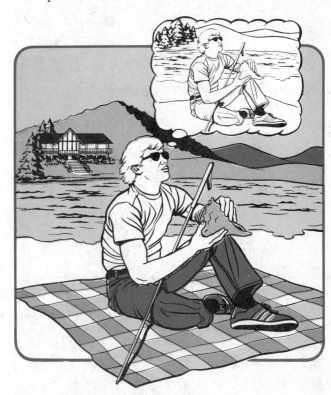

Figure 14-2: A blind person organizes information received from other senses into a mental picture of his environment.

Try to remember three things when dealing with the blind:

- Do NOT shout or speak loudly. Being blind does not mean a person cannot hear.
- Do NOT change the words you would normally use in speaking to a patient. People often become upset if they use the words "see" or "look" when they are with a blind person. Blind people also use these words. Your blind patients will know that you are not trying to embarrass them.
- Keep in contact through speech or touch.

Should you have to move a blind patient who can walk on his own, lead him while he holds on to your arm. The best placement for this patient would be standing slightly behind you, off to your side. Alert the blind patient of steps and other hazards. *Never* push the blind patient, always lead him.

The Non-English Speaking Patient

Establishing patient confidence and carrying out a useful patient assessment can be extremely difficult if your patient does not speak English. If a by-

ask if there is pain. Throughout the entire process, speak to the patient. He may understand more English than is at first apparent.

If you are an EMT whose service area includes communities of non-English speaking individuals, learn a few simple phrases to help you gain patient confidence and provide emergency care. In many cases, the people in the community would welcome the opportunity to help you and other EMTs learn their language as it applies to the emergency situation. The following chart is a guide to help you work with others to develop needed foreign language skills for your area. Additional help may be sought from the American Red Cross. They have a multilanguage book for the EMT.

BEHAVIORAL PROBLEMS

In an emergency, most patients will behave in a manner considered to be "normal" for the situation. However, using the term "normal" forces you to imply that certain medical and philosophical judgments have been made. It is more appropriate to say that the patient is behaving in a "typical" manner or behaving "as expected." This provides you with a very broad method of initially assessing patients. Based on your training and experience, you will be able to classify patients, simply stating that they are either *"behaving as expected,"* or *"behaving in an unusual manner."*

At the scene of accident or illness, you may have to provide care for:

- Stress reactions
- Emotional emergencies
- Psychiatric emergencies

Stress Reactions

An emergency is a stressful situation. You should expect that most distressed patients will display certain emotions such as fear, grief, and anger. These are typical **stress reactions** at the accident scene and are reactions to serious illness.

The emergency patient initially displays a mixture of emotions. As you begin to take control of the situation and start to treat him as an individual, his reactions to stress tend to change. In the vast majority of cases, *personal interaction* will inspire confidence in your ability to help. The patient will begin to calm down and may even begin to feel that he can cope with the emergency.

The inexperienced EMT may rush the patient interview, becoming too concerned with the physical assessment. True, it is critical that an EMT detect and attempt to correct life-threatening problems, but these aspects of care must be accomplished in a calm professional manner.

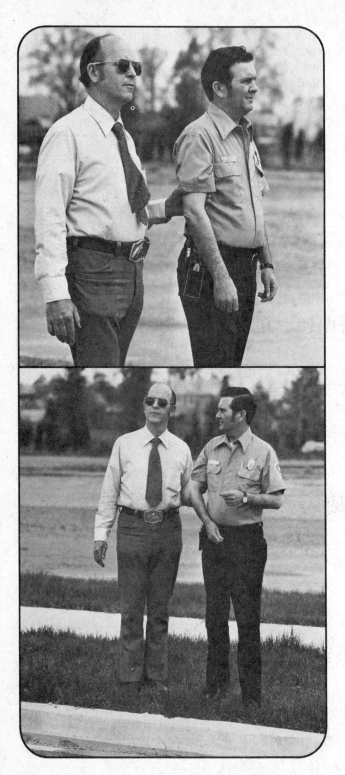

Figure 14-3: A blind person is led, not pushed.

stander can be of help, use him to help you communicate with the patient. If no such help is on hand, point to yourself and say your name. Let the patient see your patch or badge. Try to find out your patient's name. Usually, if you point to yourself and say your name and then point to the patient, he will understand and respond with his name. Point to the part of a patient's body you need to touch or examine. Use gestures to indicate there may be pain, or to

ENGLISH	FRENCH	GERMAN	SPANISH	ITALIAN
Hello	Bonjour	Guten tag	Hola!	Pronto
My name is	Je m'appelle	Ich heisse	Mi nombre es	Io mi chiamo
I am an emergency technician	Je suis infirmier	Ich bin Medicin-Techniker fur Notsälle	Yo soy un enfermero	Io sono un technico per il pronto soccorso
I am here to help you	Je vais vous aider (Je suis ici pour vous aider)	Ich bin hier um ihen zu helfen	Estoy aqui para ayudarle	Sono qui per aiutarti
Do you understand?	Comprenez vous?	Verstehn Sie?	Me Comprende?	Comprendi?
I do not understand	Je ne comprend pas	Nein, Ich verstehe Sie nicht	No comprendo!	No, non capisco
What is your name?	Comment vous appelez-vous?	Wie hessen Sie?	Cual es su nombre? (Some se llama usted?)	Come si chiama?
Mr.	Monsieur	Herr	Señor	Signore
Mrs.	Madame	Fräu	Señora	Signora
Miss	Mademoiselle	Fräulein	Señorita	Signorina
Are you sick?	Êtes-vous malade?	Sind Sie krank?	Esta usted enfermo?	Sei malato?
Are you injured?	Êtes-vous biessé	Sind Sie verietzt?	Esta usted lastimado?	Sei ferito?
Are you a diabetic?	Êtes-vous Diabetique?	Sind Sie zuckerkrank?	Esta usted diabetico? (diabetica)	Sei tu diabetico?
Yes/No	Oui/Non	Ja/Nein	Si/No	Si/No
Do you have a doctor?	Connaissez-vous un docteur?	Haben Sie einen Haus-Arzt?	Tiene usted su doctor?	Come si chiama il tuo dottore?
Who is your doctor?	Qui est votre docteur?	Wer ist lhr Arzt?	Quien es su doctor?	Chi é il tuo dottore?
Where do you live?	Où Habitez-vous?	Who wohnen Sie?	Donde vive usted?	Dove abiti?
What is your telephone number?	Quel est votre numéro de téléphone	Was ist Ihre Telefon-Nummer?	Cual es el número de su telefono?	Quale é il tuo numero du telefono?
Do you have a priest?(Rabbi? Minister?)	Connaissez-vous un prêtre? (un rabbin, un pasteur?)	Kennen Sie einen Pfarrer?(Rabiner, Paster)	Conoce usted un sacerdote?(Rabbi, pastor)	Hai un prete? (Rabbino, ministro)
I need to examine you for injuries	Jai besoin de voir vos blessures	Ich muss Sie für Verietzung untersuchen	Tengo que examinario por lastimaduras	Devo farti una vista per la tua ferita
Is that all right?	D'accord?	Sind Sie einverstanden?	Esta de acuerdo?	Va bene?
I am going to measure your blood pressure.	Je vais-mesurer votre tension artérielle	Ich nehme Ihren Blutdruck	Le voy a tomar la presión arterial	Devo misurarti la pression del sangue
I need to adjust your clothing	J'ai besoin d'ajuster vos vêtements	Ich muss Ihre Kleidung lockern	Necesito quitarle parte de la ropa	Devo sbottonarti il tuo vestito
I am going to touch the injury site. It may cause pain. Do you understand?	Je vais toucher l'endroit de vos blessures Cela peut faire un peu de mal. Comprenez-vous?	Ich werde lhre Wunde anfassen. Es wirt lhnen vielleicht weh tun. Versthen Sie Das?	Le voy a tocar parte lastimada y talvez le cause algun dolor. Me comprende?	Ora debbo toccare la tua ferita. Forse produce dolore. Comprendi?
Does this hurt?	Cela fait mal?	Tut das weh?	Le duele esto?	Fa male?
Can you move your foot? (leg, hand)	Pouvez-vous remuer le pied? (la jambe, la main)	Können sie Ihren Fuss bewegn? (lhre hand)	Puede usted mover el pie? (la mano)	Puoi muvere il tuo piede? (mano)
Can you feel that?	Pouvez-vous sentir celà?	Fühlen Sie das?	Siente usted algo cuando le toco?	Senti dovoti tocco?
I have finished the examination. Can I go ahead with emergency care procedures?	J'ai fini mon examination. Puis-je continuer avec les premiers soins?	Ich habe die Untersuchung durchgeführt kann ich jetzt mit der Notfürsorge-behandlung beginnen?	He terminado de examinario. Puedo comenzar con los tratamieto de emergencia?	Ho finito l'esame, ora debbo eseguire le pratiche per la procedura d'emergenza?
Don't move!	Ne bougez pas!	Seien sie still!	No sa mueva!	Non ti muovere!

As you begin an interview, be prepared to spend some time with the patient. Let him know that you are there to help. If you rush through conversations, the patient may feel he has lost control of the situation. He also may believe that you are concerned about the problems and not him as an individual.

Whenever you care for a distressed emergency patient who is acting in a manner you would expect:

- Act in a calm manner, giving the patient time to gain control of his emotions
- Quietly and carefully evaluate the situation
- Keep your own emotions under control
- Honestly explain things to the patient
- Let the patient know that you are listening to what he is saying
- Stay alert for sudden changes in behavior

Basically, you are applying *crisis management* techniques to help the patient deal with stress. If the patient does not begin to interact with you, or if he does not calm down, then you must assume he is having a more serious problem than an expected stress reaction.

Emotional Emergencies

We use the term **emotional emergency** to indicate situations where the patient is not acting as expected. However, he is responding to people around him and is not showing any indications of being dangerous to himself, or to others. He may be extremely frightened compared to most patients in a similar situation. Perhaps he is unable to calm his excited stage after an accident. At first, you may assume the patient's behavior is a typical stress reaction to the emergency. However, you find that the patient does not calm down during the interview and the beginning of care procedures. You must reconsider the stress of the emergency and try to establish some level of *personal interaction*. Once this is tried and the patient's behavior is still a concern, you may conclude that his behavior appears to be unusual.

Each patient is a unique individual. His behavior may be related to an undetected illness or injury, or he may simply need more time to cope with the emergency and respond to your efforts. What you observe could be part of a mental illness, but you cannot draw such a conclusion. At this point in assessment, all you can say is that you believe the patient is acting in an unusual manner and seems to be experiencing some kind of emotional emergency.

The emotional emergency may be an independent problem, or it may be the result of an accident, injury, illness, or disaster. As an independent event, the display of emotions may be due to a psychiatric problem. Before you jump to the conclusion that the patient has a "psychological" problem, or that the patient is "abnormal," consider your role as an EMT. A simple observation and some knowledge of terminology is not enough for you to reach any immediate conclusions. You must be able to rule out stress reactions, physical injury, and illness.

As an EMT, use terms such as excited, fearful, confused, overactive, unpredictable, agitated, aggressive, and detached. Avoid terms like mentally ill, psychotic, phobic, paranoid, manic, neurotic, and schizophrenic. Also avoid going to the other extreme by using terms like crazy, nuts, wacko, loony, and other nonprofessional words often associated with mental illness and emotional problems.

Often, the patient characterized as having an emotional emergency simply needs more time to cope with the stress of an emergency. *Personal interaction* is your main course of action for a patient with an emotional emergency. For this type of patient, you will have to spend more time talking with him and listening than would be necessary for most stress reaction patients. The patient may improve if he feels that he has more control over the situation. Give him time to answer your questions. When appropriate, let him decide which arm will be used for the blood pressure determination and how he would like to be positioned for transport.

Psychiatric Emergencies

As an EMT, you cannot make a medical diagnosis. Therefore, you cannot declare a patient to be mentally ill, or state that he is having a psychiatric emergency. Once you believe that apparent illness, injury, stress reactions, and emotional emergency are not the sources of a behavioral problem, then, in basic EMT-level emergency care, you can assume that a patient may be having a **psychiatric emergency** if he:

- Tries to hurt himself
- Tries to hurt others
- Withdraws, no longer responding to people or to his environment
- Continues to express rage and hostility
- Continues to act depressed, sometimes crying and expressing feelings of worthlessness
- Apparently wishes to take no actions to help himself or to allow himself to be helped.

This can be only an assumption, since you cannot detect all possible illness and injury in the field. Also, the patient may not be responding to your attempts at personal interaction at the scene, but he may respond very well to your efforts or those of another professional once he arrives at the medical facility.

If you arrive at the scene to find a patient displaying violent behavior, you cannot rule out illness or injury as the cause; however, you should immediately assume that this is a possible psychiatric emergency and not a stress reaction.

The assessment and care of the patient having a possible psychiatric emergency requires you to stay calm and to act in a strictly professional manner. Carefully observe the patient; listen to what he is saying. Detect whatever symptoms and signs are evident, making certain throughout the entire process of care that you can eliminate the possibilities of head injury, stroke, insulin shock, drug reactions, high fever, and other such medical emergencies.

Talk to the patient and let him talk to you. Make certain that he knows that you hear what he is saying. Do NOT threaten the patient or argue with him. Try to provide reassurance by telling him that you are there to help. Speak in a calm, direct manner, keeping eye contact whenever possible. Again, this is the method of *personal interaction*, your first line of action in trying to care for a patient having a possible psychiatric emergency. Do NOT leave the patient alone. Unless life-threatening illness or injury requires you to act differently, spend additional time talking with the patient. You are the first professional to begin both the physical and mental health care of the patient. The more *reassurance* you can provide for the patient, the easier it will be for the emergency department staff to continue with his care.

Aggressive Behavior

When a patient acts as if he may hurt himself or others, your first concern must be YOUR OWN SAFETY. In such cases, alert the police. Should a patient become violent, wait for police assistance. Do NOT put yourself in danger by taking any action that may be considered threatening by the patient. To do so may bring about hostile behavior directed against you or others.

DO NOT TRY TO RESTRAIN A PATIENT. In most localities, an EMT cannot legally restrain a patient, move him against his will, or force him to accept emergency care. You cannot restrain a patient even when his family asks you to do so. The restraint and forcible moving of patients is only within the jurisdiction of law enforcement officers. Once the patient is under control, the police can order you to transport the patient to the appropriate medical facility, or the order can come from a physician. A physician can order a patient to be restrained; however, the physician is not empowered to order you to do this if taking such actions may place you in danger.

REMEMBER: Each EMS System has its own standard operating procedures for dealing with aggressive patients and patients who may hurt themselves or others. Always follow your local guidelines.

If you help the police or a physician restrain a patient, make certain that the restraints are *humane* ones. Handcuffs and plastic ''throwaway'' criminal restraints should not be used because of the soft tissue damage they can inflict. Initially, the police may have to use such restraints; however, these types of restraints can be replaced with leather cuffs and belts. An ambulance should carry leather cuffs, a waist-size belt, and at least three short belts. Do NOT remove police restraints until you and the police are certain that the leather restraints will hold the patient. Once leather restraints are placed on a patient, do NOT remove them, even if the patient appears to be acting rationally. The removal of restraints is the concern of the emergency facility staff and the police.

NOTE: Never secure a patient to a stretcher in a position that will not allow the patient to be turned in case of vomiting. The patient must be secured so that his wrists and ankles remain secured, but his body can be turned.

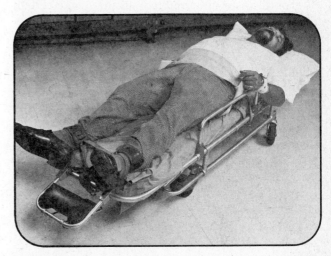

Figure 14-4: The patient can be secured to the stretcher in such a manner that he can be moved onto his side without loosening wrist and ankle restraints.

Attempted Suicide

Each year in this country, some 20,000 people commit suicide. Many more suffer both physical and emotional injuries in suicide attempts. Anyone can become suicidal if emotional distress is severe, regardless of age, sex, race, ethnic origin, or economic and social status.

People attempt suicide for many reasons, including the death of a loved one, financial problems, a terminated love affair, poor health, loss of esteem, divorce, fears of failure, and alcohol and drug abuse. They attempt to end their lives by any of a variety of methods. Most often, they try to do so with sedatives and hypnotic drugs. Less common are those individuals who attempt to die by hanging, jumping from high places, ingesting poisons, gas inhalation, wrist-cutting, self-mutilation, or by self-inflicted knife or gunshot wounds.

Providing Care for Attempted Suicide

Whenever you find yourself having to care for a patient who has attempted or is about to attempt suicide, your first concern is your OWN safety. Make certain the scene is safe and the patient does not have a weapon. *Unless you are a trained law enforcement officer following standard operating procedures, you have no business dealing with someone who has a weapon.* Should you see that a patient has a weapon, withdraw carefully, if you can. Do not frighten him with any sudden moves. Do not threaten him in any way. Above all, do not try to be a hero and attempt to seize the weapon.

If you cannot withdraw to safety, your best course of action is to try to talk to the individual and keep him engaged in conversation until additional help arrives. Again, do not do anything foolhardy that will result in you getting hurt.

For all cases of attempted suicide, make certain that the police are alerted. If your own safety is secure, establish visual and verbal contact with the patient as soon as possible. Talk with the patient in a calm, professional manner. Make certain the patient knows you are listening to what he is saying. Make no threats and offer no indication of using force.

Do not argue with the patient or criticize him. Do not point out that he is not making sense or that he contradicts something he said earlier. Never joke about the patient's situation. Ask if you can help. If he seems in doubt, tell him that you wish to help him. Ask if he is hurt or in pain. Stay calm and keep face-to-face contact whenever possible. Keeping the patient in a conversation is probably the only way you can get him to relax and grant you his confidence.

Do NOT leave the patient alone. Unless there is a physical emergency that must be cared for, sit down and spend some time with the patient. Talk with him, but do not try to direct all of the conversation. It is likely that the patient has a need to tell you his story. You should provide reassurance but not pity. As you gain the patient's confidence, tell him you wish to help and explain what questions he must answer and what must be done as part of the physical assessment. Let the patient know that you think it would be best if he went with you to the hospital. Tell him how you need his cooperation and help. If the patient indicates increasing fear or aggression, do not push the issues of the examination or transport. Instead, try to re-establish the conversation, and give the patient more time before you tell him again that going to the hospital is a good idea.

Victims of Crime

As in all aspects of emergency care, your first concern must be your own safety. If you arrive at the scene and a crime is in progress or the criminal is still active at the scene, do NOT attempt to provide care. Wait until the police arrive and they tell you that the scene is safe.

Your first priority at the controlled crime scene is to provide emergency care. While doing so, you must try to preserve the *chain of evidence* that will go from the crime scene to the courtroom. Touch only what you need to touch. Do not use the telephone unless the police tell you that you may. Unless you have police permission, do not move the patient unless he is in danger, or if he must be moved to provide proper care (example: to a hard surface for CPR).

When approaching a crime victim, clearly identify yourself and state that you are an Emergency Medical Technician trained to help. Otherwise, the patient might think you are the criminal returning to the scene. Do not burden the patient with questions about the crime. Keep to your duties involving the care of the patient. Remember, one of the most important things you can do when caring for the crime victim is to provide emotional support and reassurance.

In cases where you are called to the scene of a domestic dispute, wait for police assistance. Domestic disputes are dangerous calls because the people involved often act unpredictably. The call to have you respond was probably placed because someone had been beaten or injured by an act of violence. If the violent person is still on the scene, he may turn his aggression toward you.

If the crime is rape, do not wash the patient nor allow the patient to wash. Ask the patient not to change clothing, use the bathroom, or take any liquids or food. To do so may destroy evidence. Obviously, you may not physically prevent anyone from doing these things, but you can explain why such activities may break the chain of evidence. The patient will probably cooperate and follow your requests. *Emotional support* is a must in cases of rape. The privacy, comfort, and *dignity* of the patient must be considered from the beginning of care. The degree of future emotional problems faced by the rape victim may well depend on how the patient is initially treated by the professionals who respond to help.

REMEMBER: As an EMT, you have a legal duty to report any situation where injury is a possible result of crime, or was received in the commission of a crime. In most localities, you should not leave the crime scene until the police have given you the permission to do so.

SUMMARY

Special patients are those who require modified approaches to care and special procedures designed to consider a specific problem. Often, the EMT will find that these patients require extra effort in terms of communication and emotional support.

What is an emergency to you may be a crisis for the patient. The patient sees the event as a crucial moment or a turning point in his life. For such situations, crisis management must be initiated by the EMT.

Your main method to employ in crisis management is personal interaction. You have to act in a calm, professional manner, talking with the patient and listening to what he says. As you provide emotional support, you must do something for the patient. Providing even the simplest of care measures is useful in helping to manage the crisis.

The stress of helping others in a crisis can affect your own emotional stability. Remember that you have been trained to provide professional-level emergency care. The patient may need many things, one of which is your professional help. Keep in mind that you do make a difference.

Problems with communication can occur when providing emergency care. When dealing with elderly patients, remember that such patients have faced other emergencies. The elderly patient may set a pace of interviewing and examination different from your normal one. The older patient knows what works, so allow him some control. During the entire process of care, it is important to remember that words have more meaning and value to the older patient. Never assume an older patient cannot hear you or think clearly. Keep in mind that you will have to provide emotional support for the patient, family, and friends.

Always make certain that a patient is able to hear you. If the patient is deaf, establish this fact and then find out if the patient can read lips or if you will have to use writing and gestures for communication. Try to maintain face-to-face contact with the deaf person.

When dealing with blind patients, do not raise your voice. Talk as you would to any patient, and keep both verbal and physical contact with the patient throughout all stages of care.

Some of your patients may not speak English. Use the help of bystanders whenever you can. If there is a large community of non-English speaking people in your locality, learn some of the basic words and phrases to help you provide emergency care.

Most patients will exhibit stress reactions during an emergency. The tend to calm down as you interact with them and begin care. Emotional emergencies are those in which the patients have an emotional reaction to a situation that you do not consider to be usual. In many cases, such patients simply take longer to cope with the emergency than do most patients. Any patients who act as if they wish to hurt themselves or others, are having a psychiatric emergency. This also applies to patients who continue to express withdrawal, rage, hostility, depression, or an unwillingness to take any action.

Personal interaction is your best approach as you provide care. Make certain that the problem is not due to an injury or medical emergency. You must eliminate the possibilities of head injury, stroke, insulin shock, drug reactions, high fever, and other problems.

In cases involving psychiatric emergencies, maintain a professional manner and talk calmly with the patient. Do NOT leave the patient alone. Indicate that you are listening to what he says, and let him tell his story. If the patient is violent, wait for police assistance. Never try to provide care for a patient who has a weapon. Do not try to illegally restrain or transport the patient.

Provide care for the victim of crime only when the crime scene is controlled and you are certain of your own personal safety. Preserve the chain of evidence whenever possible. Touch only what you need to touch, and move the patient only when care or safety requires that he be moved.

Emotional support is a must in cases of rape. Consider the privacy, comfort, and dignity of the patient as soon as you begin care. Explain to the patient why she should not change clothes, wash, go to the bathroom, or take any liquids or food.

As an EMT, you have a legal duty to report any situations where injury may be due to crime or may have been received during the commission of a crime.

In all special care situations, your safety comes first.

SECTION TWO: MULTIPLE PATIENT AND DISASTER MANAGEMENT

OBJECTIVES By the end of this section, you should be able to:

1. Define "polytrauma." (p. 340)
2. Define triage and classify various illnesses and injuries as to priority. (p. 340-1)
3. Relate given signs to specific illnesses and injuries. (p. 341-3)
4. Define disaster and disaster plan. (p. 344)
5. List and define the SEVEN periods of a disaster. (p. 345)
6. Describe the impact of a disaster on EMS personnel and what can be done to reduce this impact. (p. 345-6)
7. Describe a model disaster scene operation. (pp. 346-7)

SKILLS As an EMT, you should be able to:

1. Initiate and conduct triage for a polytrauma emergency.
2. Apply assessment skills to triage.
3. Provide triage, emergency care, and transport as defined by your locality's disaster plans.

TERMS you may be using for the first time:
Triage—a process used to sort patients in terms of priority for care and transport, based on the severity of illness and injury.
Disaster—any emergency involving illness and injury that taxes the resources of an EMS System.
Disaster Plan—a prearranged plan that describes how the various services will respond and what they will do in cases of specific types of disasters in their locality.

MULTIPLE PATIENT SITUATIONS

The term **multitrauma** can mean that a patient has more than one injury. **Polytrauma** is used to indicate that there is more than one patient. This term also is applied to multiple patient situations where there are injuries and medical emergencies. To avoid confusion, use the terms "multiple patients" or "multiple casualties."

Most of the care you provide as an EMT will be delivered to one sick or injured patient at a time. There also will be cases, such as the typical motor vehicle accident, where you and your partner may have to provide care for two or more patients simultaneously. Once you have more patients than EMTs and other trained providers at the scene, deciding who receives care first and who is transported first can become a problem. There may be a time when you respond to an accident and find a number of patients—perhaps a large number—with injuries ranging from minor to lethal. Along with patients who are injured, you may also have to consider those who have had a medical emergency, either immediately before the accident, or one triggered by the accident.

TRIAGE

The process of **triage** is used to sort patients into categories of priority for care and transport, based on the severity of injuries and medical emergencies. The sorting of patients begins as soon as trained personnel reach the sick and injured persons. Through careful triage, the patients can be placed into one of three categories: highest priority, second priority, and lowest priority.

Each EMS System has its own form of triage. The following is an example based upon what is typically in use:

- *Highest Priority:*
  1. Respiratory arrest, airway obstruction, and severe breathing difficulties
  2. Cardiac arrest (remember that respiratory arrest is usually detected first)
  3. Uncontrolled severe bleeding
  4. Severe head injuries
  5. Open chest wounds

6. Open abdominal wounds
7. Severe shock
8. Burns involving the respiratory tract
9. Severe medical problems (including heart attack, stroke, heatstroke, poisoning, and abnormal childbirth)
10. Unconsciousness

• *Second Priority:*
1. Severe burns
2. Injuries to the spine (including cervical spine)
3. Moderate bleeding
4. Conscious patients with head injuries
5. Multiple fractures

• *Lowest Priority:*
1. Minor bleeding
2. Minor fractures and minor soft tissue injuries
3. Moderate and minor burns
4. Obvious mortal wounds where survival is not expected
5. Obvious death

Not everyone agrees with the above classification. Variations do occur, but they tend to be minor. Your instructor will tell you of any variations for your area.

Some EMS Systems have modified this procedure and now have four categories. In their triage, the obviously dead patients (as in decapitation) are placed in the fourth category, making the dead victim the lowest priority. Typically, this type of triage is listed as highest priority, second priority, delayed priority, and lowest priority.

Triage priorities can change depending on the number of patients, types of injuries, and number of emergency care providers at the scene. For example, cardiac arrest is a high priority emergency. However, if there are many patients with life-threatening problems and few emergency care providers, the cardiac arrest patient may become a lowest priority patient. This may be necessary to prevent many patients from dying while a rescuer tries to save one. Many people find this philosophy to be objectionable. They fail to understand that there are limits as to what the EMS System can do in certain polytrauma situations.

Identification Procedures

If there are adequate personnel for a polytrauma emergency, triage stops when you find a patient in respiratory arrest, severe respiratory distress, cardiac arrest, or with life-threatening bleeding that requires immediate care. If the first person you check is in respiratory arrest, you cannot go on to the next pa-

tient, planning to return when triage is completed. You must care for life-threatening emergencies as you find them.

One factor that may require modification in any triage is that patients do not always remain stable. You may have to update your triage. If the scene includes a large number of patients, you also will find yourself having to modify care procedures. For example, your highest priority patient may be classified as such because he is unconscious. However, when you assess another patient, you may note that a patient formerly classified as having moderate bleeding is in need of immediate care. You will have to come back to monitor the unconscious patient, but you cannot provide continuous monitoring while the other patient bleeds.

Every ambulance and rescue unit should carry tags that can be used during the triage phase of a disaster operation. While identification systems vary, an effective program uses **colored tags**. Red tags identify highest priority patients, green tags second priority, and white tags lowest priority. When highly visible colored tags are used, emergency care personnel easily can see who should be treated first. These tags are usually designed to show information such as vital signs at the time of the survey, known and suspected injuries, and changes in the patient's condition during transport. Since triage must be accomplished without delay, tags should be designed so that they can be filled out quickly. Tags should always be affixed conspicuously to the patients.

Triage and Patient Assessment

The primary and secondary surveys, including patient and bystander interviews, are critical in determining care and order of care when you have more than one patient. Vital signs and other highly significant signs must be assessed and quickly related to possible problems, injuries, or illnesses. There is no time for the EMT to try to remember how certain symptoms and signs relate to injury and illness. No time can be set aside to check charts in textbooks. The EMT must know how to conduct a proper patient assessment and how to relate his findings to specific illnesses and injuries.

As an EMT, you must be able to apply the following information to the assessment and care of patients:

• Pulse (vital sign)
  Rapid, full: fear, overexertion, heatstroke, high blood pressure, early stages of internal bleeding
  Rapid, thready: shock, blood loss, heat exhaustion, diabetic coma (some cases), falling blood pressure

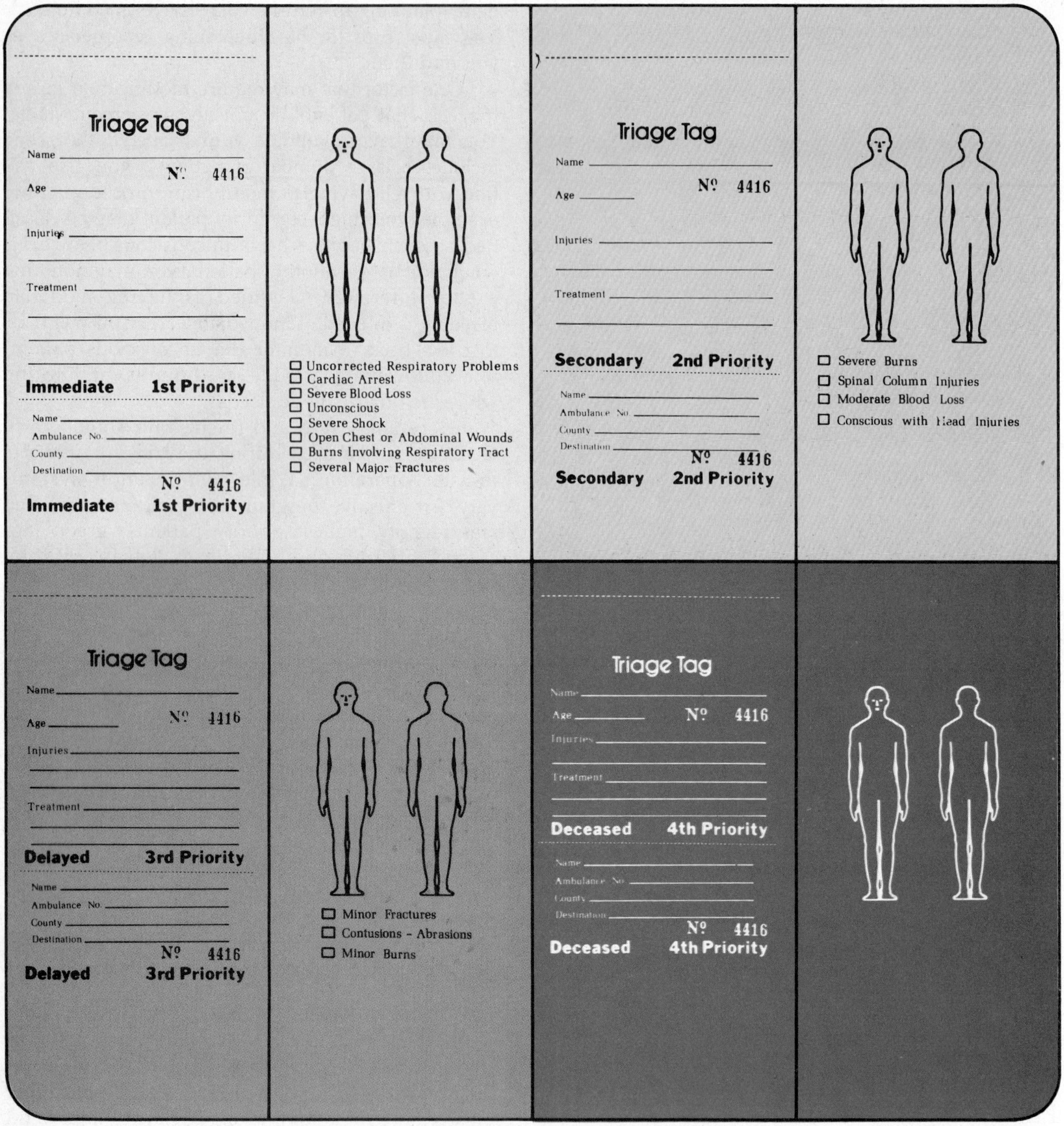

Triage Tag

Name _____
No. 4416
Age _____

Injuries _____
_____

Treatment _____
_____
_____
_____

Immediate   1st Priority

Name _____
Ambulance No. _____
County _____
Destination _____
No. 4416

Immediate   1st Priority

□ Uncorrected Respiratory Problems
□ Cardiac Arrest
□ Severe Blood Loss
□ Unconscious
□ Severe Shock
□ Open Chest or Abdominal Wounds
□ Burns Involving Respiratory Tract
□ Several Major Fractures

Triage Tag

Name _____
No. 4416
Age _____

Injuries _____
_____

Treatment _____

Secondary   2nd Priority

Name _____
Ambulance No. _____
County _____
Destination _____
No. 4416

Secondary   2nd Priority

□ Severe Burns
□ Spinal Column Injuries
□ Moderate Blood Loss
□ Conscious with Head Injuries

Triage Tag

Name _____
No. 4416
Age _____

Injuries _____
_____

Treatment _____

Delayed   3rd Priority

Name _____
Ambulance No. _____
County _____
Destination _____
No. 4416

Delayed   3rd Priority

□ Minor Fractures
□ Contusions - Abrasions
□ Minor Burns

Triage Tag

Name _____
No. 4416
Age _____

Injuries _____

Treatment _____

Deceased   4th Priority

Name _____
Ambulance No. _____
County _____
Destination _____
No. 4416

Deceased   4th Priority

Figure 14-5: Examples of triage systems in use.

Slow, full: stroke, skull fracture

No pulse: cardiac arrest

- Respiration (vital sign)

  Rapid, shallow: shock, heart problems, heat exhaustion, insulin shock, congestive heart failure

  Deep, gasping, labored: airway obstruction, congestive heart failure, heart problems, lung disease, lung injury from excessive heat, chest injuries, diabetic coma

Snoring: stroke, fractured skull, drug or alcohol abuse, partial airway obstruction

Crowing: airway obstruction, airway injury due to excessive heat

Gurgling: airway obstruction, lung disease, lung damage due to excessive heat

Coughing blood: chest wound, rib fracture

- Blood Pressure (vital sign)

  High: chronic hypertension, head injury, severe pain, drug withdrawal

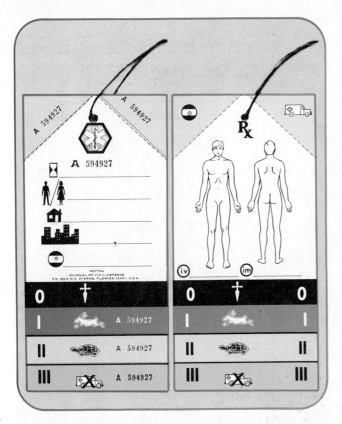

Figure 14-6: Typical triage tags used to identify highest priority, second priority, and lowest priority patients.

Low: chronic hypotension, shock, internal bleeding, chest injury, drug abuse

- Skin temperature (vital sign)

    Cool, moist: shock, bleeding, body is losing heat, heat exhaustion

    Cool, dry: exposure to cold

    Cool, clammy: shock, heart attack

    Hot, dry: heatstroke, high fever

    Hot, moist: infectious disease

- Skin color

    Red: high blood pressure, heatstroke, diabetic coma

    Cherry red: carbon monoxide poisoning

    White, pale, ashen: shock, heart attack, excessive bleeding, heat exhaustion, fright, insulin overdose or insulin shock

    Blue: heart failure, airway obstruction, lung disease, certain poisonings

- Pupils of the eyes

    Dilated, unresponsive to light: cardiac arrest, unconsciousness, shock, bleeding, heatstroke, certain types of drugs (LSD, uppers)

    Constricted: damage to the central nervous

system, certain types of drugs (heroin, morphine, codeine)

    Unequal: stroke, head injury

    Lackluster: shock, coma

- State of consciousness

    Confusion: fright, anxiety, illness, minor head injury, alcohol or drug abuse, mental illness, epilepsy

    Stupor: moderate to severe head injury, alcohol or drug abuse, stroke

    Brief unconsciousness: minor head injury, fainting, epilepsy

    Coma: stroke, anaphylactic shock, severe head injury, poisoning, drug or alcohol abuse, diabetic coma, heatstroke

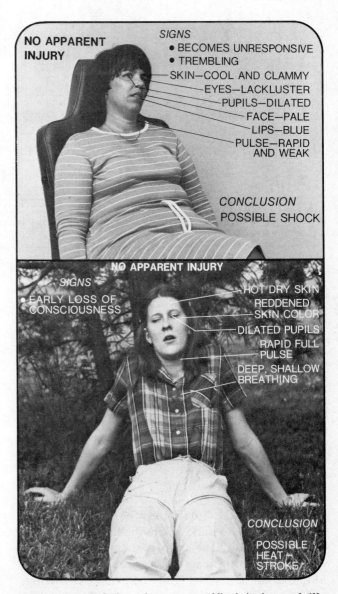

Figure 14-7: Relating signs to specific injuries and illnesses.

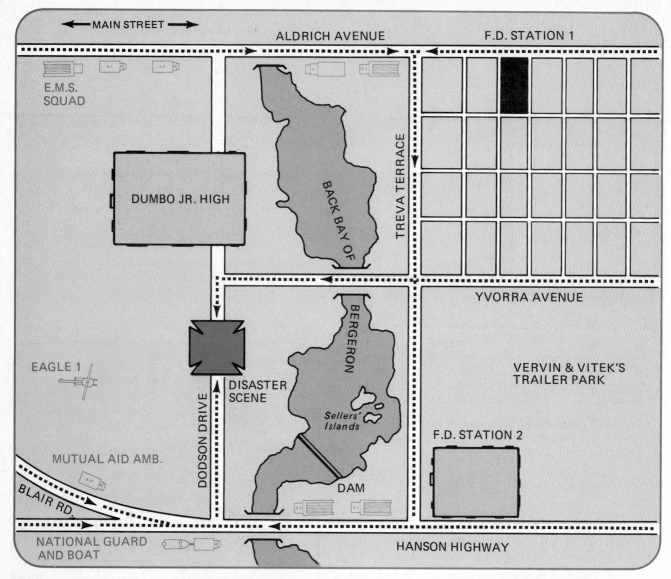

Figure 14-8: An efficient, complete response to a disaster requires prior planning, involving all appropriate agencies.

- Paralysis or loss of sensation

    One side of body: stroke, head injury

    Upper limbs: spinal injury in neck

    Lower limbs: spinal injury along back

    Upper and lower limbs: spinal injury in neck and possibly along back

    No pain, obvious injury: spinal cord or brain damage, shock, hysteria, drug or alcohol abuse

DISASTERS

Fires, floods, hurricanes, earthquakes, and tornadoes come to mind when one thinks of a disaster. So too do airplane crashes, train wrecks, or any accident in which many people are injured. To the EMS System, a **disaster** is any occurrence involving, or having the potential to cause, many injuries. To be a true disaster, the event must tax the resources of the local EMS System and rescue support systems.

To provide prompt and efficient care during a disaster, the personnel involved must be trained for such an event and have practiced the techniques and procedures to be used during the disaster. In addition, a **disaster plan** should be developed for each possible disaster that may occur within a community. A disaster plan worked out in advance will allow for all agencies, personnel, and support services to work together to meet the needs of the patients and the community. When a disaster occurs, the EMS System must know each aspect of disaster management:

- Who is in authority for the overall plan.
- Who controls each aspect of the management of the particular disaster.
- How is transportation and communication set up and regulated.

- What needs to be done.
- Where specific procedures should be done.
- Who is needed to do a particular job or procedure.
- What are the support services, where are they located, and how can they be reached.
- Who are additional sources of help.

Phases of a Disaster—
How People React

Calvin J. Frederick has proposed that any disaster can be divided into phases based on the way individuals and the community respond to it. The phases of disaster are called *periods*. They can vary according to the type of disaster; however, most include the following:

1. WARNING PERIOD—Some disasters give warning of their approach. When the onset of a disaster is sudden, as with earthquakes and airplane crashes, people respond better to the sudden emergency than they do when warned in advance. Apparently, many people are not able to cope with the anxiety and apprehension that intensifies as a known disaster approaches. For these people, the warning phase is a period of ALARM, not a period of action. During this phase, you may have to interact with "helpless" people, giving them specific tasks to do for their own safety and emotional stability.

2. THREAT PERIOD—This is a critical decision-making time for many individuals. People have to ask if the threat is real, and if so, when will the disaster materialize. A person may find himself thinking: "Will I be killed or hurt?," "Will my family be killed or hurt?," "Will I lose everything?," "Can I escape?" These and a host of other questions precipitate decisions that are important to survival. Making such decisions can bring about an emotional crisis for some people, particularly for those individuals who find day-to-day decision-making difficult.

3. IMPACT PERIOD—When the disaster strikes, people quickly realize its magnitude as they see injury, death, and destruction. Some people panic, but this is rare. On the other hand, some wander aimlessly about, unable to cope with the problem or even to follow the directions of others. A few individuals step forward to assume leadership, and it is these few that the others follow after a disaster strikes.

4. INVENTORY PERIOD—During this phase of a disaster, people try to assess what has happened to them, producing a great variety of emotional responses. Depending on a number of factors, survivors exhibit fear, anger, sorrow, depression, anxiety, apprehension, and other emotions. Most people make a quick recovery after feeling the impact of their inventory, but some carry emotional scars for the rest of their lives.

Immediately after a disaster, people tend to feel isolated and overwhelmed by the event. Observers have noted that some men stand and stare, some women hug themselves and display a rocking motion, and children have been seen to display regressive behavior (an eight-year-old child may temporarily act like a five-year-old, etc.). Most individuals try to engage themselves in some sort of purposeful activity. Once people begin to help with rescue and start to clean up the damage, their feelings of isolation and of being overwhelmed tend to fade.

5. RESCUE PERIOD—During this postdisaster phase, the survivors help each other to cope. Shock is still a problem, but in some people apathy and withdrawal are noted. Most of these individuals come out of their apathy and withdrawal once they join others in helping to rescue victims, provide comfort to others, and to reestablish shelter and other needs.

6. REMEDY PERIOD—The morale of survivors picks up during this period as they work together with rescue personnel to get the community back on its feet. A spirit of cooperation usually prevails. The period of remedy is often the longest postdisaster phase.

7. RESTORATION PERIOD—In this final phase, the individuals of a community regain the stability that they enjoyed prior to the disaster. How long it takes for a community to reach equilibrium depends on the nature of the disaster, the degree of destruction, and the amount of help available.

The Impact on EMS Personnel

During a disaster, emergency care personnel have to cope with their own fears, and their worries about the safety of their families, friends and property. Added to this emotional stress are the effects of seeing destruction, providing care for the injured and sick, and having to deal with the dead victims of the disaster. Throughout the entire emergency operation, emergency personnel have to keep their emotions in check, trying to cope with the stresses they are experiencing. Include the factors of exhaustion and exposure to environmental elements, and you have the potential for severe emotional crisis.

The problem of emotional disturbance in rescue workers was never given much thought in the past. Today, it is considered a real threat to mental health, enough so that crisis intervention teams who work with rescuers' problems are now a part of most disaster planning. Three things are now done to help reduce stress on emergency personnel:

1. EMS personnel are given work schedules for the disaster operation. These schedules contain regular rest periods.
2. Rescue efforts are organized so that someone in authority can constantly watch rescuers for signs of emotional distress and physical fatigue. If a supervisor sees that one of the workers may be having emotional problems or is physically exhausted, he can require the worker to take a longer than usual rest period. Following the rest period, the worker can be assigned to a less stressful task.
3. Rescuers are encouraged to eat and sleep whenever they can, and to engage in conversations with other workers. Talking helps, but individuals should avoid using "gallows humor" as a safety valve for dealing with stress. What seem to be harmless jokes about the disaster, fellow workers, and superiors may upset some workers at the time. Many rescuers report that this type of humor continues to bother them long after the disaster is over.

Remember that you can never fully predict how you will act in a disaster. If you are mentally prepared for what will happen in a disaster, and for what you will be doing during disaster operations, the chance of you becoming an emotional casualty is reduced. Realize that you will do a more effective job as a provider of emergency care if you:

• Attend crisis intervention training programs.
• Participate as both rescuer and victim in disaster training programs.
• Know the forms of disaster most likely to strike your community.
• Know how your community's resources will be mobilized at the time of disaster, and know what help is immediately available.

Disaster Scene Operations

Each locality has its own standard operating procedures for disaster operations. The following is a general example of the operations at a disaster scene.

1. A command post is established in a safe area. This is usually the first ambulance to arrive, though it may be replaced later by another vehicle.

2. Communications are established with hospitals, medical facilities, dispatchers, and other emergency service units. This requires a multichannel radio transmitter.

3. Hazard control must begin as soon as possible. There must be close coordination between rescue personnel, EMTs, firefighters, and law enforcement officers. If the scene is not safe, triage and patient care will have to be delayed.

4. The EMTs on the first ambulance to arrive automatically become triage officers. They continue this duty until a qualified triage officer arrives, for example, a physician from a nearby major medical facility. If a triage team arrives with this person, the EMTs can begin patient care; otherwise, they should continue to assist with triage.

5. Extrication may be difficult or delayed. Those doing the extrication must work closely with the EMTs so that triage and care can begin as soon as possible and so that patients are not injured during disentanglement operations.

6. When possible, patients are removed from wreckage according to the severity of their injuries, but this is not always practical.

7. A triage point or points should be set up in a safe area. At least one of these triage points should be in the immediate area of the command post. Triage areas are to be located so that all patients are "funneled" through triage before they are taken to ambulances for transport.

8. A staging area is set up for incoming ambulances. These ambulances are not to go to the triage areas. This will reduce congestion and allow for quicker transport.

9. All ambulance drivers should stay with their vehicles. EMTs should report to the triage officer. When reporting, the EMTs should carry portable equipment with them, such as trauma kits, spine boards, splints, folding stretchers, and other removable supplies and equipment.

10. The ambulance supplies and equipment should be placed in a supply pool near the treatment area. A rescue worker must be placed in charge of this equipment. When possible, ambulances can be directed to this equipment pool prior to reporting to their staging point.

11. Incoming EMTs should be assigned to patient care activities.

12. Volunteers can and should be used to help free EMTs, rescuers, firefighters, and police from tasks that take them away from their main duties.

13. A second triage area should be set up to determine the order of transport for treated patients. This area must be set up so that all patients go

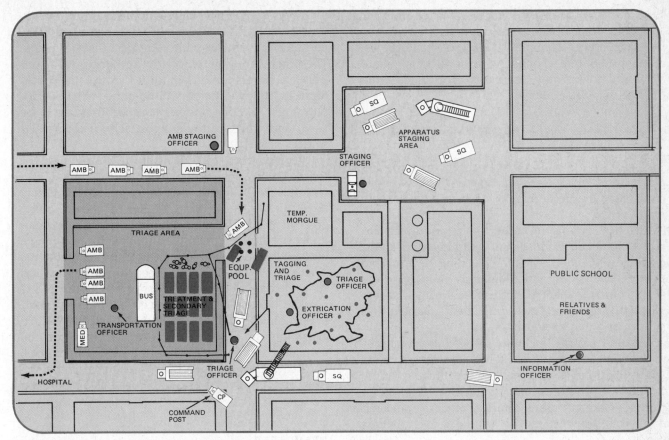

Figure 14-9: The disaster scene.

from initial triage and care through the transport triage. The patient must be brought through this second triage before ambulances are called from the staging area.

14. Patients should be readied for transport and ambulances should be called, as needed, from the staging area.

15. The command post should determine the hospital to which a particular ambulance should go. When a hospital reaches its capacity, the command post can be notified.

16. Patients should be transported with an EMT providing care.

17. As ambulances discharge their patients at a medical facility, they need to call the dispatcher or command post to see if they should return to the scene. Upon returning to the scene, they should report directly to the staging area and let the command post know they have arrived.

18. A special care area should be set up to receive relatives and friends of the disaster victims. Someone must be placed in charge of this area and must make certain that only reliable information is passed on to those waiting to hear about friends and relatives. Emergency care should be available at the information center in case a friend or relative has a medical emergency.

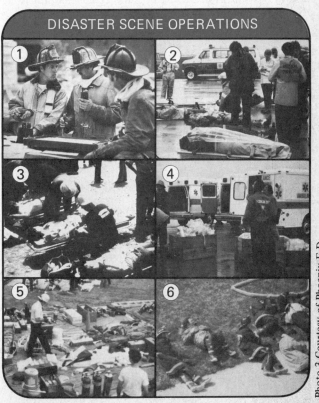

DISASTER SCENE OPERATIONS

Figure 14-10: Disaster scene operations.

Photo 3 Courtesy of Phoenix F.D.

19. Since dead victims will not be removed from the scene until all the injured patients have been transported, a temporary morgue should be established out of sight. Someone must stand guard to prevent unauthorized persons from disturbing the bodies.

SUMMARY

Triage is a method of sorting patients into categories for receiving care and transport. The sorting is done based on the severity of patients' illnesses and injuries.

Highest priority includes respiratory arrest, airway obstruction and severe breathing difficulties, cardiac arrest, life-threatening bleeding, severe head injuries, open chest and abdominal wounds, severe shock, burns involving the respiratory tract, severe medical problems (including heart attack and stroke), and unconsciousness.

Second priority includes severe burns, injuries to the spine, moderate bleeding, conscious patients with head injuries, and multiple fractures.

Lowest priority includes minor bleeding, minor fractures and soft tissue injuries, moderate and minor burns, obvious mortal wounds, and obvious death.

Patient assessment is very important during triage. Vital signs and other key signs are used. Pulse, respiration, blood pressure, skin temperature, skin color, pupils, state of consciousness, paralysis, and loss of sensation are used in making assessments.

A disaster is any emergency that taxes the resources of the EMS System. To be an effective EMT, you must be familiar with your local disaster plans. These plans indicate who is in authority, who controls and carries out certain duties, how communications and transportation will be done, what specifically must be done and what procedures are to be used, and what are the support services and other sources of help.

People react to a disaster in many different ways. Often, specific behavior can be associated with the period of the disaster. As an EMT you may have to give people directions for their own safety, give them specific tasks for their safety and emotional stability, and help the survivors by assuming a leadership role. Remember that your own emotional health can be affected. Take needed rest periods and set aside time to talk with fellow rescue workers.

The disaster scene will need a command post, multichannel radio communications established, triage points and areas for care, transport triage points, a staging area for ambulances, an equipment pool, an area to receive friends and relatives of the victims, and a protected area to be used as a temporary morgue.

REMEMBER: A disaster taxes the resources of the EMS System. Disaster management depends on all personnel performing the right task at the right time. If you are in the first ambulance to arrive, your actions during the first few minutes of operation may well influence the outcome of the disaster.

15 preparation and response

OBJECTIVES By the end of this chapter, you should be able to:

1. Explain what is meant by the term "self-preparation." (p. 350)
2. List the categories included in the daily inspection of an ambulance. (p. 351)
3. Define "central dispatch" and relate this system to the universal number (911) concept. (p. 351)
4. Describe TWO types of dispatching systems that may be used in place of a 911 central dispatch system. (p. 351, 2)
5. List the information that can be gained by the dispatcher and relayed to the squad prior to response. (p. 351-3)
6. Describe what you should do when receiving a call from the dispatcher. (p. 353)
7. Define "emergency driving" and "defensive driving." (p. 353)
8. Give FIVE examples of emergency vehicle operations regulations typically imposed by state government. (p. 353-4)
9. Describe, in your own words, the physical and mental qualities of a good ambulance driver. (p. 354)
10. Indicate the proper use of sirens, horns, and warning lights. (p. 354-5)
11. Define "stopping distance" in terms of reaction distance and braking distance. (p. 355)
12. List at least SIX factors that can be the cause of hazardous road conditions. (p. 356)
13. Define "hydroplaning" and state how this problem can be avoided when driving an ambulance. (p. 356)
14. Describe the special driving techniques needed for:
    - Skids on wet or icy roads
    - Driving in fog
    - Driving through pools of water
    - Tire blowout
    - Steering failure
    - Brake failure
    - Accelerator failure
    - Objects in the roadway
    - Animals in the roadway
    - People in the roadway. (pp. 356-7)
15. Describe how emergency driving techniques change when driving at night. (p. 357-8)
16. List SIX varieties of two-vehicle accidents in which the ambulance may be involved. (p. 358)
17. Describe how to avoid each of these two-vehicle accidents when driving an ambulance. (p. 358-60)
18. Describe the SEVEN factors that can affect a response. (p. 360-1)
19. Justify the need for alternate routes to the emergency scene. (p. 360-1)
20. Describe arriving at the emergency scene in terms of traffic, the roadway, and known hazards. (p. 361-2)
21. State the procedures to follow when parking the ambulance on a roadway. Include any cautions that pertain to the ambulance headlights. (p. 361, 2)
22. Define a "danger zone" and relate this term to the parking of the ambulance at the scene of:
    - Downed electrical wires
    - Damaged utility poles
    - Vehicle fires
    - Explosives
    - Hazardous materials. (pp. 362, 3)
23. Describe what you should do if you cannot complete a response to an emergency. (p. 362)

SKILLS   As an EMT you should be able to:

1. Properly conduct a daily inspection of the ambulance.
2. Receive information from a dispatcher.
3. Drive an ambulance according to the laws of your state.
4. Use emergency and defensive driving skills to avoid accidents while driving the ambulance.
5. Make correct use of the warning devices found on the ambulance.
6. Properly position an ambulance, taking into consideration the traffic, the roadway, and known hazards.

TERMS   you may be using for the first time:

Central Dispatch—one dispatch headquarters that receives all emergency calls and relays information to the needed services (fire department, rescue squad, police department, etc.).

Universal Number Calling—one-number calling, where the number 911 is used to gain access to central dispatch.

Reaction Distance—the number of feet a vehicle travels from the time a driver decides to stop until his foot applies pressure to the brake pedal.

Braking Distance—the number of feet a vehicle travels from the start of braking action until it comes to a full stop.

Stopping Distance—the number of feet a vehicle travels from the moment a driver decides to stop until the vehicle actually stops. It is the total of reaction distance and braking distance.

Hydroplaning—during wet driving conditions, a film of water develops between the tires and the road surface, causing the tires to ride on the water rather than the road surface.

Danger Zone—the area at the emergency scene in which rescue personnel, patients, and bystanders may be exposed to hazards such as fire, dangerous chemicals, explosion, downed electrical wires, or radiation.

PREPARATION

An effective response is one in which the ambulance arrives quickly and safely with the EMTs ready for immediate service. Such a response is a joint effort. The ambulance driver must be skilled in the operation of the vehicle, completely alert, and able to react to a wide variety of conditions. The attending EMTs must utilize the response time to plan tentative emergency care activities, based on the information provided by the dispatcher.

Before an effective response can be rendered, there must be adequate preparation. Each link in the chain of the EMS System must be ready to do its job in providing care before the emergency occurs. You must prepare yourself and the ambulance before receiving the dispatcher's call.

SELF-PREPARATION

You should be ready for duty at the beginning of the shift. This means that you will have to be on time, ready to receive a call from the dispatcher. You should be dressed in your uniform and have gathered any equipment or reporting forms required for you to have on hand prior to a response.

Physically, you should be rested and alert. You should have eaten before your time of duty and, if the meal was a large one, you should have allowed enough time for any feelings of heaviness or sleepiness to have passed. You should have refrained from the use of alcohol for at least two hours prior to reporting for your shift. If you are ill, you should make arrangements with the personnel officer for another EMT to cover your duties. Even if the nature of your illness is not infectious, you should not report. There is too great a tendency to make improper judgments and to render substandard care when ill.

Mentally, you should be prepared to respond and provide care. Every EMT needs a moment to collect his thoughts before beginning a shift. Remember that you have been trained to provide proper care. Keep in mind that you *do* make a difference.

THE AMBULANCE

Every ambulance that may be used during a shift should be inspected by the EMTs when they report for duty. Even when another person has inspected the ambulance, you should carry out your own inspection. The EMTs in the prior shift and others who may have inspected the vehicle and its equipment should not be insulted by your actions. When you inspect your own ambulance, you are providing the other individuals with backup that helps prevent errors and shows a professional interest in your squad's ability to provide the best care.

Your daily inspection of the ambulance should include:

- Body exterior—look for any damage to the body of the ambulance that needs repair. Be alert to any damage that may affect response. Pay careful attention to damage at the wheelwells that may prevent turning of the wheels, or may puncture tires. Follow local procedures if the exterior needs cleaning.
- Tires and wheels—check for damage, severe wear, and proper inflation. Be certain to check spare tires.
- Glass and mirrors—look for broken windows and mirrors. Be sure that all mirrors can be properly aligned.
- Doors and windows—check to see that each window and door will open and close properly and that all latches and locks are operational.
- Body interior—check for damage to all driver and patient compartment interior surfaces and upholstery. Be certain that the ambulance interior is clean and that any needed decontamination has been completed.
- Fuel tank—check the level of fuel. Some EMS Systems require the fuel tanks to be filled after each response. Most require refilling when the primary tank shows half empty.
- Temperature controls—check the operation of the heater or air conditioner, depending on the season, and check all vents.
- Communications equipment—check ALL communications equipment to be certain it is operational.
- Warning devices—check the siren, horn, and visual warning signals to be sure all are operational.
- Lights—in addition to the visual warning devices, test the high/low headlights, turn signals, brake lights, backup lights, spot or scene lights, and marker lights.
- Gauges—check for warnings indicating possible problems with the oil pressure, alternator, or battery.
- Brakes—depress the brake pedal to test for pressure; test the parking brake.
- Cooling system—check the water/coolant level, the fan belts, and all hoses.
- Equipment and supplies—make certain that you have all the equipment and supplies on your inventory list. Check to see that all equipment is clean and ready for use. Check all oxygen delivery and suctioning equipment.

When possible, speak directly to the crew who last used the ambulance. Find out if they experienced any problems. Check the run reports to see if any equipment was used that may need replacing or repair.

If anything is wrong, correct the problem according to local guidelines. Do NOT delay reporting any damage to the ambulance or its equipment. Make certain you record this damage on your vehicle inspection checklist.

ACTIVATING THE SYSTEM

THE DISPATCHER

In most communities, someone seeking help from the EMS System can telephone an emergency number to reach a dispatcher. The trend in recent years has been for communities to have a single central dispatching facility. Calling this facility gives the citizen access to the community's ambulance service, rescue squad, fire department, police department, or any other appropriate emergency service. The dispatcher receiving the call can obtain information, decide what services are needed, and then contact these needed services.

Many communities have adopted the central dispatch system, utilizing the universal number concept. Citizens can gain immediate access to all emergency services by dialing 911. This improves the speed by which a person can contact the central dispatch facility. The person does not have to look up a special telephone number for the service he thinks he will need, or for the central dispatch facility. Studies have shown that the public can be quickly educated to the 911 concept and remember this simple number in times of emergency.

The majority of communities that do not use a central dispatch facility provide separate dispatch centers for police, ambulance and rescue, and fire services. Many of these communities place ambulance and rescue services under the number of the fire services dispatch facility. When multiple dispatch centers are used, *cross-communication capabilities* should exist to minimize delays in cases where the wrong center is called.

Information Obtained by the Dispatcher

There are a number of ways in which dispatchers collect and disseminate information about calls for help. A trained dispatcher will ask the following questions to elicit information from a caller:

1. Do you have an emergency?
2. What is the nature of the emergency?
3. What is the exact location of the injured/sick person?

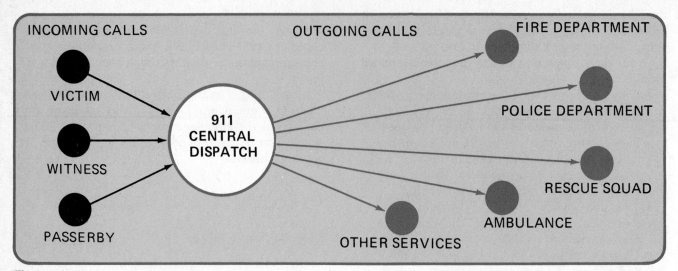

Figure 15-1: When all requests for assistance follow a direct route from caller through central dispatch to the proper agency, an efficient flow of information helps assure the proper prompt response.

4. Can you tell me the injured/sick person's name and age?
5. What is your name?
6. What number are you calling from?
7. Will you be at that number if we need more information?

The exact location of the sick or injured person is critical. Dispatchers will gain as much information as possible. They must ask for the building number, the street name with the direction designator (north, south, east, or west), and the development or subdivision name. If the location is an apartment, the number of the apartment must be obtained. When dispatchers transmit this information, they also will transmit the nearest cross street to allow for a quicker response to the correct building number.

The questions asked to obtain information about a traffic accident may vary slightly. The dispatcher will ask the following questions to learn as much about the accident scene as possible:

- What is the exact location of the accident?
- How many and what kinds of vehicles are involved?
- How many people do you think are injured?
- How serious do these injuries appear to be?
- Do the victims appear to be trapped?
- Is traffic moving?
    How many lanes are open?
    How far is traffic backed up?
- Are there any apparent hazards?
    Are any of the vehicles on fire?
    Are any electrical wires down?
    Do any of the vehicles appear unstable?
    Are there any trucks that may be carrying a hazardous cargo?

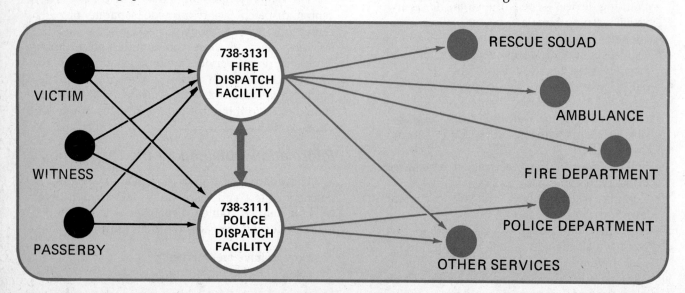

Figure 15-2: Many communities are served by separate dispatching facilities. Direct telephone and radio links between the centers help reduce the problems caused by misdirected calls.

Determining the exact location of the accident may be a problem. In urban areas, the nearest street address or the names of the streets at the nearest intersection are usually obtained. In rural areas, however, the problem of information gathering may not be as simple, especially when the caller is not familiar with the area. The name of the nearest crossroad, a nearby store, or a visible landmark such as a water tower may provide points of reference needed to determine the caller's location. In some cases, the dispatcher may have to contact the local telephone company to pinpoint the location of the caller's telephone.

It takes very little time to gather this information. What is learned will allow for the proper services to be alerted, activities to be planned before arrival at the scene, and a prompt response to the call.

THE RESPONSE

THE DISPATCHER'S CALL

The call from the dispatcher will include all the information needed to initiate a prompt and efficient response. This is how the call might sound:

> "Ambulance Company 11—an emergency call for a 34-year-old male who has fallen. Respond to the Acme Paper Products Company Warehouse located at 123 Maple Avenue. The cross street is Madison."

The message is repeated to lessen questions about its contents. The information received should be written on the form provided by your EMS System. How you respond to the dispatcher is a matter of local protocol. In many areas, you need to identify your station, confirm that you have received the call, and repeat the address to which you will be responding. The dispatcher will provide you with the time so that records will show your time out from the station or squad house.

DRIVING THE AMBULANCE TO THE SCENE

There is no way that this or any other textbook can make you an ambulance driver. Only after proper classroom instruction followed by practical road sessions will you be a trained driver.

During your training to become an ambulance driver, you will be taught **emergency driving**. You will learn the specific state laws that regulate the operation of an emergency vehicle. Your training will include the proper techniques of handling the vehicle and the proper use and limitations of the audible and visual warning devices that are pro-

vided on the ambulance. As part of your training, you will be taught how to avoid accidents, the factors that can affect response time, and how to complete an entire emergency response.

As part of emergency driving, you will learn defensive driving skills. **Defensive driving** teaches you how to prevent accidents by staying alert for problems caused by other motorists, or by road conditions and hazards. You learn to assume that other drivers make mistakes and how to avoid situations where their mistakes will involve you in an accident. You learn to assume that there will be hazards encountered along the response so that you are prepared for them.

THE DRIVING TASK

The driving task can be successful only when the ambulance arrives on the scene of an illness or injury promptly and safely. There are four components to the driving task: the *driver*, the *vehicle*, the *road*, and the *other drivers*.

Understanding the Law

Every state has statutes that regulate the operation of emergency vehicles. While the wording of different statutes may vary, the intent of the laws is essentially the same. Emergency vehicles are generally granted certain *privileges* with respect to speed, parking, passage through traffic signals, and direction of travel. But the laws also clearly state that if an emergency vehicle operator does not drive with regard for the safety of others, he must be prepared to pay the consequences of his actions.

Every person who drives an ambulance, regardless of whether he does it for pay or as a volunteer, must fully understand the laws of his state. Basically, the laws are:

1. The ambulance driver must be a licensed driver who has successfully completed emergency and defensive driving training.

2. The privileges granted under the law to the operation of an emergency vehicle apply when the vehicle is responding to an emergency or is involved in emergency transport of a patient. When the ambulance is in use for non-emergency purposes, the same laws applying to all other motor vehicles apply to the operation of the ambulance.

3. Even though certain privileges are granted during an emergency, the ambulance driver is not relieved from the duty to drive with regard for the safety of all persons. The privileges granted do not provide immunity to the driver in cases of reckless driving or disregard for the safety of others.

4. Privileges granted during emergency driving only apply if the driver is properly using warning devices as directed by state or local law.

5. During emergency operations, the driver may:

- Park or stand the vehicle anywhere that does not damage personal property or endanger lives.

- Proceed past a red stop signal, flashing red stop signal, or stop sign, but only after stopping the vehicle and proceeding with all necessary caution. This also shall apply to warnings at railroad crossings, where a complete stop is required.

- Exceed the speed limit, by 5 to 10 mph, as long as life and property are not endangered.

- Pass in no-passing zones, after providing an appropriate signal to other drivers, noting the way is clear, and exercising the necessary caution to avoid endangering life and property.

- With the proper caution and signals, disregard the regulations governing direction of travel and turning in specific directions. You must stay in your lane until the lane of oncoming traffic is clear.

The Driver

The most important component of the driving task is the driver. This person must be physically and mentally capable of controlling the ambulance. An ambulance should not be operated by a person with uncorrected defective vision. Nor should any ambulance be operated by a person with a heart condition or other impairment that might disable him while driving. The operator of an ambulance should not have any physical disability that prevents proper steering, shifting gears, or operating foot pedals.

An ambulance driver must not attempt to drive while taking certain medications. Any medication that can induce drowsiness or sleep must not be taken, including most cold remedies, pain killers, and tranquilizers. Medical stimulants must be avoided. ''Pep pills'' can interfere with concentration.

An ambulance driver should never attempt to drive after drinking alcohol. Alcoholic beverages dull reflexes and impede judgment. Remember that it takes at least one hour for the body to process 3/4 of an ounce of alcohol.

The operator's mental condition is an important consideration in driving an ambulance. The driver must be able to devote full attention to the driving task. He should be able to control personal problems, and he should not drive when he is upset. The driver should have a healthy attitude toward both his own abilities and those of other drivers using the road. He must have confidence, but not be overconfident. Feelings of superiority could bring about an accident.

An emergency vehicle operator must appreciate the importance of cooperation. There must be cooperation between the public and the EMS System. There must be coordination and cooperation between the various branches of emergency services.

The Vehicle

The ambulance must be in optimum operating condition, receiving scheduled preventive maintenance, and inspection. As noted earlier, preparation includes a daily inspection of the vehicle and its equipment and supplies.

The Use of Warning Devices

Remember, many of the privileges granted for emergency driving require the vehicle's warning devices to be in use. More often than not, the problem is not caused by failure to use the devices, but by some drivers misusing them. They tend to rely too much on the ability of a siren and flashing lights to clear the road ahead. When using such devices, they overlook hazards and take unnecessary chances. Safe emergency vehicle operation can be achieved only when the proper use of warning devices is coupled with sound emergency and defensive driving practices.

The Siren   Although the siren is the most common audible warning device, unfortunately it is also the most misused. In some cases, the sound of the siren may cause the patient to suffer increased fear and anxiety. This may worsen his condition as stress builds. It is not uncommon for the patient's pulse to quicken as the siren is applied. The siren sound also can adversely affect the driver. Tests have shown that inexperienced drivers increased their driving speed from 10 to 15 miles per hour when exposed to the continuous sound of a siren. In some reported cases, drivers using a siren were unable to negotiate curves that they could pass through easily when not using the siren.

Each local EMS System has its own regulations for the use of the siren. When you feel that you have to use the siren, do so with these suggestions in mind:

- Use the siren sparingly, and only when you must. The more you use a siren, the greater is the chance that the public will become indifferent to the device.
- Never assume that all motorists will hear your signal.

- Remember that some motorists will hear your signal, yet remain completely indifferent to it.
- Be prepared for the erratic maneuvers of other drivers. Some people panic when they suddenly hear a siren.
- Do not pull up close to a vehicle and then sound your siren. Such action may cause the driver to jam on his brakes. Use the horn when you are close to another vehicle.
- Never use the siren indiscriminantly, and never use it to scare someone.

The Horn. All ambulances must be equipped with a horn. Experienced ambulance drivers find that in many cases use of the horn clears traffic as quickly as the siren. The guidelines offered for the use of sirens also apply to the use of an ambulance horn.

Visual Warning Signals. There is a general agreement among EMS Systems that all visual warning devices should be in use when responding and transporting patients. If warning lights are used all the time, people will be so accustomed to them that they may disregard the signals during emergencies. Since the use of warning devices is regulated by law, be familiar with the emergency driving laws of your state.

The vehicle headlights can be used to warn motorists in the daytime. Often bright headlights can be seen for a greater distance than colored lights that may blend with signs, buildings, foliage, and the taillights of vehicles traveling in the opposite direction.

The vehicle headlights should be on whenever the vehicle is in use. The exception is when the vehicle is parked facing oncoming traffic. Studies in Pennsylvania have shown that the chances of an accident are reduced by 50% if the vehicle headlights are used.

REMEMBER: Audible and visual warning devices ask the drivers of other vehicles to clear the way for the ambulance. They cannot demand clearance, and certainly they cannot physically clear the road.

Stopping Distance

Stopping distance is the number of feet that a vehicle travels from the time that the driver decides to stop until the vehicle actually stops. It is dependent on several factors, including the speed and condition of the vehicle, road conditions, and the alertness of the driver.

Stopping distance is the total of reaction distance and braking distance. **Reaction distance** is the number of feet the vehicle travels from the moment a driver decides to stop until his foot applies pressure

to the brake pedal. **Braking distance** is the number of feet that the vehicle travels from the start of the braking action until the vehicle comes to a complete stop. Table 15.1 shows the stopping distances for various vehicles.

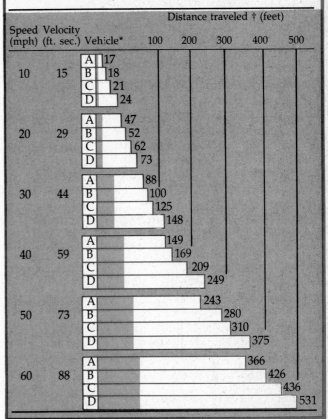

Table 15.1: The Stopping Distances of Standard Passenger Cars and Trucks on Dry, Clean, and Level Pavement

Speed (mph)	Velocity (ft. sec.)	Vehicle*	Distance traveled † (feet)
10	15	A	17
		B	18
		C	21
		D	24
20	29	A	47
		B	52
		C	62
		D	73
30	44	A	88
		B	100
		C	125
		D	148
40	59	A	149
		B	169
		C	209
		D	249
50	73	A	243
		B	280
		C	310
		D	375
60	88	A	366
		B	426
		C	436
		D	531

* (A) Standard passenger cars, (B) Light 2-axle trucks, (C) Heavy 2-axle trucks and buses, (D) 3-axle trucks and combinations.

† ▉ Driver reaction distance—based on a reaction time of ¾-second, a typical reaction for most drivers under most conditions.

☐ Vehicle stopping distance—based on provisions for the Uniform Vehicle Code for 20 mph.

The use of excessive speed increases the probability of accident. Speed reduces the chance of avoiding a hazardous situation because of the increase in stopping distance. Consider a 5-mile response trip for an ambulance. At 60 miles per hour the distance can be covered in 5 minutes. At 50 miles per hour it will take the ambulance 6 minutes to cover the 5 miles. However, at 60 miles per hour it will take more than 425 feet to bring the ambulance to a complete stop, while at 50 miles per hour the stopping distance will be less than 300 feet. The one minute gained in response time is not worth the greater risk of accident brought about by the increase in stopping distance.

The Road

Little can be done by the ambulance driver to ensure that road conditions are always the best. Many hazards can confront the driver. The majority of these hazards are weather related; however, other sources do exist. The most common road-related dangers encountered during an ambulance run include:

- Wet, slippery surfaces
- Slippery surfaces due to ice or snow
- Slippery surfaces due to oil slicks (especially dangerous during the first few minutes of a rainfall)
- Poor traction on gravel and dirt roads
- Poor handling and tire hazards due to poorly maintained roads
- Poor handling due to high-crowned roads, flat curves, or curves that are banked in the wrong direction
- Sudden hazard and tire damage due to debris in the roadway

Special Driving Techniques

Driving at the speed appropriate for road and weather conditions is the best technique for avoiding most problems associated with road conditions. A thorough knowledge of all road surfaces within the ambulance service area will help to reduce the chance of accident due to road hazards. Appropriate speed, knowledge of the road surfaces, and a few special driving techniques are necessary for the successful completion of the driving task.

NOTE: Whenever you must slow the ambulance, bring it to a stop, or pull off the road surface, warn other drivers by using the four-way flashers. If you cannot bring the vehicle to a stop, warn other drivers by honking the horn. If you must strike an object or another vehicle, avoid head-on collisions. Attempt to sideswipe the object, or strike an object that will absorb some of the impact.

Hydroplaning   Hydroplaning is a danger associated with wet road surfaces. This condition is caused by a combination of speed, wet roads, and worn tires. When a vehicle reaches higher speeds, there is a tendency for a film of water to develop between the tires and the road surface. The tires ride on the water rather than the road surface, making steering virtually impossible. The use of appropriate speed and tires with adequate tread tend to greatly reduce the chance of hydroplaning. If you are driving an ambulance and it begins to hydroplane, the solution to the problem is to *slow down*. Slowing should be gradual. Do NOT jam on the brakes.

Slippery Surfaces   Problems with slippery surfaces can be avoided if appropriate speed is used and the proper tires are used on the vehicle. Most

ambulance tires are designed for all-weather use. However, studded snow tires have been found best for ice and snow driving. When glare ice is a problem, these studded tires should be placed on the front wheels as well as the rear ones.

When slowing on any slippery surface, you should avoid locking the ambulance wheels. To do so will take away your ability to steer the vehicle and may promote skidding. By pumping the brakes, you will retain the rolling friction that exists between the wheels and the road, permitting you to brake and steer at the same time. If the ambulance begins to skid on a slippery surface, steer in the direction of the skid to bring the vehicle back to a straight course. Do NOT jam on the brakes.

Standing Water   Under certain road conditions or at certain types of accidents, you may have to drive the ambulance through large pools of water. When possible, avoid the pool; if you cannot, slow down and turn on the wipers before entering the pool. Since the brakes may become wet, tap them lightly several times as you leave the pool. This will help dry out the brakes. If the brakes remain wet, the ambulance will usually pull to one side as the brakes are tapped. If this is the case, remain at a slow rate of speed and pump the brakes until the vehicle stays on a straight course.

Poor Visibility   If you are driving under conditions of poor visibility such as fog, slow down but do not decelerate quickly. Make certain that any vehicles behind you are aware of your reduction of speed. Watch carefully for slowed or stopped vehicles ahead. Do NOT attempt to pass slower moving vehicles or to force them off the road. Turn on the low beam headlights and the wipers to improve visibility. It is recommended that you use the ambulance's four-way flashers to reduce the chance of accident with another vehicle, especially if you are traveling at less than 10 miles per hour below the speed limit. These flashers must be turned on if you stop on the road surface or pull off to the side of the road.

NOTE: Other drivers may not be able to determine that you wish to turn when the vehicle's four-way flashers are in use. With some vehicles you will have to turn off the four-ways to allow the turn signal to be recognizable.

Tire Blowout   With proper inspections, tire blowout is a rare happening on an ambulance. If you should experience a tire blowout while driving an ambulance, hold the steering wheel firmly and allow the vehicle to slow down. Slowly apply the brakes to avoid wheel locking, and bring the vehicle to a complete stop. When possible, slow to a near stop and pull off the road surface before coming to a complete stop. If you develop careless habits in how you hold the vehicle's steering wheel, you may not be able to regain control of the ambulance during a tire blow-out.

Steering Failure   Complete steering failure is very rare. Most steering problems associated with ambulance driving involve the loss of power steering. When power steering is lost, steering becomes very difficult. You will have to tightly grasp the steering wheel, allow the vehicle to slow down, and come to a full stop after pulling off the road surface. Should you experience a complete steering failure, do NOT apply the brakes. To do so may cause the ambulance to pull sharply to one side. Instead, allow the vehicle to come to a stop. During this process, continue to try the steering wheel. Sometimes steering can be regained. If need be, slowly pump the brakes. With some ambulances, stopping can be aided by applying the parking brake. Do NOT use this brake unless this method has been tested by your EMS System on the ambulances used in your service.

Brake Failure   Brake failure is one of the most serious problems that can face the ambulance driver. During a brake failure, you must take swift action to avoid accidents. Do NOT pull out into oncoming traffic. A head-on collision can be the most serious accident possible in an ambulance. Shift to the ambulance's lowest gear and apply the parking brake. Pump the brake pedal as rapidly as you can, attempting to regain brake pressure. Alert traffic directly ahead by using the siren and horn, and all other traffic by turning on the four-way flashers. Once the vehicle has slowed down, let it coast to a stop off the road surface.

Accelerator Failure   Accelerator failure can take one of two forms. If the engine fails to respond to the accelerator, shift to neutral (this must be done in case the failure suddenly self-corrects), turn on the four-way flashers, bring the vehicle to a full stop off of the road surface, and turn off the engine. If the accelerator on the ambulance becomes stuck, it is best to take the same action as you would for a nonresponsive accelerator. Do NOT try to release the pedal while you are driving, or while the vehicle is in gear.

Objects in the Roadway   Objects in the roadway may be difficult to avoid. Again, excessive speed increases the chance of accident. The avoidance of an object is accomplished by a combination of braking and steering; therefore, do not jam on the brakes and lock the wheels. Many drivers react by steering to the left. This takes may take them into oncoming traffic. When you are trying to avoid an object in the road and there is oncoming traffic, attempt to steer to the right.

Animals in the Roadway   Animals in the roadway are commonly seen. In urban areas, dogs and cats are usually the problem. Larger animals such as deer and horses may be seen in rural areas.

It may seem cruel, but you may have to hit smaller animals. If you jam on the brakes, you may loose control of the ambulance. If you try to steer around the animal, you may hit another moving vehicle, a parked vehicle, or even a person along the side of the road. When transporting a patient, keep in mind that he may not be able to tolerate the additional stress brought about by a sudden stop or a rapid swerve of the ambulance.

Whenever you see an animal that may wander onto the road surface, slow down! Tap the horn several times. Application of the siren may frighten the animal, causing it to jump into the path of the ambulance. BE ON THE ALERT FOR CHILDREN RUNNING AFTER THE ANIMAL. If you can steer the ambulance around the animal without risk to life or property, steer in the opposite direction to which the animal is running.

Large animals such as horses, deer, and cattle should be avoided by combined steering and braking actions. Collision with a large animal may produce as much damage as striking another motor vehicle. Remember to steer in the opposite direction of a running animal. If you see a horse and rider, slow down. While still at a distance, tap the horn to alert the rider. Do NOT use the siren. If the horse and rider are on a bridge or overpass, proceed with caution at a slow speed.

People in the Roadway   People in the roadway usually move to the nearest spot off the road. However, some people react to an oncoming vehicle by running out into the roadway. Of course, you must do all you can to avoid hitting someone who is in the path of the ambulance, short of having a head-on collision with another moving vehicle. Prevention, through the appropriate use of speed and staying alert at all times, is your best course of action.

Drive at a slow speed in residential areas. You will probably have to travel slower than the posted speed limit to avoid children who may run out into the street to see the ambulance.

REMEMBER: Most accidents associated with the roadway can be prevented. Excessive speed is the primary cause of ambulance roadway accidents.

Night Driving   Your chances of having a fatal accident increase at night. The reasons for this are many. Some of the drivers could be fatigued and less alert, less able to react, and more likely to make mistakes. There are drivers who do not see well during nighttime driving. Some may have problems because of the reduced light, while others are temporarily blinded by the headlights of other vehicles. This may be due to uncorrected vision problems, poor diet, liver disease, or simply a case of poor night vision. Motorists under the influence of alcohol or drugs are more likely to be driving at night.

They present the greatest nighttime hazard to the crew of the ambulance.

Dawn and dusk are the two most hazardous times to be driving. The lighting is such that many individuals have problems with contrast and depth perception. Always turn on the ambulance headlights when taking the vehicle out at dawn or dusk.

When making a nighttime ambulance run:

- Make certain that the headlights, tail lights, and turn signal lights are working. Check the dash lights to be sure that you can read all the instruments. At night, keep these lights dim so that they do not reflect on the windshield.

- Make certain that the windshield and side window glass is clean.

- Use your warning lights in accordance with local regulations and guidelines.

- Drive defensively. Assume the other drivers will make mistakes. Give them more room on the road and more time to make decisions.

- Drive more slowly than you would during a daytime run.

- Do not use the high beams if a vehicle is less than 300 feet in front of you, or an approaching vehicle is within 500 feet (do NOT flick your lights to let other motorists know they have on their high beams).

- Do not stare into the headlights of other vehicles and do not continually focus on one object. Keep your eyes moving.

COMMON AMBULANCE ACCIDENTS

Ambulances, like any other vehicles, can become involved in a variety of accidents. A driver who attempts to turn a corner at too great a speed may lose control of his ambulance; the ambulance may strike a tree, a utility pole or perhaps a parked car. Or the ambulance may leave the roadway, plunge down an embankment, and roll over. Seldom do accidents like these occur without producing injuries to the occupants—the emergency medical technicians and their patients.

However, most fatalities, injuries and the greatest property damage occur when an ambulance is involved in a collision with another vehicle. There are six varieties of such two-vehicle collisions in which an ambulance may be involved: 1) with a vehicle ahead; 2) with a vehicle behind; 3) with an approaching vehicle; 4) with a vehicle at an intersection; 5) with a vehicle being passed; and 6) with a vehicle that is passing. The first five types usually occur when the ambulance is responding to a call for help. The sixth, along with backing accidents, usually occurs when the ambulance is returning to quarters.

An Accident With the Vehicle Ahead

Drivers of passenger cars can react to the approach of an ambulance from behind in many ways. One operator may pull his vehicle to the right, as he is supposed to do. Another operator, when he sees and hears the approaching ambulance, may pull his vehicle sharply to the left. Still another operator may simply jam on his brakes and stop in the middle of the roadway.

Staying alert is the first step in avoiding a collision with the vehicle ahead. Watch for signs that indicate what the driver ahead intends to do. A flashing turn signal, for example, or a lighted brake lamp indicates a driver's intention. Movement into another lane also serves as an indicator for a following ambulance driver. However, don't be lulled into a false sense of security by these signals or movements. Drivers sometimes do just the opposite of what they have signaled. Carefully watch the driver who has not signaled or initiated any movement at all. He may not have heard or seen your approach, and he may be the one who jams on his brakes when he sees that you are behind him. Be prepared for anything. Stay alert!

Do not concentrate solely on the vehicle immediately ahead of you. Watch the line of vehicles for some distance ahead. Look for the drivers who apparently do not see you. Look for unmarked intersections. Be alert for motorists who suddenly change lanes as they near those intersections. When approaching a controlled intersection, try to time your arrival at the intersection with the changing of the traffic signal. Having the green light gives you an added measure of safety.

Stay a safe distance from the vehicle ahead. Ambulance drivers have a tendency to drive dangerously close behind other vehicles. If the car or truck ahead stops suddenly, a rear-end collision is almost inevitable. Maintaining one vehicle length for every 10 miles an hour of speed between your ambulance and the vehicle ahead gives you room to stop or maneuver if the other driver decides to brake suddenly.

As soon as you see a hazard developing, apply your brakes. A good driver reduces stopping distance by keeping a foot poised over the brake pedal when he senses a potentially dangerous situation, such as at an intersection. When it is necessary to brake suddenly, do not jam on the brakes. Pump them so that the wheels do not lock and contribute to an uncontrolled skid. In some cases the best defensive action may be to steer around an obstacle. A well-trained and experienced driver can change lanes in a relatively short distance, even in a heavy truck. A sudden change of lane is accomplished without braking.

An Accident With the Vehicle Behind

A motorist who tailgates is asking for trouble. One who tailgates an ambulance is inviting disaster. Why a driver tailgates an ambulance is a matter for conjecture. However, the reasons for tailgating are not as important as what can be done about this dangerous condition.

When you operate a passenger car, there are a number of actions to prevent tailgating. You can slow down and pull to the right, thus encouraging the tailgater to pass you. You can increase the distance between your vehicle and the one ahead. Then if the vehicle ahead has to stop suddenly, you won't have to. Accordingly, you won't have to worry about the tailgater hitting you. If these tactics fail, you can always pull over, stop and let the tailgater go around you. But when you are operating an ambulance on an emergency response, these actions are not feasible. You can, however, reduce the danger of collision with the following vehicle by properly using directional signals, making the driver behind fully aware of your intentions and, when you must stop, braking smoothly.

An Accident With an Approaching Vehicle

This type of accident is the most deadly, even at low speeds. When two vehicles hit squarely head on, the occupants continue moving forward even though their vehicle has stopped. Even when such collisions occur slightly off-center, the results can be disastrous—the vehicles have a tendency to spin after impact, doors fly open and occupants are thrown out.

Head-on collisions often occur on straight roads when the driver or an ambulance steers into an oncoming traffic lane to pass around slower vehicles. If you are caught in traffic, stay in the correct lane, slow down and give the vehicles ahead of you an opportunity to pull to the right. The time lost in this defensive action will be insignificant.

A head-on collision may occur on a straight road when a driver attempts to steer his vehicle too quickly back onto the roadway at high speed after his right front wheel has dropped off the pavement. A violent twisting of the steering wheel to the left causes the vehicle to move sharply across the roadway, and the high speed prevents the driver from recovering control of the vehicle before he enters the lane of oncoming traffic. If your wheel drops off the pavement, don't panic and above all, do *not* jam on the brakes. You may lose control of your vehicle completely if you do. Slow down and keep the ambulance on a straight path. When there is an opening in traffic—and there is no oncoming traffic—steer back onto the pavement slowly with the wheels held at a sharp angle.

Centrifugal force contributes to head-on collisions on curves. When a roadway curves to the right, there is a tendency for your vehicle to drift into oncoming traffic. On a left-hand curve, you face the possibility of another vehicle drifting into your lane. At higher speeds the drift is more pronounced and unless this drifting is corrected, a head-on crash is almost inevitable. Slow down as you enter a curve. If the road curves to the right, keep your vehicle close to the right edge of the roadway. On a left-hand curve, stay in the middle of the lane. Do not brake in a curve; if your speed is high enough this may cause a dangerous skid. Steer around the curve and apply power as you approach the straightaway.

An Accident at an Intersection

One-third of all traffic accidents occur at intersections. Following some simple suggestions will reduce the possibility of such a collision.

Know where you are going to turn. This will eliminate the need for a sudden stop or swerve which may contribute to an accident. Complete familiarity with the response district and the routes to any area within the district is the responsibility of every ambulance driver.

Slow down for the intersection. (Remember that a good driver removes his foot from the accelerator and holds it over the brake pedal whenever he perceives a potentially dangerous situation.) Signal your intention to turn; look in both directions; when it is safe to turn, go!

Be especially watchful for other emergency vehicles that may reach the intersection at the same time that you do. In intersections controlled by a traffic signal, the emergency vehicle that has the green light in its favor generally proceeds through the intersection first. At intersections without traffic signals a vehicle usually yields to the vehicle on its right.

A word of caution: When stopping at an intersection before making a left turn, keep your wheels in a straight line. Then if you are hit from behind, your vehicle will be pushed in a relatively straight line instead of being forced into oncoming traffic.

An Accident With a Vehicle Being Passed

There are few instances when an ambulance does not have to pass a vehicle that is traveling in the same direction. Some simple guidelines about passing can ensure your arrival at the location of the sick or injured person.

Check oncoming traffic before starting to pass. Bear in mind that if your vehicle and an approaching vehicle are both traveling at 55 miles per hour, the distance between vehicles is closing at slightly less than 2 miles per minute!

Check the traffic ahead moving in the same direction as your vehicle. While it may be safe to pass, it may not be safe to reenter the traffic lane. If traffic is congested, your action may cause another driver to stop short, which may in turn cause a rear-end collision, or your reentry into the lane may force another vehicle off the road.

Signal your intention to pass. Move into the adjacent lane. Alert other motorists to your actions by the horn or other device. Signal your return into the traffic lane. Return to the lane when it is completely safe to do so.

An Accident With a Passing Vehicle

As mentioned before, this type of accident usually occurs when an ambulance is being driven back to quarters.

A competent, defensive ambulance driver helps another motorist to pass, just as he expects other motorists to help him pass.

Watch for oncoming traffic. When a motorist behind you signals his intention to pass your ambulance, pull to the right as far as you safely can. If he seems hesitant to pass—and if it is safe to do so—wave him on. When he passes you, he will have to move back into line. If necessary, slow down so that

he has plenty of room to reenter the lane safely.

These are the kinds of accidents that ambulances may become involved in while responding to and returning from calls. Remember that for every type of accident there is a defense. A healthy attitude toward the operation of an ambulance and a knowledge of basic defensive driving techniques will certainly help to reduce the number of accidents that ambulances are involved in each year. However, mere handling and maneuvering of an ambulance does not always constitute defensive driving. Most defensive drivers learn accident prevention skills in a class taught by a qualified instructor. The National Safety Council, through its various state affiliates, offers defensive driving courses throughout the United States at a very modest cost. All ambulance operators should take advantage of this service and learn these driving techniques.

FACTORS THAT AFFECT RESPONSE

Most ambulance drivers find that operating an ambulance offers more of a challenge in reality than is depicted in films and on television. Experienced drivers know that certain factors affect not only the selection of a route to the emergency scene, but also their driving habits.

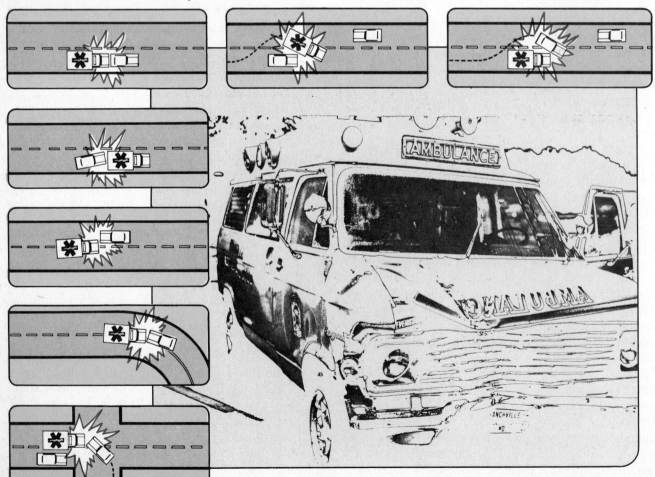

Figure 15-3: Types of ambulance accidents.

Day of the Week

This has a direct bearing on the flow of traffic within a given area. Weekdays are the days of heaviest traffic flow because people are commuting to and from work. On Saturday, commuter traffic generally diminishes, but traffic increases around urban and suburban shopping centers. Sunday traffic is generally minimal, although superhighways and interstate roads may be crowded in the late afternoon and evening.

Time of Day

Not too many years ago daily traffic patterns were predictable. Morning traffic moved from the suburbs to the city, where most of the people worked. In the evening the traffic pattern was reversed as people returned to the suburbs. Emergency vehicle operators were reasonably sure that if they opposed the flow of traffic, their way would be relatively unimpeded. They also knew that travel in the same direction as the main flow of traffic would be difficult.

Today the situation is far different. With the advent of satellite towns, massive shopping centers and huge industrial parks and office complexes, traffic over major arteries tends to be heavy in both directions at any time. Ambulance operators can expect blocked intersections, packed roads, and crawling traffic during commuter hours, regardless of the direction in which they travel.

Weather

Rain and fog reduce driving speeds and increase response times. Icy roads increase response times even more. A heavy snowfall can temporarily prevent any response.

Detours

Traffic can be seriously slowed by construction and road maintenance. Detours and lane restrictions may last only a few hours, or may be in force for months. A detour often affects the operation of emergency vehicles less than the closing of lanes on a road. When several lanes are merged into one, there is often no way for an ambulance to detour around traffic, or to even pull off the road in favor of an alternate route. Thus there is no escaping the traffic jam. Neither siren-sounding nor light-flashing can move cars out of the way when there is no place to go.

Railroads

Although the replacement of railroad crossings with bridges and underpasses has greatly reduced vehicle traffic obstructions, traffic still can be completely blocked by long, slow-moving freight trains, especially in rural areas. In small towns such a train can effectively block all roads and can isolate a part of the town. Obviously, an ambulance or other emergency vehicle cannot pass a crossing until the train clears it.

Bridges and Tunnels

While bridges and tunnels usually aid traffic flow, they can also be the reason for major traffic jams, especially during commuter hours. When traffic stops on a bridge or in a tunnel, often there is just no room for an ambulance to pass.

Schools

Schools contribute to traffic slowdowns. The reduced speed limits in force during school hours slow the flow of vehicles. Crossing guards also disrupt the flow of traffic, and it is a natural reaction of drivers to slow down when an area is congested with children.

School buses also slow traffic. When a bus makes frequent stops along a two-lane road, traffic can back up behind the bus for a considerable distance. Vehicles on the road cannot resume normal speed until the bus turns off or allows the traffic to pass.

REMEMBER: Emergency vehicles attract children, who often venture out into the street to see them. The driver of every emergency vehicle should slow down when approaching a school or playground.

When it appears that an ambulance will be delayed in reaching a sick or injured person because of these or other factors, the driver should consider taking an alternate route.

Alternate Routes

Ambulance drivers must constantly monitor road conditions in their service areas, and evaluate the effect that changing conditions will have on an ambulance's response. Maps of the area should always show troublesome traffic spots, such as schools, bridges, tunnels, railroad crossings, and other similar permanent impediments. Maps also should show temporary problem areas, such as detours and construction sites. Whenever possible, alternate routes should be established around both permanent and temporary impediments.

POSITIONING THE AMBULANCE

Parking the ambulance at a sick or injured person's location may involve little more than positioning the vehicle in a driveway, at a space along the curb, at a plant loading dock, or in any other place that is provided for a vehicle. Parking at the scene of a traffic accident may not be so easy. The accident scene may be one of total chaos.

Before you can consider solutions to any of the medical problems that an accident has created, you must first ensure the safety of your equipment. Seek a safe place for the ambulance, taking into consideration the following factors:

- The traffic
- The roadway
- Known hazards

The Traffic

Traffic at an accident scene can be affected in many ways. On a two-lane road the flow of traffic may be completely blocked by wreckage. At an intersection of 2 two-lane roads, the flow of traffic in all four directions may be blocked if the wreckage is in the center of the crossroad. If wreckage blocks only one lane of a four-lane road, the flow of vehicles may be restricted to one lane on one side, while traffic on the other side is unaffected. The ways in which traffic may be affected by an accident are virtually unlimited.

The Roadway

To ensure the safety of the ambulance, the driver should park completely off the road. If a service road or parking lot adjoins the roadway, the ambulance should be placed there. Perhaps a driveway enters the road where the accident has occurred. In that case the unit should be positioned in the driveway. If there is no other way that the ambulance can be taken off the road, it should be parked along the shoulder.

There are times when the ambulance will have to be parked on the roadway. Perhaps there is no shoulder or any other available space off the roadway. There are two schools of thought about positioning an ambulance or other emergency vehicle when it has to remain in the traffic lane. Some officials maintain that it should be located beyond the wreckage (in relation to the direction of traffic movement). However, most officials favor placing the unit between the wreckage and oncoming traffic, not less than 50 feet from the involved vehicles.

This is the best position to utilize the vehicle's warning lights (but does not reduce the need for other warning and signaling devices).

If the ambulance's brakes are locked and chocks are wedged against the tires, there is an added measure of safety for rescuers and victims from speeding cars that may not be able to stop. On busy highways, emergency care and rescue personnel need all

such protection.

CAUTION: Headlights on the ambulance should be turned off if it has to face oncoming traffic. Even lowbeam lamps can cancel the effectiveness of flashing and revolving warning lights. The headlights may also blind or confuse oncoming drivers.

Hazards

Typical hazards at the accident scene include:

- Downed electrical wires
- Damaged utility poles
- Vehicle fires
- Explosives
- Hazardous materials

The dispatcher may be able to alert you to possible hazards created by the accident. Even when you think you know what hazards will be at the scene, approach the accident zone with caution. Be on the alert for hazards and potential hazards. When a hazard exists at the scene, establish a **danger zone** and park the vehicle outside of this zone. The size of the danger zone varies as to the hazard at the scene. Scansheet 15-1 explains proper ambulance parking for various hazards. Many unfortunate incidents involving EMS personnel at the scene of accidents could be avoided if danger zones were established before the EMTs attempted to render care.

FAILURE TO RESPOND

Once you acknowledge the dispatcher's call, you are legally bound to respond. You may not be able to complete a response because of mechanical problems with the ambulance, a flat tire, traffic accidents, or traffic jams. At the first indication of something being wrong with the ambulance, or the first indication that something may prevent or delay your response, you MUST CALL THE DISPATCHER. This will allow for another ambulance and crew to respond to the call for help.

SUMMARY

Always make certain that you and the ambulance are ready to respond at the beginning of your shift. Perform a daily inspection of the ambulance.

In most communities, citizens can activate the EMS System by phoning a central dispatch facility. In many cases, the universal number 911 is used. The majority of communities that do not use a central dispatch facility have separate dispatch centers for various emergency services. These centers have cross-communication capabilities.

HAZARDS

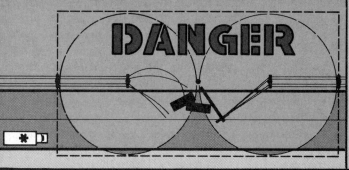

IN ACCIDENTS INVOLVING DOWNED ELEC-TRICAL WIRES AND DAMAGED UTILITY POLES, THE DANGER ZONE SHOULD EXTEND BEYOND EACH INTACT POLE FOR A FULL SPAN AND TO THE SIDES FOR THE DISTANCE THAT THE SEVERED WIRES CAN REACH. STAY OUT OF THE DANGER ZONE UNTIL THE UTILITY COM-PANY HAS DEACTIVATED THE WIRES, OR UNTIL TRAINED RESCUERS HAVE MOVED AND ANCHORED THEM.

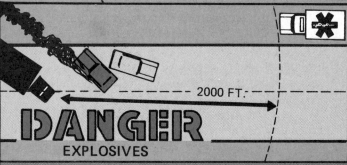

IF NO OTHER HAZARDS ARE INVOLVED — HAZARDS SUCH AS DANGEROUS CHEMICALS OR EXPLOSIVES — THE AMBU-LANCE SHOULD BE PARKED NO CLOSER THAN 100 FEET FROM A BURNING VEHICLE.

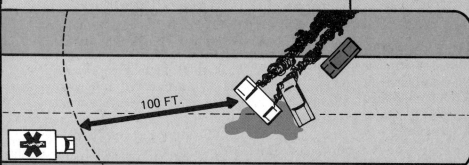

WHEN HAZARDOUS MATERIALS ARE EITHER INVOLVED IN OR THREATENED BY FIRE, THE SIZE OF THE DANGER ZONE IS DICTATED BY THE NATURE OF THE MATERIALS. IF EXPLO-SIVES ARE PRESENT, IT MAY BE NECESSARY TO PARK THE AMBULANCE 2000 FEET FROM THE ACCIDENT.

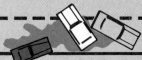

THE AMBULANCE SHOULD BE PARKED UPHILL FROM FLOWING FUEL. IF THIS IS NOT POSSIBLE, THE VEHICLE SHOULD BE PARKED AS FAR FROM THE FUEL FLOW AS POSSIBLE, AVOIDING GUTTERS, DITCHES, AND GULLIES THAT MAY CARRY THE SPILL TO THE PARKING SITE.

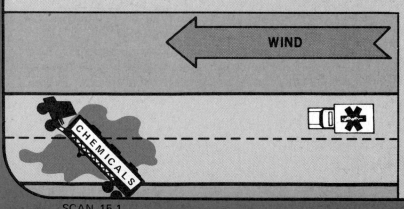

LEAKING CONTAINERS OF DANGEROUS CHEMICALS MAY PRODUCE A HEALTH AS WELL AS A FIRE HAZARD. WHEN CHEMI-CALS HAVE BEEN SPILLED, WHETHER FUMES ARE EVIDENT OR NOT, THE AM-BULANCE SHOULD BE PARKED UPWIND. IF THE HAZARDOUS MATERIAL IS KNOWN, SEEK ADVICE FROM EXPERTS THROUGH THE DISPATCHER OR CHEMTREC (SEE CHAPTER 13).

SCAN 15-1

A trained dispatcher will be able to gather required information to relay to the ambulance crew what is needed for a prompt and efficient response. Usually, the information relayed from the dispatcher will tell the EMTs if there is an emergency, the age and sex of the patient, what has happened, and the exact location of the emergency. Traffic problems and any apparent hazards at the scene also may be provided.

Driving the ambulance to the scene may require emergency driving techniques, employing warning devices, and using the privileges granted by special state laws. Any response requires defensive driving skills. When driving defensively, you should assume other drivers will make mistakes and that hazards may be encountered during the response.

Privileges are granted to ambulance drivers by state emergency vehicle laws. However, the driver still has the duty to drive with regard to the safety of all persons. Many of the privileges apply only during an emergency response and transport. Some of these privileges only apply if warning devices are in use.

As long as there is no danger to life or property, you may park the ambulance anywhere, proceed with caution through red stop signals and signs, safely exceed the speed limit, pass with caution in no-passing zones, and with proper caution and signals, disregard regulations concerning direction of travel and turning in specific directions.

The driving task involves the driver, the ambulance, the road, and other drivers. The most important component of the driving task is the driver. This person must be physically and mentally capable of controlling the ambulance. The ambulance driver must appreciate the importance of cooperation.

The ambulance must be in optimum operating condition, receiving scheduled inspections and maintenance. Warning devices should be used in accordance with local guidelines and regulations. The siren should be used sparingly, and only when needed. Never assume that another motorist has heard the siren or will pay attention to it. Some motorists panic when they suddenly hear a siren. The same basic rules for the use of the siren apply to the use of the ambulance horn. Visual warning lights and headlights should be used in accordance with state guidelines and regulations.

Stopping distance is the number of feet traveled from the time a driver decides to stop until the vehicle comes to a complete stop. It is the sum of the reaction distance and the braking distance.

Road surfaces may be slippery due to water, ice, snow, or oil. Hydroplaning also can occur on wet surfaces. The problems of slippery surfaces and hydroplaning can be avoided if appropriate speed is used and the vehicle has the proper tires for the road conditions. If hydroplaning occurs, slow the vehicle. If the ambulance skids on a slippery surface, steer in the direction of the skid. There are many hazards associated with the roadway and the road surface. See the specifics in this chapter. Remember that most problems can be avoided by using appropriate speed and staying alert.

The six basic ambulance accidents involving the ambulance and another vehicle include those with: a vehicle ahead, a vehicle behind, an approaching vehicle, a vehicle at an intersection, a vehicle being passed, and a vehicle that is passing. To avoid such accidents, drive with appropriate speed and stay alert. Properly employ warning devices when they are needed. Do not concentrate solely on the vehicle immediately ahead of you. Exercise caution when passing and when approaching an intersection. Keep in mind that other motorists may not grant you the right-of-way. As soon as you see a hazard developing, apply the brakes, but do not lock the wheels. Most problems will require a combination of braking and steering to be avoided.

The seven major factors affecting response include: day of the week, time of day, weather, detours, railroads, bridges and tunnels, and schools. Consider these factors when planning a response. Always have an alternate route for a response.

When arriving at the scene, position the ambulance according to the traffic, the roadway, and any possible hazards. If hazards are present establish a danger zone and park the vehicle outside this zone. Stay at least 100 feet from a burning vehicle. If explosives are involved, you may have to park 2000 feet from the scene. Stay uphill from fuel leaks and upwind from spilled chemicals. The danger zone around downed wires should extend beyond each intact pole for a full span and to the sides for the distance that the severed wires can reach.

If you are unable to complete a response to the scene, or there are indications that there will be problems or delays, immediately call the dispatcher.

16 controlling the scene and gaining access

OBJECTIVES By the end of this chapter, you should be able to:

1. List some of the problems associated with gaining access to buildings. (p. 367)

2. List the minimum protective gear you should wear if you are to enter a burning building, if this is considered part of your standard operating procedures. (p. 367)

3. Describe the precautions to take if you find yourself in a burning building. (p. 367-8)

4. Select the tools of choice for opening locked gates, doors with padlocks and hasps, and locked hinged single, hinged double, sliding glass, tempered glass, and overhead doors. (p. 369, 70)

5. Describe the procedures for opening locked gates and the various doors listed above. (p. 369, 70)

6. Select the tools of choice for opening locked double-hung, sliding, casement, awning-type, and factory-type windows. (p. 369, 71-2)

7. Describe the procedures for opening the various windows listed above, including the procedures for breaking window glass. (p. 369, 71-2)

8. List the TEN phases of a vehicle rescue operation. (p. 373)

9. Compare and contrast the primary situation assessment and the secondary situation assessment. (p. 375-6)

10. List some of the sources of information for locating patients at a motor vehicle accident. (p. 376)

11. Describe the use of flares, define "accident zone," and state the basic rule of thumb for flare placement. (p. 376-7)

12. Describe the procedures for the emergency moving of downed wires, if you have been fully trained in the procedures and carry the necessary safety equipment. (p. 377-80)

13. Describe how to fight a fire in the vehicle engine compartment when the hood is open and when the hood is closed (compared to fighting a spilled fuel fire), if you have been specifically trained in fire fighting and carry the necessary equipment. (p. 380)

14. Describe the principles behind the stabilization of a vehicle. (p. 380-1)

15. Compare and contrast gaining access and disentanglement. (p. 373)

16. Indicate the tools of choice and list, step by step, the basic procedures to gain access through vehicle doors. (p. 383-4)

17. Indicate the tools of choice and list, step by step, the basic procedures to gain access through vehicle windows. (p. 385-6)

18. Indicate the tools of choice and list, step by step, the basic procedures to gain access through the body of a vehicle. (p. 382, 7)

SKILLS   As an EMT, you should be able to:

1. Control hazards at the emergency scene, doing only what you have been trained to do and using the required safety equipment.
2. Protect yourself if you find that you are in a building that is on fire.
3. Reach patients trapped in buildings by gaining access through locked doors and windows, doing only what you have been trained to do.
4. Reach patients trapped in vehicles by gaining access through locked doors, through windows, and through the vehicle body (optional), doing only what you have been trained to do.
5. Effectively evaluate an emergency and summon the appropriate services to aid in scene control and gaining access.

TERMS   you may be using for the first time:

Extrication—any actions that disentangle and free patients from entrapment.

Disentanglement—creating a pathway through wreckage and removing wreckage from the patient to allow for proper care and the preparation for removal and transfer.

Packaging—completing the care procedures needed (dressing, bandaging, splinting, immobilizing) for transfer to the ambulance.

Transfer—moving the packaged patient to the ambulance for transport, or moving him from the ambulance to the emergency department.

Tempered Glass—specially hardened plate glass. When processed as safety glass, it will shatter into small pieces with rounded edges.

Laminated Glass—glass made from bonding two sheets of plate glass to a plastic layer. When shattered, the plastic layer will hold most of the pieces.

Mastic—a material used to set windshields, rear windows, and stationary windows in motor vehicles.

A-posts, B-posts, C-posts—the first, second, and third roof pillars from the windshield of a vehicle.

REACHING THE SICK AND INJURED

In most ambulance responses, there is little or no trouble in reaching the patient. The police will control the scene, if needed. You may have to do no more than knock on a door, report to a security guard, or walk over to a vehicle to begin assessment and care. However, there will be times when you must control hazards at the scene. A common hazard is traffic at the motor vehicle accident scene. If you arrive before the police, you may have to begin traffic control before you can reach the patients.

Gaining access to patients at times can be a major problem, often more challenging than the care you will have to render once you reach the patient. Locked gates, doors, and windows in buildings may prevent you from reaching the patient. The locked doors of a motor vehicle with rolled up windows may stop you from gaining access. The results of impact may jam doors, or obstruct your entry through a door or side window. Unless you are trained in gaining access and have the needed tools in the ambulance, you may have to wait until the fire service or a special rescue squad unit arrives. If the patient has a life-threatening problem, this delay may lead to the death of the patient.

To solve the problem of scene control and gaining access, many EMS Systems send the police to all calls for help. This frees the EMTs to provide assessment and basic emergency care. These systems usually send the fire service to all motor vehicle accidents and any other scene where fire and problems with gaining access may occur. Again, this frees the EMTs to provide assessment and care.

There will be times when you must initiate the procedures of gaining access. Remember to radio for help. There is no sense in trying to gain access, only to fail and then have to call for the appropriate services to respond. When you must gain access, do only what you have been trained to do, wear the appropriate safety gear, and use the proper tools.

REMEMBER: Your first priority at an emergency scene is your own safety. Your first responsibilities are patient assessment and basic EMT-level emergency care. When other trained personnel are at the scene, let them control the scene and do the procedures required to allow you to gain access.

CAUTION: Do only what you have been trained to do! If you are not trained in firefighting, you have no business trying to fight fires. If you are not trained in electrical hazards, don't try to move downed lines.

GAINING ACCESS TO PATIENTS TRAPPED IN BUILDINGS

When you respond to render care for a patient in a building, there usually is no problem in scene control or gaining access. However, you may be faced with:

- Hazards—usually fire or structural hazards
- Animals—usually a pet or guard dog
- Locked doors and windows

Fire

Do NOT enter burning buildings unless you are trained to evaluate the fire scene, to fight structural fires, have the needed equipment, and have the needed personnel. NEVER enter a burning building alone. NEVER enter a burning building without the proper helmet, coat, gloves, boots, and breathing apparatus.

Positive pressure breathing apparatus (or self-contained demand regulator breathing apparatus in some systems) is a must for fire rescue. You must receive *special* training to use this equipment. Do NOT read about the apparatus that you carry on your ambulance and think you know how to use it. You must know how to test the apparatus and how to apply it properly. You MUST know what to do if the apparatus should fail.

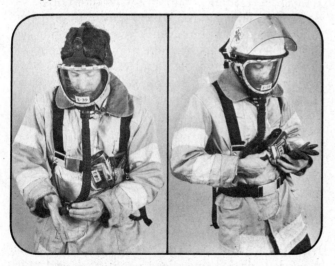

Figure 16-1: An EMT ready for service at the fire scene.

Ambulances are usually called to a fire scene. Circumstances may result in an ambulance arriving on the scene first, as, for example, when the unit responds while in transit. Thus it is wise for EMTs to learn a little about fire behavior.

You may arrive on the scene of a structural fire ahead of the apparatus and have someone tell you a person is trapped in the building. Think about the dangers of entering the building. Don't allow motivation to overcome common sense. A condition

known as "backdraft" may be imminent in a building that is on fire. **Backdraft** is an explosion that results when oxygen is suddenly admitted to a fire that is not burning freely. A fire in a generally confined area (such as a tightly sealed building) generates large amounts of heated, flammable gases that are deficient in oxygen. The gases rise and are trapped within the building because there is no way for them to escape. When air is admitted to the structure, the gases flash explosively.

If you arrive at the scene of a structural fire before firefighting units, look for a reliable sign of a backdraft condition. Grayish-yellow smoke puffs from openings such as poorly fitted windows, ventilators, and spaces under the eaves. The distinctive-colored smoke may even be sucked back into the building through the same openings from which it issued. If such a smoke condition is evident, backdraft is imminent. Not even protected firefighters will enter through the door or ground-level windows when the possibility of a backdraft explosion is high. Instead, they will first ventilate the structure at its highest point so that the potentially explosive gases can escape.

If you suspect that there is fire on the other side of a door that opens toward you, don't simply fling it open. As soon as you turn the handle and release the latching mechanism, pressure from the heat and smoke on the other side may force the door to open violently. You may be subjected to a sudden (perhaps fatal) blast of lung-searing heat.

Instead, feel the door at the top. **If the door is hot, don't open it.** A dangerous condition exists on the other side. If the upper part of the door is not hot, open the door carefully after bracing it firmly at the bottom with your foot. If the door opens away from you, still feel the upper portion first. **If the door is hot, don't open it.**

While entering or leaving a smoke-filled room, *crawl on your hands and knees.* In this position you are below dangerous heated gases and the bulk of the smoke. You also will be above toxic, heavier-than-air gases that may have been generated by burning plastics and natural materials.

If you do enter a building that is on fire, you may have a problem leaving because of the spread of fire or heavy smoke conditions, especially in hotels and other structures with many rooms.

Consider this situation: you reach a person in a room and are cut off by heat and smoke. The top of the door to the room is hot—a signal that you should not open the door.

Seal the opening around the door as much as possible with wet towels and bedding. Don't overlook the often large openings at the bottom of the door. Plug all openings through which smoke may enter the room, such as air conditioning vents, air return openings and heating ducts. If smoke enters

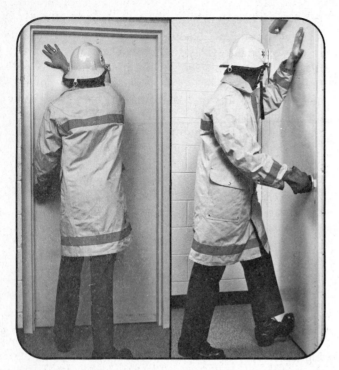

Figure 16-2: The procedure for opening a door when there may be fire on the other side. If the door is hot, do not open it!

the room, kneel with the patient at the bottom of the window opening. If the window is a double-hung sash type, open the window at the top as well as the bottom to let fresh air enter at the bottom, while smoke leaves through the upper opening.

Another survival technique is to make a tent at the window opening with blankets, other bedding, or drapes. Simply slip behind the drapes and hold your head out the window into the fresh air.

When trapped in a room, phone for help. If possible, hang sheets or other highly visible materials

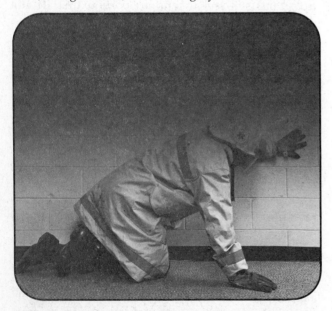

Figure 16-3: Moving along a smoke-filled passageway in this manner avoids lighter-than-air smoke and heavier-than-air gases.

out the window. Above all, *don't panic*. In many fire situations panic kills more people than smoke and flames do.

Structural Hazards

Be alert for weak ceilings and floors in any building. Be extra cautious in abandoned buildings. Reaching an injured person may be exceedingly difficult if the building has been vandalized or is filled with debris. Open shafts present extreme hazards, especially at night. Often they house elevator assemblies that are removed when the building is vacated. Incomplete stairways present another problem. Wood staircases are often torn up by vandals. Glass, broken pipes, loose wires, sharp metal objects, remnants of machinery, and a variety of other hazards may impede progress as you attempt to reach your patient.

These problems are compounded at night. Even with a powerful handlight, you may be in extreme danger. Even though it means a delay in reaching an injured person, call the fire department or rescue squad and request lights before entering a strange, abandoned building at night.

Animals

Do NOT believe that you can learn to handle animals by reading a simple set of directions. Pet dogs may attack you. Guard dogs, if properly trained, will hold you so that you cannot gain access, or leave! A poorly trained guard dog may attack you, inflicting serious injury. Unless you have been trained in animal control, call the dispatcher so that he may alert the police, fire service, special rescue unit, or animal control board to respond trained personnel.

Opening Locked Gates and Doors

If a gate is locked, there may be another gate that is open, or someone at the scene may have a key. You may, with care, be able to climb a low fence. In the case of locked doors, make certain that they are locked. Remember to both push and pull. Look to see if there is a key "hidden" near the door. Your partner can look for other doors or someone with a key while you ready yourself for forcible entry. If the locked door is to a private residence, a neighbor may have the key.

Whenever you have to cut through or break chains and locks, or whenever you have to force your way through a locked door, wear protective gear. The minimum is goggles and gloves. It is recommended that you wear a full face shield and helmet, gloves, and a protective coat.

Padlocked Gates. You may have to cut padlocks, chains, or cut away a section of chain link fence. The tool of choice is the long-handled bolt cutter. Remember that locks, chains, and certain types of chain link fence are made to withstand the cutting action of a hacksaw.

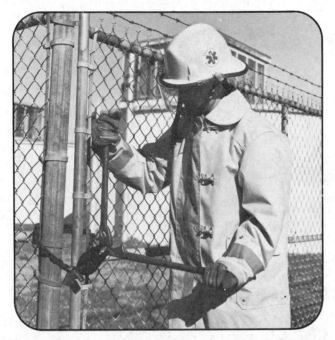

Figure 16-4: Using a long-handled bolt cutter to gain access through a padlocked gate.

Locked Doors. The procedures for locked doors are shown in Scansheet 16-1. You will need a prying tool, an ax, or a combination tool such as the Pry-Axe. For more information on tools, see page 374.

Your first impulse with certain types of doors may be to break the glass and reach in to unlock the door. This may work for some doors, provided they do not have special locks that require key operation on both sides of the door. If the door is made of plate glass, breaking the glass can be very dangerous. An improper blow could send the tool bouncing back into your face. **REMEMBER:** Almost every forcible entry generates flying particles. Make certain that you are well protected.

Opening Locked Windows

There are several types of windows: double-hung, sliding, casement, awning-type, and factory-type. The first four are found in virtually any occupancy, while the factory-type is common in industrial buildings.

In many cases, it will be possible to pry open double-hung and sliding windows. It is usually a waste of time prying casement, awning-type, and factory-type windows. With these windows, you will have to break a pane of glass and reach in to unlock the window.

New key-operated wedge locks and other ''burglar-resistant'' locks are being installed with increasing numbers on residential windows. Most of these are fixed in place with one direction screws. In the majority of cases, these devices will not stand up to direct prying or a hard blow from a hammer or ax. **CAUTION:** Protect yourself when breaking window glass. Do NOT attempt to break fixed plate glass windows except as a last resort. If you must, use a sharp tool and hammer or the pike of an ax directed as close to the frame as possible in a lower corner.

The techniques for opening locked windows are shown in Scansheet 16-2.

Security

When forcibly entering a building (or a room or apartment) to reach a sick or injured person, remember that the area is now vulnerable to other persons once you leave. If you cannot secure the property, or if no one can remain there, call the police. Give the dispatcher the address and the circumstances.

GAINING ACCESS TO PATIENTS IN VEHICLES

Often, control at the motor vehicle accident scene will not be the concern of the EMT. The police will be at the scene and have authority over control procedures. There will be times when you respond to a motor vehicle accident and arrive before the police. In such cases, you must assure your own safety and use the proper warning devices.

Reaching a person injured in a motor vehicle accident may involve nothing more than opening a door, or it may be necessary to use a variety of tools and appliances on doors, windows, or even the body of the vehicle. When gaining access to patients trapped in a motor vehicle:

1. Assure your own safety.

2. Do what you can to protect the patients, or take an entry route that reduces the chance of harming them.

3. Gain entry by the quickest, yet safest way possible. Delay elaborate procedures with special tools until you have provided the needed care for life-threatening problems.

Extrication

The term **extrication** refers to all activities that disentangle and free a patient from entrapment. Too often, the extrication aspect of vehicle rescue is stressed in training sessions, while other aspects of the rescue are given far less consideration. There are

BUILDINGS-OPENING LOCKED DOORS

TOOLS USED TO OPEN LOCKED DOORS

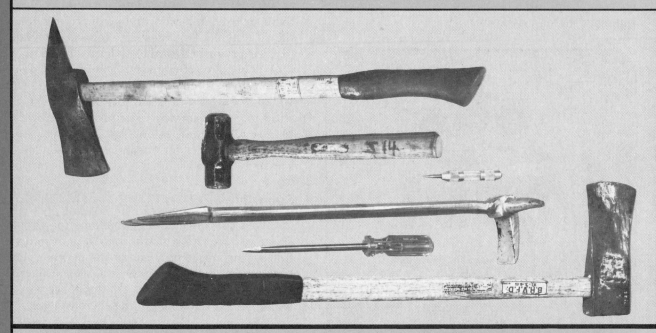

DOORS WITH PADLOCKS AND HASPS

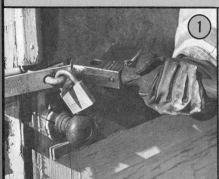

1 INSERT POINT OF TOOL INTO EYE OF LOCK AND PULL BACK, OR. . .

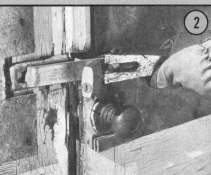

2 PLACE CLAW BETWEEN LOCK SHACKLE AND HASP STAPLE. PRY OR TWIST TO BREAK AWAY THE THE HASP, OR . . .

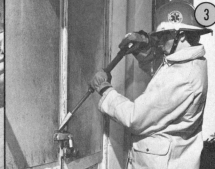

3 DRIVE CLAW END OF TOOL BETWEEN HASP AND DOOR. PRY HASP AWAY

HINGED SINGLE DOORS

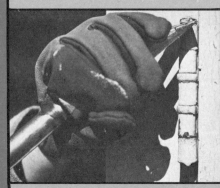

DOOR OPENS OUTWARD. DRIVE OUT EXPOSED HINGE PINS WITH PRY BAR, AX, OR SCREWDRIVER

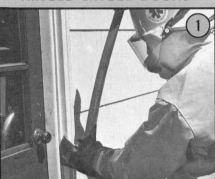

1 DOOR OPENS INWARD. USE AX OR PRY BAR TO BREAK AWAY THE RABBET STRIP

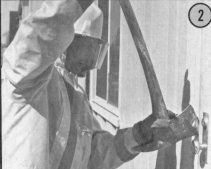

2 WEDGE CLAW OR AX HEAD BETWEEN DOOR AND JAMB AND PRY

SCAN 16.1A

BUILDINGS-OPENING LOCKED DOORS (cont'd)

DESTRUCTION OF A CYLINDER LOCK

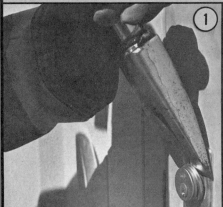

①

INSERT CLAW OVER LOCK RIM, FLUSH WITH DOOR—RAM IT BEHIND CYLINDER. CONTINUE UNTIL CYLINDER IS KNOCKED AWAY

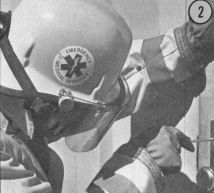

②

INSERT A FLAT-BLADE SCREWDRIVER AND TURN TO OPERATE THE LOCK

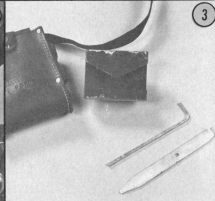

③

SPECIAL KITS ARE AVAILABLE FOR REMOVAL OF CYLINDER LOCKS

HINGED DOUBLE DOORS

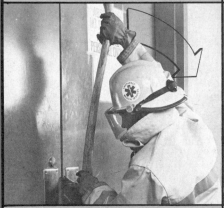

INSERT THE CLAW OF A TOOL OR AN AX BLADE BETWEEN DOORS AND PRY

SLIDING DOORS

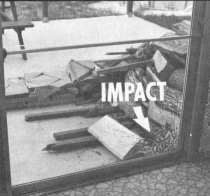

IMPACT

INSERT CLAW TOOL OR AX BLADE BETWEEN DOOR & FRAME. TWIST. IF SECURING DEVICE, BREAK GLASS IN LOWER CORNER. USE PIKE OF AX OR CENTER PUNCH & HAMMER

OVERHEAD DOORS

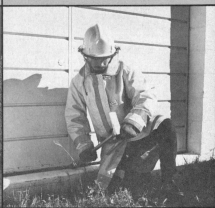

INSERT PRYING TOOL UNDER DOOR AT ITS CENTER AND PRY UPWARD. IF THIS FAILS, BREAK PANEL NEAR LOCKING MECHANISM. OPERATE THE LOCK BY HAND

TEMPERED GLASS DOORS

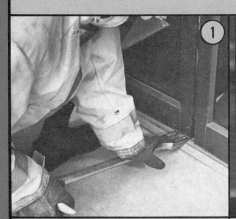

①

INSERT CLAW BETWEEN DOOR FRAME & FLOOR—PRY UPWARD TILL BOLT SEPARATES FROM KEEPER

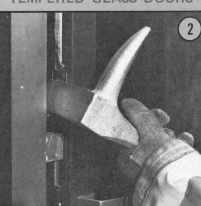

②

INSERT THE CLAW BETWEEN THE DOORS AND PRY

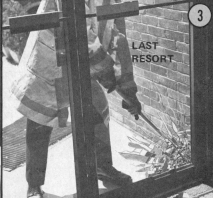

③

LAST RESORT

BREAK THE GLASS. USE CENTER PUNCH AND HAMMER OR PIKE OF AN AX. STRIKE EXPOSED EDGE OR LOWER CORNER NEAR FRAME

SCAN 16.1B

BUILDINGS-OPENING LOCKED WINDOWS

CAUTION! FORCING OPEN A WINDOW MAY RESULT IN SHATTERING THE GLASS. WHENEVER YOU ARE REQUIRED TO BREAK GLASS, LOOK TO SEE IF ANYONE IS DIRECTLY UNDER THE WINDOW

BREAKING WINDOW GLASS

- WEAR PROTECTIVE GEAR
- WHEN PRACTICAL, USE AN AX OR COMBINATION TOOL
- STAND TO ONE SIDE, BREAK GLASS WITH FLAT PART OF TOOL
- REMOVE LOOSE PIECES BEFORE REACHING IN TO UNLOCK WINDOW
- IF YOU HAVE TO CRAWL THROUGH OPENING, REMOVE ALL PIECES OF GLASS STILL IN THE FRAME

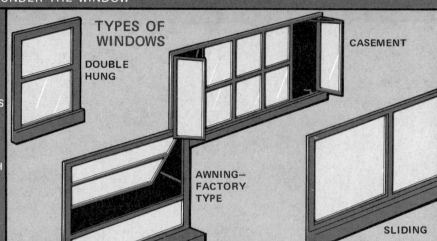

TYPES OF WINDOWS — DOUBLE HUNG — CASEMENT — AWNING—FACTORY TYPE — SLIDING

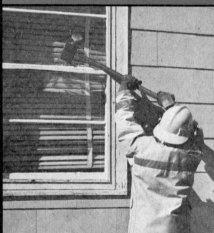

THE SAFE WAY TO BREAK OUT WINDOW GLASS WITH AN AX

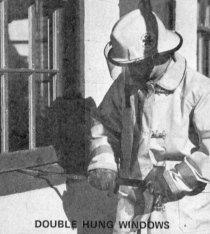

DOUBLE HUNG WINDOWS

FORCE CLAW UNDER LOWER SASH—PRY UPWARD. IF THIS FAILS, BREAK A PANE, REACH IN, UNLOCK WINDOW

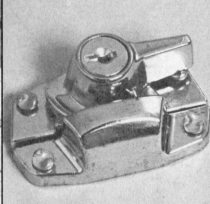

SPECIAL LOCKS

BREAK THE GLASS, FORCE CLAW UNDER LOCK, PRY UPWARD

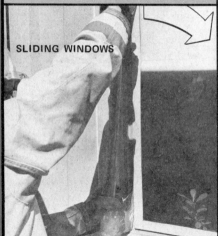

SLIDING WINDOWS

FORCE CLAW OR AX BLADE BETWEEN SLIDING PORTION AND FRAME & PRY. IF THIS FAILS, BREAK PANE, UNLOCK THE WINDOW

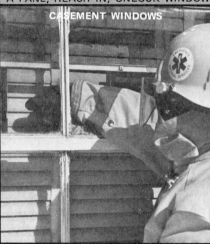

CASEMENT WINDOWS

BREAK A PANE, REACH IN, OPERATE CRANK TO OPEN WINDOW

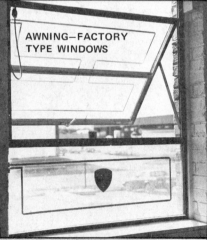

AWNING—FACTORY TYPE WINDOWS

A TYPICAL TOP-HINGED WINDOW. BREAK PANE AND UNLOCK THE WINDOW MANUALLY

SCAN 16-2

10 distinct phases of a vehicle rescue operation. As an EMT, you may be involved in all of these phases; however, your main duties are to perform patient assessment and to provide basic EMT-level emergency care.

THE 10 PHASES OF A VEHICLE RESCUE OPERATION

Analyses of motor vehicle accident scene activities show that the operations of emergency service personnel can be grouped into 10 phases of activity.

- PREPARATION. This process refers to the indefinite period before an accident call during which the system of people and machines is prepared for service. Officers and squad personnel continue to train, equipment is serviced, and the vehicle is kept ready to respond.

- RESPONSE. The second phase begins when an alarm is received. It continues while the unit responds and ends when the unit is safely parked at the scene of the accident.

- ASSESSMENT. In this phase the officer in charge 1) assesses the need for service, 2) assesses the capabilities of the emergency service unit to control the situation, and 3) locates the accident victims.

- HAZARD CONTROL. Two types of hazards may be encountered at the scene of a motor vehicle accident, traffic and non-traffic. In almost every accident these hazards must be controlled before patients can be reached.

- SUPPORT OPERATIONS. There may be a need for flood-lighting, patient protection, special rescuer protection, fire prevention, and warning and signaling operations.

- GAINING ACCESS. It is during this phase of activity that an opening is made in the wreckage large enough for an EMT to pass through with a life-support kit.

- PATIENT ASSESSMENT AND EMERGENCY CARE. This phase begins when an EMT reaches the patient and initiates the primary survey or begins talking with the patient. The emergency care phase does not end until the patient is transferred to the care of the emergency department personnel.

- DISENTANGLEMENT. This procedure can be regarded as the ''extrication'' phase of a vehicle rescue operation. The phase has two parts. First, rescuers make a pathway through the wreckage by which other rescuers and tools may reach the patients. The pathway also will serve as a means of egress. Second, the rescuers remove wreckage from the patient so that he can be removed.

- REMOVAL AND TRANSFER. This is another two-part operation. Once properly packaged, the patient is 1) removed from the wreckage and 2) transferred to the waiting ambulance.

- TERMINATION. The final phase of accident scene activities begins when all patients have been transferred to ambulances. The phase ends when the system of people and machines is once again in quarters and ready for service.

The EMT in a Vehicle Rescue Operation

If your ambulance arrives first on the scene of an accident, you may have to perform activities typically done by firefighters or specialized rescue personnel. Using the tools and appliances that are carried on your vehicle, you may have to:

- Initiate traffic control measures
- Work around downed electric wires (if trained to do so)
- Extinguish a fire in the wreckage (if trained to do so)
- Stabilize the vehicle
- Gain access to trapped persons by entering through the doors, windows, or even the body of the vehicle.
- Disentangle patients from seat belts, steering wheels, seats, or other parts of the vehicle in which they may be trapped.
- Remove the patients from the wreckage and transfer them to the ambulance.

Attitude and Personal Safety It may sound obvious, but when you think of your responsibilities at the scene of a motor vehicle accident, think positively! In the majority of accidents, access to trapped persons was gained quickly and with no more than basic hand tools. You can control almost every situation with basic tools and techniques.

Let's consider personal safety. Fix in your mind the image of firefighters properly dressed for dangerous duty. They wear: a specially designed helmet; a wrap-around shield or coverall-type goggles; a multi-layered coat that resists both penetration by sharp objects and fire; waterproof, slip-resistant gloves; and rubber boots that probably have steel insoles and shin guards. Moreover, they may be wearing canvas and rubber turnout pants for additional lower body protection, and coat and pants may be made with a special fire resistant material.

How will you be protected at the scene of an accident? Obviously, a firefighter's gear offers the utmost protection from accident scene hazards. Many EMTs find that this gear limits their mobility, however, and they choose articles of clothing lighter and less cumbersome. A construction-type helmet offers excellent protection without the height, length, and weight of an ordinary fire helmet. Keep it *strapped* on. Coverall-type goggles provide excellent eye protection. A fringe benefit of chemical or mechanical safety goggles is that they can be held securely on a helmet by the elastic strap. Use only the better-grade goggles that are vented and keep fogging to a minimum. Select gloves that are light but strong. Ordinary garden gloves often fit the needs of EMTs, and are not as bulky as those firefighters often wear. A short turnout coat offers adequate protection. Few EMTs wear boots; instead many wear either high-top or low quarter-style work shoes with steel toe protectors.

Whatever your choice of protective gear, wear it! A rescuer is of little value when an on-the-scene mishap causes him to become one of the victims.

Equipment

There are over 600 tools and appliances that could be useful in a vehicle rescue operation. Because of the size, weight, or cost of some tools, however, or because some of them require an external power supply, many are not practical for inclusion in ambulances. The following is a list of tools recommended for ambulances in Federal Specification KKK-A-1822-A, as well as a few that expand the capabilities of EMTs in vehicle rescue efforts.

- The *12 in. adjustable wrench* can be used for a variety of disentanglement operations when disassembly is required.

- The *12 in. Phillips screwdriver*—another disassembly tool—also can be used to break tempered glass when other sharp-pointed tools are not available.

- The *12 in. regular blade screwdriver* also is a disassembly tool. It can be used to make an opening in sheet metal as, for example, in the door or roof of a car.

- The *hacksaw* is used for numerous cutting operations, e.g., cutting through a vehicle's corner posts so that the top can be removed.

- The *vise-grip pliers* facilitate grasp; they also are useful for breaking away the plastic covering of a steering wheel so that the core can be cut more easily with the bolt cutter or a hacksaw.

- The *5-pound hammer* provides force; however, the 15 in. hammer should be replaced with two other hammers: short-handled, 2½-pound hammer is an excellent tool for making openings in doors and roofs with cutting tools. A long-handled sledgehammer is used in conjunction with a flat-head ax to cut away a section of a vehicle's roof.

- The *flat-head fire ax* can be used to cut a roof section and is also a valuable tool for clearing brush in an off-the-road accident situation.

- The *24-in. wrecking bar* can be replaced by a combination tool like the *pry-axe*, which can be used in a number of vehicle rescue operations.

- The *51-in. pinch point bar* gives leverage and is essential in displacing and prying operations, such as forcing a jammed door.

- The *bolt cutter* is an ideal tool for breaking padlocks, cutting chains, and severing the rim of a steering wheel. It is strongly recommended that the cutter have handles at least 36 in. long. It is virtually impossible to cut case-hardened lock shackles and the cores of steering wheels with smaller cutters.

- *Shoring blocks* are used to support an unstable vehicle and also can be used to prevent the collapse of hood and trunk sections when a hand winch is being used.

- The *folding pointed shovel* is useful in removing debris.

- The *double action tin snips* can be used to remove metal trim that is close to a victim. They can also be used to cut seat belts.

- The two *manila ropes* that are specified stabilize a vehicle, raise or lower equipment, raise or lower stretchers or facilitate the grasp of rescuers who must move stretcher patients up or down steep grades.

- The *hand winch*, commonly called a "comealong," increases the pulling ability of an EMT to two tons. Rescuers use hand winches to widen door openings, stabilize vehicles, pull wreckage away from poles and walls, displace steering columns, and perform other tasks.

- The *aluminized blanket* offers patients a degree of protection from flash fires and flying particles of glass and metal. An asbestos blanket was originally included among recommended items. An aluminized blanket should be used instead because asbestos absorbs spilled fuel. Moreover, when asbestos is heated by a fire and then comes into contact with water that is used to extinguish the flames, steam is produced. Patients supposedly being protected by the blanket may be seriously scalded.

- *Porta-power hydraulic tools* for opening jammed doors, moving floor pedals, and other duties requiring spreading and lifting. They are manually-powered.

Other tools and appliances may be carried; however, the above list will allow most ambulance crews to handle most "ordinary" rescue operations. See Appendix 2.

The Door and Windshield Kit Most ambulances are equipped with a door and windshield kit containing hacksaws, punches, hammers, wrenches, screwdrivers, pliers, prying bars, knives, and other hand tools that may be useful in gaining access. The tools in this kit and a few basic power tools will allow you to gain access to most patients trapped in motor vehicle accidents.

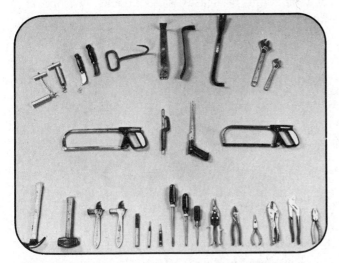

Figure 16-5: A typical door and windshield kit.

The Importance of a Proper Assessment

The scene of a serious vehicle accident is often a nightmare of sights and sounds that tax the emotional stability of even the most experienced EMTs. Inexperienced EMTs often jump from the ambulance and wish to rush to the assistance of accident victims without regard for their own safety. Unfortunately this basic desire to help may place an entire rescue operation in danger. Independent activity—with little regard for a sequence of operations or a team effort—can have serious consequences. For example, an EMT may be electrocuted if he brushes against a downed wire that he overlooked in his rush to aid the injured. He may spend valuable time trying to remove persons only slightly injured, while persons with life-threatening problems go unattended. He may aggravate injuries or cause death by attempting to pull from the wreckage those persons who require immobilization. Or, he may injure himself while trying to accomplish difficult extrication procedures while in a highly emotional state.

Assessing the Situation

An Emergency Medical Technician makes a two-part assessment of the patient to determine the extent of injuries, the primary and the secondary surveys.

Likewise, an on-the-scene assessment of a vehi-

cle accident situation has two parts. First the EMT should make a **primary assessment** to determine if the services of emergency service units are needed. Then he should determine by a **secondary assessment** if the immediately available resources are sufficient to control the situation.

The Primary Assessment for Need It is a natural reaction for people who witness an accident to call for help. The problem is that in many instances they overreact. To determine if services are needed, you must answer two questions: Are there injuries? Are people or property endangered? The second of these questions embraces the objectives of all fire, rescue, and ambulance services, namely, to protect life and property.

If a car leaves the road, grazes a tree and comes to rest in a field away from the road, an accident has occurred. That no one was injured does not make the accident any less real. But if no injuries have been produced and there are no dangers to spectators or to property, it may not be the kind of accident that requires the services of emergency units.

There are often less-than-obvious dangers present, however. Perhaps the vehicle's gas tank was punctured and is leaking fuel. Passing cars may create a traffic problem. Spectators standing about the accident scene may be threatened by passing vehicles. Although no one was injured and there are no requirements for extrication, there may still be a need for emergency units.

The Secondary Assessment for Capabilities Are there sufficient rescuers in the responding force to cope with the accident situation? Are the rescuers properly trained and equipped?

Even when you can answer all of these questions affirmatively, you will not be able to determine whether the responding force is sufficient to cope with the problem until you complete your assessment.

Consider the following factors in the secondary assessment:

- The number and kinds of vehicles involved.
- The number of persons injured and the apparent extent of their injuries.
- Traffic and non-traffic hazards.
- Apparent extrication problems.

A trained EMT is able to call for assistance logically, properly, and strictly on the basis of information that he has gathered in the secondary assessment of the situation. Some of the kinds and sources of specialized aids include:

- Additional ambulances when many people are injured.
- Heavy rescue vehicles for severe extrication problems.
- Fire apparatus either when vehicles are on fire

or when there is danger of fire.

- Wreckers to pull apart accident vehicles.
- Utility company crews to remove downed wires.
- Helicopter ambulances to move seriously injured persons.
- A medical team to assist when the removal of injured persons will be delayed.
- A scuba team when vehicles are partially or completely under water.
- The humane society for accidents involving animals.
- Clergymen to meet an accident victim's religious needs.

Resources may be limited in many communities. Keep in mind these points: 1) you must know where community resources are and how to contact them quickly; 2) you must be willing to call for resources; and 3) you must be willing to use them. A vehicle accident may produce dangerous situations that will test the capabilities of the most proficient and experienced EMT.

Locating Accident Victims

Once the EMT in charge has completed his assessment of the situation, he must be sure that he has located all of the accident victims. The likelihood of one or more victims being away from the wreckage—even far away—is very real. Spectators may pull accident victims away from the wrecked vehicles. Passers-by may take victims to nearby houses, or even to hospitals. The probability of victims being moved from the immediate scene increases in bad weather.

Moreover, injured persons may walk away from the scene in a dazed state. It is not uncommon for an injured person to leave the wreckage and seek help for someone who is trapped within the wreckage. Nor is it uncommon for those injured persons to fall unconscious along the roadway.

Whatever the case, injured persons must be located and cared for before their condition deteriorates.

Information about the number and location of accident victims can be obtained from various sources. If they are conscious and coherent, *occupants* of the involved vehicles are the best sources of information about the number of persons in the vehicles at the time of the crash. If possible, get the names of all persons so that a comparison can be made between names and numbers. Frame your questions, however, so that they do not cause apprehension to injured persons. Make no reference to the severity of injuries and, above all, do not ask questions or make statements in such a way that

suggests that some of the victims are not accounted for. Learning that a family member or friend is lost may cause an injured person to become emotionally unstable or to slip into deep shock.

Witnesses are not always reliable. However, you should ask if they saw anyone walk away from the wreckage, or if they saw someone assist any of the victims either to a car or to a nearby building.

The involved vehicles themselves often offer clues as to the number of persons in a vehicle at the time of an accident. Briefcases, school books, lunchboxes, toys, luggage, clothing, and a multitude of other items may be tossed about within vehicles at the time of an accident. Such objects are clues. If a vehicle has infant clothing and toys scattered about, you should assume that an infant was in the car at the time of the crash.

If any sources of information lead you to believe that there were people in the accident vehicles other than those immediately accounted for, be prepared to search areas around the wreckage, including:

- Roadways
- Ditches and gulleys
- Ravines
- Tall grass and crops
- Nearby buildings
- Hospitals

The Hazard Control Phase of Vehicle Rescue Operations

The ambulance squad responding to a vehicle accident may find itself confronted with a variety of hazards, including *traffic hazards, downed electrical lines, vehicle fires, and unstable vehicles.*

Traffic Hazards

Accidents invariably produce some sort of traffic problem. Traffic slowdown caused by curious drivers, lane blockage by wreckage, and drivers attempting to steer through or close to the accident can produce potential problems. If the ambulance arrives before police assistance, you must take action to control the scene to protect rescuers and patients.

The ambulance, with its warning lights, serves as the first form of control. Flares or special warning lights must be placed to alert other drivers to the accident and to help establish the accident zone. The *accident zone* is the area around the crashed vehicles included in a circle with a radius of 50 feet. As noted in Chapter 15, this may have to be extended if a safety zone is needed due to hazards.

Factors in placing warning devices include:
- The posted speed of the roadway
- The required stopping distance for passenger cars

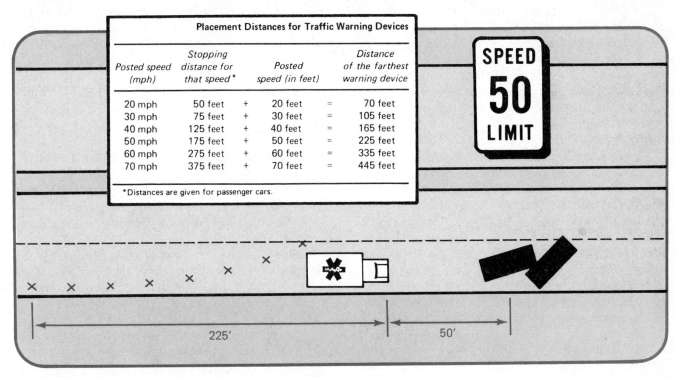

Placement Distances for Traffic Warning Devices			
Posted speed (mph)	Stopping distance for that speed*	Posted speed (in feet)	Distance of the farthest warning device
20 mph	50 feet +	20 feet =	70 feet
30 mph	75 feet +	30 feet =	105 feet
40 mph	125 feet +	40 feet =	165 feet
50 mph	175 feet +	50 feet =	225 feet
60 mph	275 feet +	60 feet =	335 feet
70 mph	375 feet +	70 feet =	445 feet

*Distances are given for passenger cars.

Figure 16-6: Placing traffic warning devices on a straight road.

- The volume of traffic
- The condition of the road surface
- The weather
- The location of the accident (straight road or curve).

There is a basic rule of thumb in warning light placement. *The farthest device should be placed at a distance from the accident zone equal to the stopping distance for the road's posted speed, plus a distance in feet equal to the posted speed.* Note that this distance is from the edge of the accident zone, not from the vehicles at its center.

Do not worry about exact distances, a close estimate is all you will need. When setting the warning devices, you will not be able to measure off the distance. Utility poles along a highway can serve as a guide since they are usually placed 100 to 125 feet apart. The important thing is to set up the devices so that motorists can slow down and stop before they reach the accident zone and do so without causing other accidents.

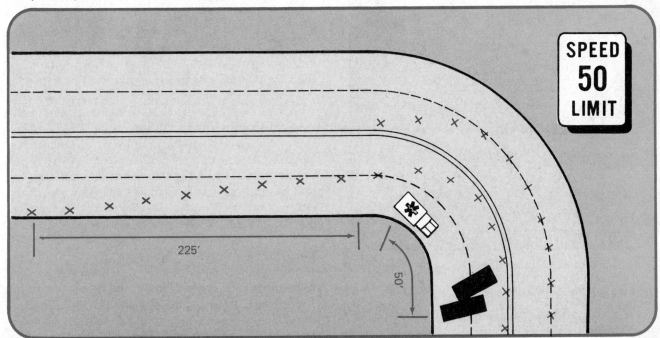

Figure 16-7: Placing traffic warning devices on a curved road.

CAUTION: Do NOT throw flares out of the ambulance while it is moving. Walk and place each flare, being alert for fuel spills and dry vegetation.

Warning devices should be placed *every 10 feet,* when possible. The important thing is to extend the first device far enough so that motorists have enough time to calmly slow down and stop. An example of proper warning device placement for an accident on a *straight road* is shown in Figure 16-6.

Traffic warning devices should be placed *ahead* of a curve. Consider the start of the curve to be the edge of the accident zone. The farthest warning device should be placed the appropriate distance from it rather than the usual 50-foot zone. This prevents motorists from having to change lanes while negotiating the curve, and gives them a chance to slow before the curve.

Igniting Road Flares With one hand, grasp the flare near the base and use your free hand to pry off the plastic cap, exposing the scratching surface. Pull the cap off to expose the ignitor. Hold the flare in one hand and the cap in the other, so that the scratching surface is against the ignitor. Move the flare away from your body sharply so that the ignitor strikes against the scratching surface. Repeat this if the flare does not ignite. Keep the flare pointed away from your body as you position it on the wire stand, or on the ground with the plastic holder in place.

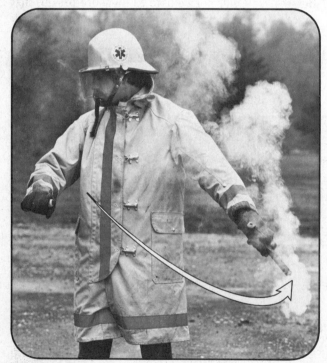

Figure 16-8: Igniting a traffic flare.

Downed Electrical Wires

CAUTION: Do NOT enter an accident zone where there are downed electrical wires. First, create a safety zone, (see Chapter 15). Do NOT attempt to move the wires unless you have been trained to do so and have the necessary equipment. Every ambulance squad, fire department, and rescue squad should work with its local power company to develop training programs.

Always keep in mind the following warnings when confronted with the problem of a downed wire.

- Never assume that a downed wire is not dangerous because the surrounding area is dark. Power distribution systems are built so that if there is a break in the line, switching arrangements cause power to be fed from another direction. Power may be restored to the area at any time.
- Never assume that guy wires are not energized. Rescuers often think that the bright, uninsulated guy wire that stabilizes a utility pole is safe. As the pole was struck and broken, the guy wire may have contacted one of the primary or secondary conductors. Likewise, telephone cables, cable television lines, fire alarm wires, street lighting wires, and any other attachment to a utility pole may be carrying the highest voltage available if the wires have been jumbled after a crash.
- Never attempt to control downed wires with makeshift equipment. Tree limbs, ordinary manila rope, and even wood ladders and firefighting appliances may actually serve as conductors if conditions are right. A lineman's clamp stick, often referred to as a ''hot stick'' offers the greatest protection for rescuers when used with a set of lineman's gloves. The clamp stick is a special device designed with one purpose in mind, namely, to handle an energized wire. A clamp stick requires using *special training* in dealing with electrical hazards.

An alternative to a clamp stick is the 100-foot length of polypropylene rope suggested in the federal specification for ambulances. The rope should be prepared with a weight on each end so that it can be easily thrown. This synthetic rope is a nonconductor, and can be used to remove an energized wire from a wrecked vehicle. Bear in mind that only synthetic rope with a high dielectric strength can be used around high voltage wires. Do not use ordinary manila rope; under certain conditions, manila rope can become an effective conductor.

Neither the clamp stick nor the weighted rope should be used unless the rescuer has a lineman's glove set that consists of a pair of rubber gloves, a pair of protective leather shells, and a pair of cotton glove inserts. The glove set should be properly stored in a marked container and should not be used for any task other than handling a downed wire. Lineman's gloves should be tested periodically by a qualified testing agency and field tested by the rescuer before each use.

REMEMBER: Ordinary firefighter's gloves and firefighting boots *do not* offer protection against electrocution. Never approach a downed wire thinking that you are protected by such equipment.

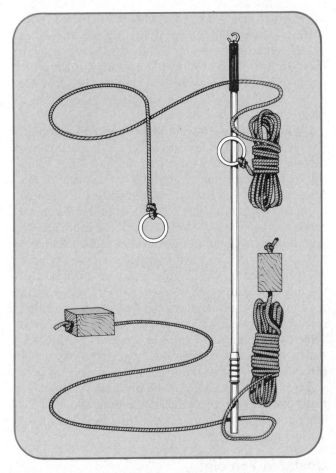

Figure 16-9: A lineman's clamp stick and two types of weighted throwing lines.

Using a Lineman's Clampstick You should be *properly protected* with a pair of approved lineman's gloves and *trained* in the use of the specialized equipment recommended for use with downed wires. To remove an energized wire from a wrecked vehicle, grasp the wire about 2 or 3 feet from its end with the clamp stick. This eliminates the problem of the wire whipping and contacting you. Move away from the wreckage in such a manner that the clamp stick is between you and the wire at all times and so that a slight tension is maintained on the wire. Then if the wire should slip from the clamp or if it arcs on something and burns through, the natural tendency for the wire to curl will cause the conductor to move away from you.

After removing the wire from the vehicle, move it to a safe place with the clamp stick. If you do not need the stick for another wire, leave it attached to the conductor that you have moved and lower it to the ground. The stick will help hold the wire in place.

If you do need the stick again, have someone carefully anchor the wire in place with a coil of rope, a roll of hose, a traffic cone or anything else that can be dropped onto the wire. If possible, post a guard near the wire to keep other rescuers and spectators away from the danger.

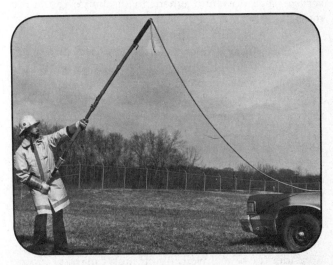

Figure 16-10: Moving a downed wire with a clamp stick.

Using a Weighted Throwing Line An energized downed wire can be moved away from a wrecked vehicle with the weighted throwing line.

Put on the lineman's gloves and leather shells and take a position about 20 feet from the wire on the side opposite from where the wire will be pulled. Uncoil the weighted throwing line until you reach the midpoint (which should be marked). Stand on the center portion and loosely coil half of the line in your hand. Toss the weighted end under the downed wire as far as you can. If the throw is short, retrieve the line and toss it again. When you are satisfied with the position of the weight, toss the other half of the throwing line over the wire.

If another EMT is working with you and has a set of lineman's gloves, have him pick up the two weights and walk in the direction that you want the wire to move. If you are working alone, walk around the wreckage and move the wire yourself. When the wire is clear of the vehicle, weight it in place and post a guard if possible.

REMEMBER: You must watch the energized wire at all times when moving it with a weighted rope. There is not as much control over the wire as there is when using a clamp stick. Curling and whipping will be much more pronounced. Utilize the full length of the doubled rope so that the greatest possible distance is maintained between you and the conductor.

Vehicle Fires

CAUTION: Do NOT attempt to fight a vehicle fire unless you have been trained to do so and have all the necessary equipment. Always call for fire service support.

Before you attempt to use a portable extinguisher, know the class of fire for which it is intended, how to hold it, how to make it ready for service, and how and where to discharge the contents.

If there is a fire in the engine compartment and the hood is open, attack the fire with short bursts of the agent. If possible, position yourself so the wind is at your back, but avoid forcing smoke, fumes and the agent into the passenger compartment. Avoid placing yourself directly in front of the vehicle. Use no more of the agent than is necessary. You may need what is left if there is a flare-up.

If the hood of the vehicle is closed (or opened only to the safety latch), resist the temptation to throw open the hood fully before operating the extinguisher. By keeping the hood closed you will restrict the flow of air to the fire. Direct the agent under the hood opening, through the grill, or even up under the wheel well. Again, don't use any more extinguishing agent than necessary.

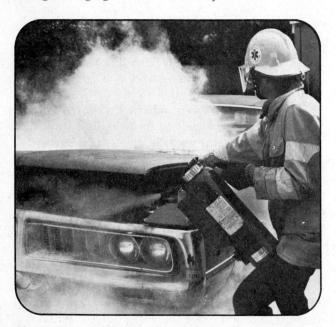

Figure 16-11: Combating an engine compartment fire.

Fighting a fire in spilled fuel with a portable extinguisher may be an exercise in futility. But when there is a fire under a vehicle in which people are trapped, you must try nonetheless. Attempt to sweep the flames away from the passenger compartment as you apply the agent. If you are able to extin-

guish the fire, be sure sources of future ignition are kept away from the vehicle.

Some persons recommend cutting the battery cable of a wrecked vehicle as a standard operating procedure. If there is no spilled fuel, cutting the battery out of a vehicle's electrical system may not only be a waste of time, it may hinder the rescue operation. Many cars have electrically operated seats, windows, trunk locks, door locks, and hood locks. Being able to operate powered seats may save you considerable time and effort if an injured driver or passenger must be removed. In cold weather, you may want to keep the heater operating during the rescue effort for at least as long as there is hot water in the heater core. Neither of these can be done if the battery cable has been cut!

When it is necessary to disconnect the battery, always work with the *negative* cable. When a positive cable is cut or pulled from its terminal, a hot spark can be produced that could ignite spilled fuel or hydrogen gas leaking from a cracked battery. The same thing can happen if the cutting tool touches a metal component as the jaws bite through the cable insulation. If you cannot disconnect the negative cable, cut it. Many newer cars have two negative cables, with one connected to the engine and one grounded to the frame or body.

In the past, fire services have recommended that rescuers remove the fuel tank caps from all accident vehicles to minimize explosions caused by heated, sealed fuel tanks. This is no longer true of all fire services. Some have reported cases of serious fires and explosions occurring when gasoline vapors have made contact with the vehicle's catalytic converter or other source of ignition. Follow local protocol on all matters involving fire.

Unstable Vehicles

Any motor vehicle involved in an accident may be unstable. This is true of a vehicle that is on all four wheels, sitting on what appears to be a level road surface. The rule is to stabilize "any vehicle—every time."

An upright vehicle may be unstable in the following situations:

- Inclined surface—the vehicle may have come to rest on a slanted surface and may roll forward or backward. Chock the wheels.

- Slippery surface—oil, ice, or snow may have produced a road surface that will allow the vehicle to slide away without warning. This often happens when a door of the vehicle is opened. Chock the wheels.

- Tilted surface—the vehicle may be on a surface that causes it to tilt to one side, or slant down a hill. Chocking the wheels may offer some degree of stability. When practical, tie strong lines to the vehicle frame (not the bumper) and then secure the lines to large trees, guardrails, or heavy, secured vehicles. Do NOT work on the downhill side of the vehicle.

- Stacked vehicles—the vehicles may be upright, but part of one vehicle may be resting on part of another vehicle. Chock the wheels of both vehicles and insert spare wheels, lumber, blocks, or any suitable materials at the scene between the road surface and the misplaced part of the vehicle. You may have to secure both vehicles with line.

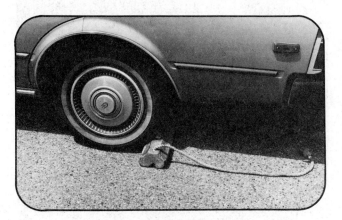

Figure 16-12: Stabilize all vehicles before attempting to gain access.

A vehicle may come to rest on its side. To stabilize this vehicle:

1. Increase the number of contact points made with the ground.
2. Spread the contact points over as wide an area as possible.

If you find a vehicle on its side, you should stabilize the vehicle by placing cribbing and wedges, spare wheels, blocks, timbers, wheel chocks, or whatever materials are available between the roof line and the road surface. If need be, place stabilizing materials between the wheels and the road surface. It may be necessary to have volunteers help hold the car in a vertical position for proper stabilization.

A bumper jack and a spare tire can be used to help stabilize a vehicle. First slide the spare tire under a wheel. There should be metal-to-metal contact, that is, the steel wheel of the wrecked vehicle should be in contact with the steel wheel of the spare tire. This eliminates the "give" that would be present if rubber tire contacts rubber tire. Next, have helpers push the car to a vertical position (onto the spare

tire). While they hold the car steady, position the bumper jack so that the lifting toe contacts the rain gutter close to the C-post. Operate the jack until the car is stable. Note: if the spare wheel is placed under the rear wheel of the wreck, position the jack near the A-post. The diagonal placement of the stabilizing devices is more effective. The procedure can be reversed. The jack can be used on a frame member after the spare wheel is positioned under a corner post. Ironically, vehicles stabilized with these makeshift devices are often more rigid than those stabilized with the recommended shoring blocks.

There are a number of ways to stabilize a vehicle. Two alternate methods of stabilization are shown in Figure 16-14.

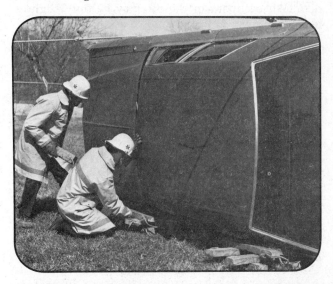

Figure 16-13: Stabilizing a car with cribbing and wedges.

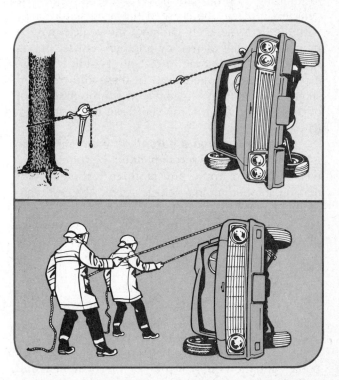

Figure 16-14: Alternate ways of stabilizing a vehicle.

Gaining Access to Trapped Patients

Do not try to assess your route of access or attempt access until the vehicle is stabilized. Generally, the access routes are considered in the following order:

1. Doors
2. Side windows and rear window
3. Windshield
4. Vehicle body—roof, floor, or trunk (very rare and time consuming)

Always try the vehicle doors to see if they will open. All the doors may not be damaged or locked. A window may be down, allowing you to unlock the door. An occupant of the car may be only slightly injured and can unlock a door.

If these efforts fail, attempting to open a locked door is your best approach unless you are certain that it will require a time-consuming effort, or cause a delay while special tools are brought to the scene.

The procedures for gaining access through vehicle doors and windows are covered in Scansheets 16-3, 16-4, and 16-5. You should always wear protective gear when trying to gain access to trapped patients. Try to use methods that will not aggravate the patient's injuries or cause more harm. Take great care if you have to break or remove glass.

Gaining Access Through the Vehicle Body

In some accidents you may have no alternative to entering through the body of the vehicle. The vehicle's top may be crushed flat against the body with the doors severely jammed, the vehicle may be pinned to a wall or tree by another vehicle, or the vehicle may have come to rest on its side with the exposed doors jammed shut. In these and other instances you will have to gain access through the roof or through the floor of the vehicle, if it is resting on its top.

Cutting Through the Roof   If your ambulance is provided with the recommended equipment, you will be able to apply any of three techniques for making an opening in a vehicle's roof. The first technique involves the air-operated cutting chisel.

Stabilize the vehicle using one of the techniques described earlier. If you use a bumper jack and spare wheel, position the jack so it will not be in the way of the cutting chisel.

With the chisel, make a starting hole in a lower corner of the roof, about 6 in. from the windshield edge. Drive the chisel up one side, across the top, and down the other side in an uninterrupted movement. Pull the resulting flap down. Cut roof supports with the chisel. Rip away the headliner and pull out any rod struts that support the headliner.

If you are using an air-cutting chisel set with an adjustable pressure regulator, set the operating pressure at 100 to 125 p.s.i. This will provide sufficient force for cutting sheet metal without excessive air consumption. You may need the remaining air supply for subsequent disentanglement operations.

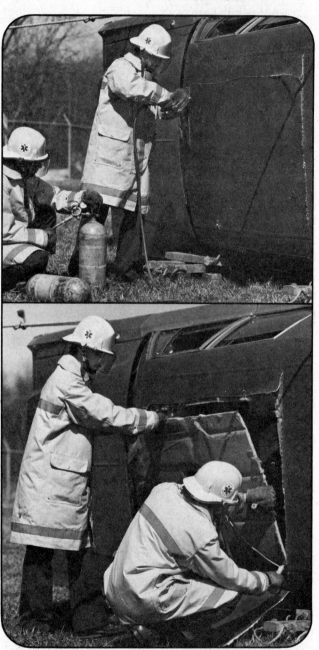

Figure 16-15: An air-operated chisel can be used to open a roof quickly.

If you do not have an air-operated cutting chisel or if the tool is being used for other rescue operations, make an opening in the roof with an ax and sledgehammer. As with most rescue efforts, a helmet, eye protection, and gloves are essential for this operation. Let's say that you are going to hold the ax while your partner wields the sledgehammer.

VEHICLES-ACCESS THRU DOORS

UNLOCKING UNDAMAGED DOORS

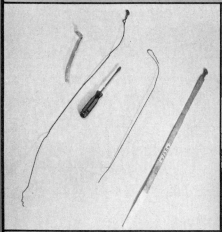

TOOLS. A. FLAT PRY BAR B. WIRE AND WASHER C. SCREWDRIVER D. WIRE HOOK E. "THIEVES' TOOL".

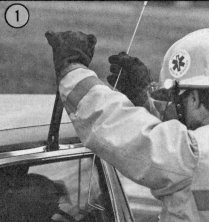

① FRAMED WINDOWS. PRY FRAME AWAY FROM VEHICLE BODY, INSERT WIRE HOOK.

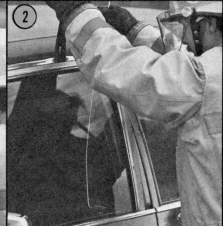

② SNAG THE LOCKING BUTTON AND PULL UPWARD.

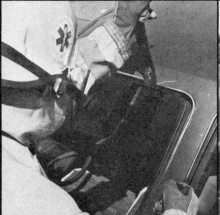

UNFRAMED WINDOWS. PRY WINDOW, INSERT SCREWDRIVER, KEYHOLE SAW BLADE, OR OIL DIP STICK TO LIFT BUTTON.

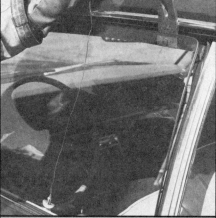

"THIEF-PROOF LOCK." INSERT WASHER ON WIRE, DROP OVER SHANK. PULL UP, ALLOWING WASHER TO CANT & GRAB.

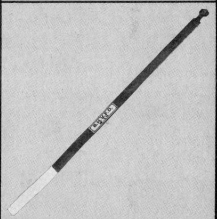

"THIEVES' TOOL." INSERT BETWEEN WINDOW & DOOR NEAR LOCKING BUTTON. PULL UP & REINSERT UNTIL LOCK DISENGAGES.

EXPOSING A LOCKING MECHANISM—NO EXPOSED LOCKING BUTTON

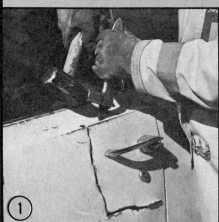

① USE SHORT HANDLE SLEDGEHAMMER & PANEL CUTTER. MAKE 3-SIDED CUT AROUND HANDLE & LOCK. . .

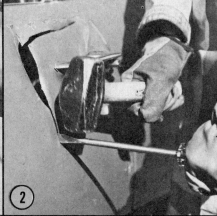

② . . .OR USE SCREWDRIVER. PULL THE METAL FLAP OPEN

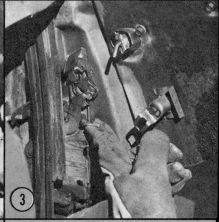

③ OPERATE RODS & LEVERS TO POP OPEN LOCK. PUSH ON PLATE BEHIND PUSH BUTTON TO OPEN DOOR

SCAN 16–3

VEHICLES-OPENING DAMAGED DOORS

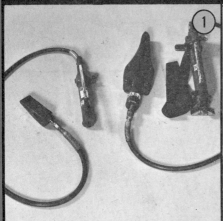

1 PULL UP LOCKING BUTTON, THEN USE PORTA-POWER TOOLS TO OPEN DOOR.

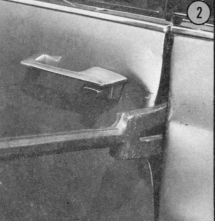

2 WIDEN THE OPENING BETWEEN DOOR EDGE AND FRAME.

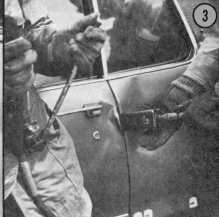

3 INSERT THE "WEDGIE" (SMALLER) TOOL.

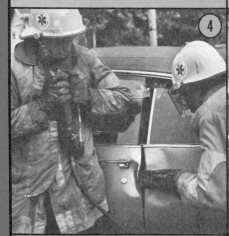

4 OPEN WEDGIE WHILE LEANING A-GAINST DOOR SO THAT IT WILL NOT SPRING OPEN.

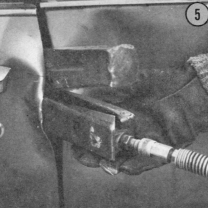

5 CRIB THE OPENING.

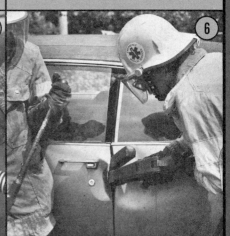

6 INSERT "SPREADER" (LARGER TOOL) AND CONTINUE TO WIDEN OPENING.

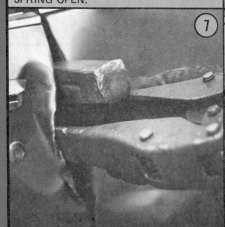

7 CRIB THE OPENING.

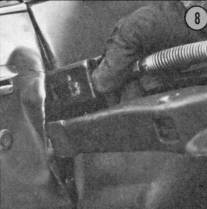

8 RESET THE WEDGIE, SPREAD, AND CRIB.

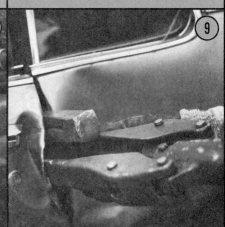

9 RESET SPREADER, SPREAD, & CRIB. CONTINUE THE CYCLE UNTIL DOOR LATCHES SEPARATE OR ARE PULLED AWAY.

NOTE: YOU CAN OPEN SOME OLDER MODEL CARS WITH A JACK AND SPREADER AND WEDGES. THIS IS TIME CONSUMING IN NEWER MODEL CARS. TRYING TO PRY OPEN A DOOR WITH A LONG BAR IS VERY TIME CONSUMING. DON'T WASTE TIME! IF OPENING THE DOOR WILL BE A LONG PROCESS, TRY ANOTHER ACCESS ROUTE.

SCAN 16-4

VEHICLES-ACCESS THRU WINDOWS

CAUTION: MAKE CERTAIN TO PROTECT YOURSELF IF YOU HAVE TO BREAK GLASS. TAKE SPECIAL CARE TO PROTECT YOUR EYES, FACE, AND HANDS. WHEN POSSIBLE, BREAK GLASS SO THAT IT WILL NOT ENDANGER PATIENT. IF PRACTICAL, REMOVE WINDSHIELD RATHER THAN BREAK GLASS.

AUTOMOBILE SAFETY GLASS

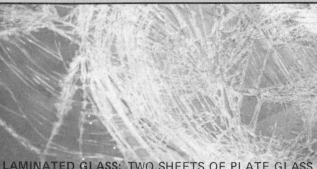

TEMPERED GLASS: SPECIALLY HARDENED PLATE GLASS THAT SHATTERS INTO SMALL PIECES WITH ROUNDED EDGES. IT IS USED IN SIDE AND REAR WINDOWS.

LAMINATED GLASS: TWO SHEETS OF PLATE GLASS ARE BONDED TO A SHEET OF TRANSPARENT PLASTIC. WHEN THE GLASS BREAKS, THE SHARDS ARE HELD IN PLACE. TYPICALLY FOUND IN WINDSHIELDS.

BREAKING VEHICLE WINDOW GLASS

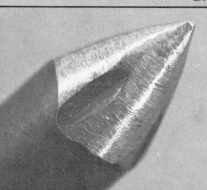

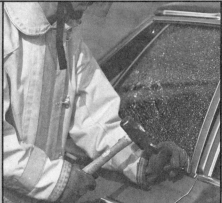

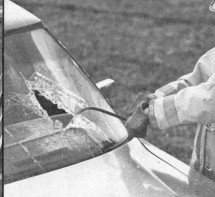

IT IS BEST TO BREAK TEMPERED GLASS WITH THE SHARPEST TOOL YOU CAN FIND. USE THIS METHOD FOR SIDE AND REAR WINDOWS.

BREAKING TEMPERED GLASS WITH A SHARP TOOL. STRIKE IN A LOWER CORNER, AS CLOSE TO THE DOOR AS POSSIBLE.

YOU CAN BREAK AND REMOVE A SECTION OF LAMINATED GLASS BY USING A BALING HOOK.

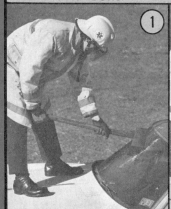

①

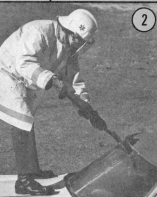

②

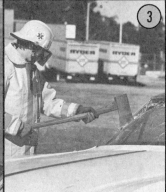

③

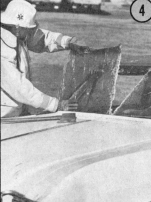

④

WORK FROM HOOD AND DRIVE AX INTO UPPER MID-POINT OF GLASS. USE ONLY ENOUGH FORCE TO HAVE THE EDGE PENETRATE.

CHOP DOWNWARD TO BOTTOM OF WINDSHIELD, CUT ACROSS TOP.

CUT DOWNWARD TIL YOU REACH BOTTOM.

DO NOT CUT ACROSS BOTTOM. PULL CUT PIECE OUTWARD FROM TOP.

SCAN 16-5A

VEHICLES-ACCESS THRU WINDOWS (cont'd)

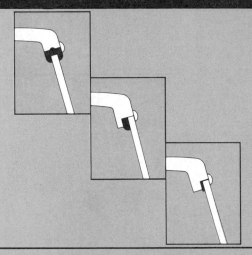

TYPES OF WINDSHIELD MOUNTINGS

U-SHAPED RUBBER CHANNEL ... PRIOR TO 1965, BUT STILL FOUND IN SOME TRUCKS AND VANS.

SOFT ADHESIVE OR THERMOSETTING PLASTIC ... 1965–1969.

MASTIC ... SINCE 1969. IF YOU CAN SEE ONLY CHROME, THE WINDSHIELD IS MOUNTED IN MASTIC. MASTIC MAKES WINDSHIELDS DIFFICULT TO REMOVE. YOU MAY HAVE TO BREAK AWAY THE GLASS.

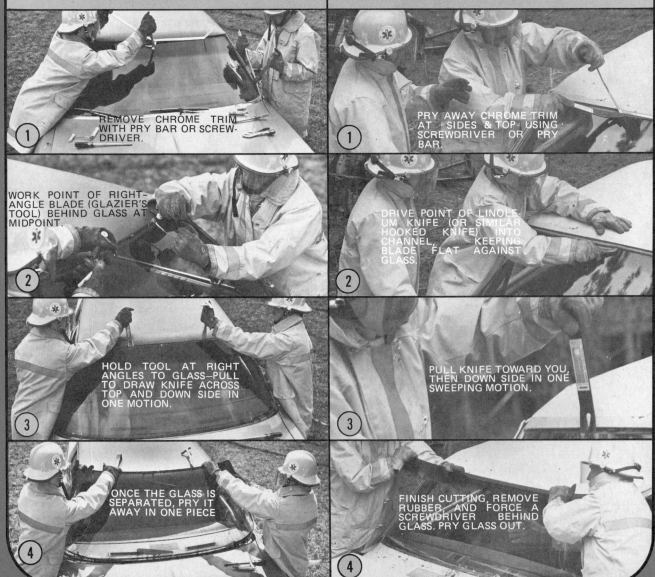

REMOVING MASTIC MOUNTED GLASS

1. REMOVE CHROME TRIM WITH PRY BAR OR SCREW-DRIVER.

2. WORK POINT OF RIGHT-ANGLE BLADE (GLAZIER'S TOOL) BEHIND GLASS AT MIDPOINT.

3. HOLD TOOL AT RIGHT ANGLES TO GLASS—PULL TO DRAW KNIFE ACROSS TOP AND DOWN SIDE IN ONE MOTION.

4. ONCE THE GLASS IS SEPARATED, PRY IT AWAY IN ONE PIECE

REMOVING CHANNEL MOUNTED GLASS

1. PRY AWAY CHROME TRIM AT SIDES & TOP USING SCREWDRIVER OR PRY BAR.

2. DRIVE POINT OF LINOLE-UM KNIFE (OR SIMILAR HOOKED KNIFE) INTO CHANNEL, KEEPING BLADE FLAT AGAINST GLASS.

3. PULL KNIFE TOWARD YOU, THEN DOWN SIDE IN ONE SWEEPING MOTION.

4. FINISH CUTTING, REMOVE RUBBER, AND FORCE A SCREWDRIVER BEHIND GLASS. PRY GLASS OUT.

SCAN 16-5B

Hold the ax in the manner shown in Figure 16-16, with the leading point of the blade about 6 in. from the windshield edge and 6 in. from the rain gutter. Instruct your partner to strike the ax repeatedly until the blade is through the metal. Then turn the ax so that the blade is as nearly parallel to the roof as possible. Thus it will not be necessary to cut through roof struts, and there will be less chance for the blade to bind in the cut. Guide the ax while your partner drives it down. Lifting and lowering the handle will cause the blade to change direction, allowing you to "steer" the ax. Make three cuts in this fashion: one down the right side, one across the top and one down the left side. You thus leave a smooth edge over which the victims can be moved once the roof flap is pulled down.

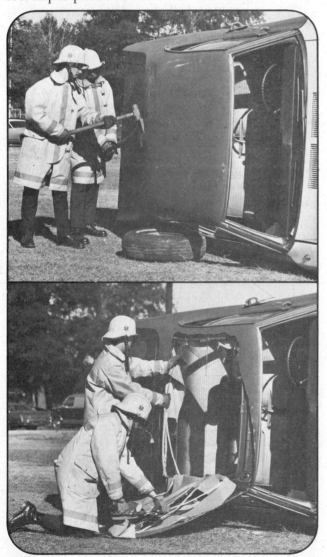

Figure 16-16: Opening a vehicle roof with an ax and sledgehammer.

Both the ax and sledgehammer are made of tool steel, but of different hardnesses. When an ax is struck repeatedly with a sledgehammer there is a tendency for the ax head to "mushroom". Fragments can break away from the head and fly for a considerable distance with enough force to penetrate an eye. Warn spectators and other rescuers of the danger of flying particles when using this technique.

Cutting with an ax also produces razor-sharp metal edges. Be careful when working around them, especially when removing victims from the vehicle. Duct tape can be applied over the edges. Many rescue units carry lengths of split fire hose to slip over dangerous metal edges.

Making roof openings is not limited to the air-cutting chisel and the ax and sledgehammer combination. In extreme circumstances an opening can be made with a flat blade screwdriver and a short sledgehammer.

Cutting Through the Floor You may arrive at an accident and find that a vehicle has come to rest on its top, with the roof crushed flat against the body.

First stabilize the vehicle. This may require a combination of cribbing, spare wheels, and bumper jacks, depending on the circumstances.

Next, locate the rear foot-well. It is easily recognized stamping in most cars. If the foot-well is provided with a rubber drain plug, pry the plug out and probe gently through the opening to be sure that no one is jammed tightly against the portion of floor that is to be cut. Use either the air chisel or the flat blade screwdriver (or a metal cutting tool) to make a three-sided cut around the foot-well. Fold the resulting flap back out of the way. Use scissors or a sharp knife to remove the carpet mat and the carpet itself. The opening should be large enough for an EMT to pass through.

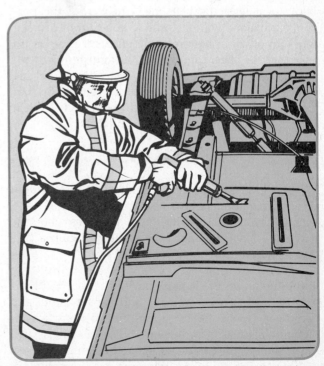

Figure 16-17: Access can be gained through the floor of an overturned vehicle.

In situations where there are several people in an overturned car, it may be necessary to lower an EMT head-first through the opening. While two persons hold him, he will be able to use his hands to move body parts sufficiently so he can be lowered completely into the interior.

REACHING PERSONS TRAPPED IN CAVE-INS (TRENCH RESCUE)

Cave-in and trench rescue are skills requiring special training. The following is an introduction to a complex problem of gaining access and providing care.

Cave-ins are not a problem associated with construction workers alone. Children can be trapped when a large pile of dirt on which they are playing suddenly shifts. Farmers may be trapped under a pile of grain or silage. Climbers may be trapped by a landslide of loose earth. Speed is important when attempting to reach a victim who is covered with dirt (or other loose material). The dirt not only covers his mouth and nose, it is also usually packed tightly around his chest, thus preventing the movement of the chest necessary for breathing. Death usually occurs quickly.

As part of an ambulance team, there may be little that you can do for a cave-in victim. Start, however, by calling for help—notify the fire department or the rescue squad. Follow local guidelines for such rescues. If you are to begin rescue activities, dig with hand tools. Try to determine the location of the victim from witnesses. Dig carefully and be alert for a shifting of the material that may in turn bury you.

If you are able to locate the patient, uncover his body to at least the belt line. Uncovering the person's face alone will not suffice. You cannot resuscitate him or assist his breathing efforts if there is no way that the chest can expand. Administer oxygen.

Do not pull the patient free. Instead, uncover his body and remove him. As you do, remember that the accident may also have produced a neck or back injury. Package the patient accordingly.

SUMMARY

The EMT's major responsibilities at the accident scene are patient assessment and basic EMT-level emergency care. However, there are times when the EMT will have to control the scene and gain access to the patient.

When gaining access to patients trapped in buildings, the EMT may have to face problems caused by hazards, animals, and locked doors and windows. As an EMT, you are not to fight fires or attempt rescues from burning buildings unless you have been trained to do so, have the equipment you will need (including positive pressure breathing apparatus), and the trained personnel at the scene to

help you. If you are in a building that is on fire, do not open a door if it is hot to the touch. Stay low in smoke-filled rooms and hallways.

You may have to forcibly enter locked buildings. Your entry may begin with having to use bolt cutters on a padlocked gate. Locked doors may require you to pry away hasps, drive out exposed hinges, destroy cylinder locks, and pry open double, sliding, and overhead doors. In all cases, make certain you wear the needed protective gear. The minimum is goggles and gloves. The primary tool for entry will be a pry bar or a combination tool.

If you must break a tempered glass door, do so with great care, using a sharp punch or pike and a hammer. Strike the glass in a lower corner, near the frame, or on an exposed edge.

You can open locked double-hung and sliding windows with a pry bar. If prying fails, break a pane of glass and reach in to unlock the window. With casement and awning- and factor-type windows, do not waste time with prying. Carefully break the glass to unlock the window.

Extrication refers to all activities that disentangle and free a patient. Remember that there is more to a vehicle rescue than extrication. The 10 phases of a vehicle rescue operation are: preparation, response, assessment, hazard control, support operations, gaining access, patient assessment and emergency care, disentanglement (clearing a path through the wreckage and removing wreckage from the patient), removal and transfer, and termination. You may have to do more than assess patients and provide care. Your first concern should be your own safety.

Learn to assess the situation at a motor vehicle accident. You will have to decide what the problems are, how many patients there are, and if supportive services are needed for the rescue.

Set up an accident zone at least 50 feet from the vehicles. Use the ambulance's warning lights and place warning lights every 10 feet for a distance equal to the stopping distance for the posted speed plus a distance in feet equal to the posted speed. This distance is from the edge of the accident zone, not from its center. If the accident occurred on a curve, extend the accident zone to include the curve.

Do NOT attempt to work with downed electrical wires unless you have been trained to do so and have the proper tested gloves and boots. Never assume that a downed wire is not energized. Never assume that guy wires are not energized. Do NOT try to control downed wires with makeshift equipment.

Do NOT try to fight vehicle fires unless you have been trained to do so and have the necessary equipment and personnel. If you are fighting an engine compartment fire and the hood is open, attack the fire with short bursts of the agent. If the hood is closed, or held by safety latch, do not open it. Direct the agent under the hood opening, through the grill, or up the wheel well.

Stabilize "any vehicle—every time." Chock wheels to insure that a vehicle will not roll or slide. If the vehicle is on its side, increase the number of contact points with the ground and spread these contact points over as wide an area as possible. Stabilize the vehicle by placing cribbing and wedges or other suitable materials between the roof line and the road surface. When necessary do the same for the wheels.

Make certain that the vehicle is stabilized before you assess your route of access or attempt access. The routes of access are: doors, side and rear windows, windshield, and the vehicle body.

You can gain access through locked doors by inserting a wire hook between the window and frame or window and vehicle and pry up the locking button. A panel cutter can be used to expose a locking mechanism when there is no way to access a locking button. The porta-power tools should be used if you have to open a damaged door.

There are two kinds of automobile safety glass: laminated (shards held by plastic layer) and tempered (pieces are small and rounded). Windshields are made of laminated safety glass. Side windows and rear windows are usually made of safety plate glass.

Whenever possible, avoid breaking glass. The fastest course of action if breaking glass is necessary is to use a sharp tool positioned in the lower corner of a side window, as near to the frame as possible. If you must break a windshield, use a baling hook, or cut out a section with an ax. A special tool can be used to remove a mastic-held windshield. Old channel mounted glass can be removed with a linoleum knife.

If you have to gain access through the vehicle roof, you can use an air-operated chisel, or use an ax blade and sledgehammer to cut away metal. An air chisel or a flathead screwdriver (or other handheld cutting tool) and hammer can be used to cut through the floor of an overturned vehicle.

In cave-in and trench rescue situations, assure your own safety. Make certain that the patient has an open airway. You will have to expose his body to the waist to prevent debris from restricting chest movements during breathing.

17
disentanglement

SKILLS As an EMT, you should be able to:

1. Properly protect a patient during disentanglement.
2. Make a pathway through the wreckage by helping to:
   - Raise a crushed vehicle roof
   - Remove the top of a vehicle
   - Widen vehicle door openings.
3. Remove wreckage from the patient by helping to:
   - Cut seat belts
   - Remove a steering wheel
   - Displace a steering column
   - Displace a vehicle floor pedal
   - Displace a dash
   - Displace a vehicle seat.

TERMS · you may be using for the first time:

Disentanglement—the process of altering or removing wreckage so that proper care can be rendered and the patient can be prepared and removed for transfer to the ambulance.

DISENTANGLEMENT

NOTE: The disentanglement skills required in the basic EMT-level course vary greatly. When disentanglement is taught, emphasis is usually placed on the use of hand tools, porta-power tools, and the hydraulic jack and spreader.

Disentanglement involves making a pathway through the wreckage of an accident and removing wreckage from patients. During the entire process, patients are protected from harm as the rescuers alter and remove the wreckage. When possible, communication with the patients should continue throughout disentanglement.

REMEMBER: As an EMT, your primary duties are patient assessment and emergency care. You should not overlook these duties in order to perform other activities at the accident scene.

There will be times when you can gain access to the patient, but there is no room to reposition the patient for care, or to provide needed care. You may find that you can provide initial care, but you are unable to remove the patient for transport due to confined space or the patient being entrapped by the wreckage. These problems must be solved by the process of disentanglement.

Usually disentanglement will be done by specially trained personnel from the rescue squad or fire service. However, if you are unable to provide basic life support, or the patient's condition is deteriorating too quickly to wait for appropriate help to arrive, you may have to begin the process of disentanglement. ALWAYS summon assistance from the rescue squad, fire service, or appropriate service needed to perform the disentanglement. Do NOT start a long process of disentanglement, only to fail and then have to call for help. Call for assistance and *then* do what you have been trained to do in the process of disentanglement.

The first series of activities described here is intended to *make a pathway in wreckage* through which properly prepared patients can be removed without danger of further injury. Making a pathway may involve nothing more than opening a door, or it may be an operation as complex as completely removing the top of a vehicle.

Activities in the second group are designed to *remove wreckage* from the victim so that he can be prepared for safe transfer to an ambulance.

REMEMBER: Personal safety is a prime consideration at all times during gaining access and disentanglement operations. Wear your helmet, eye protection, gloves, and whatever body protection is available.

PATIENT PROTECTION

Disentanglement activities often expose trapped persons to diverse hazards, produced by either the accident or the disentanglement operations themselves. Particles of broken glass and sharp metal edges are common in accident vehicles.

During the disentanglement operation, you should explain to the patient what is being done and:

1. Protect trapped accident victims with blankets, clothing, or even dressing and bandaging materials, taking particular care to shield their eyes.

2. Make sure that there is adequate ventilation under protective coverings. This is especially important when gasoline-powered tools are being used nearby.

3. If it appears that the disentanglement operations will cause patients to come into contact with

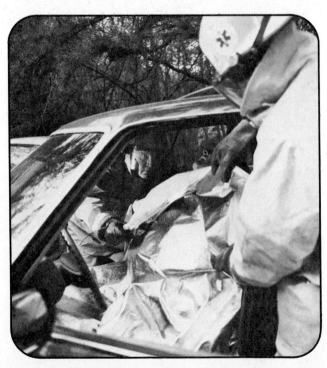

Figure 17-1: Protecting the patient with a rescue blanket.

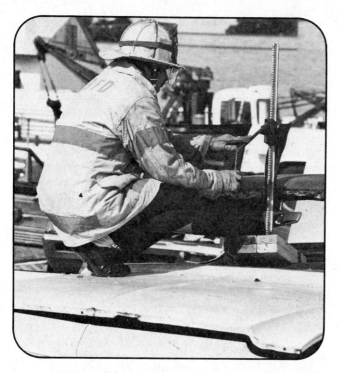

Figure 17-2: A bumper jack can be used to raise a roof that has been partially crushed.

metal parts or the tools being used, provide some sort of rigid protection such as that offered by a spine board.

4. Always have someone stand by with the ambulance fire extinguisher.

MAKING A PATHWAY THROUGH THE WRECKAGE

There is a two-fold purpose in making a pathway through vehicular wreckage. First, the pathway allows other rescuers with tools and appliances to reach the patients. Second, the pathway is the route by which patients can be removed from the wreckage once they are disentangled.

Raising a Crushed Roof

In a rollover-type accident, the roof of a passenger car, pickup truck, or even a heavy truck may be crushed to the point that the people inside are encased in the wreckage. You may be able to gain access to them by prying a door open or by raising a corner of the crushed roof. To extricate victims without causing additional harm, it may be necessary to raise the roof so that either other doors can be opened, or the vehicle's top can be removed altogether. Selecting a suitable tool for raising a crushed roof is usually influenced by how severely the roof has been damaged.

Hand Tools If the roof is not jammed tightly against the body of the vehicle, it may be possible to wedge the toe and foot plate of a bumper jack, a small hydraulic jack, or a screw jack between the body and the roof line.

If you can find a space in which a lifting device can be positioned, raise the portion of the roof directly behind the A-posts first. If you can adequately expose the posts, it may be possible to cut them and fold back the roof without doing any additional jacking.

Power Tools The hydraulic jack and spreader unit offers a distinct advantage over other jacks when the roof line is very close to the body; the wedge or spreader unit can be inserted into a small opening. As was suggested for the procedure with hand tools, first efforts with power tools should be directed toward raising the portions of the roof directly behind the A-posts.

1. Lift the roof section as far as you can with the wedge or spreader unit. Before releasing pressure and removing the lifting device, however, have an assistant position shoring blocks and wedges in the opening. They will prevent the metal that is under stress from collapsing when the wedge or spreader is removed.
2. If the hydraulic jack kit is provided with accessories, replace the wedge or spreader unit with a ram that has been fitted with an appropriate facepiece (such as a V-block or wedge) and a foot plate. Alternately raise and block the roof section until the post can be cut or the door can be opened.
3. If an accessory ram is not available, continue to raise the roof section with the wedge or spreader unit. It will be necessary to place a shoring block under the wedge or spreader each time that it is opened fully and then closed.

Removing the Top of a Vehicle

Once the top is raised as far as possible with whatever lifting device is available, it may be possible to force doors open. However, if patients have or may have spinal injuries or extremity fractures, it will be virtually impossible to immobilize them effectively prior to removal. In these situations it is far better to remove or fold back the vehicle's top, thus providing an almost unrestricted work space. Top removal is not a lengthy operation that requires special equipment or extraordinary skill.

This procedure is often the first choice of rescuers when they need more work space within a wrecked vehicle. With practice, the entire procedure can be done in 10 to 15 minutes. This is usually faster than attempting to create more space by other procedures, such as displacing a seat.

Hand Tools   A hacksaw can be used to cut through roof pillars. The task can be accomplished quicker when two (or more) hacksaws are available. Cuts can be made simultaneously by two rescuers, or one hacksaw can be held ready should the blade of the other saw break during the cutting operation. Two blades may be placed in the saw, positioned to allow for cutting in both directions of the sawing stroke. In some cases, cutting oil may have to be applied to the blade to facilitate its sawing action. A number of replacement blades should be on hand.

The easiest way to rid a vehicle of its restrictive roof is to cut the forward and middle pillars (the A-posts and B-posts, respectively) and then fold the roof back just ahead of the rear pillars (the C-posts). Before this can be done, however, the windshield must be either removed or broken in one of the ways described in the section on gaining access. Once the glass has been removed, the roof can be cut and folded in the following manner.

1. Use a short pry bar or a flat-bladed screwdriver to strip plastic and chrome trim from around the posts that must be cut. Pull away any rubber weather stripping and scrape off any gummy sealant. This takes only a few seconds, but the effort may save valuable minutes and prevent a great deal of aggravation. Chrome trim is difficult to cut; plastic and rubber tend to clog saw blades, as do the soft sealing materials.

2. Cut the A-post first, then the B-post of the same side. Hold the hacksaw firmly and make smooth, even cuts while exerting steady downward force. Do not rush; attempting to cut fast causes movement that contributes to broken saw blades. Excessive downward force also causes blades to break.

3. As you cut, have someone support the roof on the same side. This prevents the saw from binding.

4. When you finish cutting through the A-post and B-post on one side, sever the corresponding posts on the other side while someone supports the roof.

5. Do not cut the C-posts; to do so makes the roof hard to handle. Instead, make a right-angle cut in the roof just ahead of the C-posts. The cut should be just as deep as the hacksaw frame will allow.

6. Direct someone to stand on the rearward portion of the roof with one foot approximately where the roof will fold. Have those people who are supporting the cut roof lift while the person on the roof dimples the metal with his foot. Thus the roof is folded back like that of a convertible, and the entire vehicle interior is exposed.

Severed pillars have sharp edges that are dangerous. Cover these edges with duct tape or adhesive bandage tape, or tape multitrauma dressings or rags over the sharp edges. Short sections of used fire hose can be easily slipped over the pillar ends to provide adequate protection.

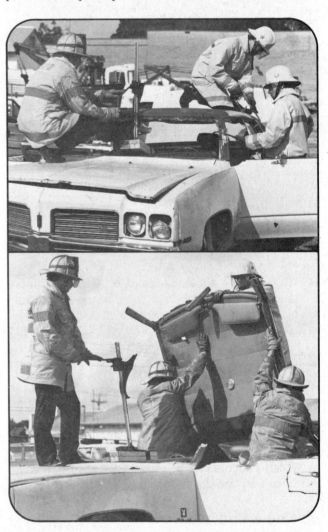

Figure 17-3: a. Peripheral cuts are made first. A bumper jack can be used to support a roof when help is limited during pillar-severing operations. b. Folding the roof back exposes the vehicle's entire interior.

Power Tools   Most ambulances do not carry the power tools needed to remove the top of a vehicle. Even when such equipment is carried, it should be used only by trained personnel. Make certain that you and the patient are adequately protected.

An air-operated chisel lends speed and efficiency to top removal operations. However, cutting time is limited by the air supply available. Backup tools (such as hacksaws) should be available for situations when the nature of damage or the number of vehicles calls for a lengthy cutting period.

A common problem with users of air-operated chisels is that when cutting roof pillars, they often bind the chisel fast in the attempt to drive it through the center of the post. Then they continue to supply air to the unit in an effort to remove the chisel. It is not unusual for an entire cylinder of air to be wasted this way.

To prevent binding an air-operated chisel, make peripheral cuts first; cut one side of the pillar first, then the other, and then sever the post by cutting through the middle.

The correct chisel bit for the air-operated chisel must be selected. The regulator must be set so that the proper air pressure is delivered to the tool. This is usually 250 to 300 p.s.i.

The procedure for removing (folding) the top is the same as when hacksaws are used. Remove or break away the windshield. Cut the A-post of one side while someone supports the roof edge, then cut the B-post. Move to the other side and cut the posts while a second person supports the roof there. Make right-angle cuts ahead of the C-posts. Direct the persons supporting the roof to lift while a third person stands on the roof and dimples the metal with his foot. You should be able to make the necessary cuts with a single cylinder of air if you operate the chisel carefully.

In many instances there are not enough people to support and fold the roof in the manner just described. Top removal can be accomplished by two rescuers and a bumper jack, if necessary. After removing the windshield, one rescuer positions the bumper jack in the opening, with the base of the jack on the vehicle's dashboard and the lifting toe under the forward roof edge. While the second rescuer severs the pillars and cuts the roof edges, the first operates the jack a few clicks at a time. This raises the roof enough to prevent binding of the cutting tool. After he finishes cutting, the second rescuer climbs onto the roof and dimples the metal while the first rescuer lifts the roof and folds it back.

Widening Door Openings

Seldom do car or truck doors open a full 90°, or at right angles to the body of the vehicle. Usually doors open to only about 75°; thus it is just about impossible to position a long spine board against the edge of a seat to remove a packaged patient. A door also should be forced past its usual fully-open position when the seat must be pulled backward, as when a person is found on the floor of the vehicle. Various techniques can be used for this task and as in many other situations, the simplest is the fastest.

Without Tools Few vehicle doors can withstand the combined pushing and pulling efforts of three rescuers. If rocking will pose no threat, follow this procedure:

1. Place a shoring block or other chock ahead of the front wheel and behind the rear wheel on the side of the vehicle where you will be working.
2. As you take a position where you can push on the open door, have two helpers position themselves where they can pull. On the count of 3, move the door. Most doors open beyond their usual limit after one or two efforts.
3. If a second push is required, wait until any rocking motion has stopped. Otherwise a rythmic movement may be created that causes the vehicle to ride over the wheel chocks. Be alert for breaking hinges.

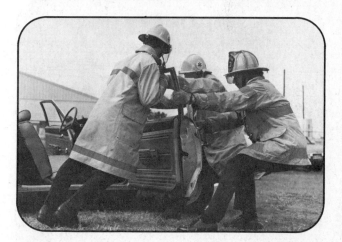

Figure 17-4: Few vehicle doors can withstand the combined pushing and pulling efforts of three rescuers.

Hand Tools The combination of a hand winch and two chains can widen a door opening when rocking is unsafe, or when the door is so badly damaged that manual efforts will not budge it.

Anchor the long chain of a two-chain set to a secure point on the vehicle frame. Using the grab hook, adjust the chain so that the ring rests on the hood just behind the front of the vehicle. Snap the fixed hook of the hand winch over the ring and rest the winch on the hood.

Don't secure the running hook of the hand winch to the door handle, likewise do not secure the hook to the window frame. Neither may be strong enough to withstand the strenuous pull that is often required when a door is severely jammed. Instead, *fasten the short chain around the door to be pulled.* Usually the chain will lay in the lip of the door; if it does there is no need to make an opening for the chain to pass through. In some cases it may be possible to run the chain through the door handle and then around the door so that it is more secure. Snap the running hook of the hand winch over the ring of the short chain.

Operate the handle of the hand winch until the door is pulled the required distance. If the hand winch is not needed for another disentanglement task, leave it in place to prevent the door from closing.

CAUTION: Never use a "cheater" bar on a hand winch during a door pulling or any other lifting or pulling operation. A cheater bar is a length of pipe slipped over the winch handle to lengthen it. Handles of hand winches are designed so that the user can achieve maximum lifting or pulling power. A length of pipe over the handle affords a greater mechanical advantage, but it also causes the device to work beyond its stated capacity. Damage to the winch and injury to the user often result when it is forced to operate beyond its capacity.

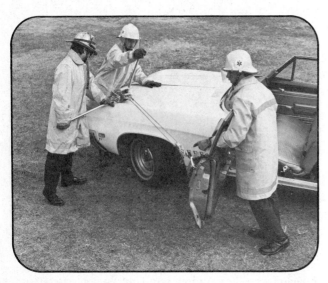

Figure 17-5: Doors that cannot be moved by hand can be pulled open with a hand winch.

Power Tools   The hydraulic jack and ram can be used with appropriate extension bars to widen a door opening. Place the foot of the ram against the door post and the V-block or wedge end of the extension bar against a suitable receptacle or opening that you have made in the door. Have someone support the assembly while you operate the hand pump.

REMOVING WRECKAGE FROM PATIENTS

First efforts should be directed toward removing or displacing items that are in direct contact with the patients.

Cutting Seat Belts

It is highly unlikely that the quick-release buckles of lap and shoulder belts will not work after an accident. If they don't work, cutting the web belt is a simple matter. Use the scissors from your belt kit, or the seat belt cutters or snips provided in the ambulance tool kit.

Be careful! Remember that sudden release from a restraining belt may cause an abdominal injury to bleed freely, or a shoulder injury to become worse.

Removing the Steering Wheel

A head-on collision may cause a manually adjusted seat to move forward on its track, pinning the driver between the seat back and the steering wheel. As the column is moved, the wheel describes an arc. However, the lower part of the wheel moves out before it moves up. As it does, it presses deeply into the patient's abdomen or rib cage. Obviously then the proper maneuver is to remove the steering wheel before attempting to displace the column.

> Before going to the trouble of cutting the steering wheel, try to move the seat backward on its track. Have another person climb onto the front seat and sit in the middle, if possible. As you operate the adjustment lever, have him push backward. Even in serious head-on collisions, the seat adjustment mechanism remains intact and the seat tracks are undamaged. If the seat can be moved back several inches, there may be no need to cut the steering wheel or displace the column.

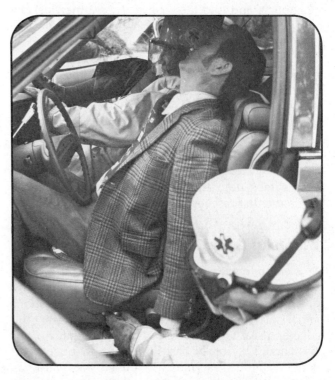

Figure 17-6: Moving a seat backward may eliminate the need for cutting a steering wheel or displacing a steering column.

Electrically operated seats do not usually move forward in a crash because of the rather complex adjustment mechanisms. However, a passenger not restrained by a seat belt may slide forward and become jammed under the steering wheel. If the car's electrical system has not been damaged or disabled, it may be possible to move the seat back by operating the adjustment switch.

If moving the seat in the usual manner is not possible, cut the steering wheel. There are two steps in this operation.

1. First break away the hard plastic covering. This covering may be too thick to accommodate the jaws of a bolt cutter. If a hacksaw is used, the plastic may quickly clog the blade. Use a pair of channel-locking pliers or vise-grip pliers to break away the plastic at points where you can cut the inner core. A simple twisting action usually causes the plastic to break and fall away. Pieces may fly, however, so take a few seconds to protect your patient's eyes and any open wounds.

2. Next cut the inner core. In some cases you may have to cut only the lower half of the wheel away. In other cases, it will be necessary to remove the wheel and the spokes that join it to the column. Whatever action is necessary, carefully support the wheel and protect the driver while you sever the core with a bolt cutter or a hacksaw. Be wary about rotating a bent wheel against the victim's chest or abdomen; it may be safer to reposition the bolt cutter or saw.

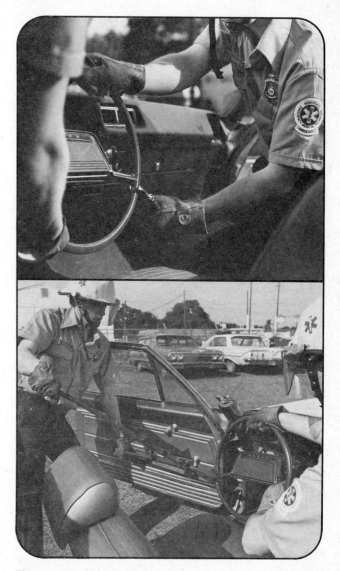

Figure 17-7: a. The core of a steering wheel can be severed more easily when the plastic covering is broken away. b. A bolt cutter expedites removal of a steering wheel.

Displacing the Steering Column

WARNING: Do NOT attempt to displace a steering column with the steering wheel in place.

NOTE: On some of the newer models, particularly with small-size cars, plastic coverings around the steering column and plastic parts of the dashboard may crack and splinter during displacement. Make certain that you and the patient are protected from splinters.

If removing the steering wheel does not provide room for packaging and removing the driver, it will be necessary to displace the steering column upward with either hand or power tools. This can be done either inside or outside the vehicle.

Displacing the Column From Inside the Vehicle

If you can work between or around the driver's legs without injuring them, it may be possible to move the column away from him from inside the vehicle.

Hand Tools An ordinary bumper jack develops sufficient force to move a steering column several inches. Position the jack on two or three shoring blocks that you have laid on the floor. The blocks prevent the jack from being pushed through a corroded area.

If you have a *contour-style jack,* simply place the neck of the curved portion under the column and operate the jack handle.

If yours is a *notch-type jack,* wrap a short chain around the hub of the wheel and the upper portion of the column. Catch the notch of the jack in the ring of the chain. Operate the jack handle until the column is moved the desired distance.

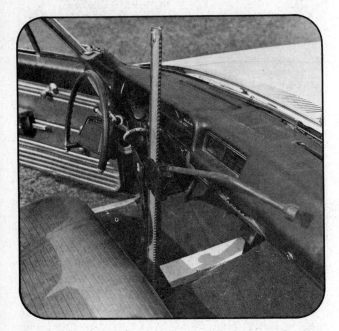

Figure 17-8: Another use for a bumper jack is to displace a steering column from inside the vehicle.

Power Tools   The hydraulic jack and ram can be used to displace a steering column from inside the vehicle when the ram is fitted with appropriate extensions. Since the area of the ram base is considerably less than the base of a bumper jack, it is important that you spread shoring blocks over the floor, especially when the vehicle is an older model.

Displacing the Column From Outside the Vehicle

One of the following techniques can be used when the driver's legs prevent displacement of the steering column from inside. The techniques require removal of the windshield, or at least making a hole through which the winch cable or chain can pass.

Hand Tools   The hand winch can be used with the chain set to displace a steering column from the outside. First secure the slip hook of the long chain to an appropriate anchor point on the frame. Adjust the chain with the grab hook so that the ring rests just behind the front of the hood. Snap the fixed hook of the hand winch over the chain ring. Rest the winch on the hood.

Wrap the short chain around the hub and upper portion of the column. The ring must be close to the column and accessible.

If the windshield has been removed, lay two shoring blocks in line with the steering column, railroad track style. Lay another block across the two at a right angle. When the winch is being operated, the cable or chain will ride over the upper block and the

upper block will slide on the two lower blocks. The blocks cause the cable or chain to pull at a more efficient angle; they also prevent the cable or chain from "biting" into the soft dash.

Lay one or two shoring blocks under the winch itself to prevent the hood from collapsing when the cable or chain is under tension.

Connect the running hook of the hand winch to the ring of the chain that is around the column.

Operate the winch handle until the column is displaced the desired distance.

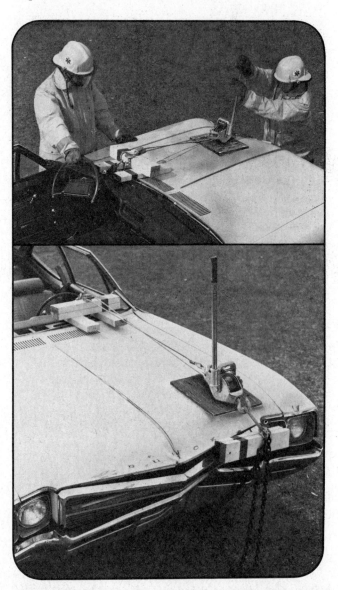

Figure 17-9: The arrangement of hand winch, chains, and shoring blocks facilitates displacing a steering column from outside the vehicle.

Displacing Floor Pedals

Brake and clutch pedals sometimes hold a driver's foot firmly against the floor of a wrecked vehicle. This usually occurs in head-on crashes when the foot is directly under the pedal. Hand and power tools can be used to displace pedals.

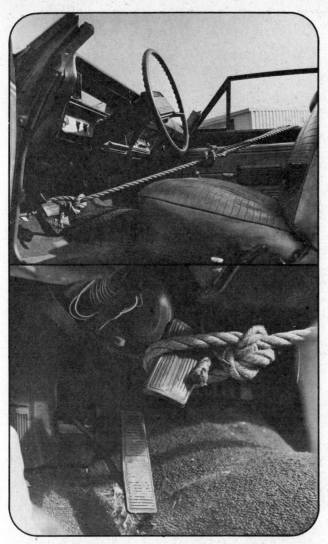

Figure 17-10: a. A length of rope may be all that is needed to displace a brake or clutch pedal. b. Two rescuers can pull back on the door to raise the pedal.

Hand Tools   A floor pedal can be displaced by a simple procedure done with a length of rope.

Form a loop in the end of a length of half-inch rope. A small bowline will do. Slip the loop over the pedal to be moved, and extend the end of the rope to the door of the side of the vehicle toward which the pedal must be pulled. Hold the door open a few inches and form a loop in the rope about three feet from the door.

If the door has a window frame, wrap the doubled rope a few times around the frame close to the door body. Keep the rope between the pedal and the door taut as you do this.

If the door has no window frame, pass the doubled rope through the door handle, or wrap it a few times around the door itself.

Hold the rope in place and with someone else helping you, pull sharply on the door. The rope will move with the door, and the pedal with the rope.

Another EMT or rescuer should protect the patient's foot at all times during a pedal-displacing operation, and those rescuers on the rope should not pull until they are assured that it is safe to do so. If a door cannot be used as a lever, pedal displacement can be accomplished by two rescuers pulling sharply on the rope.

Displacing the Dash

One of the more difficult tasks for EMTs working with hand tools is displacing a crushed dash. Even rescue squad personnel with special power tools have trouble moving dashboards when victims are flush or nearly flush against the crumpled metal. You can move a dash with limited equipment at hand and a little patience.

NOTE: Dashboard displacement can be very difficult to accomplish on some small models. The plastic materials of the dash may crush, break and splinter, or crack.

Hand Tools   A hand winch can often be used to move a crushed dash. Rig the winch in the manner suggested for displacing a steering column. Although finding a suitable place to secure the hook may be a problem, you may be able to work a small pry bar behind the crushed parts of the dash to provide an anchor point for the chain or cable hook.

Displacing Seats

In some accident situations the driver or passenger is found on the floor of the vehicle, ahead of the seat. With the seat in place it may be impossible to move him without aggravating a spinal injury or worsening fractures. Even when there are no such injuries, it will be difficult to remove the patient without first moving the seat.

Stabilizing the patient in place is the first requirement. This can be done by two helpers carefully supporting him, or by placing a long spine board between the patient and the seat and having the helpers hold it in place.

Hand Tools   A hand winch and chain set can be used to pull a seat back. Rig an anchor chain to a frame member as you would in preparation for displacing a steering column or widening a door opening, except that the hand winch is positioned on the trunk deck. The rear window of the vehicle will have to be removed or broken away. Adjust the chain so that the ring rests on the trunk lid. Snap the fixed hook of the hand winch over the ring.

Run the winch chain or cable through the rear window opening, and snap the hook over the ring of the short chain that has been wrapped around the lower seat near either side.

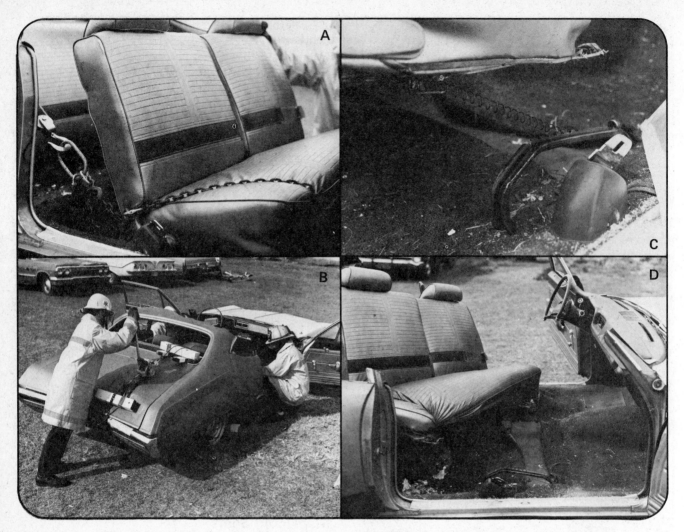

Figure 17-11: a. The chain is placed so that the seat may be pulled freely on its track. b. A hand winch may be used to pull the seat back. c. To prevent injury, care should be given to cut the seat adjusting spring. d. When the seat has been pulled back completely, there is sufficient space to render emergency care.

Position shoring blocks under the winch and at any point where the cable or chain may snag.

While another EMT or rescuer depresses the seat adjustment mechanism, operate the winch handle until the seat breaks free. If necessary, repeat the operation on the other side of the seat, thus freeing the seat altogether.

CAUTION: As a manually-operated seat moves back, a spring will come into view. This is part of the seat adjustment mechanism. It should be cut as soon as it becomes visible so that it does not break loose.

Power Tools   A hydraulic jack can be used to remove a seat from its supports one side at a time. Place the foot of the ram against the door frame and the wedge or V-block end of the unit against the seat support. If no accessory ram is available, attempt to force the seat upward and off its support with the wedge or spreader. Know that this technique may not be successful, however, because of the limited force available with the spreading appliances. An air-operated chisel can be used to cut the seat support or to cut the seat bolts from underneath.

SUMMARY

Disentanglement involves altering and removing wreckage so that appropriate care can be rendered, the patient can be made ready for transfer to the ambulance, and the patient can be moved for transfer. The activities of disentanglement involve making a pathway in the wreckage and removing wreckage.

Remember that the major duties of an EMT at an accident are patient assessment and care. Call for the help you will need to disentangle a patient. Do only what you have been trained to do in disentanglement operations.

Personal safety of the rescue workers and the patient is the prime concern during disentanglement. Take special care to guard the patient's eyes and to assure adequate ventilation.

Making a pathway through the wreckage can be done by raising the vehicle's roof, removing or folding back the top of the vehicle, or by widening door openings.

A jack or a hydraulic jack and spreader can be used to raise a roof. The operation should begin with that portion of the roof directly behind the A-posts. Once raised, the top of a vehicle can be folded back or removed by cutting through the roof pillars using a hacksaw. Cut the A-posts and the B-posts, but not the C-posts. Right angle cut the roof just ahead of the C-posts so that the roof can be folded back. An air-operated chisel can be used for roof removal.

It is possible to widen door openings without tools. The door of a properly shored vehicle can be opened and then widened by the combined pushing and pulling efforts of three rescuers. A hand winch and two chains can be used to pull the door beyond its normal open position. The short chain must be fastened around the door, not to the handle or window frame. The hydraulic jack and ram, with extension bars, can be used to widen door openings.

Removing wreckage from the patient may involve cutting seat belts, removing the steering wheel, displacing the steering column, displacing floor pedals, displacing the dashboard, and displacing seats.

Before cutting a steering wheel, carefully try to move the seat backward on its track. If this fails, break away the plastic covering of the steering wheel using channel-locking or vise-grip pliers. Cut away the inner core with a bolt cutter or hacksaw.

Never attempt to displace a steering column without first cutting away the steering wheel. A bumper jack or a hydraulic jack and ram can be used to displace the column from inside the vehicle. From outside the vehicle, use a hand winch.

One end of a rope can be tied around a floor pedal and the other end secured to the door on the side of the vehicle to which the pedal must be pulled. Two rescuers can pull back on the door to raise the pedal.

Displacing a dashboard is a very difficult, time-consuming task. This can be done with a winch using the same basic procedure as used for displacing a steering column.

A seat can be displaced using a hand winch set on the deck of the trunk. The seat is pulled backward. A hydraulic jack and ram can be used to remove the seat from its supports one side at a time. An air-operated chisel can be used to cut seat supports or seat bolts.

18 *moving and transferring patients*

OBJECTIVES By the end of this chapter, you should be able to:

1. Define ''emergency move,'' ''nonemergency move,'' and ''transfer.'' (p. 404)

2. Give THREE reasons why you may have to perform an emergency move. (p. 404)

3. Give FOUR reasons why you may have to perform a nonemergency move and state the SIX rules that must be followed if a nonemergency move is to be performed. (p. 404)

4. Describe the one-rescuer assist, the piggyback carry, the cradle carry, the pack strap carry, and the fireman's carry. (p. 406)

5. Describe the two-rescuer assist, the extremity carry, and the three-rescuer carry. (p. 407)

6. Describe the shoulder drag, the foot drag, the clothes drag, the incline drag, the fireman's drag, and the blanket drag, and state which of these is the superior method of moving a patient. (p. 408)

7. List at least SIX patient-carrying devices and give an example of when you would use each device. (p. 405, 9)

8. Define ''packaging.'' (p. 409)

9. Describe how to use a wheeled ambulance stretcher, stating how to prepare the device, move the patient (bed- and ground-level), cover and secure the patient, and transfer and load the patient. (p. 411-4)

10. Describe how to use a stair chair. (p. 411, 6)

11. Describe when and how to use a scoop-style stretcher. (p. 416-8)

12. Describe the three-rescuer lift and the blanket lift in relation to moving a patient into a basket stretcher. (p. 418-9)

13. Describe, step by step, how to secure a patient to a short spine board and remove him from a vehicle. (p. 421-4)

14. Describe how to apply a Kendrick extrication device. (p. 422, 5)

15. In addition to the log-roll, list FOUR methods of placing a patient on a long spine board, indicating when each method may be used. (p. 425-7)

SKILLS As an EMT you should be able to:

1. Decide when an emergency or nonemergency move is necessary.

2. Carry out one-, two-, and three-rescuer moves.

3. Package patients for transfer and transport.

4. Use the wheeled ambulance stretcher to transfer patients.

5. Use the stair chair, scoop-style stretcher, and basket stretcher to transfer patients.

6. Apply a short spine board to a patient found in a vehicle or confined space and move the patient to a long spine board.

7. Move a patient to a long spine board by the four-rescuer straddle slide and a rope sling.

8. Move a patient to a long spine board when he is found under the dashboard or between the front and rear seat of an automobile.

TERMS you may be using for the first time: **Transfer**—the orderly moving of a patient to the ambulance for transport.

Packaging—the orderly sequence of operations used to ready a patient for a move and to secure the patient to a patient-moving device for transfer.

BASIC PRINCIPLES OF MOVING PATIENTS

There are three types of moves used at the emergency scene. Dangers at the scene may require you to move a patient quickly, perhaps prior to assessment and care. This type of move is an **emergency move.** There are also **nonemergency moves,** like the moving of a patient to a cooler environment when he has apparent heat cramps. The third move is when you take the patient from the scene to the ambulance for transport. This type of move is called a **transfer.**

EMERGENCY AND NONEMERGENCY MOVES

When To Move A Patient

There are times when you must move a patient quickly, using an emergency move. This type of move may have to take place before assessment can begin or be completed. The patient may need basic life support, wound care, or splinting of fractures; however, the move must still be made without delay. An emergency move should take place when:

- *The scene is hazardous*—Hazards may make it necessary to move a patient quickly in order to protect both you and the patient. This may occur when the emergency scene involves uncontrolled traffic, fire or threat of fire, possible explosions, possible electrical hazards, toxic gases, or radiation.

- *Care requires repositioning*—You may have to move a patient to a hard, flat surface to provide CPR, or you may have to move a patient to reach life-threatening bleeding.

- *You must gain access to other patients*—You may have to quickly move an assessed patient with minor problems to reach a patient who needs life-saving care. This is seen most often in motor vehicle accidents.

It may become necessary to perform a nonemergency move of a patient. Such a move may be called for when:

- *Factors at the scene cause patient decline*—If a patient is RAPIDLY declining due to heat or cold, he may have to be moved. Should the patient appear to be allergic to something at the scene, he may have to be moved to reduce the chances of developing anaphylactic shock.

- *You must reach other patients*—When there are other assessed patients at the scene requiring care for life-threatening problems, you may have to move another patient to have the space needed to provide care. The patient being moved may need certain care procedures to avoid additional pain and injury before being moved.

- *Care requires moving the patient*—This is usually seen in cases where there are no injuries or severe medical problems. Problems due to extreme heat or cold (heat cramps, heat exhaustion, hypothermia, and frostbite) are good examples.

- *The patient insists on being moved*—You are not allowed to restrain a patient. Explain to the patient why he should not move or be moved. If he tries to move himself, you may have to assist him. A patient may become so insistent that stress worsens his condition. If this type of patient can be moved, and the move is a short one, you may have to move him in order to reduce the stress and provide care.

Nonemergency moves should be carried out in such a way as to prevent additional injury to the patient and to avoid discomfort and pain. The following rules are to be followed for a nonemergency move:

1. The patient should be conscious.
2. The patient assessment should be completed.
3. All vital signs should be within normal range and stable.
4. There should be no serious bleeding or wounds.
5. There must be ABSOLUTELY no signs of spinal injury, no injuries associated with spinal injury, and the mechanism of injury should not indicate any chances of such an injury.
6. All fractures must be immobilized or splinted.

Types of Moves

None of these moves protects the patient's spine or provides adequate protection for unsplinted fractures. In an emergency move, you will have to use the most efficient method for the amount of time you have to move the patient. The most commonly used moves include:

- *One-Rescuer Moves*

  One-Rescuer Assist—patient is conscious and can walk with assistance.

  Piggyback Carry—patient is conscious, can stand, and has no fractures of the extremities.

  Cradle Carry—patient may be conscious or unconscious.

  Fireman's Carry—conscious or unconscious patient with no fractures of the extremities.

  Pack Strap Carry—this does not require any equipment. Use on the conscious patient with no fractures of the extremities.

  One-Rescuer Drags—conscious or unconscious patient with no fractures of the body part being held during the drag.

- *Two-Rescuer Moves*

  Two-Rescuer Assist—patient is conscious and can walk with assistance.

  Extremity Carry—conscious or unconscious patient with no fractures of the extremities.

  Fireman's Carry with Assist—conscious or unconscious patient with no fractures of the extremities.

- *Three-Rescuer Move*

  Three-Rescuer Carry—conscious or unconscious patient, free of fractures of the extremities.

The most common emergency moves are presented in Scansheets 18-1 through 18-3. All of these can be used for nonemergency moves, depending on the situation. If the rules for a nonemergency move are met, the one- or two-rescuer assist should be practical to use. A cradle carry or two-rescuer extremity carry may be useful in some cases.

TRANSFERRING THE PATIENT

Usually the transfer of a sick or injured patient involves little more than placing the patient on the wheeled ambulance stretcher and moving it a short distance to the ambulance. The process becomes more complicated when you believe the patient may have spinal injuries. For such cases, extrication collars and spine boards become part of the process. If a traction splint has been applied to a patient, special care must be taken to assure that the splint will continue to immobilize the extremity and no additional injury occurs to the patient.

Transfer to the ambulance is accomplished in four steps, regardless of the complexity of the operation. The steps include:

1. Selecting the proper patient-carrying device.
2. Packaging the patient for transfer.
3. Moving the patient to the ambulance.
4. Loading the patient onto the ambulance.

PATIENT-CARRYING DEVICES

Commonly used patient-carrying devices include:

- Wheeled Ambulance Stretchers (Cots)—existing as two- and multi-level devices with a number of options. Most have adjustable head rests. Some also allow for the patient's feet to be elevated (*Trendelenburg* position) for cases of shock. The patient can be secured to the device and then wheeled or carried.

- Portable Stretchers—these devices may or may not have wheels. They are made of folding U-frames and a canvas or vinyl nylon coated fabric body. Most have foldaway legs and wheels that fit into receptacles in the ambulance floor.

- Collapsible Stretchers (Stair Chairs)—a folding chair with safety straps. Most models have two rear leg wheels. Stair chairs are useful when transferring a patient down stairs or through narrow spaces. These devices are not recommended for use with unconscious or disoriented patients.

- Spine Boards—existing as long and short boards used to help immobilize possible spinal injury patients. If a short spine board is used, the patient and the short board also must be secured to a long spine board. There are modifications of the short board, including short boards for bucket seats, and newer devices meant to replace the short spine board in certain situations, including the Kendrick extrication device (K.E.D.).

- Scoop-Style (Orthopedic) Stretchers—devices for picking up seriously injured patients with a minimum of body movement. To use this type of stretcher effectively, you must have access to the patient from all sides.

- Basket (Stokes) Stretchers—wire and plastic devices generally used to move patients from high places by ladder or rope, or to move patients up or down a hill, or over debris and obstacles. The typical basket stretcher has four-point suspension bridles, patient-security straps, and an adjustable footrest (providing additional security for vertical moves).

- Pole Stretchers—the least-used patient-carrying devices, made up of two poles and a fabric body.

EMERGENCY MOVES-ONE RESCUER

THE ONE RESCUER ASSIST

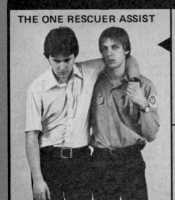

PLACE PT'S ARM AROUND YOUR NECK, GRASPING HIS HAND IN YOURS. PLACE YOUR OTHER ARM AROUND PT'S WAIST. HELP PT WALK TO SAFETY. BE PREPARED TO CHANGE MOVEMENT TECHNIQUE IF LEVEL OF DANGER INCREASES.

PLACE ONE ARM ACROSS PT'S BACK WITH YOUR HAND UNDER HIS FAR ARM. PLACE YOUR OTHER ARM UNDER HIS KNEES AND LIFT. IF PT IS CONSCIOUS, HAVE HIM PLACE HIS NEAR ARM OVER YOUR SHOULDER.

THE CRADLE CARRY

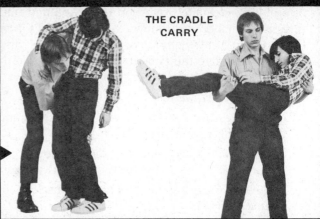

THE PIGGY BACK CARRY

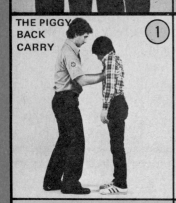

(1) ASSIST THE PT TO STAND

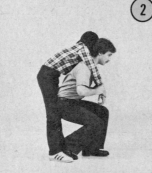

(2) PLACE HIS ARMS OVER YOUR SHOULDER SO THEY CROSS YOUR CHEST. BEND OVER AND LIFT PATIENT.

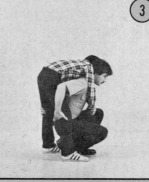

(3) WHILE HE HOLDS ON WITH HIS ARMS, CROUCH AND GRASP EACH THIGH. USE A LIFTING MOTION TO MOVE HIM ONTO YOUR BACK.

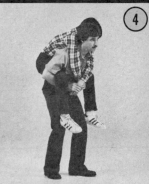

(4) PASS YOUR FOREARMS UNDER HIS KNEES AND GRASP HIS WRISTS.

THE PACK STRAP CARRY

HAVE PT STAND — TURN YOUR BACK TO HIM, BRINGING HIS ARMS OVER YOUR SHOULDERS TO CROSS YOUR CHEST. KEEP HIS ARMS STRAIGHT AS POSSIBLE, HIS ARMPITS OVER YOUR SHOULDERS. HOLD PT'S WRISTS, BEND, AND PULL HIM ONTO YOUR BACK.

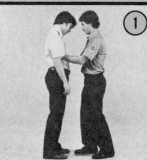

(1)

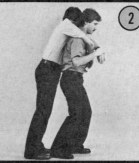

(2)

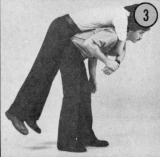

(3)

THE FIREMAN'S CARRY

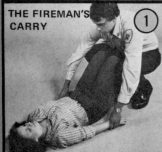

(1) WHEN POSSIBLE, HAVE PT BEND HIS KNEES. STEP CLOSE TO PT — GRASP WRISTS.

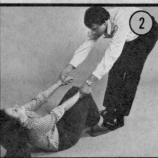

(2) PLACE YOUR FEET AGAINST HIS FEET AND PULL PT TOWARD YOU. BEND AT WAIST AND FLEX KNEES.

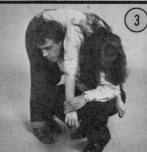

(3) DUCK & PULL HIM ACROSS YOUR SHOULDER, KEEPING HOLD OF ONE OF HIS WRISTS. USE YOUR FREE ARM TO REACH BETWEEN HIS LEGS AND GRASP THIGH.

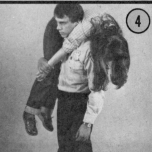

(4) WEIGHT OF PT FALLS ONTO YOUR SHOULDERS. STAND UP. TRANSFER YOUR GRIP ON THIGH TO PT'S WRIST.

SCAN 18-1

EMERGENCY MOVES-ONE RESCUER DRAGS

CAUTION: ALWAYS PULL IN DIRECTION OF LONG AXIS OF PATIENT'S BODY. DO NOT PULL PATIENT SIDEWAYS. AVOID BENDING OR TWISTING THE TRUNK IF AT ALL POSSIBLE

THE SHOULDER DRAG
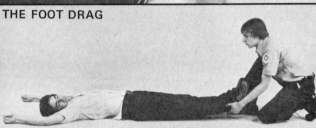

THE CLOTHES DRAG
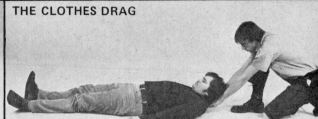

THE FOOT DRAG
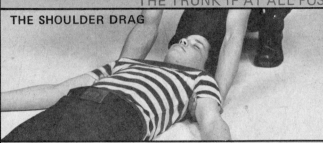

THE INCLINE DRAG. . . ALWAYS HEAD FIRST
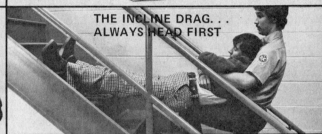

THE FIREMAN'S DRAG

PLACE PT ON HIS BACK AND TIE HANDS TOGETHER WITH SOMETHING THAT WILL NOT CUT INTO HIS SKIN. STRADDLE THE PATIENT, FACING HIS HEAD CROUCH, PASSING YOUR HEAD THRU HIS TRUSSED ARMS AND RAISE YOUR BODY. THIS WILL IN TURN RAISE PATIENT'S HEAD, NECK, AND UPPER TRUNK CRAWL ON YOUR HANDS AND KNEES, DRAGGING THE PERSON.

①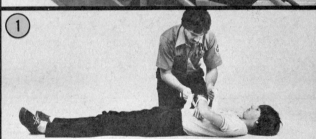

②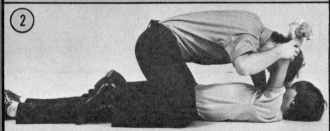

③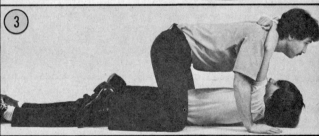

① **THE BLANKET DRAG** GATHER HALF OF THE BLANKET MATERIAL UP AGAINST PT'S SIDE
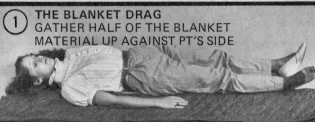

② ROLL THE PATIENT TOWARD YOUR KNEES SO THAT YOU CAN PLACE THE BLANKET UNDER HIM
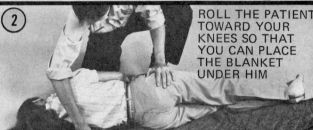

③ GENTLY ROLL THE PATIENT BACK ONTO THE BLANKET
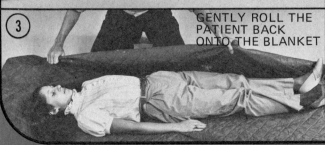

④ DURING THE DRAG, KEEP THE PT'S HEAD AS LOW AS POSSIBLE
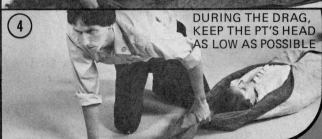

SCAN 18-2

EMERGENCY MOVES-2 & 3 RESCUER

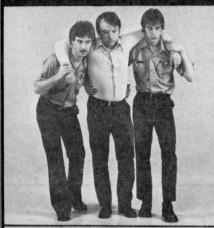

TWO-RESCUER ASSIST. PT'S ARMS ARE PLACED AROUND SHOULDERS OF BOTH RESCUERS. THEY EACH GRIP A HAND, THEN PLACE THEIR FREE ARMS AROUND PT'S WAIST. HELP HIM WALK TO SAFETY.

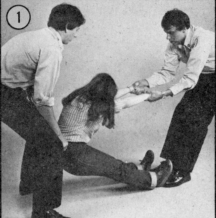

FIREMAN'S CARRY WITH ASSISTANCE HAVE SOMEONE HELP LIFT PATIENT.

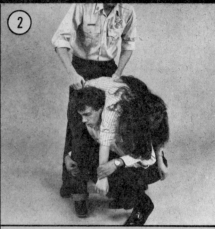

THE SECOND RESCUER HELPS TO POSITION THE PATIENT.

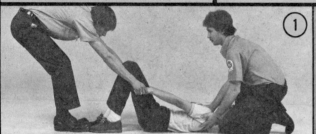

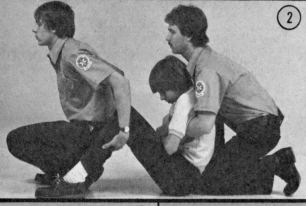

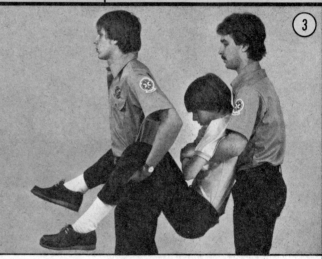

THE TWO-RESCUER EXTREMITY CARRY. PLACE PT ON BACK, WITH KNEES FLEXED. KNEEL AT PT'S HEAD — PLACE YOUR HANDS UNDER HIS SHOULDERS. HELPER STANDS AT PT'S FEET AND GRASPS HIS WRISTS. HELPER LIFTS PT FORWARD WHILE YOU SLIP YOUR ARMS UNDER PT'S ARMPITS AND GRASP HIS WRIST. HELPER CAN TURN, CROUCH DOWN AND GRASP PT'S KNEES. DIRECT HELPER SO YOU BOTH STAND AT THE SAME TIME AND MOVE AS A UNIT WHEN CARRYING PT.

THE THREE-RESCUER CARRY

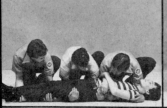

KNEEL ON KNEE TOWARDS PT'S FEET — ARM POSITIONS: NECK & UPPER BACK, WAIST & HIPS, KNEES & ANKLES.

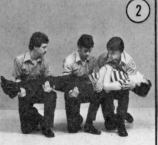

THE HEAD-END RESCUER DIRECTS ALL RESCUERS TO LIFT PT TO THEIR KNEES.

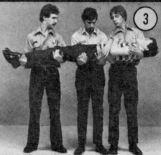

THE HEAD-END RESCUER DIRECTS ALL RESCUERS TO MOVE TO A STANDING POSITION.

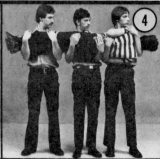

ON ANOTHER SIGNAL, ALL RESCUERS ROLL PT TO THEIR CHESTS. MOVEMENT OF PT CAN TAKE PLACE BY RESCUERS WALKING FORWARD OR SIDESTEPPING

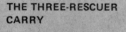

be used to transfer a patient with no spinal injury. The choice of device often depends on the pathway from the patient to the ambulance. For example:

- *Unrestricted movement*—the wheeled ambulance stretcher.
- *Confined or narrow spaces*—the folding ambulance stretcher, the folding stair chair, long spine board (must have footrest if moving patient over stairs).
- *High place; no stairs or elevator*—the basket stretcher, pole stretcher (rarely used).
- *Obstacles and inclines*—the basket stretcher.

Selecting the Proper Carrying Device—Possible Spinal Injury

When the patient has a possible spinal injury, the patient-carrying device selected must provide rigid, straight-line neck and back immobilization. Selection of the device may depend on the position of the patient, or how the patient will have to be moved. For example:

- Patient on the ground or floor—scoop-style stretcher or a long spine board. Once immobilized on either of these devices, the patient can be placed on a wheeled or folding ambulance stretcher.
- Patient supine in a vehicle—long spine board. The scoop-style stretcher can be used if the seats are removed.
- Patient seated in vehicle—short spine board or similar device (e.g., K.E.D.) is used to immobilize the patient before he is removed from the vehicle. The patient and short board must then be secured to a long spine board. The patient and boards are then moved as a unit onto the wheeled or folding ambulance stretcher, or placed into a basket stretcher. It is possible to carry the patient and boards as a unit to the ambulance.
- Transfer from high place—the long spine board is used to immobilize the patient and both are placed as a unit into a modified basket stretcher.

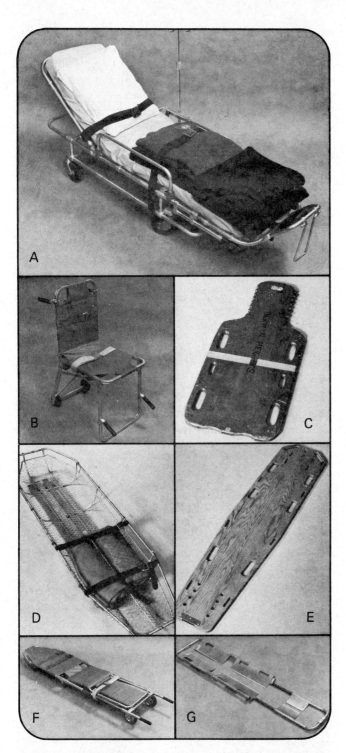

Figure 18-1: Patient carrying devices; A. wheeled, B. folding stair chair, C. short spine board, D. basket, E. long spine board, F. folding, G. scoop.

The well-equipped ambulance carries a wheeled ambulance stretcher, spine boards, and other patient-carrying devices as space permits. A folding ambulance stretcher, a collapsible stretcher, and a scoop-style stretcher are commonly carried.

Selecting the Proper Carrying Device—No Spinal Injury

Almost any of the patient-carrying devices can

PACKAGING THE PATIENT

Packaging refers to the sequence of operations required to ready the patient to be moved and to combine the patient and the patient-carrying device into a unit ready for transfer. A sick or injured patient must be packaged so that his condition is not aggravated. Necessary care for wounds and fractures should be completed. Impaled objects must be stabilized. All dressings and splints must be checked before the patient is placed on the patient-carrying device. The properly packaged patient is covered and secured to the patient-carrying device.

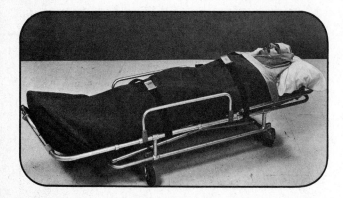

Figure 18-2: The patient properly positioned, covered, and secured.

Covering the Patient

Covering a patient helps to maintain body temperature, prevents exposure to the elements, and helps assure privacy. A single blanket or perhaps just a sheet may be all that is required in warm weather. A sheet and blankets should be used in cold weather. When practical, cuff the blankets under the patient's chin, with the top sheet outside. Do not leave sheets and blankets hanging loose. Tuck them under the mattress at the foot and sides of the stretcher. In wet weather, a plastic cover should be placed over the blankets during transfer. This can be removed once in the ambulance to prevent the patient from overheating.

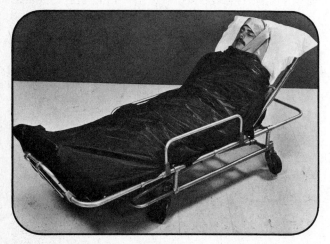

Figure 18-3: A plastic cover prevents blankets from becoming soaked in wet weather.

If a scoop-style stretcher is used, you will have to fold a blanket once or twice lengthwise and carefully tuck the blanket under the patient. Do NOT move a patient with possible spinal injury in order to tuck in a blanket. Cover the patient as best you can, place the patient and scoop-style stretcher on a wheeled ambulance stretcher, and then apply full covering. The same directions apply when using the long spine board.

When a basket stretcher is used, line the basket with a blanket prior to positioning the patient. If this is not done, cover the patient as you would in the case of the scoop-style stretcher.

A patient being transferred on a stair chair should be covered. Have the patient sitting upright with his hands folded over his lap and his legs together. Drape a sheet and then a blanket over the patient's body and shoulders. Carefully tuck in the sheet and blanket all around.

In cold or wet weather cover the patient's head, leaving the face exposed. If the nature of the patient's injuries allow you to do so:

1. Place a towel flat under the patient's head.
2. Pull the outermost edge of the towel up and over the patient's head so that it covers the forehead, but not the eyes.
3. Draw the corners of the towel diagonally to the patient's chest, allowing the towel to drape each side of the patient's head.

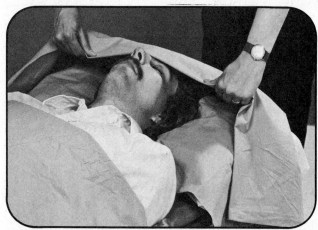

Figure 18-4a: The edge of the towel is laid over the patient's forehead.

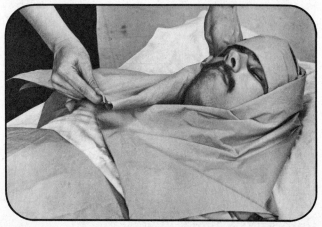

Figure 18-4b: The top corners of the towel are drawn diagonally to the patient's chest.

Securing the Patient

All patients, including those receiving CPR, must be secured to the patient-carrying device. This is typically done by fastening body straps. If the device has side rails, as in the case of the wheeled ambulance stretcher, the rails should be locked in place before securing the straps.

THE WHEELED AMBULANCE STRETCHER

This is the most commonly used patient-carrying device. The principles of transfer that apply to this device also apply in general to all others.

Preparing the Stretcher

Elevate the stretcher to bed-level if it is a two-level or multi-level device. Unfasten the safety straps; tuck them under the mattress or otherwise make sure they do not become tripping hazards. Lower the rail on the loading side of the stretcher. Remove the blankets and the top sheet; place them on a clean surface nearby. Place the pillow in the appropriate position.

Transferring the Patient

In some cases, a patient may stand and help place himself on the stretcher. When the patient with *no* spinal injury is in a vehicle, wreckage, or debris, you may have to adapt a standard patient moving technique to transfer him to the stretcher. An example would be to modify the cradle carry for someone seated and turned sideways in the front of an automobile. The patient *with* spinal injury should be secured to a long spine board before being transferred to the stretcher. The long board and the secured patient are lifted as a unit and secured to the wheeled ambulance stretcher.

The transfer of a bed-level or ground-level patient may require you to use special lifting techniques. There are three techniques commonly used to transfer the bed-level patient to a wheeled ambulance stretcher: **the direct carry method, the draw sheet method,** and **the slide transfer method.** For the transfer of a ground-level patient, a **modified direct carry method** is used. These methods are shown on Scansheet 18-4A and 18-4B. Regardless of the method used, protect yourself. Do not position yourself too far from the patient and do not strain to lift the patient. You must protect yourself from lower back strain and hernia. Also, you must be certain not to lose your balance and possibly injure yourself, your partner, or the patient.

Covering and Securing the Patient

As noted earlier, all patients should be covered and secured to the patient-carrying device. A top sheet and blankets, as required by weather, are to be applied over the patient's body. The side rails should be locked in the up position and the body straps should be fastened.

Moving and Loading the Patient

Regardless of the method used to move a patient, you and your partner should walk naturally at a smooth, fairly slow pace.

Use the pull handles to roll and maneuver the stretcher. Roll the stretcher at a safe, constant speed. Turn corners slowly and squarely to minimize discomfort to the patient. Lift the stretcher over thresholds and rugs. Use caution when maneuvering the stretcher; bumps from a wheeled stretcher can cause unsightly and costly damage to walls and furniture. Roll the stretcher to within three feet of the ambulance loading door.

The wheeled stretcher can be carried by the end carry method or the side carry method. The **end carry** is most widely used, with the **side carry** used to load the patient into the ambulance. The techniques of carrying and loading a patient secured to a wheeled ambulance stretcher are shown in Scansheet 18-5.

FOLDING STAIR CHAIRS

These devices are useful for narrow corridors, narrow doorways, small elevators, and for taking a patient up or down stairs. *They should not be used for patients who are unconscious or disoriented. They should not be used when a patient has a possible spinal injury or fractures of the lower extremities.* When a folding stair chair is not available, a strongly constructed desk chair may be used to move the patient.

Preparing a Stair Chair

The chair is unfolded and secured by positive locking devices (not on all chairs). The safety straps are unfastened and positioned so that they do not become tripping hazards. Sheets and blankets should not be draped over the chair prior to positioning the patient.

Transferring the Patient

The direct carry method can be modified when a bed-level patient must be moved into a stair chair. The first part of the technique is the same as for transfer of a patient to a wheeled stretcher. When it is time to move the patient from the bed, however, the foot-end EMT slides his arm under the patient's thighs rather than under the midcalf. This maneuver allows the lower part of the patient's legs to drop down into a sitting position as he is eased into the chair.

WHEELED AMBULANCE STRETCHERS-
Transferring the patient

THE BED-LEVEL PATIENT: DIRECT CARRY METHOD

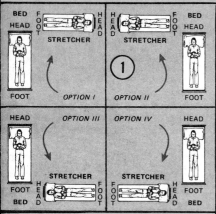

STRETCHER IS PLACED AT 90° ANGLE TO BED, DEPENDING ON ROOM CONFIGURATION.

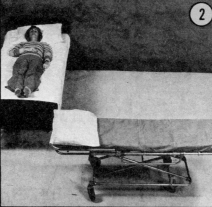

THE PT SHOULD BE SUPINE. WHEN POSSIBLE, THE HANDS SHOULD BE FOLDED ON CHEST & LEGS HELD STRAIGHT TOGETHER.

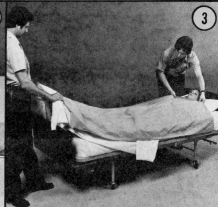

THE AMBULANCE STRETCHER TOP SHEET IS PLACED OVER PT AND ANY BED COVERING IS REMOVED FROM UNDER THIS TOP SHEET.

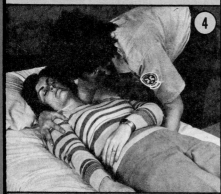

THE HEAD-END EMT CRADLES PT'S HEAD & NECK BY SLIDING ONE ARM UNDER PT'S NECK TO GRASP SHOULDER.

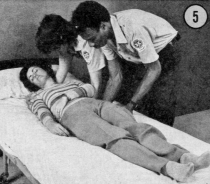

FOOT-END EMT SLIDES HIS HAND CLOSEST TO PT'S FEET UNDER PT'S HIP AND LIFTS SLIGHTLY. HE THEN SLIDES HIS OTHER ARM UNDER PT'S SACRUM. THE HEAD-END EMT CAN NOW SLIDE HIS FREE ARM UNDER SMALL OF PT'S BACK.

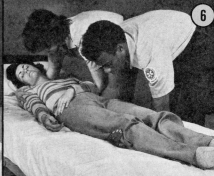

FOOT-END EMT MOVES HIS HAND FROM PT'S HIP TO A POSITION UNDER PT'S KNEES.

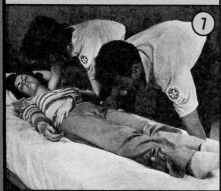

FOOT-END EMT MOVES HIS ARM FROM UNDER PT'S KNEES TO A POSITION UNDER MID-CALF AREAS.

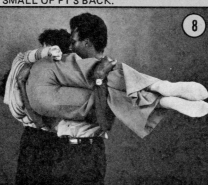

EMTS SLIDE PT TO EDGE OF BED & BEND TOWARD HIM WITH THEIR KNEES SLIGHTLY BENT. THEY CURL PT TO THEIR CHESTS & RETURN TO A STANDING POSITION. THE PT IS LIFTED, CRADLED IN THEIR ARMS.

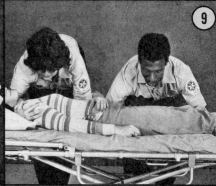

EMTS EACH TAKE A STEP BACKWARD, TURN WITH PT, AND WALK SLOWLY TO STRETCHER. THEY EACH PLACE ONE FOOT AGAINST A WHEEL, FLEX AT KNEES, AND GENTLY LOWER PATIENT TO THE MATTRESS.

NOTE: IF WHEELED STRETCHER IS A SINGLE-LEVEL UNIT, EMTS WILL HAVE TO STOP ONE STEP FROM STRETCHER, STEP FORWARD WITH LEFT FOOT & BEND RIGHT KNEE TO THE FLOOR. EACH EMT SHOULD SWING HIS LEFT KNEE TO A POSITION OUTSIDE HIS LEFT ARM. BOTH EMTS CAN NOW ROLL FORWARD AND PLACE PT GENTLY ONTO MATTRESS

SCAN 18-4A

WHEELED AMBULANCE STRETCHERS-
Transferring the patient(cont'd)

BED-LEVEL PATIENT: DRAW SHEET METHOD

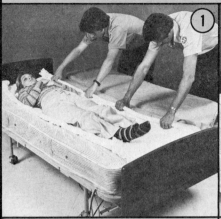

BOTTOM SHEET OF BED IS ROLLED FROM BOTH SIDES OF BED TOWARD PT. THE STRETCHER, WITH ITS RAILS LOWERED, IS PLACED PARALLEL TO BED, TOUCHING SIDE OF BED.

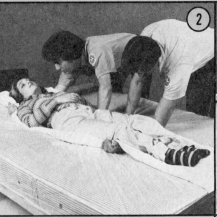

EMTS PULL ON DRAW SHEET TO MOVE PT TO SIDE OF BED. THEY EACH USE ONE HAND TO SUPPORT PT WHILE THEY REACH UNDER HIM TO GRASP DRAW SHEET.

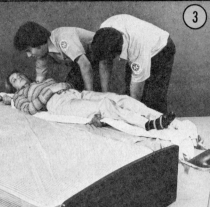

EMTS SIMULTANEOUSLY DRAW PT ONTO STRETCHER.

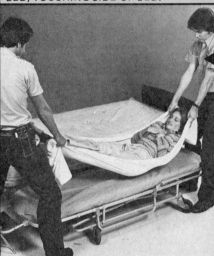

HAMMOCK-STYLE MOVE. WHEN WHEELED STRETCHER IS A SINGLE-LEVEL MODEL, IT IS NECESSARY THAT EACH EMT FORM A "HANDLE" FROM ROLLED SHEET ON EACH SIDE OF PT AND THEN LOWER PT HAMMOCK-STYLE ONTO STRETCHER.

THE SLIDE TRANSFER METHOD. THIS IS A VARIATION OF DRAW SHEET METHOD. HEAD-END EMT SUPPORTS PT'S HEAD & NECK WITH ONE ARM & PT'S WAIST WITH HIS OTHER ARM. FOOT-END EMT SUPPORTS PT ABOVE & BELOW BUTTOCKS. EMTS SLIDE PT ONTO STRETCHER WITH AN UPWARD DRAWING MOTION.

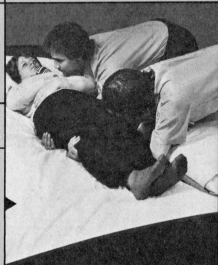

TRANSFERRING THE GROUND-LEVEL PATIENT

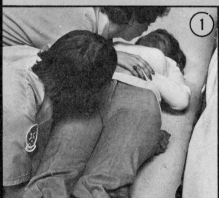

STRETCHER IS SET IN ITS LOWEST POSITION & PLACED ON OPPOSITE SIDE OF PT. EMTS DROP TO ONE KNEE, FACING PT. RESCUER'S ARMS ARE POSITIONED AS THEY ARE FOR A DIRECT CARRY.

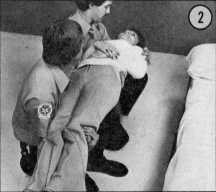

EMTS LIFT PT TO THEIR KNEES.

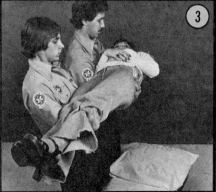

THEY STAND AND CARRY PT TO STRETCHER, DROP TO ONE KNEE, AND ROLL FORWARD TO PLACE PT ONTO MATTRESS.

SCAN 18-4B

WHEELED AMBULANCE STRETCHERS-
Moving & loading patient

MOVING THE PATIENT

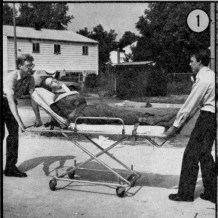

1 USE PULL HANDLES TO ROLL AND MANEUVER THE STRETCHER.

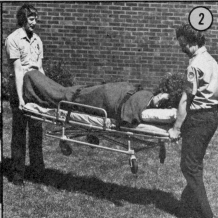

2 END CARRY WITH PALMS UP AND ARMS SLIGHTLY FLEXED IS THE USUAL METHOD OF MOVING A STRETCHER PT.

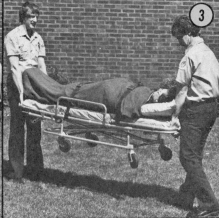

3 ALTERNATE END CARRY FOR PT INVOLVES ARMS STRAIGHT AND PALMS DOWN.

LOADING THE AMBULANCE

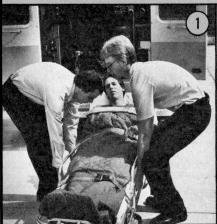

1 MAKE SURE STRETCHER IS LOCKED IN ITS LOWEST LEVEL BEFORE LIFTING ONTO AMBULANCE.

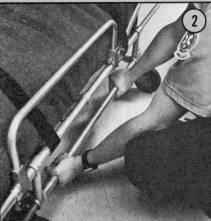

2 EMTS SHOULD POSITION THEMSELVES ON OPPOSITE SIDES OF STRETCHER. BEND AT KNEES AND GRASP LOWER BAR OF STRETCHER FRAME.

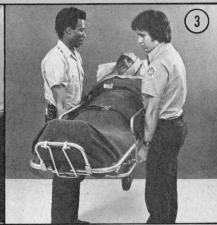

3 BOTH EMTS COME TO FULL STANDING POSITION WITH BACKS STRAIGHT.

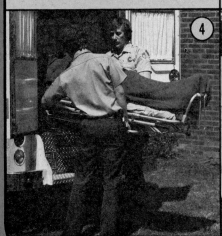

4 OBLIQUE STEPPING MOVEMENTS ARE USED TO MOVE STRETCHER ONTO AMBULANCE.

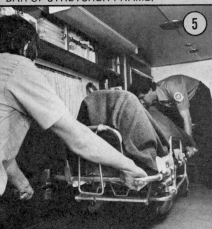

5 STRETCHER IS MOVED INTO SECURING DEVICE.

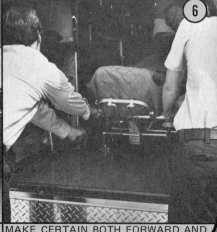

6 MAKE CERTAIN BOTH FORWARD AND REAR CATCHES ARE ENGAGED TO HOLD STRETCHER.

SCAN 18-5

When transferring a ground-level patient, a modification of the direct carry method can be used. There also are two other methods that can be used effectively.

The Extremity Transfer. This technique can be used to move a patient from the floor or ground to a stair chair or to any other patient-carrying device, for that matter. This method is not to be used, however, when the patient has a spinal injury or extremity fractures.

1. One EMT assumes a head-end position, while the other EMT takes the foot-end position.
2. The EMTs assist the patient to a sitting position.

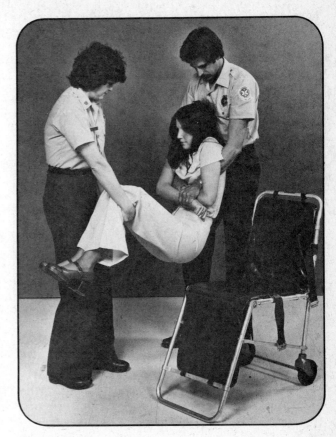

Figure 18-6: On a signal from the head-end EMT, both lift the patient.

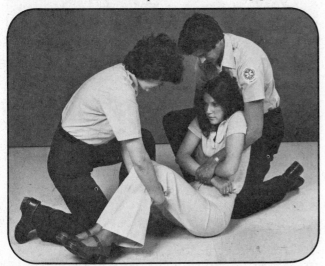

Figure 18-5: The EMTs assist the patient to a sitting position.

3. The head-end EMT reaches under the patient's armpits and grasps the patient's wrists, holding the arms to the patient's chest.
4. The foot-end EMT flexes the patient's knees and slides his hands into position under the knees.
5. Simultaneously, on the command of the head-end EMT, both EMTs move to a standing position, lifting the patient.
6. They carry the patient to the chair and lower him onto it.
7. The patient is draped with a sheet and blanket placed over his body and shoulders.
8. The patient is secured to the chair with three straps. One is fastened around the chest and the back of the chair. A second strap is placed across the thighs and around the seat of the chair. The third is fastened around the patient's legs and the lower portion of the chair.

The Chair Lift. This method can be used when it is desirable to limit the number of times the patient is lifted as, for example, when the patient is quite heavy.

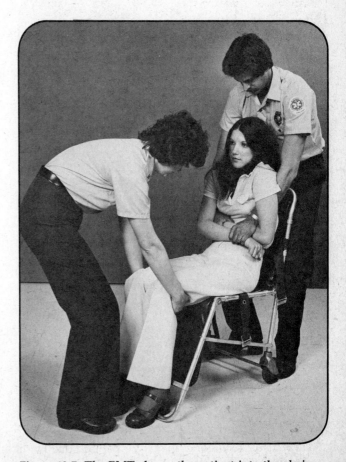

Figure 18-7: The EMTs lower the patient into the chair.

1. The patient is positioned on his back. One EMT kneels at the patient's hips and the other EMT positions himself at the patient's feet.

2. The EMT at the hips uses both hands to raise the patient's hips.

3. The foot-end EMT lifts the patient's legs and slides the chair under the patient.

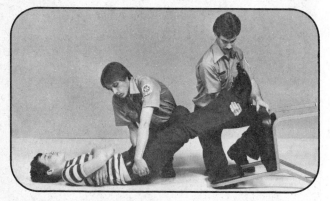

Figure 18-8: While one EMT lifts the patient's hips, the other EMT slides the chair in place.

4. The chair is positioned under the patient so that he is placed in a seated position.

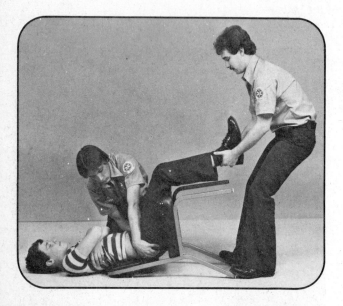

Figure 18-9: The chair is positioned under the patient.

5. The EMTs simultaneously lift the patient and chair into an upright position.

6. The patient is covered and secured to the chair by three straps, using the same procedure as explained in the extremity transfer.

NOTE: This technique may not be possible with some stair chairs because of their construction.

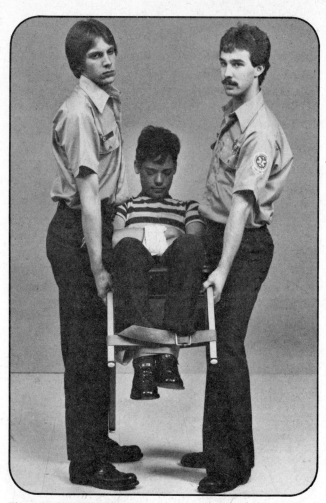

Figure 18-10: The EMTs lift the patient and chair into an upright position and make ready for the carry.

Moving a Stair Chair

A loaded stair chair is fairly easy to carry and maneuver, especially if the chair is on wheels. As with the ambulance stretcher, stair chairs should be rolled whenever possible; this reduces the risk of back strain for the EMTs and injury to the patient. The following procedure is suggested when a stair chair must be carried over level ground.

When the chair and patient are to be moved, one EMT must be behind the chair to tilt the chair back. This must be done carefully if the chair has wheels. The other EMT should stand at the patient's feet, with his back to the patient. As the chair is tilted back, he should crouch and grasp the chair by its legs. The two EMTs should lift the chair simultaneously and carry the patient to the wheeled stretcher. The patient should be transferred to the wheeled stretcher as soon as possible and before he is loaded onto the ambulance.

If the patient and chair must be carried down stairs, the foot-end EMT should face the patient while carrying the chair. A third person should support the foot-end EMT while the chair is being moved down the steps. If the chair has wheels, they should not be allowed to touch the steps.

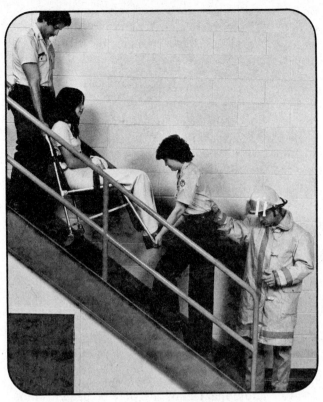

Figure 18-11: Moving a stair chair down steps.

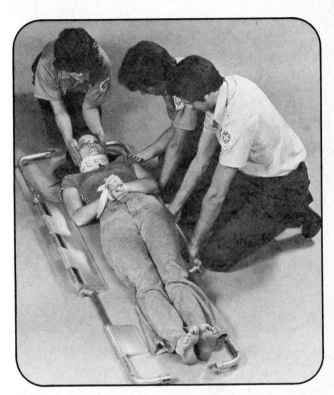

Figure 18-12: One EMT carefully supports the patient's head while half of the stretcher is positioned.

SCOOP-STYLE (Orthopedic) STRETCHERS

The scoop-style stretcher can be used to lift and carry most patients; however, *its main use is in cases of possible spinal injury.*

Preparing the Patient with Possible Spinal Injury

An extrication or rigid collar should be secured to the patient as soon as possible. Someone should continue to support the head after the collar is applied and throughout the stretcher application procedure. The patient should be placed in a supine position, as anatomically straight as possible. His arms should be secured in place, with roller bandage applied to hold the wrists together.

Preparing the Stretcher

ALWAYS adjust the length of the stretcher to fit the height of the patient. Separate the stretcher halves and place one half on each side of the patient. If the stretcher is the folding type, make sure the pins are properly set.

Applying the Stretcher

Slide the stretcher halves under the patient one at a time. This may be difficult since the stretcher may snag on clothing, grass, or debris. If necessary, roll the patient as a unit to either side to allow for proper positioning of the parts. Mate the latch parts and make certain that the stretcher halves are securely locked together. Latching should be done from head to feet. Adjust the head support.

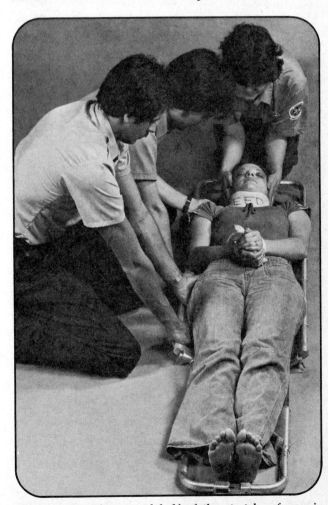

Figure 18-13: The second half of the stretcher frame is locked into the first.

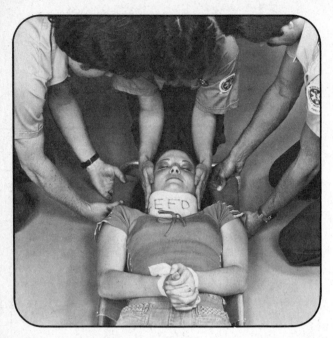

Figure 18-14: The vinyl head support is properly positioned.

Covering and Securing the Patient

The patient is covered with a blanket folded to size. The head is secured to the stretcher by a cravat, then the stretcher straps are fastened across the chest, hips, and legs.

The Velcro at the head end of folding scoop-style stretchers may not remain secure. To guard against this, tape the patient's head.

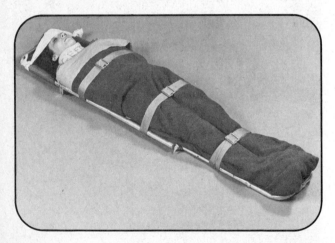

Figure 18-15: A patient properly positioned, covered, and secured on a scoop-style stretcher.

Moving the Patient

Lift the patient and stretcher by the end-carry method. The patient should be moved to the wheeled ambulance stretcher as soon as possible. The scoop-style stretcher provides rigid support for the spine. For this reason, and to avoid aggravating possible spinal injuries, it should not be removed

once the patient is on the wheeled stretcher. The patient and scoop-style stretcher should be secured as a unit to the wheeled stretcher by using two or three straps.

BASKET (Stokes) STRETCHERS

WARNING: Do NOT attempt to move a patient in a basket stretcher by rope or ladder unless you have been specifically trained in the techniques used for such moves.

The basket stretcher can be used to move patients from high places or over rough terrain. The basket should be lined with blankets prior to positioning the patient.

Transferring the Patient to the Stretcher

If the patient has no spinal injury, modifications of the direct carry and extremity transfer methods can be used by two EMTs to transfer a bed-level or ground-level patient to a basket stretcher. The draw sheet method also can be used to transfer a bed-level patient who has no spinal injury, provided the draw sheet can support the patient's weight while he is being lowered into the stretcher hammock-style.

Two additional techniques may be used to transfer a floor- or ground-level patient to a basket stretcher when he is heavy or when two EMTs cannot accomplish the transfer by themselves. Each technique requires additional personnel, however.

The Three-Rescuer Lift. This is a modification of the lift that was used for the three-rescuer carry covered earlier. Once the patient is brought to knee-level, he can be placed in the basket stretcher.

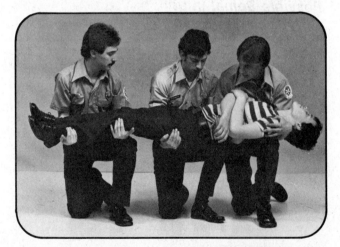

Figure 18-16: The EMTs raise the patient to their knees so that he can be placed in the stretcher.

The Blanket Lift. In this procedure, the blanket serves as the basket liner as well as the lifting mechanism. This lift can be done with four rescuers; however, it is best done with five. Four people can do the lifting, while the fifth one positions the stretcher. This procedure is shown in Scansheet 18-6.

THE BLANKET LIFT

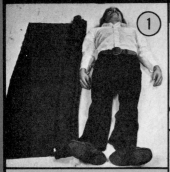

1. LAY ONE THIRD OF THE BLANKET ALONGSIDE PT AND LOOSELY FANFOLD REMAINDER NEXT TO HIM.

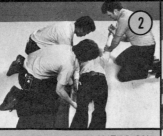

2. PLACE TWO RESCUERS ON FAR EDGE OF BLANKET, SINGLE RESCUER ON OTHER SIDE OF PT. THIS RESCUER EXTENDS OVER HEAD OF THE PT THE ARM OF THE SIDE ON WHICH PT WILL BE ROLLED.

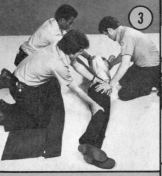

3. TWO RESCUERS LOG-ROLL PT ONTO THAT SIDE, AWAY FROM BLANKET.

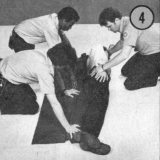

4. WHILE SINGLE RESCUER HOLDS PT, OTHER TWO RESCUERS PUSH BLANKET FOLDS AGAINST PT'S BACK.

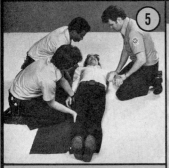

5. TWO RESCUERS ROLL PT ONTO BACK. SINGLE RESCUER REPOSITIONS PT'S ARM ALONG HIS SIDE.

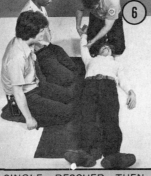

6. SINGLE RESCUER THEN EXTENDS THE PT'S OTHER ARM OVER THE HEAD.

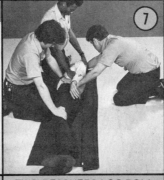

7. TWO RESCUERS LOG-ROLL PT TOWARD THEM ONTO UNFOLDED BLANKET.

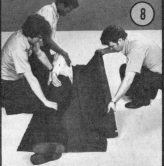

8. TWO RESCUERS HOLD PT, SINGLE RESCUER UNFOLDS BLANKET.

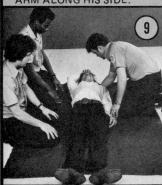

9. TWO RESCUERS ROLL PT ONTO HIS BACK ON UNFOLDED BLANKET.

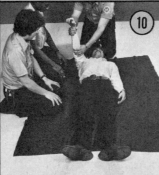

10. SINGLE RESCUER REPOSITIONS PT'S ARM ALONG HIS SIDE.

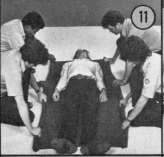

11. FOUR RESCUERS POSITION THEMSELVES, TWO ON EACH SIDE OF PT. ROLL BLANKET SIDES TOWARD THE PT.

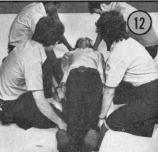

12. FOUR RESCUERS GRIP BLANKET IN LINE WITH TOP OF HEAD, LOWER BACK, UPPER THIGH, AND MIDCALF.

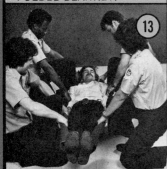

13. ON SIGNAL, RESCUERS LEAN BACK TO LIFT PT 8" FROM GROUND.

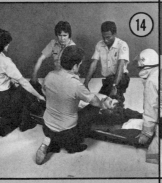

14. A FIFTH RESCUER SLIDES BASKET STRETCHER IN PLACE UNDER PT.

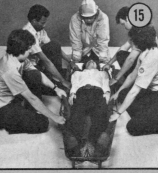

15. ON SIGNAL, ALL RESCUERS LEAN FORWARD TO GENTLY PLACE PT INTO BASKET.

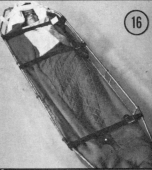

16. COVER AND SECURE PT BEFORE MOVING STRETCHER.

SCAN 18-6

Covering and Securing the Patient

If no blanket is in place, cover the patient and tuck in the blanket as best you can without aggravating possible spinal injuries. Provide a head covering in cold weather.

Fill the voids between the patient's body and the sides of the basket with rolled blankets or pillows. Secure the patient's head with a cravat and fasten the body straps. If the basket has a foot rest, make sure that it is in the proper position.

Moving a Basket Stretcher

The basket stretcher can be moved in a variety of ways, including:

- *Over level ground*—two rescuers can use the end-carry method, with both rescuers facing the patient. A four-rescuer carry can be done with one rescuer positioned at the head, the foot, and the center of each side. The foot-end rescuer can face in the direction of travel.

- *Over debris or rough terrain*—six rescuers, three per side, should carry the basket. These rescuers may have to change position during the carry in order to avoid obstacles.

- *Uphill*—there are three procedures:

  1. Two lines of rescuers can be formed and the basket can be passed from hand to hand.
  2. Six rescuers can be used, with the rescuers changing position to avoid obstacles.
  3. Two guide ropes can be secured at the top of the hill and used to slide the stretcher up the hill. The ground must be slippery for this procedure to be successful.

Lowering a Basket Stretcher

Rope can be used to lower a basket with a 4-point suspension bridle. There are four ways in which a basket stretcher can be lowered by rope:

- *Direct Horizontal Lower*—This requires three rescuers to maintain strain on the lowering line, two rescuers to ease the stretcher over the railing or ledge, and two rescuers on the ground to pull on tag lines to keep the stretcher from rotating. The stretcher is lowered in a horizontal position.

- *Direct Vertical Lower*—This method cannot be used with some types of plastic stretchers because the plastic can pull away from the frame. The same number of rescuers in the same position is used as during the horizontal lower.

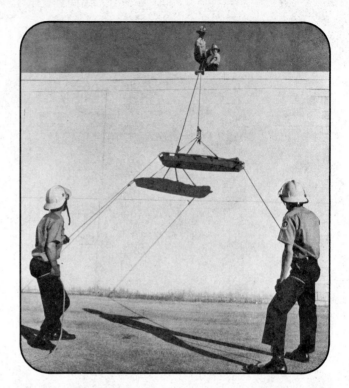

Figure 18-17: The direct horizontal lower.

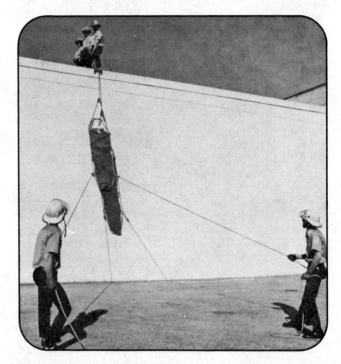

Figure 18-18: The direct vertical lower.

- *Ladder Slide*—The basket can be in a horizontal or vertical position.

- *Friction Lower*—A lowering rope can be passed over several rungs of a ladder to create friction to give better control. This added control means fewer rescuers are needed during the move.

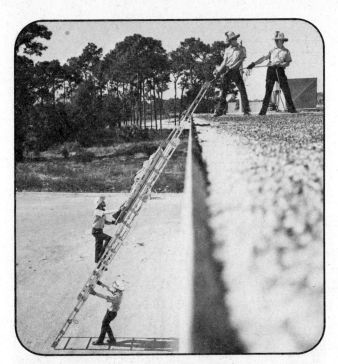

Figure 18-19: The vertical ladder slide.

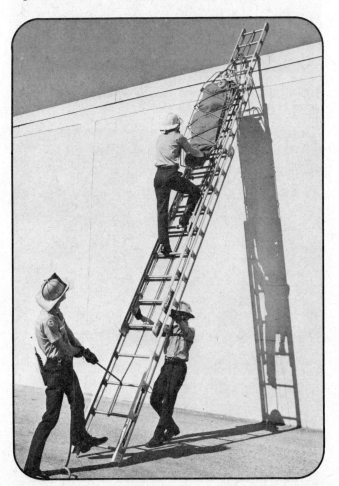

Figure 18-20: A friction lower allows easy lowering of a basket stretcher with a minimum of rescuers.

SHORT SPINE BOARDS

All unconscious trauma patients and all patients with possible spinal injuries should be rigidly immobilized. Patients found in a seated position, like those found in some automobile accidents, and patients who have to be moved to a seated position before they can be extricated and moved, should be secured to a short spine board and then transferred to a long one. Modified short spine boards may be used for special situations, such as when a patient is found seated in a short-backed bucket seat. New devices, such as the Kendrick extrication device, may be used in place of the short board.

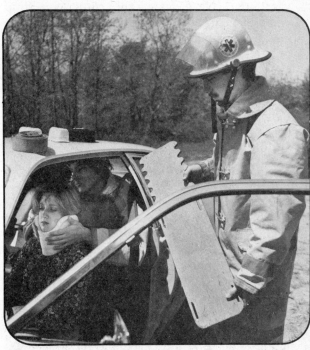

Figure 18-21: A short spine board modified for use in cars with bucket seats.

Preparing the Patient

Before the short board or similar device can be used, an extrication or rigid collar MUST be applied to the patient. Remember that manual stabilization of the head and neck has to be done before the collar is applied. Maintain this stabilization throughout the application of the collar, the short spine board, and the long spine board.

Applying the Short Spine Board

The procedure for applying a short spine board is shown in Scansheet 18-7. There are several methods that can be used for strapping the patient to the board. Some EMS Systems have studied and tested each of these methods and have received physicians' approval for the method they have selected. The procedure shown in Scansheet 18-7 is the most widely accepted. Use the method outlined in your system's local protocol.

There are four special warnings that must always be considered when applying a short spine board to a patient:

1. **WARNING:** You must push the spine board as far down into the seat as possible. If you don't, the board may shift and the patient's cervical spine may compress during application of the short spine board. To provide full cervical support, the top of the board must be level with the top of the patient's head.
2. **WARNING:** Never place a chin cup or chin strap on the patient. Such devices may prevent the patient from opening his mouth if he has to vomit.
3. **WARNING:** The patient's head must be firmly secured to the short spine board after the application of an extrication or rigid collar.
4. **WARNING:** Some short spine boards have buckles with release mechanisms that can be accidentally activated during patient transfer operations. This is especially true of ''quick-release'' buckles. These buckles must be taped closed after the final adjustment of the straps.

An alternate method of securing the patient to the short spine board calls for securing the torso first and the head last. This procedure offers greater stability in maintaining board position throughout the strapping process. In addition to board stability, the torso-to-head securing procedure may help prevent compression of the cervical spine.

A quick-release strap is placed across the patient's abdomen and through the lower strap holes of the board. This strap secures the lower end of the board and keeps the board at the proper height in relation to the top of the patient's head.

The patient's upper torso is secured to the board by using another quick-release strap that crosses from the shoulder strap hole to the bottom strap hole. This strap crosses the patient's chest and is buckled just below the clavicle. Thin padding should be placed under the buckles to assure patient comfort.

NOTE: You may have to use the strapping method shown in Scansheet 18-7 if the patient has suffered abdominal injuries or displays diaphragmatic breathing.

The head is secured last, after padding is placed between the board and collar to maintain the head in a neutral position. A three inch wide cravat can be used to secure the lower head and neck. It should be positioned at the midline of the collar and applied so that its ends travel along the wings of the collar and are tied on the top notch of the board. A second cravat is used to secure the top of the patient's head. It is tied to the lower notches on top of the board.

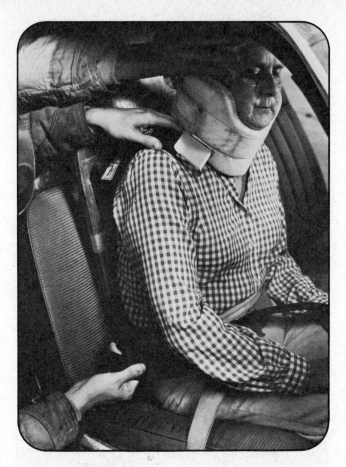

Figure 18-22: The patient can be secured to the short spine board from lap to chest.

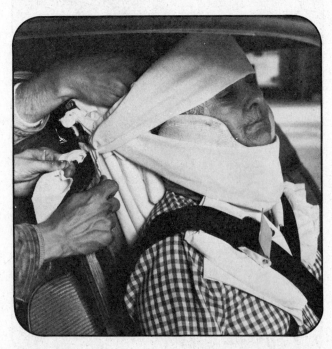

Figure 18-23: The patient's head can be secured after strapping the torso.

THE KENDRICK EXTRICATION DEVICE

The **Kendrick extrication device (K.E.D.)** is a flexible piece of equipment useful for immobilizing

APPLYING A SHORT SPINE BOARD

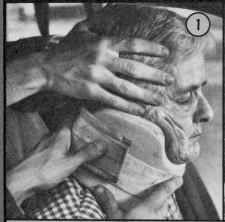

1 IMMOBILIZE PT'S HEAD BY HAND. APPLY EXTRICATION OR RIGID COLLAR.

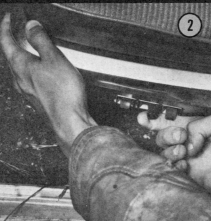

2 CAREFULLY MOVE SEAT AS FAR TO REAR AS POSSIBLE TO PROVIDE WORKING ROOM.

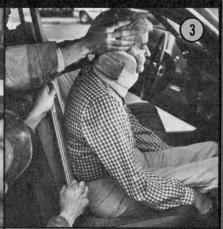

3 EMT STABILIZING HEAD DIRECTS SLIGHT REPOSITIONING OF PT TO FACILITATE INSERTION OF BOARD. HEAD, NECK, & BACK MUST BE MOVED AS A UNIT.

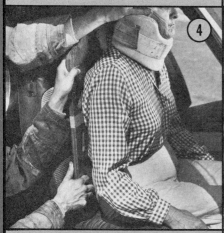

4 POSITION BOARD BEHIND PT, AS FAR DOWN INTO SEAT AS POSSIBLE.

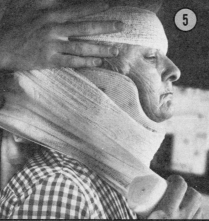

5 SECURE PT'S HEAD TO BOARD WITH WIDE SELF-ADHERING BANDAGE, LARGE STRIPS OF ADHESIVE TAPE, OR VELCRO STRAPS (IF BOARD IS SO EQUIPPED).

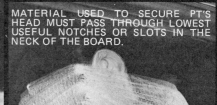

MATERIAL USED TO SECURE PT'S HEAD MUST PASS THROUGH LOWEST USEFUL NOTCHES OR SLOTS IN THE NECK OF THE BOARD.

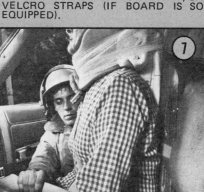

6 INSERT TONGUE OF ONE STRAP THROUGH UPPER SLOT OF ONE SIDE OF THE BOARD.

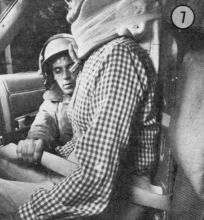

7 PASS STRAP ACROSS PT'S CHEST AND PULL IT THROUGH OPPOSITE LOWER STRAP SLOT FROM INSIDE TO OUTSIDE.

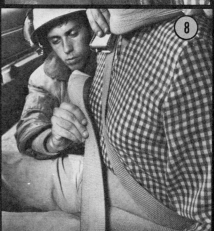

8 CARRY STRAP OVER AND AROUND PT'S THIGH, KEEPING IT AS CLOSE TO GROIN AS POSSIBLE WITHOUT CAUSING INJURY OR DISCOMFORT

SCAN 18-7A

APPLYING A SHORT SPINE BOARD   (cont'd)

⑨ BRING STRAP UP FROM OUTSIDE OF THIGH AND PASS TONGUE OF STRAP THROUGH THE BUCKLE.

⑩ INSERT TONGUE OF SECOND STRAP THROUGH OPPOSITE UPPER STRAP SLOT.

⑪ PASS STRAP ACROSS PT'S CHEST & THROUGH OPPOSITE LOWER STRAP SLOT.

⑫ CARRY STRAP OVER & AROUND PT'S OUTER THIGH. KEEP IT AS CLOSE AS POSSIBLE TO GROIN WITHOUT CAUSING INJURY OR DISCOMFORT.

⑬ DRAW BOTH STRAPS UP SNUGGLY SO PT IS FIRMLY STRAPPED TO BOARD.

PROPER PLACEMENT OF TWO BODY STRAPS. KEEP BUCKLES HIGH ENOUGH ON CHEST TO APPLY CPR, IF NEEDED.

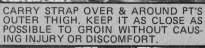

⑭ BANDAGE PT'S HANDS TOGETHER & TURN HIM GENTLY SO THAT LEGS ARE ON THE SEAT.

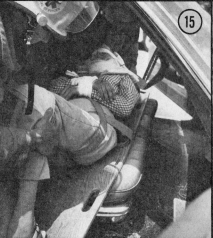

⑮ A THIRD PERSON CAN PLACE LONG SPINE BOARD ON THE SEAT. GENTLY LOWER PT ONTO LONG SPINE BOARD.

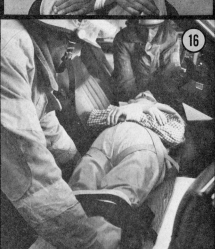

⑯ SECURE PT AND SHORT BOARD AS A UNIT TO THE LONG BOARD. REMOVE PT. PLACE ON WHEELED STRETCHER.

SCAN 18-7B

patients with possible injury to the cervical spine. This device can be used when the patient is found seated in a bucket seat, a short compact car seat, a seat with a contoured back, or in a confined space. The K.E.D. is also useful when the short spine board cannot be inserted into a car because of obstructions.

The use of a K.E.D. eliminates problems caused by straps and buckles. The device will immobilize the patient's head without the use of a confining chin strap.

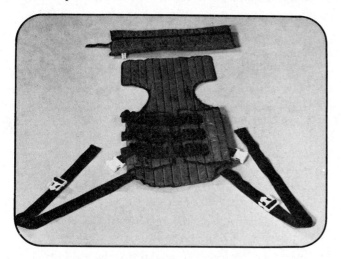

Figure 18-24: The Kendrick extrication device.

To apply a Kendrick extrication device:

1. Have one rescuer apply manual stabilization of the patient's head and neck. Stabilization is maintained throughout the entire application procedure.
2. Apply an extrication or rigid collar.
3. Slip the body portion of the K.E.D. behind the patient, with the smooth side toward his back. Straighten the K.E.D. so that the patient is centered within the device.
4. Pull the leg straps down so they are clear of the device.
5. Position the K.E.D. so that it is placed firmly under the patient's armpits.
6. Fasten the bottom chest strap.
7. Fasten the middle chest strap.
8. Pass the leg straps under the patient's legs and cross them at the crotch. Avoid discomfort or injury to the patient's groin. Pull each strap over to the opposite side of the patient and connect to the appropriate fastener.
9. Secure the patient's head with the Velcro head straps.
10. Fasten the top chest strap.
11. Check all straps before moving the patient.
12. Two rescuers are required to lift the patient. They should grasp the handles of the

K.E.D., located under the patient's armpits, and lock their other hands under the patient's thighs.

NOTE: Once the patient is extricated, the upper chest strap can be loosened if the patient is uncomfortable when breathing or displays signs of difficult or inadequate breathing.

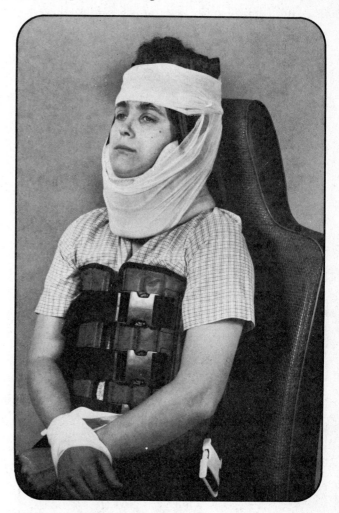

Figure 18-25: The K.E.D. applied to a patient.

LONG SPINE BOARDS

The basic procedures for using the long spine board were presented in Chapter 10. Here, we will consider some of the transfers that may be used when it is not possible to log-roll the patient.

The Four-Rescuer Straddle Slide

This is another technique for moving a person with a spinal injury onto a long board. Three rescuers handle the patient; the fourth slides the board in place.

1. One rescuer (usually one of the EMTs) maintains an open airway and applies manual traction at

the same time with the modified jaw-thrust.

2. The other EMT applies an extrication collar.

3. The head-end EMT stands, faces the patient, spreads his legs, bends at the waist, and supports the head.

4. The second EMT faces and straddles the patient. Bending at the waist, he grips the patient's sides just below the armpits.

5. A third person also faces and straddles the patient. Bending at the waist, he places his hands under the patient's waist. (The legs of the three rescuers must be spread sufficiently to allow passage of the long board between them).

6. The fourth person positions the board at the patient's head in line with his body.

7. On a signal from the head-end EMT, all rescuers lift the patient sufficiently to allow the fourth rescuer to slide the board under him. The smooth, wedge-shaped end of the board will slide under the patient's legs even though they are not lifted from the ground or floor.

8. On a signal from the head-end EMT, all rescuers gently lower the patient onto the board.

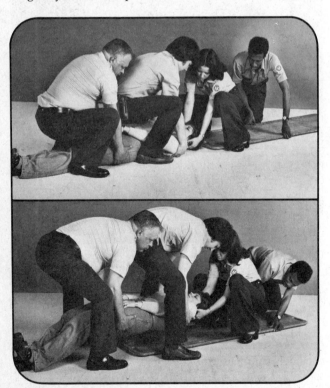

Figure 18-26: The four-rescuer straddle slide.

Transferring a Patient with a Rope Sling

In some accident situations, it may not be possible for rescuers to position themselves around a patient during the transfer effort. He may be under a vehicle or a piece of machinery or in a pocket of debris. A one-inch diameter rope sling or loop can be used to great advantage in situations like these. Rope slings are especially efficient when there are only two EMTs.

1. Manually stabilize the head and neck, and apply an extrication or rigid collar. The head and neck are manually stabilized until the patient is secured to the long spine board.

2. Slip the rope sling over the person's chest and under his arms.

3. Slide the steel rings down the rope. Position them as close to the person's head as possible. This will assure that a straight pull is made, and the doubled rope will help to support the person's head.

4. As you slightly raise the person's head and shoulders, have your partner slide the end of the board under them.

5. Exert a smooth, steady pull on the rope to move the person onto the board. Keep your hands as close to the board as you can to assure that the person's spine is kept straight.

6. Continue to pull on the rope until the person is completely on the board.

It may be necessary to angle the board slightly to move the patient onto it, for example, when an accident victim must be pulled through the window of an overturned car. The door frame and the curved portion of the roof will prevent a straight pull.

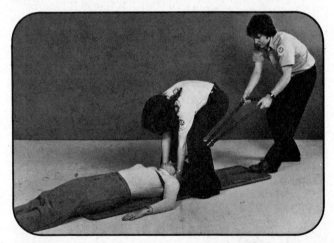

Figure 18-27: Moving a patient onto a long spine board using a rope sling.

Transferring a Patient From Under the Dashboard of a Vehicle

An accident victim may be found between the front seat and the dashboard. If proper tools are available, the front seat should be removed or displaced to the rear while the patient is protected. Working room is thus provided, and the patient can be moved directly onto a long board without difficulty. It also may be possible to lift him with a scoop stretcher.

If tools are unavailable to remove or displace the seat, the patient can be transferred to a seat-level long board by four persons. Rescuers should first force both front doors of the vehicle beyond their normal range of motion to provide an unobstructed work area on each side.

1. One rescuer (usually one of the EMTs) takes up a position at the patient's head. While he maintains an open airway and applies manual traction by the modified jaw-thrust, the other EMT applies an extrication collar.
2. After applying the collar, the second EMT positions himself outside the vehicle at the patient's feet.
3. Two other rescuers climb into the area behind the front seat, and reach over and grasp his clothing at the shoulder, chest, waist, and thigh. If the patient is in a loose garment that cannot be easily grasped, the rescuers reach over and place their hands under the patient's body.
4. On a signal from the head-end EMT, all rescuers lift the patient, keeping his back and legs against the front of the seat.
5. They slide the patient onto the long board in a face-up position and remove him from the vehicle.

Transferring a Patient From Between the Front and Rear Seats of a Vehicle

This technique is essentially the same as the one just described. In this case, however, the two assisting rescuers lean over the back of the front seat to lift the patient onto a board laid on the rear seat.

SUMMARY

The specific procedures covered in this chapter should be studied in a step-by-step fashion.

Patients can be moved during emergency moves, nonemergency moves, and transfer to the ambulance.

You may have to perform an emergency move of a patient if the scene is hazardous, if care requires repositioning the patient (e.g., CPR), or if you must gain access to other patients in need of basic life support.

Sometimes it is necessary to perform a nonemergency move of a patient to prevent the decline of his condition, to reach other patients, to provide better patient care, or because the patient insists on being moved.

For a nonemergency move, the patient must be conscious, fully assessed, and have normal, stable vital signs. He should have no serious wounds, bleeding, or any indications of spinal injury. All fractures must be immobilized.

Many one-rescuer moves exist for use on the conscious patient, including: the one-rescuer assist (patient can walk with assistance); the piggyback carry; the cradle carry; the fireman's carry; and the pack strap carry. The fireman's carry can be used for the unconscious patient.

One-rescuer drags can be used on both conscious and unconscious patients. The blanket drag is superior to all other drags.

Two rescuers can perform the two-rescuer assist on conscious patients who can walk with assistance. The two-rescuer extremity carry can be used for both conscious and unconscious patients. Three rescuers can use the three-rescuer carry for conscious and unconscious patients.

When using a patient-carrying device, the patient must be covered and secured to the device. The scoop-style stretcher and spine boards offer protection for possible spinal injuries.

The most common patient-carrying device used is the wheeled ambulance stretcher. The bed-level patient can be transferred to the stretcher by the direct carry method, the draw sheet method, or the slide transfer method. The ground-level patient can be transferred by a variation of the direct carry method. The stretcher can be wheeled or end-carried after covering and securing the patient. The patient is loaded by using the side carry technique.

Folding stair chairs are useful to move patients through narrow corridors and doorways, up or down stairs, and in small elevators. The patient should be conscious and responsive. There should be no indications of spinal or lower extremity injuries.

The scoop-style stretcher can be used for patients with possible spinal injury. An extrication or rigid collar should be applied before using the stretcher.

Basket stretchers are useful when moving patients from high places, down ladders, or across rough terrain. They can be hand-carried or lowered by ropes, depending on the situation. The blanket lift is a useful way of moving a patient into the basket stretcher.

Patients with possible spinal injury found seated in a motor vehicle, or those who must be moved to a seated position before removal from a vehicle, should be secured to a short spine board or Kendrick extrication device. An extrication or rigid collar should be applied before applying the board or K.E.D.

After a patient is secured to a short spine board, he must be moved and secured to a long spine board.

In addition to the log-roll method, the four-rescuer straddle can be used to place a patient on a long spine board. The patient can be transferred to the long spine board by a rope sling. Special techniques are employed to transfer a patient to the long spine board when he is found under the dashboard, or between the rear and front seats of a vehicle.

19 transport and termination of activities

OBJECTIVES By the end of this chapter, you should be able to:

1. Define "transport." (p. 430)
2. List and describe the ELEVEN steps to settle the patient for transport. (pp. 430-3)
3. List, in the correct order, the EIGHT essential elements of ambulance–hospital radio communications during transport. (p. 434)
4. Describe the attending EMT's activities during transport. (p. 435)
5. Describe what should be done if the patient develops cardiac arrest during transport. (p. 435)
6. Define "handoff." (p. 436)
7. Describe an orderly handoff of a patient at the emergency department. (p. 434, 6-7)
8. List the activities to be carried out at the medical facility to make the ambulance ready for service. (p. 437-9)
9. Describe how to make up a wheeled ambulance stretcher. (p. 438-9)
10. List the activities to be carried out en route to quarters to make the ambulance ready for service. (p. 439)
11. List the procedures done in quarters to make the ambulance ready for service. (p. 439-40)
12. Describe what the EMT should do to ready himself for the next response. (p. 440)

SKILLS As an EMT, you should be able to:

1. Physically and mentally ready a patient for transport.
2. Take vital signs and provide needed basic EMT-level emergency care during transport.
3. Relay, by radio, patient information to the emergency department.
4. Conduct an orderly handoff of the patient.
5. Carry out all activities necessary at the medical facility, en route to quarters, and in quarters to ready the ambulance and crew for service.

TERMS you may be using for the first time:

Transport—the prompt and safe moving of the patient from the emergency scene to a medical facility, providing emergency care and gathering patient information while en route.

Handoff—the orderly transfer of care from the EMTs to the emergency department staff.

Germicide—a chemical that will kill microorganisms associated with disease.

TRANSPORT

Transport includes more than the movement of a patient to a medical facility. Transport must be prompt, yet safe. During transport, vital signs are taken, emergency care is provided, and when possible, additional patient information is obtained. As part of the EMT's duties during transport, ambulance–hospital radio communications are established to provide information to the emergency department staff and to inform them of any changes in the patient's condition.

BEFORE THE AMBULANCE MOVES

Efforts of emergency medical technicians should be directed toward "settling the patient in" for the trip to the hospital.

Patient compartments are equipped with positive locking devices that prevent the ambulance cot from moving about while the vehicle is in motion. It is unlikely, but in haste, an EMT may engage the forward part of the cot in the hook of the fastener bar and fail to engage the rear catch completely. An unfastened stretcher can create havoc in the patient compartment, and both patient and EMT may be injured before the ambulance can be brought to a stop. Before closing the rear door, make sure the cot is *securely* in place.

The need to move a patient from an upper floor or over rough terrain requires that he be firmly strapped to a stretcher while on his back. Even an uncomplicated movement of the wheeled ambulance stretcher for a short distance may have to be done with the patient in the supine position. This does not mean, however, that he must be transferred to the hospital in that position. Rather, positioning should be dictated by the nature of his injury or illness.

The unconscious patient, or the patient with a low level of awareness, must be positioned to allow for drainage of fluids from the nose and mouth. In many cases, the coma (lateral recumbent) position can be used. Security straps have to be placed so that the patient is safely in position during transport. If the patient is in the traumatic coma position, he has been secured to a long spine board. Check to be certain that the patient is adequately strapped to the board and that the board is secured to the stretcher.

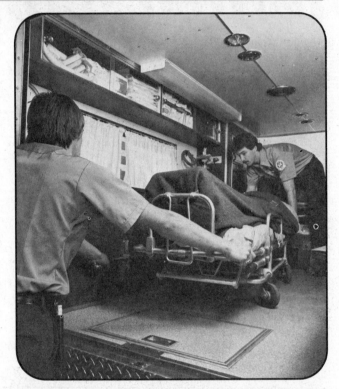

Figure 19-1: Make sure that the cot is secured in place.

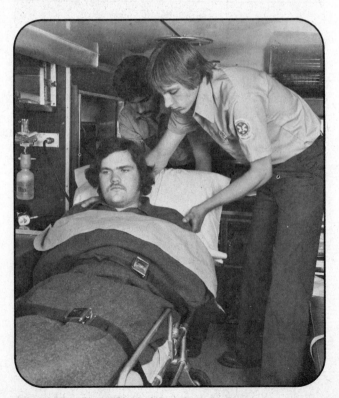

Figure 19-2: Properly position the patient.

If the patient is immobilized on a long spine-board, the board and patient may be rotated to allow for drainage. However, this may be done *only* if the patient is properly secured to the board and the board can be effectively propped and secured for transport.

A patient with a heart condition or respiratory difficulty should be transported in a position that allows him to breathe freely. If the patient is likely to develop cardiac arrest, position a short spine board or similar device between him and the ambulance cot prior to startup. (If the patient is alert and apprehensive, do not add to his stress by placing the short board.) Thus, if arrest occurs, there will be no need to locate and position the board. Riding on a hard board may not be comfortable for a patient, but temporary discomfort is better than permanent injury from delayed resuscitation efforts.

Security straps applied when a patient is being prepared for transfer to the ambulance may tighten by the time he is loaded into the vehicle. Adjust straps so that they hold the patient safely in place, but are not so tight that they interfere with circulation or respiration, or cause pain.

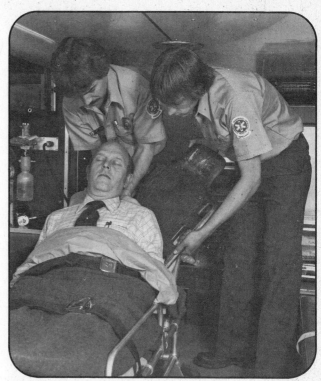

Figure 19-4: Allow for respiratory and cardiac complications.

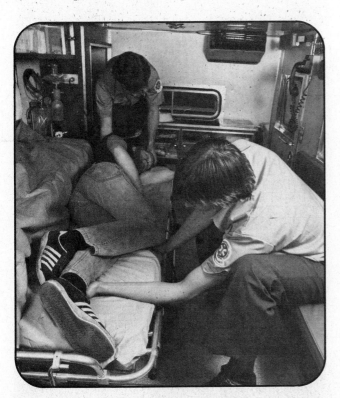

Figure 19-3: Position the patient to allow for proper drainage. Take care not to aggravate existing injuries.

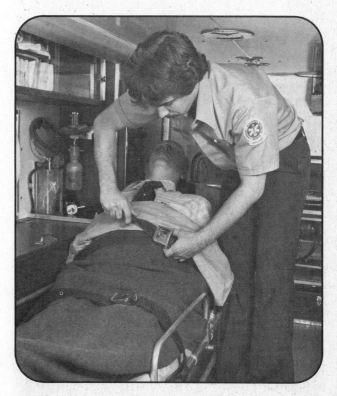

Figure 19-5: Adjust constricting straps.

As with straps, clothing may interfere with circulation and breathing. Loosen ties, belts, and any clothing around the neck. Straighten clothing that is caught under safety straps. Remember that clothes bunched at the crotch can be painful to the patient.

Be certain that a conscious patient is breathing properly once you have positioned him on the ambulance stretcher. If the patient is unconscious, with an airway in place, make sure he has adequate air exchange once you have moved him into the position for transport.

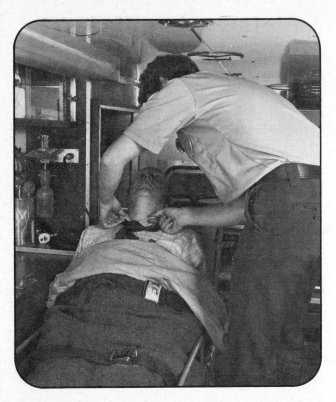

Figure 19-6: Loosen any constricting clothing.

Even properly applied bandages can loosen during transfer to the ambulance, especially if body movement is considerable. Severe bleeding can *resume* when the pressure of a bandage is removed from a dressing. If the wound site is covered with a sheet or blanket, lack of bandage pressure may go unnoticed until the patient slips into deep shock.

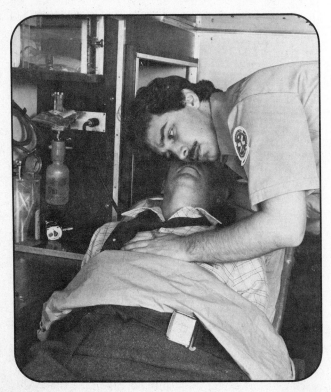

Figure 19-7: Continually monitor the patient's airway.

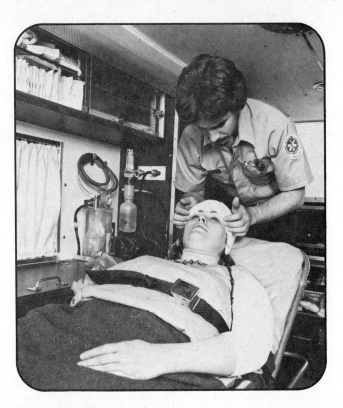

Figure 19-8: Check bandages.

Immobilizing devices also can loosen during movement to the ambulance. Inspect the bandages that hold board splints in place. Test air splints with your fingertip to see that they have remained properly inflated during transfer to the ambulance. Inspect traction devices to see that proper tension is still maintained. Safe adjustment of splinting devices is virtually impossible when an ambulance is pitching about during the trip to the hospital. Check the splinted patient for distal pulse, skin color and temperature at the fingertips or toes, capillary refilling, and neurological activity.

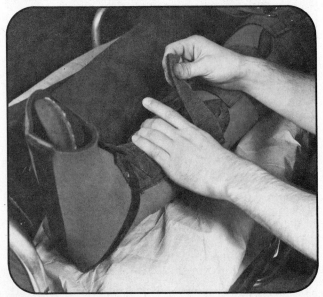

Figure 19-9: Check all splints and determine changes in distal pulse, circulation, and neurological activity.

Once the patient is properly positioned and you have made all necessary adjustments in straps, clothing, and bandages, record blood pressure, pulse, and respiratory rates. Accurate measurements of vital signs may not be possible if the trip to the hospital is particularly rough. Vital signs should be taken no less than every five minutes. In severe cases of shock, you may have to begin to take another set of vital signs immediately after completing the first set and continue this cycle throughout transport.

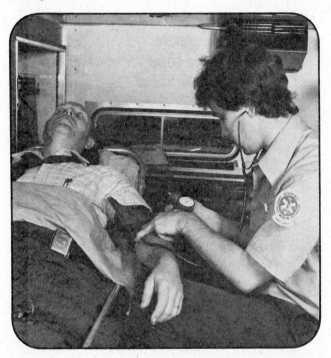

Figure 19-10: Determine and record vital signs.

A member of the patient's family or a friend may be transported with the patient. Local regulations determine if this person is to ride in the driver or patient compartment. Follow all local guidelines, including the use of safety belts for passengers. **CAUTION:** Under no circumstances should smoking be allowed in an ambulance!

Entry of a passenger into the patient compartment should be delayed until the patient is properly positioned because of the need for working space. You will have to move around in the patient compartment as you adjust the stretcher level, loosen straps, straighten clothing, and do whatever else has to be done to ensure a safe and comfortable trip. This may not be possible with another person in the compartment.

Carefully consider the emotional state of a relative or friend of the patient before you allow him to enter the patient compartment. If the person appears to be under control, and if his presence will not interfere with patient care activities, he should be allowed to come along. If he appears to be in a highly emotional state, perhaps he should be taken

to the hospital by some other means—by police car, for example. An emotional person may become irrational in the presence of a seriously ill or injured friend or relative, and you may spend more time restraining him than working with your patient. For the same reason, the passenger's emotional state should certainly be considered before he is allowed to ride with the driver.

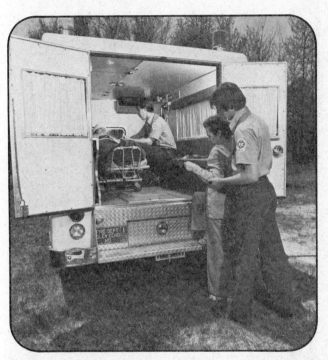

Figure 19-11: Delay entry of a passenger until the patient is properly positioned.

If a purse, briefcase, overnight bag or other personal item is to accompany the patient, make sure it is loaded into the ambulance.

Apprehension often mounts in a sick or injured person after being loaded into an ambulance. Not only is he confined, he may also be separated from family members or friends who have comforted him to this point. Now is the time for a few kind words and a reassuring hand. Remember that a favorite toy can do much to calm a frightened child. When you are satisfied that the patient is ready for transportation, signal the driver to proceed.

EN ROUTE TO THE MEDICAL FACILITY

Your primary concern while en route is to provide basic life support and basic EMT-level emergency care. This includes providing emotional support for the patient and any loved ones in the patient compartment. The driver will have to provide care and support for any passengers in the driver's compartment.

If the patient is conscious and emergency care activities will not be compromised, obtain any patient information not collected at the scene. This will

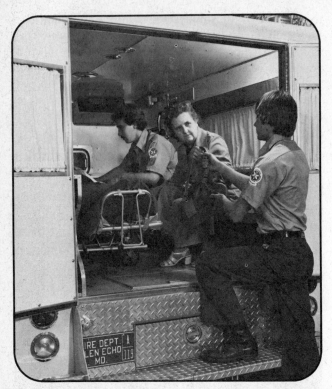

Figure 19-12: Account for the patient's personal effects.

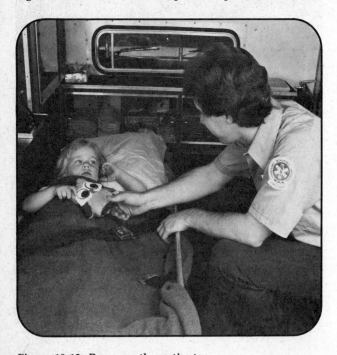

Figure 19-13: Reassure the patient.

allow you to complete your report, provide useful information to the emergency department staff, and may temporarily take the patient's mind off his troubles.

Communications While En Route

Ambulance–hospital radio communications are part of your duties during transport. Ambulance–hospital radio communications should be conducted in accordance with local protocol. These communications are usually sent directly to the emergency department. The first call should be an informational message that includes:

1. The hospital identification
2. Ambulance or rescue identification
3. A brief description of the situation
4. A review of the subjective interview
5. A review of the objective examination, including vital signs
6. The suspected medical problem or injuries
7. The emergency care being provided
8. The estimated time of arrival at the medical facility

An example of such a message is as follows:

"Mercy Hospital, this is Johnstown squad three. We are transporting a man who has fallen approximately 20 feet from a ladder onto a concrete driveway. The patient is a 34-year-old male who complains of headache and severe pain in the right leg. He was unconscious for a short time after the fall. He is a patient of Dr. Robert Johnson. The patient appears to be confused and is obviously in pain. Vitals are BP 140/90, pulse 85 and strong, respirations 26 and normal. Positive findings are a contusion of the back of the head, and swelling and point tenderness over the right femur. I suspect a fracture of the right femur shaft and a concussion. We have applied a traction splint. We will arrive at your location in approximately 10 minutes."

In about 45 seconds, you can transmit the information needed by the emergency department staff personnel so that they can begin to plan a definitive course of treatment before seeing the patient.

If the patient has an injury or illness that requires special emergency care procedures (as in poisoning), solicit this information by radio from the emergency department or the proper agency (such as the poison control center).

Remember that changes in vital signs indicate a change in the patient's condition. Radio the emergency department if the patient worsens or improves.

ON ARRIVAL AT THE MEDICAL FACILITY

Make an orderly transfer of the patient to the care of the emergency department personnel.

The Handoff

It is usually the emergency department nurse to whom the EMT most directly relates, either through the ambulance–hospital radio communication system or in face-to-face contact in the hospital. The

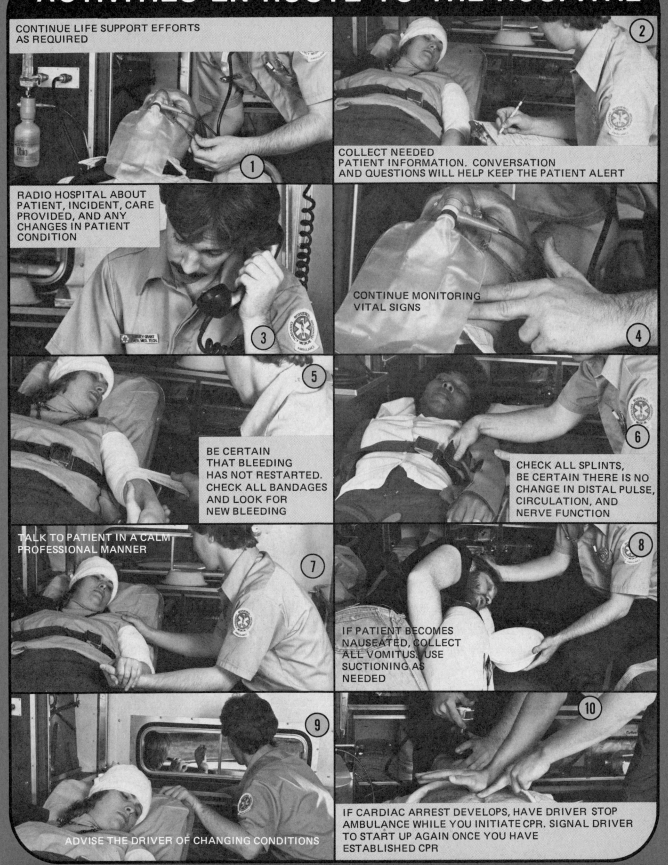

ACTIVITIES EN ROUTE TO THE HOSPITAL

CONTINUE LIFE SUPPORT EFFORTS AS REQUIRED ①

② COLLECT NEEDED PATIENT INFORMATION. CONVERSATION AND QUESTIONS WILL HELP KEEP THE PATIENT ALERT

RADIO HOSPITAL ABOUT PATIENT, INCIDENT, CARE PROVIDED, AND ANY CHANGES IN PATIENT CONDITION ③

CONTINUE MONITORING VITAL SIGNS ④

⑤ BE CERTAIN THAT BLEEDING HAS NOT RESTARTED. CHECK ALL BANDAGES AND LOOK FOR NEW BLEEDING

⑥ CHECK ALL SPLINTS, BE CERTAIN THERE IS NO CHANGE IN DISTAL PULSE, CIRCULATION, AND NERVE FUNCTION

TALK TO PATIENT IN A CALM PROFESSIONAL MANNER ⑦

⑧ IF PATIENT BECOMES NAUSEATED, COLLECT ALL VOMITUS. USE SUCTIONING AS NEEDED

⑨ ADVISE THE DRIVER OF CHANGING CONDITIONS

⑩ IF CARDIAC ARREST DEVELOPS, HAVE DRIVER STOP AMBULANCE WHILE YOU INITIATE CPR. SIGNAL DRIVER TO START UP AGAIN ONCE YOU HAVE ESTABLISHED CPR

SCAN 19.1

following are steps that you might take to see that "handoff" is accomplished smoothly and without incident. **Handoff** is the transition from prehospital to hospital emergency care. It is a crucial period during which your primary concern must be the continuation of patient care activities.

In a routine admission or when an illness or injury is not life-threatening, first check to see what is to be done with the patient.

If emergency department activity is particularly hectic—as it is when many seriously injured people are admitted at the same time—it might be better to leave your patient attended in the relative security and comfort of the ambulance while you find out where he should be taken. Otherwise the patient may be subjected to distressing sights and sounds and perhaps be in the way. Under no circumstances simply wheel a nonemergency patient into the hospital, place him on a bed or gurney, and leave him!

Keep in mind that the staff may be treating other seriously injured or ill persons, so suppress the urge to demand attention for *your* patient. Report his condition and continue emergency care procedures until someone can assume the responsibility for the patient. When directed, transfer the patient to a bed or gurney.

staff member all information about the patient and his illness or injury. Remember to relate any changes in the patient's vital signs and level of consciousness noted during the initial emergency care and subsequent transfer and transport activities.

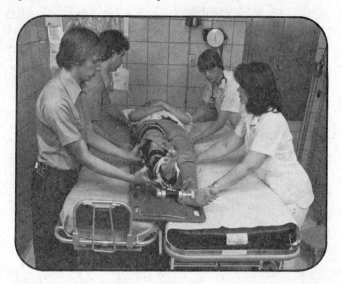

Figure 19-15: Assist the emergency department staff as required.

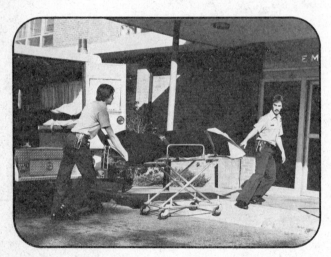

Figure 19-14: Transfer at the emergency department.

All EMTs can and should participate in the early emergency department care of the sick and injured. Even when the emergency department staff has taken over completely, it is often beneficial for the EMTs to remain in the area to be of assistance. The experience not only promotes better patient care, but also fosters improved communications and understanding between EMTs and emergency department personnel. Working with the staff gives an EMT the opportunity to learn more about definitive measures, while the staff can evaluate the EMT's abilities.

As soon as you are free from patient care activities, either orally or by written report, transfer to a

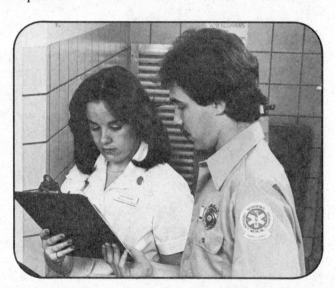

Figure 19-16: Transfer patient information.

If a patient's valuables or other personal effects were entrusted to you, transfer them to a staff member and have that person give you a written receipt. Space often is provided on the report form for this purpose. While the procedure may be irksome to the staff member, it gives you a measure of protection.

Leaving the Hospital

This task is not as formal as it sounds. Simply ask the emergency department nurse or physician if your services are still needed. In rural areas where some hospital services are not available, it may be necessary to transfer seriously injured or ill persons to other facilities. If you leave and have to be recalled, valuable time is lost. Or a person's condition may be such that he will not be admitted, and you may have to take him home. If you are recalled in this case, it is *your* time that is taken up.

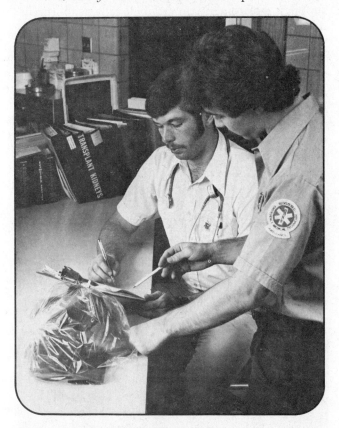

Figure 19-17: **Transfer personal effects.**

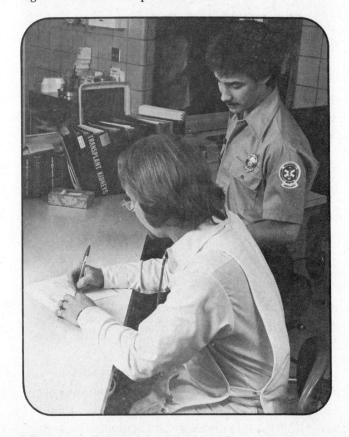

Figure 19-18: **Release from the hospital.**

TERMINATION OF ACTIVITIES

An ambulance run is not over until the personnel, ambulance, and equipment are ready for the next response. The functions of EMTs in the termination of activities are much more involved than merely changing linens and cleaning the passenger compartment. Diverse tasks must be accomplished at the medical facility, during the return to quarters, and after arrival at the ambulance station.

AT THE MEDICAL FACILITY

Activities should be directed toward making the ambulance ready for service should another call be received prior to the return to quarters.

Time, equipment, and space limitations preclude vigorous cleaning of the ambulance while it is parked at the hospital. However, every effort should be made for rapid preparation of the ambulance for the next patient. Clean up blood, vomitus, and other body fluids and wipe down equipment that may have been splashed. Remove and dispose of bandage wrappings, contaminated dressings, open but unused dressings, and similar items. Sweep away dirt that may have been tracked into the patient compartment; when the weather is inclement, sponge up mud or water from the floor. Use a deodorizer to neutralize odors of vomitus, urine, or feces. Various sprays or concentrates are available for this purpose.

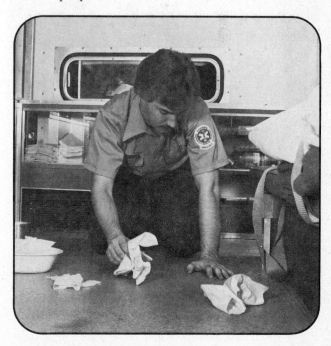

Figure 19-19: **Clean the ambulance interior as required.**

Used bag-valve-mask units, oxygen masks, nasal cannulas, and other parts of respiratory-assist and inhalation therapy devices become reservoirs of infectious agents. To minimize cross-infection, many ambulance squads use disposable masks and other items with which the patient comes into direct contact. But some squads use nondisposable items that must be cleaned and disinfected after each use. Cleaning should not be limited to a quick inefficient rinsing in a hospital sink. It should be a rigorous procedure carried out after the ambulance is returned to quarters. Place used nondisposable items in a plastic bag and seal it. Replace the items with similar ones carried in the ambulance as spares.

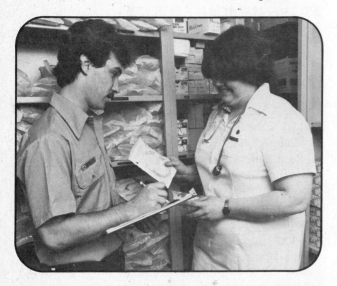

Figure 19-20: Replace respiratory equipment as required.

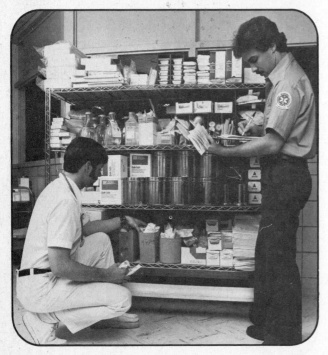

Figure 19-21: Replace expendable items according to local policies.

Many larger medical facilities allow ambulance squads to replace expendable items from hospital storerooms (e.g., sterile dressings, bandaging materials, towels, disposable masks, caps, gowns, sterile

water and IV saline solutions). If this is the policy in your area, replace items on a one-for-one basis, but do not take advantage of the program. Abuse of a supplies replacement program usually leads to its discontinuation.

Another policy of larger medical facilities is to allow the exchange of items like splints and spine boards. Crews are not delayed at the hospital, and ambulances can return to quarters fully prepared for the next run.

When equipment is available for exchange, quickly check it for completeness and operability. By checking equipment before you leave the exchange facility, you assure that your unit is properly prepared for the next run. If you *do* find a piece of equipment that is faulty or incomplete, complete the proper report form and notify someone in authority so that the device can be repaired or replaced.

Making Up the Ambulance Stretcher

The following procedure is one of many that can be used to make up a wheeled ambulance stretcher.

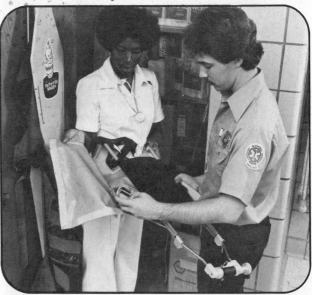

Figure 19-22: Exchange equipment according to local policies.

- Remove unsoiled blankets and place them on a clean surface.
- Remove the pillow case and place the pillow on a clean surface.
- Remove all soiled linen and place it in the designated receptacle.
- Raise the stretcher to the high-level position, if possible; this makes the procedure easier. The stretcher should be flat.
- Lower the side rails and unfasten straps.
- Clean the mattress surface with an appropriate detergent if necessary.
- Turn the mattress over; rotation adds to the life of the mattress.

- Center the bottom sheet on the mattress and open it fully. If a full-sized bed sheet is used, first fold it lengthwise.
- Tuck the sheet under each end of the mattress and then under each side; form square corners.
- Place a disposable pad, if one is used, on the center of the mattress.
- Place the slip-covered pillow lengthwise at the head of the mattress.
- Open the top sheet fully; fold it lengthwise first; then fold it in half and place it at the foot of the mattress.
- Fully open the blanket. If a second blanket is used, open it fully and match it to the first blanket. This task should be done with an EMT at each end of the stretcher.
- Fold the blanket(s) lengthwise to match the width of the stretcher; fold one side first, then the other.
- Tuck the foot of the folded blanket(s) under the foot of the mattress.
- Tuck the head of the folded blanket(s) under the head of the mattress.
- Buckle the safety straps and tuck in excess straps.
- Raise the side rails and foot rest.
- Use the securing strap to hold the pillow.

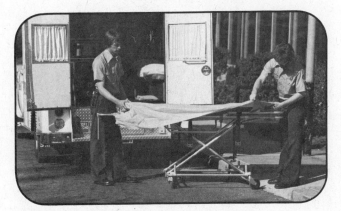

Figure 19-23: Make up the wheeled stretcher.

The stretcher is now ready for the next patient.

It must be reemphasized that this is one of many techniques for preparing a wheeled ambulance stretcher for service. Whatever the method, it should meet the following objectives:

- All linens, blankets and pouches should be stored neatly on the stretcher.
- Preparation for the next call should be done as soon as possible.

- All linen and blankets should be folded or tucked so that they will be contained within the stretcher frame.
- Replace the cot in the ambulance.
- Check for equipment left in the hospital. Make sure that any nondisposable patient care items have been replaced.

EN ROUTE TO QUARTERS

Emphasis should be on a safe return. An ambulance driver may practice every suggestion for safe vehicle operation while en route to the hospital and then totally disregard those suggestions during the return to quarters. Defensive driving must be a full-time effort.

Radio the dispatcher that you are returning to quarters and that you are (or are not) available for service. Valuable time is often lost when a dispatcher, trying to locate and alert a backup ambulance, does not know that a ready-for-service unit is on the road. Be sure to notify the dispatcher if you must stop and leave the ambulance unattended for any reason during the return to quarters.

If the patient just delivered to the hospital had a communicable disease—or if it was not possible to neutralize disagreeable odors while at the hospital—make the return trip, weather permitting, with the windows of the patient compartment partially open. If the unit has sealed windows, use the air-conditioning or ventilating system to air the patient compartment.

Local policy usually dictates the frequency with which the ambulance fuel tank is refilled. Some squads require drivers to refuel after each run regardless of distance traveled. In other squads the policy is to refuel when the gauge reaches a certain level. There should be enough fuel that the ambulance can travel to an emergency and to the medical facility without running low.

IN QUARTERS

Direct your attention to cleaning and disinfecting, replenishing materials and supplies, maintaining the ambulance, finishing reports, and caring for yourself. An example of an EMT's termination activities in quarters is shown in Scansheet 19-2.

TERMINATION OF ACTIVITIES: IN QUARTERS

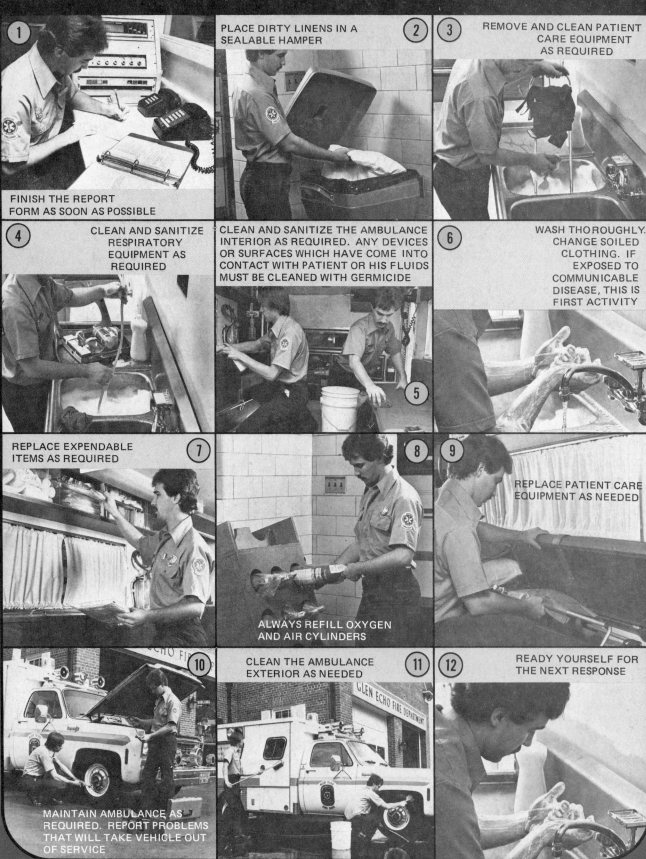

1 FINISH THE REPORT FORM AS SOON AS POSSIBLE

2 PLACE DIRTY LINENS IN A SEALABLE HAMPER

3 REMOVE AND CLEAN PATIENT CARE EQUIPMENT AS REQUIRED

4 CLEAN AND SANITIZE RESPIRATORY EQUIPMENT AS REQUIRED

5 CLEAN AND SANITIZE THE AMBULANCE INTERIOR AS REQUIRED. ANY DEVICES OR SURFACES WHICH HAVE COME INTO CONTACT WITH PATIENT OR HIS FLUIDS MUST BE CLEANED WITH GERMICIDE

6 WASH THOROUGHLY. CHANGE SOILED CLOTHING. IF EXPOSED TO COMMUNICABLE DISEASE, THIS IS FIRST ACTIVITY

7 REPLACE EXPENDABLE ITEMS AS REQUIRED

8 ALWAYS REFILL OXYGEN AND AIR CYLINDERS

9 REPLACE PATIENT CARE EQUIPMENT AS NEEDED

10 MAINTAIN AMBULANCE AS REQUIRED. REPORT PROBLEMS THAT WILL TAKE VEHICLE OUT OF SERVICE

11 CLEAN THE AMBULANCE EXTERIOR AS NEEDED

12 READY YOURSELF FOR THE NEXT RESPONSE

SCAN 19.2

SUMMARY

Transport is the prompt and safe moving of a patient to a medical facility, providing emergency care while en route. Needed patient information can be gathered and communications with the emergency department can be made during this time.

Before the ambulance moves, you should secure the cot in place, properly position the patient, allow for respiratory or cardiac emergencies, adjust constricting straps, loosen constricting clothing, check the airway, bandages, and splints, determine and record vital signs, check for personal effects, and reassure the patient. If a relative or friend of the patient is to be transported, follow local protocol and assure the safety of this passenger.

En route to the hospital, continue basic life support and basic EMT-level care as required, take patient information when practical, radio the emergency department, monitor vital signs at least once every five minutes, check bandages and splints, collect vomitus and suction when required, and advise the driver of changing conditions. Talk to the responsive patient in a calm professional manner.

If cardiac arrest develops, have the driver stop the ambulance while you initiate CPR. Signal the driver to start up again once CPR has been properly established.

Communications while en route should provide the emergency department staff with a brief description of the situation, a review of the subjective interview and the objective examination (including vital signs), the suspected medical problem or nature of the injury, the emergency care rendered, and the estimated time of arrival. Alert the staff of any changes in the patient's condition while en route.

Make an orderly transfer of the patient, patient information, and the patient's personal effects upon arrival at the medical facility. Unload and transfer the patient in accordance with local guidelines. The handoff of the patient occurs only when the staff assumes the responsibility for care of the patient. Assist the staff as required. Obtain a release before leaving the medical facility.

The termination of activities for an ambulance run takes place at the hospital, while en route to quarters, and while in quarters. Before leaving the hospital, clean the ambulance as required, replace respiratory equipment and expendable items (local policy), and exchange equipment in need of repair (local policy). Make up the wheeled ambulance stretcher.

Radio the dispatcher and return to quarters, airing the patient compartment as needed and replenishing the fuel supply.

When in quarters, complete the report, dispose of dirty linens, remove and clean patient care and respiratory equipment as required, clean and sanitize the ambulance interior as required, care for yourself, replace needed items and replenish oxygen and air cylinders, replace patient care equipment, maintain the ambulance as needed, clean the exterior as required, and ready yourself for the next response.

20
communications and reports

OBJECTIVES By the end of this chapter, you should be able to:

1. Define "communications." (p. 444)

2. List four ways to improve your oral communication skills. (p. 444)

3. State the four basic components of an emergency communications system. (p. 444)

4. List at least FOUR ways in which this communications system may be expanded. (p. 444-5)

5. Give TEN rules to follow in regard to ambulance radio communications. (p. 445)

6. State when you can use codes in a radio communication. (p. 445)

7. List the information that can be gained from an accurate and complete ambulance run report. (p. 445, 8)

SKILLS As an EMT, you should be able to:

1. Present oral reports in a calm professional manner.

2. Conduct proper radio communications.

3. Complete all reports required by your system.

TERMS   you may be using for the first time:

Communications—all conversations, radio transmissions, and written reports that are part of an EMT's official duties.

Base Communication Station—the transmitter/receiver station at the dispatch center. It usually has the ability for two-way communications with the ambulance and the hospital, to put the hospital in communication with the ambulance, connect phone and radio communications, and to bring in communications with other appropriate services.

Transmitter/Receiver—a two-way radio.

Remote Center—the transmitter/receiver system at the emergency department. Usually, the transmissions go through the dispatch base station and are relayed to the ambulance.

Ambulance Repeater Station—a station that will retransmit between the ambulance radio and portable 2-way units so that portable transmitter/receivers can be used by the EMTs when they are at the scene but away from the ambulance.

COMMUNICATION

In emergency care, communication means more than radio transmissions. Being able to talk with people is an important trait of an EMT. You must be able to talk with bystanders at the scene so that they will give you information and let you take charge. An efficient patient assessment may depend on your ability to ask a patient questions and listen to his statements. Personal interaction is one of the most important things in gaining patient confidence and it is the main approach that you take when dealing with patients having stress reactions, emotional emergencies, or psychological emergencies.

Your ability to communicate with others is very important when interacting with the members of the EMS System. On a typical ambulance run, you may have to talk with the dispatcher, other members of the ambulance crew, First Responders, other EMTs responding to the scene, and the emergency department staff. You must be able to speak clearly and calmly, using the correct terminology to allow for effective oral communication. You also must be able to listen to others. The ability to listen to others so that they have confidence in you as a member of the patient care team is a major skill you must develop as an EMT.

To improve your skills in oral communications while on duty:

1. Use correct terminology whenever possible. Do not use layperson's terms or slang.

2. Do not use a term unless you know its meaning.

3. Use complete sentences when you speak.

4. Speak calmly using a neutral tone.

In addition to oral communications skills, you will have to develop written skills as they apply to your duties as an EMT. Just as listening is an important part of oral communication, reading is a major element in written communications skills. Make certain that you read reports and memoranda. Too many people scan over documents, missing important information.

Your written reports are very important. Make certain that they are filled in correctly, they are complete and accurate, and the correct terminology has been used.

RADIO COMMUNICATIONS

We have covered radio communications between the EMT and the dispatcher, and the ambulance and the emergency department (Chapters 14 and 18). We also have stressed that you should make use of radio communications with the dispatcher to obtain the help you need at an accident, or when hazardous materials are at the scene. In this chapter, the radio communications system and some general considerations about its use will be covered.

The Emergency Communications System

The basic communications system includes:

1. The dispatcher base station

2. The ambulance transmitter/receiver

3. The emergency department remote center

4. Telephone line backup.

With these components, the ambulance can send and receive messages from the dispatcher and the emergency department.

This system can be expanded in many ways, including:

- Portable transmitter/receivers—to allow EMTs at the scene to communicate with each other, and to send and receive messages while they are at the scene but away from the ambulance.

- Ambulance repeater stations—to retransmit between the two-way radio and the portable units.

- Biotelemetry—to send to the emergency department an electrocardiogram (ECG) while it is being taken at the scene.

- Telephone patches—done via the dispatcher base station to allow radio communications to be connected with telephones.

Ambulance Communications Procedures

The Federal Communications Commission has allocated certain frequencies for emergency medical use. They have ruled, ''Except for test transmissions, stations licensed to ambulance operators or rescue squads may be used only for the transmission of messages pertaining to the safety of life or property and urgent messages necessary for the rendition of an efficient ambulance or emergency rescue service.'' This means that you are to use the ambulance radio for official use only. Your calls are to relate to your duties and they are to be carried out in a professional manner.

When using the radio:

1. Do not try to transmit if other EMS personnel are using the channel or the dispatcher is sending to you.
2. Speak into the microphone using normal voice volume. Keep the tone of your voice neutral, and slow down your rate of speech.
3. Speak clearly, making an effort to pronounce each word distinctly.
4. Be brief, using the correct terms and phrases needed to make your message understood. Know what you are going to say before you press the transmit key.
5. Avoid using codes and abbreviations, unless they are part of your system and will be understood by the person receiving the message.
6. Receive a full message from the sender. Do not attempt to cut him off so that you can send.
7. Do not use slang or profanity.
8. Do not use individuals' names. Use unit, dispatch, and hospital identifications.
9. Politeness is understood to be part of every radio transmission. Do not use ''please,'' ''thank you,'' and other such terms.
10. If you do not understand something that is said while receiving, ask for a repeat. NEVER pretend to understand what was said.

Codes

Many EMS Systems use some form of code in their radio communications. Do NOT use a code unless it is part of your system. If the code is not used by the emergency department, then you have wasted time and a transmission.

One of the most popular codes being used is the ''10-Code.'' Efficient use of this code helps to reduce transmission time. Table 20.1 gives some examples

of this code. The codes from 10-1 to 10-34 should not be altered. Codes 10-35 to 10-39 are reserved. Codes from 10-40 and up can be used according to local assignment.

Table 20.1: Examples from the 10-Code

10-1	Signal weak
10-2	Signal strong
10-3	Stop transmitting
10-4	Affirmative
10-7	Out of service
10-8	In service
10-9	Repeat
10-10	Negative
10-17	Enroute
10-18	Urgent
10-20	Location
10-22	Disregard
10-26	Estimated time of arrival
10-30	Danger
10-33	Emergency (help)

REPORTS

Reports can be oral or written. When you radio the emergency department from the scene or during transport, this is an oral report. Upon arrival at the medical facility, you will be giving an oral report to the emergency department staff. Your report is to be brief yet accurate and complete, and presented in a calm professional manner. The information you give in oral reports becomes part of the patient's medical record.

Written reports are very important in an EMS System. They help keep track of patient information, provide the emergency department with this information, serve as part of the medical record, and supply information on personnel and equipment usage and needs.

In Chapters 1 and 3, certain aspects of the written report were covered. Written reports may involve:

- Patient assessment and care forms (also called field or street forms)
- Special assessment forms (e.g., neurological)
- Ambulance run reports
- Release forms when consent is not granted
- Release forms for patients' possessions
- Vehicle inspection forms

Many systems have combined most of these forms so that one report will cover all the needed information. An example of such a form is shown in Figure 20-1 and 20-2.

Montgomery County-Fire/Rescue Services

COMPLETED BY FIRST DUE UNIT   EMERGENCY MEDICAL INCIDENT REPORT

L O C A T I O N   I N F O R M A T I O N

A | 5 | 0 | Incident No. | Time | Date | Station Run No. | Change ☐
| 1 | 2 | 3 | 7 | Out: | On Scene: | In: | | Delete ☐

B Incident Type | Action Taken | Occupant
| | 10 | 11 | | 12 |

C Address · Location | | City
| 13 | | 45 |

D Census Tract | District | Property Classification | Complex | Individual
| 46 | 50 | 51 | 52 | 53 | 54 | 55 | 57 |

COMPLETE FOR EACH UNIT RESPONDING

U N I T   I N F O R M A T I O N

K | 6 | 0 | Incident No. | Suf. | Unit | Assigned Station | Responded From | Disposition | ☐ 22 = No Service | ☐ Transfer Station No.
| 1 | 2 | 3 | 7 | 8 | 9 | 13 | 14 | 15 | 16 | 17 | ☐ 11 = In Serv. W/Respond | ☐ 33 = Serv. Rend. | ☐ 44 = Serv. Refused | 18 | 19

L Unit Operation
☐ 1 = None   ☐ 4 = First-Aid/Rescue   ☐ 7 = Other
☐ 2 = Search/Rescue ☐ 5 = Investigation   ☐ 8 = Med Amb
☐ 3 = Extinguishment ☐ 6 = Ventilation/Salvage ☐ 9 = Medic

Personnel on Unit
ON UNIT | Pd. | Vol. | AT SC. | Pd. | Vol. | AT ST. | Pd. | Vol.
20 | 21 | 22 | | 23 | 24 | 25 | 26 | | 27 | 28 | 29 | 30

U Observations Upon Arrival
Loc ☐ 1 ☐ 4 | Pupils | Moisture | Patient Code on Arrival | Paramedic
☐ 2 ☐ 5 | ☐ Dilated Fixed ☐ Responsive | ☐ Dry Skin ☐ Normal | 1 2 3 4
☐ 3 ☐ 6 | ☐ Unequal ☐ Constricted | ☐ Moist.

V Color | Temp | Other | Patient Code Enroute | Base Physician
☐ Normal ☐ Pale | ☐ Hot ☐ Normal | ☐ Vomiting ☐ Hemorrhaging | 1 2 3 4
☐ Cyanotic ☐ Flushed | ☐ Cold | ☐ Convulsing

W Chief Complaint and Onset | Hx | Allergies

X Treatment Before Arrival | Pts Physician | Next of Kin

Y IV | | Medication
Time | Solution | Amount | Site | Treatment | Drug | Amount | Route

| Time | Pulse | Resp | BP | | | | |
| EKG | | | | | | | |

| Time | Pulse | Resp | BP | | | | |
| EKG | | | | | | | |

| Time | Pulse | Resp | BP | | | | |
| EKG | | | | | | | |

| Time | Pulse | Resp | BP | | | | |
| EKG | | | | | | | |

| Time | Pulse | Resp | BP | | | | |
| EKG | | | | | | | |

Q | 2 | 0 | Age | Sex | Male (M) | Part of Body Affected | Nature of Illness or Injury
| 1 | 2 | 14 | 16 | Female (F) | 17 | 18 | 19 | 20 | 22

R Treatment Performed | Disposition | Hospital | Transported
| 23 | 24 | 25 | 26 | 27 | Routine (R) or Emergency (E) | 28

S Name | Notifications
| ☐ Police ☐ Next of Kin

T Address

EMS-100 (REV. 1/1/78)

HOSPITAL COPY

Figure 20-1: Side A of a standard report form.

EKG STRIPS — PT. HISTORY/OBSERVATION

Incident Number	Supp.

PAID	PERSONNEL	VOLUNTEER	
NAME	POSITION	NAME	POSITION

I, _____HEREBY REFUSE TREATMENT AND/OR TRANSPORT

DATE: _____ TIME: _____

SIGNATURE: _____

Figure 20-2: Side B of a standard report form.

Regardless of the forms used by your system, you will be asked to provide information that is required by all systems. Someone reading your report will be able to tell:

- An ambulance run occurred, and the date it occurred
- If it was an emergency run
- Who ordered the run (e.g., the dispatcher)
- Who made the run
- Time out of quarters
- Location of the scene and arrival time
- Assessment of the patient
- Care rendered
- Changes in the patient's condition
- Time leaving the scene
- Destination and time of arrival
- A transfer was completed
- Time back in quarters

Remember, the report must be accurate and complete, using the proper terms (correctly spelled). The report should be completed in quarters, as soon as possible.

SUMMARY

Communication involves both oral and written skills. In all communications involving EMT duties, you are to be brief yet accurate and complete. You must use the correct terminology, written or spoken, so that it can be understood. You must communicate orally in a calm professional manner.

The basic components of an EMS radio communications system are the dispatcher base station, the ambulance transmitter/receiver, and the emergency department remote center. Telephone back-up should be part of the system.

Radio communications should be limited to official use. Keep your transmission as brief as possible. Make sure you know what you are going to say before you go on the air. Make your transmission as accurate as possible. Do not interrupt someone else using the channel or the dispatcher. Remember to wait for the person who is transmitting to finish before you start your own transmission.

Use codes only if they are part of your system and the person receiving knows the code.

Your written reports should be accurate, complete, and finished as soon as possible. You should use correct terminology in your reports. The patient information in your report becomes part of the patient's medical record.

appendices

APPENDIX 1
EMT Skills

As an EMT, you will be expected to perform your duties in a calm professional manner. You must be able to apply the knowledge gained in your course to carry out the duties of an EMT-A. You must be able to perform the activities of preparation, response, gaining access, patient assessment, basic EMT-level emergency care, disentanglement, moving and transfer, transport, termination of activities, and communications and reporting. You must be able to carry out all EMT-level patient assessment and emergency care procedures.

The major skills of an EMT include being able to:

☐ Perform assigned duties in accordance with the law
☐ Properly inform patients and gain actual consent
☐ Correctly apply implied consent
☐ File the proper reports for special patient situations
☐ Apply anatomical knowledge directly to patient assessment and care procedures
☐ Use correct medical terminology in communications and reports
☐ Present proper identification at the emergency scene
☐ Relate mechanisms of injury to accident patients in order to detect possible injuries
☐ Open an airway
☐ Determine adequate breathing
☐ Determine a carotid pulse
☐ Detect and control profuse bleeding
☐ Use direct pressure, pressure dressings, elevation, pressure points, the blood pressure cuff, and tourniquets to control bleeding
☐ Use anti-shock garments for internal bleeding (optional)
☐ Complete a primary survey
☐ Gather information from bystanders
☐ Conduct a subjective patient interview
☐ Determine radial pulse rate, rhythm, and character
☐ Determine respiratory rate and character
☐ Determine blood pressure by auscultation
☐ Determine blood pressure by palpation
☐ Determine relative skin temperature
☐ Determine changes in skin color, including the indications of cyanosis
☐ Determine pupil size, equality, and reactivity
☐ Detect distal pulse and nerve activity during assessment of the upper and lower limbs
☐ Detect cervical and lower back point tenderness

☐ Use a stethoscope to determine equal air entry in the lungs
☐ Conduct an objective physical examination
☐ Complete a secondary survey
☐ Accurately record information gained during the patient assessment
☐ Detect and record changes in vital signs
☐ Detect and record changes in a patient's condition
☐ Clear partially and fully obstructed airways using back blows, manual thrusts, finger sweeps, and suction equipment for conscious patients, patients observed to have lost consciousness, and unconscious patients
☐ Establish respiratory arrest
☐ Provide mouth-to-mouth, mouth-to-nose, mouth-to-stoma, and mouth-to-mouth and nose (infants) ventilation
☐ Provide respiratory resuscitation while in transport
☐ Establish cardiac arrest
☐ Locate the CPR compression site on infants, children, and adults
☐ Deliver external chest compressions at the proper rate and depth
☐ Provide proper interposed ventilations, at the correct rate, for infants, children, and adults
☐ Provide one-rescuer CPR
☐ Provide two-rescuer CPR
☐ Carry out position changes during two-rescuer CPR
☐ Perform CPR while moving patients
☐ Provide CPR while in transport
☐ Deliver interposed ventilations by bag-valve-mask, pocket face mask, and positive pressure resuscitator (in manual mode)
☐ Select and insert an oropharyngeal airway
☐ Select and insert a nasopharyngeal airway
☐ Take apart, clean, reassemble, and test fixed and portable suction devices
☐ Take apart, clean, reassemble, and test bag-valve-mask ventilators
☐ Provide ventilations with a bag-valve-mask ventilator, with and without supplemental oxygen
☐ Set up the equipment for oxygen therapy
☐ Provide supplemental oxygen to the breathing patient, selecting the proper delivery device and flow
☐ Provide supplemental oxygen to the breathing COPD patient, selecting the proper delivery device and flow
☐ Provide oxygen to nonbreathing patients by using the bag-valve-mask ventilator with supplemental oxygen, the pocket face mask with supplemental oxygen, and the positive pressure resuscitator
☐ Provide oxygen using the demand valve resuscitator in the patient demand mode
☐ Transfer patients receiving oxygen to the ambulance

and from the ambulance to the emergency department

☐ Provide oxygen while in transport

☐ Determine when patients need supplemental oxygen based on symptoms and signs

☐ Detect external bleeding

☐ Control external bleeding

☐ Estimate external blood loss

☐ Detect possible internal bleeding based on symptoms, signs, and mechanism of injury

☐ Estimate possible internal blood loss

☐ Detect shock based on symptoms and signs

☐ Detect anaphylactic shock based on symptoms and signs

☐ Treat for shock

☐ Position patients to prevent fainting

☐ Detect soft tissue injuries and determine their type

☐ Expose, clear, dress, and bandage open wounds

☐ Use occlusive dressings for open chest wounds, open abdominal wounds, and bleeding from major neck veins

☐ Preserve and transport avulsed and amputated tissues

☐ Provide care for wounds to the scalp, face, eyes, nose, ears, mouth, and neck

☐ Provide care for an object impaled in the eye

☐ Provide care for an avulsed eye

☐ Provide care for an object impaled in the cheek

☐ Provide care for a nosebleed

☐ Provide care when there are clear or bloody fluids flowing from the nose and/or ears

☐ Wash debris from the eyes

☐ Provide care for acid and alkaline burns of the eyes

☐ Provide care for light burns of the eyes

☐ Provide care for heat burns of the eyes

☐ Remove contact lenses from a patient's eyes

☐ Provide care for unconscious patients' eyes

☐ Stabilize an impaled object

☐ Provide care for soft tissue wounds of the chest that do not puncture the thoracic cavity

☐ Detect possible internal abdominal injury

☐ Care for open and closed abdominal injury

☐ Place, apply, deflate, and remove anti-shock garments for cases of abdominal injury as to local protocol (optional)

☐ Detect and care for injuries to the pelvis and groin

☐ Identify injuries to the extremities based upon symptoms and signs

☐ Provide soft tissue injury care to the extremities

☐ Straighten mildly angulated closed fractures of the humerus, radius, ulna, femur, tibia, and fibula

☐ Straighten angulations of the elbow, knee, and ankle in accordance with local protocol

☐ Utilize slings and swathes, upper extremity rigid board splints, lower extremity rigid board splints, air-inflated splints, pillow splints, and traction splints

☐ Provide care for fractures and dislocations of the pectoral girdle

☐ Provide care for fractures of the humerus

☐ Provide care for fractures and dislocations of the elbow

☐ Provide care for fractures of the forearm and wrist

☐ Provide care for fractures of the hand and fingers

☐ Provide care for pelvic fractures

☐ Provide care for anterior and posterior hip dislocations

☐ Provide care for fractures of the femur

☐ Provide care for fractures and dislocations of the knee

☐ Provide care for fractures of the leg and ankle

☐ Provide care for fractures of the foot

☐ Evaluate nerve and vascular function for the upper and lower extremities, before and after splinting

☐ Make and utilize noncommercial splints for emergency situations

☐ Transfer and transport splinted patients

☐ Apply patient assessment techniques to detect possible cranial fractures and facial fractures

☐ Apply patient assessment techniques to detect possible brain injury

☐ Apply patient assessment techniques to detect possible spinal injury

☐ Apply patient assessment techniques to detect possible blunt trauma to the chest, fractured ribs, and flail chest

☐ Detect and provide care for pneumothorax

☐ Detect and provide care for pneumothorax with tension pneumothorax

☐ Detect and provide basic life support for traumatic asphyxia

☐ Detect and provide basic life support for possible hemothorax, hemo-pneumothorax, and cardiac tamponade

☐ Provide basic care for possible fractured skull and facial bones

☐ Provide basic care for possible brain injury

☐ Apply an extrication collar

☐ Immobilize possible spinal injury patients to a long spine board

☐ Use the four-rescuer log roll when placing patients on a long spine board

☐ Position patients for drainage

☐ Apply cravats for possible rib fracture

☐ Correct paradoxical respirations in cases of flail chest

☐ Apply patient assessment techniques to detect possible angina pectoris, impending AMI, AMI, mechanical pump failure, and congestive heart failure

☐ Provide basic care for and transport patients with possible heart disorders

☐ Assess patients for stroke

☐ Provide proper care and positioning for possible stroke patients

☐ Assess patients for possible respiratory distress and for chronic obstructive pulmonary disease

☐ Care for patients in respiratory distress, including those with COPD

☐ Evaluate and care for hyperventilation as a condition and as a sign

☐ Distinguish between possible diabetic coma (diabetic ketoacidosis) and insulin shock (hypoglycemia)

☐ Provide proper care for patients having diabetic emergencies

☐ Use medical identification devices to collect patient information

☐ Care for patients having convulsive seizures

☐ Detect and provide basic care for acute abdomen

☐ Detect and provide basic care for patients with possible infectious diseases

☐ Provide care, protecting yourself from infectious disease

☐ Exercise proper personal hygiene after contact with patients who may have an infectious disease

☐ Ready the ambulance and its equipment and supplies after transporting patients who may have an infectious disease

☐ Detect possible cases of poisoning

☐ Call the poison control center, provide patient information, and carry out orders given by the staff at the center

☐ Administer Syrup of Ipecac and activated charcoal and water

☐ Collect vomitus at the scene and in transport

☐ Provide initial basic care for snakebites

☐ Detect and care for possible alcohol abuse and withdrawal

☐ Detect and care for possible drug abuse and withdrawal

☐ Evaluate a woman in labor

☐ Use all items in the sterile emergency obstetric pack

☐ Prepare an expectant mother for delivery, including the use of sheets or towels to properly cover her

☐ Assist a woman in the delivery of her baby

☐ Provide postdelivery care for the newborn, including proper airway and umbilical cord care

☐ Provide resuscitative measures for newborns in respiratory and cardiac arrest

☐ Assist a woman in the delivery of the placenta

☐ Provide postdelivery care for the mother, including emotional support and care for postdelivery bleeding

☐ Collect and transport the afterbirth

☐ Provide basic care for predelivery, delivery, and postdelivery complications, including the proper administration of oxygen

☐ Provide basic care and needed life support procedures for abnormal deliveries, including breech and premature birth.

☐ Administer oxygen properly for the newborn, when required, using the "tent method"

☐ Accurately record a birth

☐ Evaluate a woman for possible eclampsia, ectopic pregnancy, and abortion, and provide the appropriate care

☐ Assist a woman with a multiple delivery

☐ Provide emotional support in cases of stillborn infants

☐ Determine if a patient is an infant or a child

☐ Conduct a primary and secondary survey on infants and children

☐ Provide basic life support to infants and children

☐ Detect and care for head injury in infants and children

☐ Control your emotions during a pediatric emergency

☐ Interview child patients

☐ Provide emotional support in cases of possible sudden infant death syndrome

☐ Relate symptoms and signs to possible child abuse

☐ Classify burns as first, second, or third degree

☐ Use the rule of nines to determine the severity of burns

☐ Provide care for thermal burns

☐ Provide care for chemical burns

☐ Provide care for electrical burns

☐ Provide care for radiation burns

☐ Provide care for cases of smoke inhalation

☐ Detect and care for heat cramps, heat exhaustion, and heatstroke

☐ Detect and care for incipient frostbite, superficial frostbite, and deep frostbite (freezing)

☐ Care for superficial and deep frostbite when transport is delayed

☐ Detect, classify as to severity, and provide proper care for hypothermia

☐ Provide care, to the level of your training, at special emergencies (electrical accidents, hazardous materials accidents, and radiation accidents)

☐ Follow local protocol to request the appropriate help when the scene involves electrical hazards, hazardous materials, and radioactivity

☐ Use appropriate patient assessment techniques at the scene of an accident involving an explosion

☐ Evaluate victims of swimming or diving accidents

☐ Solve basic problems faced in reaching patients in water- and ice-related accidents

☐ Apply resuscitative measures to near-drowning patients

☐ Work as a member of a team to turn patients in the water and place them on a long spine board (optional)

☐ Determine if patients may be having a possible stress reaction, emotional emergency, or psychiatric emergency

☐ Use personal interaction for cases of stress reaction, emotional emergency, and psychiatric emergency

☐ Initiate crisis management when appropriate

☐ Conduct efficient interviews with elderly patients

☐ Establish effective communications with deaf patients

☐ Provide care and comfort for blind patients

☐ Establish some form of communication with nonEnglish speaking patients

☐ Provide proper care for aggressive patients, when your own safety is assured

☐ Provide proper care for patients attempting suicide, when your own safety is assured

☐ Provide care at the controlled crime scene, helping to preserve the chain of evidence

☐ Provide care for rape victims, considering their emotional needs, privacy, comfort, and dignity, but preserving the chain of evidence

☐ Initiate and conduct triage

☐ Provide care when triage is in effect

☐ Apply basic assessment skills to triage

☐ Follow local protocol when providing care in a situation controlled by a disaster plan

☐ Reduce stress on rescuers during a disaster

☐ Properly conduct a daily inspection of the ambulance

☐ Receive information from a dispatcher

☐ Drive an ambulance in accordance to the laws of your state

☐ Use emergency and defensive driving skills to avoid accidents while driving the ambulance

☐ Correctly use warning devices found on the ambulance

☐ Properly position an ambulance, taking into consideration the traffic, the roadway, and known hazards

☐ Control hazards at the emergency scene, doing only what you have been trained to do and using the required safety equipment

☐ Protect yourself if you find that you are in a building that is on fire

☐ Reach patients trapped in buildings by gaining access through locked doors and windows, doing only what you have been trained to do

☐ Reach patients trapped in vehicles by gaining access through locked doors, through windows, and through the vehicle body (optional), doing only what you have been trained to do

☐ Effectively evaluate an emergency and summon the appropriate services to aid in scene control and gaining access

☐ Properly protect patients during disentanglement

☐ Make a pathway through the wreckage by helping to:

- Raise a crushed vehicle roof
- Remove the top of a vehicle
- Widen vehicle door openings

☐ Remove wreckage from the patient by helping to:

- Cut a seat belt
- Remove a steering wheel
- Displace a steering column
- Displace a vehicle floor pedal
- Displace a dash
- Displace a vehicle seat

☐ Decide when an emergency or nonemergency move is necessary

☐ Carry out one-, two-, and three-rescuer moves

☐ Package patients for transfer and transport

☐ Use the wheeled ambulance stretcher to transfer patients

☐ Use the stair chair, scoop-style stretcher, and basket stretcher to transfer patients

☐ Apply a short spine board to patients found in a vehicle or confined space and move them to a long spine board

☐ Move patients to a long spine board by the four-rescuer straddle slide and a rope sling

☐ Move patients to a long spine board when found under the dashboard or between the front and rear seat of an automobile

☐ Physically and mentally ready patients for transport

☐ Take vital signs and provide needed basic EMT-level care during transport

☐ Relay, by radio, patient information to the emergency department

☐ Conduct an orderly handoff of patients

☐ Carry out all activities necessary at the medical facility, en route to quarters, and in quarters to ready the ambulance and crew for service

☐ Present oral reports in a calm, professional manner

☐ Conduct proper radio communications

☐ Complete all reports required by your system

APPENDIX 2
Ambulance Supplies and Equipment

Basic Supplies

Patient Protection

- Two pillows
- Four pillow cases
- Four sheets
- Two spare sheets
- Four blankets (number may vary according to climate)

Patient's Personal Needs

- Four towels
- Six disposable emesis bags
- Two boxes of tissues
- One bedpan
- Four towels

Patient Monitoring

- Two sphygmomanometers
- Two stethoscopes
- One thermometer (oral type)

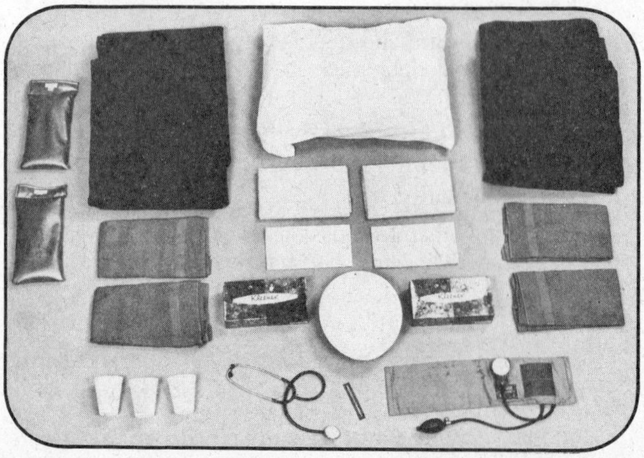

Figure A2-1: Basic ambulance supplies.

Equipment for the Transfer of Patients

- One wheeled stretcher
- One folding ambulance stretcher
- One folding stair chair
- One scoop-style (orthopedic) stretcher

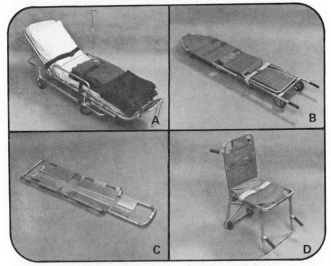

Figure A2-2: Patient carrying devices—wheeled (a); folding (b); scoop-type stretchers (c); folding stair chair (d).

Equipment for the Transfer of Newborns It is not suggested that an incubator be carried on all ambulances. All ambulance units should be able to acquire an incubator without delay, however, from a local hospital. The incubator should be provided with these items:

- A crib
- Three hot water bottles
- One quilted pad
- One baby blanket

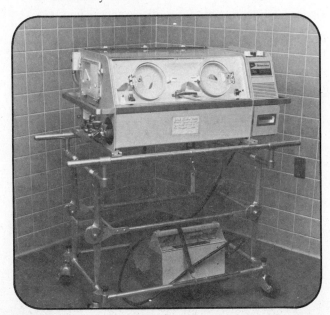

Figure A2-3: A transport incubator.

- Two diapers
- One room thermometer
- One rubber suction bulb with trap
- Three umbilical clamps and/or tape
- One rubber suction bulb
- One funnel with tube
- One portable oxygen cylinder
- One bottle of 70% alcohol

Equipment for Airway Maintenance

Airways

- Oropharyngeal airways in sizes for adults, children, and infants
- Nasopharyngeal airways for adults and children

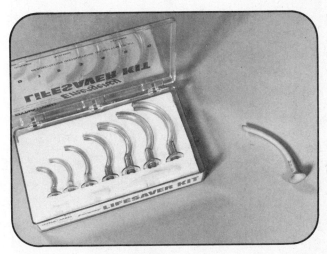

Figure A2-4: Adjunct airways.

Suction Equipment

- One fixed suction system
- One portable suction system

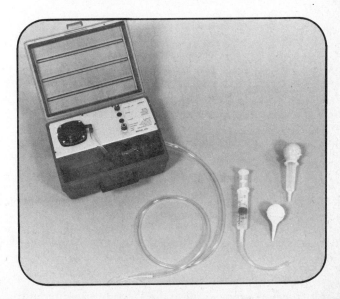

Figure A2-5: Suction equipment.

Artificial Ventilation Devices

- Two manually operated, self-filling bag-valve-mask units (one adult's and one child's)
- One pocket face mask
- One manually triggered oxygen supply device
- One positive pressure demand valve resuscitator (may be a combination device having manual mode)

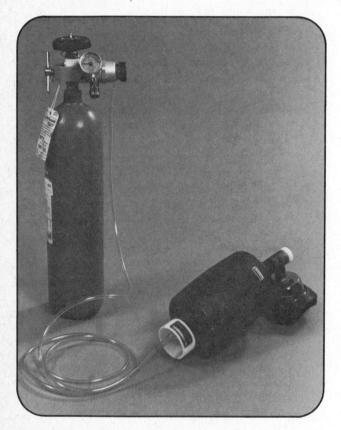

Figure A2-6: Equipment for ventilation.

Oxygen Therapy Equipment

- One fixed oxygen delivery system
- One portable oxygen delivery system

The above should include supplies of tubing, nasal cannulas, and various masks.

Equipment for Cardiac Compressions

There are no devices that are recommended for mechanical chest compression during CPR efforts. It is suggested, however, that some device be carried to assist in manual CPR efforts.

Spine boards that are generally carried on ambulances for the immobilization of neck and back injuries can be used to great advantage during CPR efforts. A short spine board offers the rigidity that is necessary for chest compression efforts to be effective.

CPR boards are available from vendors of emergency care supplies. These devices offer rigidity and

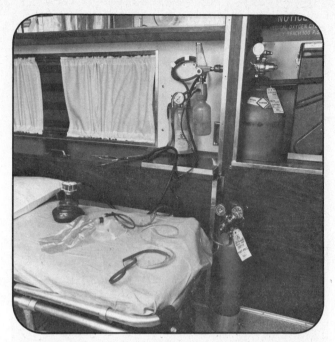

Figure A2-7: Oxygen delivery equipment.

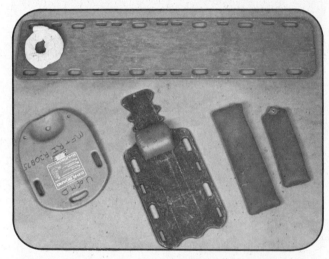

Figure A2-8: Equipment for cardiac compressions.

at the same time properly place the patient's head in the backward-tilt position that is recommended for airway maintenance.

Supplies for Immobilizing Fractures

- A rigid, hinged, half-ring, lower extremity traction splint with limb-support straps, a padded ankle hitch, and a traction strap with buckle, or. . .
- A telescoping traction splint unit
- A number of other immobilization devices should be carried, depending on the policy established by the unit medical director. Typically, the ambulance should carry: upper extremity padded board splints; lower extremity padded board splints; and air-inflatable splints.

- Triangular bandages
- Long and short spine boards, or in place of short spine boards, vest-type immobilization devices.
- Six web straps with aircraft style buckles
- Two sand bags

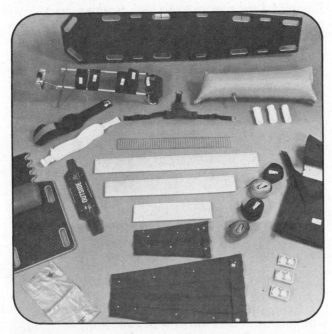

Figure A2-9: Supplies for immobilizing fractures.

Supplies and Equipment for Treating Shock

- A pneumatic counterpressure device (anti-shock garment, MAST unit) with inflation equipment
- Aluminum survival blankets

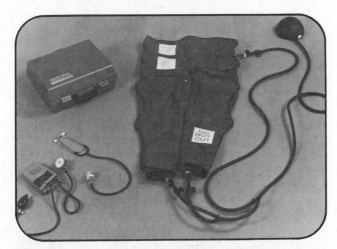

Figure A2-10: Anti-shock garment.

Supplies for Dressing and Bandaging Wounds

- Sterile gauze pads in a variety of sizes

- Sterile universal dressings approximately 10 × 36 in. when unfolded
- Soft, self-adhering roller bandages in various widths
- Sterile, nonporous, nonadherent occlusive dressings
- Wide adhesive tape
- Safety pins
- Bandage shears

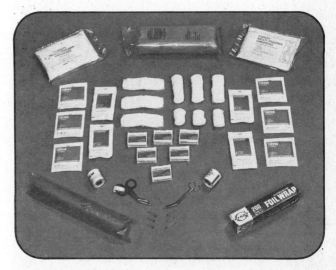

Figure A2-11: Supplies for dressing and bandaging.

Supplies for Childbirth

A sterile childbirth kit is recommended.

- One pair of surgical scissors
- Three umbilical cord clamps or umbilical tapes
- One rubber bulb syringe
- Twelve 4 by 4 in. gauze pads

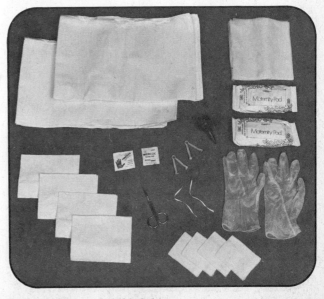

Figure A2-12: A childbirth kit.

- Five towels
- Four pairs of surgical gloves
- One baby blanket
- Sanitary napkins
- Two large plastic bags

Supplies for Treating Acute Poisoning

- Syrup of Ipecac
- Activated charcoal
- Drinking water
- Equipment for oral administration
- Equipment for irrigating the eyes
- Constriction bands for snakebite

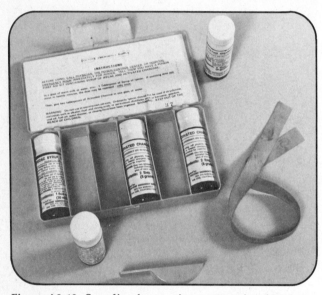

Figure A2-13: Supplies for treating acute poisoning.

Trauma (Jump) Kit

Many items on the list of recommended emergency care supplies and equipment can be carried in a kit. Thus, they become immediately available to an

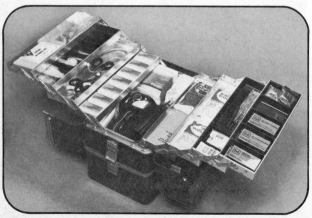

Figure A2-14: Specially prepared trauma kit.

EMT when patient care activities must be undertaken away from the ambulance. Prepared kits are commercially available, or one can be fashioned with a fishing tackle box, a soft-sided airline bag, or even a gym bag.

Special Equipment for Physicians and Qualified Paramedics

Some ambulances are provided with locked kits of supplies and equipment that can be used by physicians and trained paramedics who either travel with the ambulance or otherwise respond to the scene. Such kits include:

- IV infusion kits
- Pleural decompression kit
- Drug injection kit
- Tracheostomy or cricothyrotomy kit
- Portable cardioscope and defibrillator
- Venous cutdown kit
- Minor surgical kit
- Sterile urinary catheters

Equipment for Gaining Access and Disentanglement

Hand Tools

- One 12 in. adjustable wrench
- One 12 in. regular-blade screwdriver
- One 12 in. Phillips-type screwdriver
- One hacksaw with a minimum of 12 spare blades
- One pair of vise-grip pliers 10 in. long
- One 5-lb. hammer with a 15 in. handle
- One 24 in. flat-head fire ax
- One 24 in. wrecking bar or combination tool
- One 51 in. pinch point bar
- One 1-1/4 in. capacity bolt cutter
- One double action tin snips

Power Tools

- One portable hydraulic jack with accessories (The jack should be rated for at least 4 tons.)
- One 2-ton capacity hand winch with a rated chain set

Miscellaneous Items

- One aluminized blanket for patient protection
- Two ropes, each 3/4 in. by 50 ft.
- One folding shovel
- Two alloy steel rescue chains (one 6' and one

12', each with a slip hook on one end and a ring and a grab hook on the other
- An assortment of shoring blocks

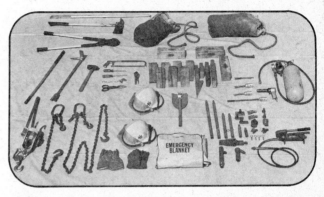

Figure A2-16: Equipment for gaining access and disentanglement

Equipment for Safeguarding Ambulance Personnel

For each EMT on the ambulance:
- A firefighter's turnout coat, preferably of fire-resistant cloth

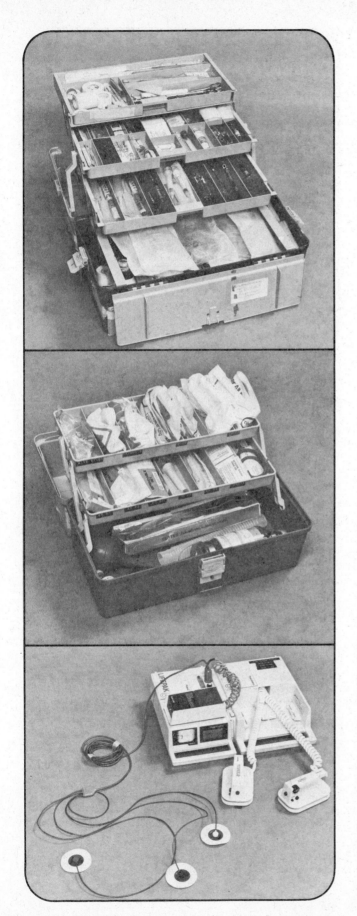

Figure A2-15: Special equipment for physicians and EMT-Ps.

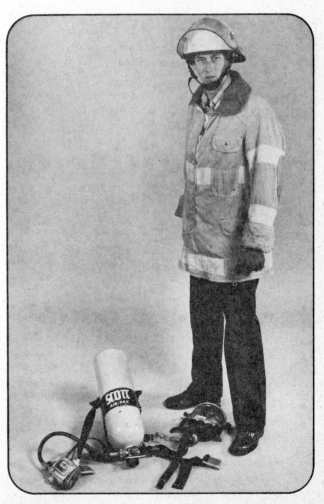

Figure A2-17: Equipment for safeguarding personnel.

- A firefighter's or construction-style safety helmet with chin strap
- A pair of coverall-type safety goggles
- A pair of leather gauntlet-type gloves

and for hazardous atmospheres:

- Two self-contained, positive pressure breathing apparatus with a minimum air supply of 30 minutes
- Two spare cylinders

Equipment for Warning, Signaling, and Lighting

- Twelve 30 min. pyrotechnic flares
- Two battery-powered hand lights
- Two 300-watt minimum portable floodlights and extension cords for 110 v. operation

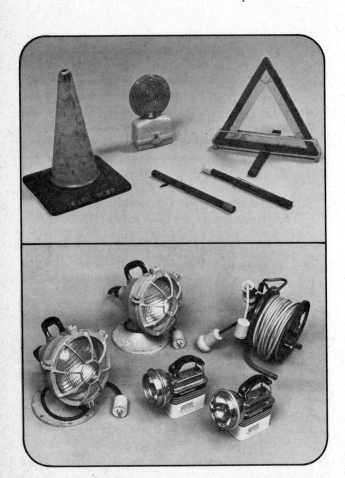

Figure A2-18: Equipment for warning, signaling, and lighting.

Equipment for Extinguishing Fire

Two 5-pound Class B:C fire extinguishers should be carried as minimum protection. An A:B:C extinguisher provides greater protection, and a 15- or 20-pound unit offers a longer extinguishing period.

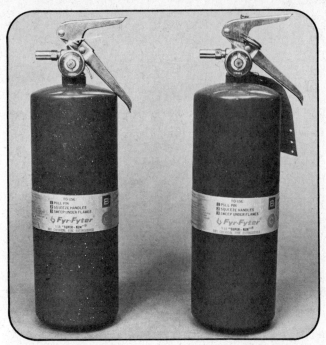

Figure A2-19: Equipment for extinguishing fire.

APPENDIX 3
Word Elements Commonly Used To Construct Medical Terms

When a dash appears after an element, the element is usually used as a prefix; i.e., it precedes other elements that combine to form the term. Likewise, when a dash appears before an element, the element is generally used as a suffix, following other elements that make up the term.

a- (absent or deficient in) AFEBRILE, without fever
ab- (away from) ABDUCT, to draw away from the midline
abdomin(o)- (abdomen) ABDOMINALGIA, pain in the abdomen
ac- (to, *see* ad-) ACCLIMATE, to become accustomed to new conditions
acid- (sour) ACIDIFY, to make sour
acou- (hear) ACOUSTIC, pertaining to sound or hearing
acr- (extremity, peak) ACROPHOBIA, fear of heights
ad- (to, the d changes to c, f, g, p, s or t when the stem begins with one of those consonants) ADDUCT, to draw toward the midline
adeno- (gland) ADENITIS, inflammation of a gland
adip(o)- (fat) ADIPOSE, fatty; fat (in size)
aer(o)- (air) AEROBIC, able to live and grow in the presence of oxygen
af- (to, *see* ad-) AFFERENT, conveying toward
ag- (to, *see* ad-) AGGREGATE, to crowd or cluster together
agra- (seizure of acute pain) PODAGRA, acute pain in the great toe
alb- (white) ALBINO, a person who has little or no normal pigmentation in his body
-algia (painful condition) NEURALGIA, pain along nerve pathways
alve- (channel, trough, cavity) ALVEOLUS, a small sac
ambi- (both) AMBIDEXTROUS, able to use both hands with equal facility, as when writing
amyl- (starch) AMYLOID, starchlike

an- (without) ANEMIA, a reduced volume of red blood cells
ana- (up, positive, excessively) ANAPHYLAXIS, the exaggerated reaction of an organism to a substance to which it has become sensitized
andr(o)- (male) ANDROID, resembling a man
angi(o)- (vessel) ANGIOCARDITIS, inflammation of the heart and blood vessels
ant- (against) ANTACID, an agent that counteracts acidity
ante- (before) ANTEBRACHIUM, the forearm
anti- (against, counter) ANTIBODY, a substance produced by one microorganism that kills or inhibits the growth of other microorganisms
ap- (to, *see* ad-) APPROXIMATE, place close to
apo- (away from, the o is dropped when the prefix is used with stems that begin with a vowel) APOPHYSIS, any swelling or outgrowth
arterio- (artery) ARTERIOGRAM, a radiograph of an artery
arthr(o)- (joint) ARTHRITIS, inflammation of a joint (or joints)
articul(o)- (join) ARTICULATED, united by joints
as- (to, *see* ad-) ASSIMILATE, to take into
at- (to, *see* ad-) ATTRACT, to draw toward
aur- (ear) AURICLE, the flap of the ear

blephar(o)- (eyelid) BLEPHARITIS, inflammation of the eyelids
-bol- (throw) EMBOLUS, a clot or other plug carried in the bloodstream
brachi- (arm) BRACHIAL, pertaining to the arm
brachy- (short) BRACHYPHALANGIA, abnormal shortness of one or more of the phalanges
brady- (slow) BRADYCARDIA, an abnormally slow heart rate
bronch- (larger air passages) BRONCHODILATOR, an agent that dilates the larger air passages
bucco- (cheek) BUCCAL, pertaining to the cheek

cac(o)- (bad; ill) CACOSMIA, a bad odor
calc- (1) (stone) CALCULUS, an abnormal hard inorganic mass (such as a gallstone)
calc- (2) (heel) CALCANEUS, the heel bone
calor- (heat) CALORIC, pertaining to heat
cancr- (cancer) CANCROID, resembling cancer
capit- (head) CAPITATE, head-shaped
caps- (container) CAPSULATION, enclosure in a capsule or container
carcin- (cancer) CARCINOGEN, a substance that causes cancer
cardi(o)- (heart) CARDIOGENIC, originating in the heart
cat(a)- (down, against, under) CATABASIS, the decline of a disease
caudi- (tail) CAUDAL, toward the tail
cav- (hollow) CAVITY, a hollow place or space
-cele (tumor, hernia, cavity) HYDROCELE, a confined collection of water
celi(o)- (abdomen) CELIOPARACENTESIS, surgical puncture of the abdominal wall
cephal(o)- (head) CEPHALIC, pertaining to the head
cerebr- (cerebrum) CEREBRAL, pertaining to the cerebrum
cervic(o)- (neck; cervix) CERVICAL, pertaining to the neck (or cervix)
cheil(o)- (lip) CHEILITIS, inflammation of the lips
cheir(o)- or chir(o)- (hand) CHEIRALGIA, pain in the hand
chole- (bile) CHOLEDOCHITIS, inflammation of the common bile duct
chondr- (cartilage) CHONDROYNIA, pain in a cartilage
chrom(o)- (color) MONOCHROMATIC, being of one color
chron(o)- (time) CHRONIC, persisting for a long time
circum- (around) CIRCUMSCRIBED, confined to a limited space
co- (with, *see* con-) COHESION, the uniting of particles
col- (with, *see* con-) COLLATERAL, a small branch to the side
colo- (colon) COLOPTOSIS, downward displacement of the colon
colp- (vagina) COLPORRHAGIA, bleeding from the vagina
com- (with, *see* con-) COMMINUTED, broken into small pieces
con- (with, becomes co- before vowels or h or w; col- before l; com- before b, m, or p; and cor- before r) CONGENITAL, existing from the time of birth
contra- (against) CONTRAINDICATED, inadvisable
cor- (with, *see* con-) CORRESPOND, to be in agreement with
core- (pupil of the eye) CORECTOPIA, abnormal location of the pupil of the eye
cost(o)- (rib) INTERCOSTAL, between the ribs

crani(o)- (skull) CRANIAL, pertaining to the skull
cry(o)- (cold) CRYOGENIC, that which produces low temperatures
crypt(o)- (concealed) CRYPTOGENIC, of doubtful origin
cut- (skin) SUBCUTANEOUS, below the skin
cyst(o)- (bladder) CYSTITIS, inflammation of the urinary bladder
-cyte (cell) LEUKOCYTE, white cell
cyt(o)- (cell) CYTOPENIA, deficiency in the cells of the blood

dacry(o)- (tear) DACRYORRHEA, excessive flow of tears
de- (from) DECAPITATION, removal of the head
dermat(o)- (skin) DERMATITIS, inflammation of the skin
-desis (a binding) SPONDYLODESIS, fusion of the spinal vertabrae
di- (two) DIPLEGIA, paralysis of like parts on either side of the body
digit- (finger, toe) DIGITAL, pertaining to the fingers (or toes)
diplo- (double) DIPLOPIA, double vision
dis- (apart) DISSECT, to cut apart
dors- (back) DORSAL, relating to the back
dur- (hard) INDURATED, abnormally hard
dys- (bad) DYSFUNCTION, impairment; abnormality

e- (out, from) EMESIS, the act of vomiting
ect(o)- (outside of, external) ECTOPIC, away from the normal position
-ectomy (excision of an organ or part) APPENDECTOMY, surgical removal of the appendix
ede- (swell) EDEMA, an abnormal accumulation of fluid
ef- (out of) EFFUSION, the escape of fluid into a part
electro- (electrical) ELECTROCARDIOGRAM, the written record of the heart's electrical activity
em- (in, on) EMPYEMA, an accumulation of pus in a cavity
-em- (blood) ANEMIA, a deficiency of red blood cells
en- (in, on, the n changes to m before b, p, m, or ph) ENCAPSULATE, to enclose within a capsule or container
encephal(o)- (brain) ENCEPHALITIS, inflammation of the brain
end(o)- (inside, within) ENDOTRACHEAL, within the trachea
enter(o)- (intestine) ENTERITIS, inflammation of the intestine
ento- (within, inner) ENTOPIC, occurring in the proper place
epi- (upon, after, in addition to) EPIDERMIS, the outermost layer of skin
erythro- (red) ERYTHROCYTE, red blood cell
eu- (normal, good) EUPHORIA, a feeling of well being
ex- (out of) EXCREMENT, waste material cast out of the body
exo- (outside, outward) EXOSKELETON, structures produced by the epidermis (hair, nails, teeth, etc.)
extra- (outside of, in addition to) EXTRACORPOREAL, outside of the body

faci(o)- (face) FACIAL, pertaining to the face
fasci- (sheet, band) FASCIA, a sheet or band of fibrous tissue
febr- (fever) FEBRILE, feverish
-ferent (bear, carry) EFFERENT, carrying away from a center
-ferous (bearing, producing) TOXIFEROUS, poisonous
fibr- (fiber) FIBRILLATION, muscular contractions due to the activity of muscle fibers
fil- (thread) FILAMENT, a delicate thread or fiber
fis- (split) FISSURE, groove
flex- (bent) FLEXIBLE, pliable; capable of being bent
-form (shape) DEFORMED, abnormally shaped
front- (forehead) FRONTAL, pertaining to the forehead
-fuge (driving away, fleeing) CENTRIFUGAL, moving away from a center
funct- (perform, serve) FUNCTION, the action of a body organ or part

galact(o)- (milk) GALACTOPYRIA, milk fever
gangli(o)- (ganglion) GANGLIOFORM, having the shape of a knot-like mass
gastr(o)- (stomach) GASTRITIS, inflammation of the stomach
gelat- (congeal) GELATINOUS, like jelly
gen- (originate, become) GENETIC, inherited
-gen (an agent that produces) ANTIGEN, a substance capable of inducing antibody formation
-genic (causing) ALLERGENIC, capable of causing hypersensitivity
genit(o)- (organs of reproduction) GENITALIA, the reproductive organs

germ- (bud) GERMINATE, to sprout

gest- (bear, carry) GESTATION, the period of development of an offspring in the uterus

gloss(o)- (tongue) GLOSSAL, pertaining to the tongue

glutin- (glue) GLUTINOUS, sticky

glyc- (sweet) GLYCEMIA, the presence of sugar in the blood

gnath(o)- (jaw) GNATHITIS, inflammation of the jaw

-gram (a written record) ELECTROENCEPHALOGRAM, a written record of the brain's electrical activity

gran- (particle) GRANULATION, the formation of small, rounded masses of tissue in wounds during healing

grav- (heavy) GRAVID, pregnant

gyn(e)(eco)(o)- (woman) GYNECOLOGIST, a specialist in diseases of a woman's genital tract

gyr- (ring, circle) GYROSPASMS, spasms of the head that result in rotating movements

helc- (sore) HELCOID, like an ulcer

hem(at)- (blood) HEMATEMESIS, the vomiting of blood

hemi- (half) HEMIPLEGIA, paralysis of one side of the body

hepat(o)- (liver) HEPATITIS, inflammation of the liver

heter(o)- (other) HETEROGENEOUS, from a different source

hidr(o)- (sweat) HIDROUS, containing water

hist(o)(io)- (tissue) HISTODYALYSIS, the breaking down of tissue

homeo- (similar, same) HOMEOSTASIS, stability in an organism's normal physiological states

homo- (same, common) HOMOGENEOUS, of the same structure

hyal(o)- (glassy) HYALINE, glassy, transparent

hydr(o)- (water) HYDROCEPHALUS, an accumulation of cerebrospinal fluid in the skull with resulting enlargement of the head

hyper- (above; beyond) HYPERTENSION, abnormally high blood pressure

hypno- (sleep) HYPNOTIC, that which induces sleep

hypo- (under, below, the o is dropped before words that start with a vowel) HYPOTENSION, abnormally low blood pressure

hyster(o)- (womb) HYSTERECTOMY, surgical removal of the uterus

-ia (state, condition) TACHYCARDIA, a condition of the heart characterized by an abnormally rapid heart rate

-iasis (state, condition) HYPOCHONDRIASIS, abnormal anxiety about one's health

iatr(o)- (physician) IATROGENIC, caused by a physician

idio- (peculiar, self) IDIOPATHIC, occurring without a known cause

il- (negative prefix) ILLEGIBLE, cannot be read

ile- (ileum) ILEITIS, inflammation of the ileum

ili(o)- (ilium) ILIAC, pertaining to the ilium

im- (negative prefix) IMBALANCE, a lack of balance

in- (negative prefix) INCURABLE, not capable of being cured

in- (in, on) INCISE, to cut with a sharp instrument

infra- (beneath) INFRACOSTAL, beneath a rib

insul- (island) INSULIN, a protein secreted by cells of the Islands of Langerhans in the pancreas

inter- (between, among) INTERCOSTAL, between two ribs

intra- (inside, within) INTRAORAL, within the mouth

-ion (process) EXTRACTION, the process of drawing out

ir- (negative prefix) IRREDUCIBLE, not susceptible to reduction

irid- (colored circle, iris of the eye) IRIDOTOMY, incision of the iris

ischi- (hip) ISCHIALGIA, pain in the ischium

iso- (equal) ISOMETRIC, of equal dimensions

-itis (inflammation) PHLEBITIS, inflammation of a vein

jact- (throw) JACTITATION, restless tossing about during an acute illness

junct- (yoke, join) JUNCTION, a meeting place

kerat(o)- (horny tissue, cornea) KERATITIS, inflammation of the cornea

keto- (ketone bodies) KETOSIS, excessive ketone bodies in the tissues or fluids

kin(e)- (movement) KINESALGIA, pain caused by muscular movement

kinesi(o)- (movement) KINESIA, motion sickness

labio- (lip) LABIODENTAL, pertaining to the lip and teeth

lact(o)- (milk) LACTATE, to secrete milk

lal- (speech) LALOPATHY, any speech disorder

laparo- (flank, abdomen) LAPAROTOMY, an incision through the abdominal wall

laryng(o)- (larynx) LARYNGOSCOPE, an instrument for examining the larynx

lepto- (slender) LEPTODACTYOUS, having slender fingers

leuk(o)- (white) LUEKEMIA, a malignant disease characterized by the increased development of white blood cells

lig- (tie) LIGATE, to tie a vessel

lingua- (tongue) SUBLINGUAL, under the tongue

lip(o)- (fat) LIPOID, fat-like

lith(o)- (stone) LITHOTOMY, an incision made in a duct or organ so that a stone can be removed

log(o)- (words, speech) LOGOSPASMS, spasmodic speech

-logy (science of) BIOLOGY, the science of living things

lumb(o)- (loin) LUMBAGO, pain in the lumbar region

-lysis (dissolution) DIALYSIS, the process of separating parts of a solution

macr(o)- (large, abnormal size) MACROCEPHALOUS, having an abnormally large head

mal- (bad, abnormal) MALADY, a disease or illness

mamm(o)- (breast, mammary gland) MAMMARY, pertaining to the breast or mammary gland

mani- (mental aberration) KLEPTOMANIAC, one who has impulses to steal

masto- (breast) MASTECTOMY, surgical removal of the breast

medi- (middle) MEDIASTINUM, middle partition

mega- (great, large) MEGACOLON, an abnormally large colon

megal(o)- (great, abnormal enlargement) MEGALOMANIA, abnormal self-esteem

-megaly (enlargement) CARDIOMEGALY, enlargement of the heart

melan(o)- (black, melanin) MELANOMA, a tumor comprised of pigmented cells

mening(o)- (meninges) MENINGITIS, inflammation of the meninges

mens- (month) MENOPAUSE, cessation of menstruation

mes(o)- (middle) MESIAD, toward the center

meta- (change, transformation) METAMORPHOSIS, a change of shape or structure

metra-, metro- (uterus) METRALGIA, pain in the uterus

micr(o)- (small) MICROSCOPE, an instrument for magnifying

mono- (one, single) MONOPLEGIA, paralysis of a single part

morph(o)- (form, shape) MORPHOLOGY, the science of form and shape

-morphic (pertaining to form or shape) POLYMORPHIC, occurring in several forms

multi- (many) MULTIPARA, a woman who has had two or more pregnancies

my(o)- (muscle) MYASTHENIA, muscular weakness

myc(o)- (fungus) MYCOSIS, any disease caused by a fungus

myel(o)- (marrow, often refers to spinal cord) MYELOCELE, protrusion of the spinal cord through a defect in the spinal column

myx(o)- (mucus, slime) MYXOID, resembling mucus

narco- (stupor) NARCOTIC, an agent that induces sleep

naso- (nose) NASO-ORAL, pertaining to the nose and mouth

necr(o)- (death) NECROTIC, dead (when referring to tissue)

neo- (new) NEONATE, a newborn infant

nephr(o)- (kidney) NEPHRALGIA, pain in the kidneys

neur(o)- (nerve) NEURITIS, inflammation of nerve pathways

norm(o)- (normal, usual) NORMOTENSION, normal blood pressure

nyct(o)- (night) NYCTALOPIA, night blindness

ob- (against, toward, the b changes to c before words beginning with c) OBTURATOR, a device that closes an opening

oc- (against, *see* ob-) OCCLUDE, to obstruct

ocul(o)- (eye) OCULAR, pertaining to the eye

odont(o)- (tooth) ODONTALGIA, toothache

-odyn- (pain) GASTRODYNIA, pain in the stomach

-oid (resembling) SPHEROID, resembling a ball or sphere

ole(o)- (oil) OLEOTHERAPY, treatment with injections of oil

olig(o)- (few, little) OLIGEMIA, lacking in blood volume

-oma (tumor) MYOMA, a muscular tumor

onco- (tumor, swelling) ONCOTOMY, excision of a tumor

oo- (egg, ovum) OOBLAST, a primitive cell from which an ovum develops

oophor(o)- (ovary) OOPHORECTOMY, a surgical removal of one or both ovaries

opthalm(o)- (eye) OPTHALMIC, pertaining to the eyes

opto- (vision, sight) OPTOMETRIST, a specialist in adapting lenses for the correcting of visual defects

or- (mouth) INTRAORAL, within the mouth

orb- (circle) ORBIT, the bony cavity that contains the eyeball

orchi(o)- (testicle) ORCHITIS, inflammation of the testicles

ortho- (straight, normal) ORTHOPEDIC, pertaining to the correction of skeletal defects

-osis (disease, abnormal condition) HALITOSIS, bad breath odor

oss- (bone) OSSIFY, to develop into bone

oste(o)- (bone) OSTEOMYELITIS, inflammation of bone or bone marrow

ot(o)- (ear) OTALGIA, earache

ovari(o)- (ovary) OVARIOCELE, hernia of an ovary

ovi-, ovo- (egg, ovum) OVIDUCT, a passage through which an egg passes

pachy- (thick) PACHYSOMIA, abnormal thickening of body parts

palat(o)- (palate) PALATITIS, inflammation of the palate

pan- (all) PANACEA, a remedy for all diseases, a "cure-all"

para- (beside, beyond, the final a is dropped before words that begin with a vowel) PARACENTESIS, surgical puncture of a cavity to allow the aspiration of fluid

path(o)- (disease) PATHOGEN, any disease-producing agent

-pen- (lack) LEUKOPENIA, a deficiency in white blood cells

pend- (hang down) PENDULOUS, hanging down loosely

pept(o)- (digestion) PEPTOGENIC, promoting digestion

per- (through) PERFUSION, the passage of fluid through an organ

peri- (around) PERICARDIUM, the sac that encloses the heart

-pexy (surgical fixation) SPLENOPEXY, surgical fixation of the spleen

phag(o)- (eating, ingestion) PHAGOMANIA, an insatiable craving for food

pharyng(o)- (pharynx) PHARYNGOSPASMS, spasms of the muscles of the pharynx

-philia (affinity for) NECROPHILIA, an abnormal interest in death

phleb(o)- (vein) PHLEBOTOMY, surgical incision of a vein

phob- (fear) PHOBIA, any persistent fear

phon(o)- (sound, speech) PHONETIC, pertaining to the voice

-phoresis (bear) DIAPHORESIS, profuse sweating

phot(o)- (light) PHOTOSENSITIVITY, abnormal reactivity of the skin to sunlight

phren(o)- (diaphragm) PHRENALGIA, pain in the diaphragm

physio- (nature) PHYSIOLOGY, the science that studies the function of living things

pilo- (hair) PILOSE, hairy

plas- (mold, shape) PLASTIC, pliant; capable of being molded

-plegia (paralysis) PARAPLEGIA, paralysis of the lower body, including the legs

pleur(o)- (the pleura) PLEUROTOMY, incision in the pleura

pneumat(o)- (breath, air, lung) PNEUMATIC, pertaining to air

pneumo- (breath, air, lung) PNEUMONIA, inflammation of the lungs with the escape of fluid

pod(o)- (foot) PODIATRIST, a specialist in the care of feet

poly- (many) POLYCHROMATIC, multicolored

post- (after, in time or place) POSTMORTEM, after death

postero- (the back, after) POSTERIOR, situated at the back

pre- (before, in time or place) PREMATURE, occurring before the proper time

pro- (before, in time and place) PROCREATION, the act of reproducing

proct(o)- (rectum) PROCTITIS, inflammation of the rectum

pseud(o)- (false) PSEUDOPLEGIA, hysterical paralysis

psych(o)- (mind) PSYCHOPATH, one who displays aggressive antisocial behavior

-ptosis (downward displacement) CARDIOPTOSIS, downward displacement of the heart

pulmo- (lung) PULMONARY, pertaining to the lungs

py(o)- (pus) PYORRHEA, copious discharge of pus

pyr(o)- (fire) PYROMANIAC, compulsive fire setter

quad- (four) QUADRIPLEGIA, paralysis of all four limbs

rachi(o)- (spine) RACHIALGIA, pain in the spine

radio- (ray, radiation) RADIOLOGY, the use of ionizing radiation in diagnosis and treatment

re- (again, back, contrary) RECURRENCE, the return of symptoms

ren(o)- (kidney) RENAL, pertaining to the kidneys

retro- (behind, backward) RETROPERITONEAL, behind the peritoneum

rhin(o)- (nose) RHINITIS, inflammation of the mucus membranes of the nose

-rrhage (excessive flow) HEMORRHAGE, profuse bleeding

-rrhea (profuse flow) DYSMENORRHEA, painful menstruation

sacr(o)- (sacrum) SACROSPINAL, pertaining to the sacrum and spinal column

sanguin- (blood) EXSANGUINATE, to lose a large volume of blood either internally or externally

sarc- (flesh) SARCOMA, a malignant tumor

scler(o)- (hard) ARTERIOSCLEROSIS, hardening of the arteries

-scop (observe, look at) MICROSCOPE, an instrument that magnifies extremely small objects

-sect (cut) DISSECT, to cut apart

semi- (half) SEMIFLEXION, moving a limb to a position halfway between flexion and extension

sens- (feel, perceive) SENSITIVE, able to respond to stimulus

sep- (rot, decay) SEPSIS, the presence of pathogenic microorganisms in the blood or tissues

sept- (fence, wall off) ANTISEPTIC, an agent that inhibits the growth of microorganisms

ser- (watery substance) SERUM, the clean portion of blood

sin- (hollow) SINUS, a cavity (as in a bone)

-sis (state, condition) PSYCHOSIS, any major mental disorder that is marked by personality changes and a loss of reality

somat(o)- (body) PSYCHOSOMATIC, both psychological and physiological

spas- (draw, pull) SPASMS, muscular contractions

spermat(o)- (sperm) SPERMACIDE, an agent that kills sperm

spers- (scatter) DISPERSE, to scatter components

sphen- (wedge) SPHENOID, wedge-shaped (as used to describe bones)

spher- (ball) SPHERICAL, round or ball-shaped

sphygm(o)- (pulse) SPHYGMOMANOMETER, an instrument used for measuring blood pressure

spin- (spine) SPINAL, pertaining to the spine

spirat- (breathe) INSPIRATION, drawing air into the lungs

splanchn- (viscera) SPLANCHNIC, pertaining to the viscera

splen- (spleen) SPLENECTOMY, surgical removal of the spleen

squam- (scale) DESQUAMATION, the shedding of skin in scales or sheets

-stalsis (contraction) PERISTALSIS, contractions that move food particles along the intestinal tract

staphyl(o)- (resembling a bunch of grapes) STAPHYLOCOCCUS, a genus of bacteria that causes infection

-stasis (maintaining a constant level) HEMOSTASIS, the control of bleeding (naturally or by surgical means)

steno- (narrow) STENOSIS, a narrowing of a passage or opening

stereo- (solid) STEREOSCOPIC, a three-dimensional appearance

-sthen- (strength) MYASTHENIA, muscular weakness

stom- (mouth, orifice) STOMA, an artificial opening

-stomy (creation of an opening) COLOSTOMY, a surgical opening between the colon and the body surface

strepto- (curved) STREPTOCOCCUS, a genus of bacteria that causes infection

-strict (draw tight) CONSTRICTED, drawn tightly together

-stringent (see strict-) ASTRINGENT, an agent that causes contraction

sub- (under, below) SUBCLAVIAN, below the collarbone

super- (above, in addition to) SUPERFICIAL, lying on or near the surface

supra- (in excess of, above, over) SUPRAPUBIC, above the pubic arch

syn- (with, together) SYNERGIST, an agent that acts with another agent

syring(o)- (tube) SYRINGE, an instrument for injecting fluids

tachy- (fast) TACHYPNEA, very rapid respirations

tact- (touch) TACTILE, pertaining to touch

teg- (cover) INTEGUMENT, the skin

tele- (far away) TELEMETRY, making a measurement at some

distance from the subject
therm(o)- (heat) THERMOGENESIS, the production of heat
thorac(o)- (chest) THORACIC, pertaining to the chest
thromb(o)- (clot, lump) THROMBUS, a solid mass of blood constituents in the heart or vessels
-tomy (incision, cutting) THORACOTOMY, incision in the chest wall
top- (place) TOPALGIA, localized pain
tors- (twist) TORTUOUS, full of twists and turns
tox- (poison) TOXIC, poisonous
trache(o)- (trachea) TRACHEOSTOMY, an opening in the neck that passes to the trachea
trans- (through, across) TRANSFUSION, the introduction of blood or blood components into active circulation
trich(o)- (hair) TRICHOSIS, any disease of the hair
-trophic (nourishment) HYPERTROPHIC, enlargement of an organ or body part due to the increase in the size of cells
-tropic (turning, changing) CHEMOTROPIC, able to change because of chemical stimulation

ultra- (beyond, excess) ULTRASONIC, beyond the audible range
uni- (one) UNILATERAL, affecting one side
-uresis (urination) ENURESIS, involuntary excretion of urine usually at night; "bedwetting"
urethr(o)- (urethra) URETHRITIS, inflammation of the uretha
-uria (condition of the urine) PYURIA, pus in the urine
uro- (urine, urinary tract) UROLOGIST, a specialist in diseases and disorders of the urinary tract

vas(o)- (vessel) VASOCONSTRICTOR, an agent that causes constriction of blood vessels
ven-, vene-, veni-, veno- (vein) VENIPUNCTURE, surgical puncture of a vein
ventr(o)- (belly, front) VENTRAL, relating to the belly or abdomen
vertebr(o)- (spine) VERTEBRAL, pertaining to the spinal column
vesic(a)- (blister, bladder) VESICLE, a small, fluid-filled blister
viscer(o)- (viscera) VISCERAL, pertaining to the viscera (abdominal organs)
vit- (life) VITAL, necessary to life

xeno- (strange, foreign) XENOPHOBIA, abnormal fear of strangers
xero- (dry) XEROSIS, abnormal dryness (of the mouth, eyes, etc.)

zo(o)- (animal) ZOOGENOUS, acquired from an animal
zyg(o)- (yoked, joined) ZYGOTE, the fertilized ovum

APPENDIX 4A
Anti-Shock Garments

Anti-shock garments are pneumatic counterpressure devices. This means that air is used to create a pressure against something. In this case, the pressure is applied against the flow of blood. Anti-shock garments also are referred to as Military Anti-Shock Trousers, Medical Anti-Shock Trousers, and MAST.

The anti-shock garment is used primarily for the patient who has developed or is certain to develop severe hypovolemic shock.

HOW ANTI-SHOCK GARMENTS WORK

The anti-shock garment is designed to correct or counteract certain internal bleeding conditions and hypovolemia (low circulating blood volume). The garment does this by developing an encircling pressure up to 120 mmHg around both lower extremities, pelvis, and abdomen. The typical pressure exerted is 100 mmHg. This pressure:

* Slows or stops venous and arterial bleeding in the areas of the body enclosed by the pressurized garment.
* Forces available blood from the lower body to the heart, brain, and other vital upper body organs.
* Prevents the return and pooling of the available circulating blood to the lower extremities.

There are a number of advantages associated with the use of an anti-shock garment other than the prevention of further blood loss and the direction of circulating blood to the vital organs. Among the advantages are:

* An anti-shock garment serves as an air splint for fractured lower extremities.
* The garment often stabilizes a patient so effectively and quickly that other persons with more critical injuries can be treated first. Patient monitoring is still required.
* When a patient is effectively stabilized with an anti-shock garment, diagnosis and preparation for surgery may be delayed for an hour or even longer, while an unstable patient often must be diagnosed and prepared for surgery in a few minutes.
* ECGs and X rays can be taken, and a Foley catheter can be inserted while a patient is in an inflated garment.

INDICATIONS FOR USE

Use of an anti-shock garment should be considered for patients with:

* Systolic blood pressure less than 80 mmHg.
* Systolic blood pressure less than 100 mmHg and exhibiting the classic signs of shock.
* Profuse bleeding from injuries to the lower extremities.
* Fractures of the pelvis or lower extremities.

In the past, anti-shock garments were recommended for patients who developed cardiac arrest. This is a controversial procedure and is currently under study. If your local protocol indicates application of anti-shock garments for cardiac arrest patients, remember that you cannot delay or stop CPR in order to apply the garment.

CONTRAINDICATIONS

NOTE: Recent findings show that pulmonary edema is the only *absolute* contraindication for the application of anti-shock garments. The decision to apply a garment is the choice of the emergency department physician or the attending physician.

A physician may choose not to order an anti-shock garment based on the following conditional contraindications:

1. Congestive heart failure
2. Heart attack
3. Cerebrovascular accident (stroke)
4. Pregnancy, unless the abdominal compartment can be left uninflated

There are additional conditional contraindications for the use of the anti-shock garment. These cases usually involve injury to the chest or abdomen and the lower extremities. The anti-shock garment can be applied for such cases only upon the orders of a physician who has been informed of the patient's problems. In such cases, the garment is applied for the lower extremity injury. The abdominal compartment is not inflated. The conditional contraindications include:

- Massive bleeding into the thoracic cavity
- Abdominal injury with evisceration
- Abdominal penetration where the object is still in the abdomen
- Injury above the level of the garment that has external bleeding that cannot be controlled with a simple pressure dressing.

The anti-shock garment may be ordered for all of the above situations, even when there is no lower extremity injury. Typically, the physician ordering the application of the garment will be concerned with severe hypovolemia, considering this to be a greater concern than the other problems suffered by the patient. Abdominal compartment inflation may be ordered for some patients, except those with abdominal evisceration or penetration.

Some EMS Systems have a protocol that does not allow for the application of anti-shock garments in cases involving injury to the head. The reason is to help prevent an increase in intracranial pressure. However, some protocols now allow application of an anti-shock garment when there is head injury and severe hypovolemia. This is justified for certain patients because the hypovolemia is a greater problem than the increased intracranial pressure. Follow your local guidelines.

NOTE: The application of anti-shock garments for patients with hypovolemia, secondary to hypothermia, may cause ventricular fibrillation. Make certain that the emergency department physician is given a full patient assessment before he orders you to apply the anti-shock garment.

APPLYING AN ANTI-SHOCK GARMENT

An anti-shock garment is to be applied in accordance with local protocol. In many localities, application requires an order from a physician. The procedure for application of the garment is shown in Scansheet A4-1.

NOTE: Take vital signs before applying an anti-shock garment. If clothing is to remain in place, all sharp and bulky objects are to be removed from the patient's pockets before applying the garment.

REMOVING AN ANTI-SHOCK GARMENT

The garment should be removed *only when a physician is present* and:

1. The physician orders the removal of the garment.
2. Intravenous volume replacement has begun.
3. Vital signs have just been monitored and recorded, noting that the patient is stable.
4. An operating room is available.

In some cases, the garment may have to remain inflated until the patient is taken into surgery. The garment should only be deflated and removed by someone trained in its use and familiar with the type of garment being used. When possible, the person who has applied the garment should be the one who removes it. Have someone continually monitor vital signs while you deflate the unit.

1. Slowly deflate the abdominal compartment.
2. Wait 20 minutes, then slowly deflate one leg compartment.
3. Wait another 20 minutes, then slowly deflate the other leg compartment.

Discontinue deflation if systolic blood pressure drops more than 10 mmHg from the previous level or if the systolic blood pressure is 110 mmHg or less. Additional intravenous infusion is needed before deflation can continue.

In some cases, you will be able to deflate the garment in less than 60 minutes. Follow the attending physician's directions. The time for deflation should not be less than 20 minutes, checking for 10 minutes of stable vital signs after deflating the abdominal compartment and after deflating the first lower extremity compartment.

WARNING: There is no indication for the prehospital removal of anti-shock garments.

APPLICATION OF AN ANTI-SHOCK GARMENT

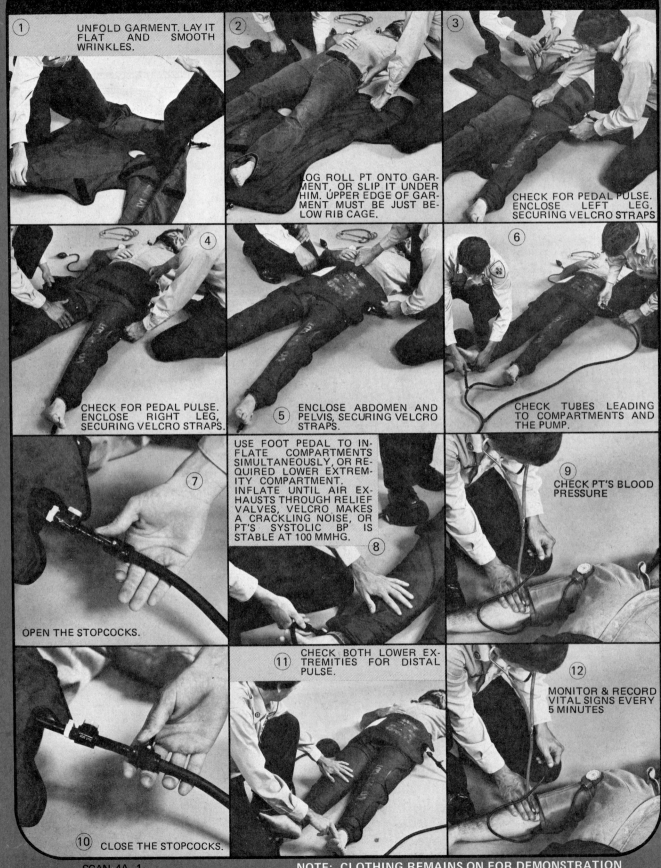

① UNFOLD GARMENT. LAY IT FLAT AND SMOOTH WRINKLES.

② LOG ROLL PT ONTO GARMENT, OR SLIP IT UNDER HIM. UPPER EDGE OF GARMENT MUST BE JUST BELOW RIB CAGE.

③ CHECK FOR PEDAL PULSE. ENCLOSE LEFT LEG, SECURING VELCRO STRAPS

④ CHECK FOR PEDAL PULSE. ENCLOSE RIGHT LEG, SECURING VELCRO STRAPS.

⑤ ENCLOSE ABDOMEN AND PELVIS, SECURING VELCRO STRAPS.

⑥ CHECK TUBES LEADING TO COMPARTMENTS AND THE PUMP.

⑦ OPEN THE STOPCOCKS.

⑧ USE FOOT PEDAL TO INFLATE COMPARTMENTS SIMULTANEOUSLY, OR REQUIRED LOWER EXTREMITY COMPARTMENT. INFLATE UNTIL AIR EXHAUSTS THROUGH RELIEF VALVES, VELCRO MAKES A CRACKLING NOISE, OR PT'S SYSTOLIC BP IS STABLE AT 100 MMHG.

⑨ CHECK PT'S BLOOD PRESSURE

⑩ CLOSE THE STOPCOCKS.

⑪ CHECK BOTH LOWER EXTREMITIES FOR DISTAL PULSE.

⑫ MONITOR & RECORD VITAL SIGNS EVERY 5 MINUTES

SCAN 4A—1

NOTE: CLOTHING REMAINS ON FOR DEMONSTRATION PURPOSES. IN ACTUAL USE, CLOTHING SHOULD BE REMOVED. MAST GARMENT CAN BE PLACED OVER TRACTION SPLINT.

THE ESOPHAGEAL OBTURATOR AIRWAY (EOA)

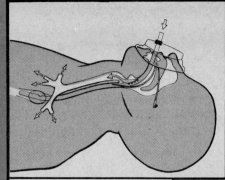

NOTE: IF YOUR MEDICAL ADVISOR HAS APPROVED THE USE OF EOA, CONTINUALLY PRACTICE INSERTION IN A MANIKIN UNTIL YOU ARE PROFICIENT. THE TUBE OF AN EOA IS PERFORATED IN THE UPPER THIRD OF ITS LENGTH. WHEN TUBE IS IN PLACE, THE INFLATED CUFF FILLS THE AREA BETWEEN TUBE AND ESOPHAGUS. AIR FORCED THROUGH PERFORATIONS IS PREVENTED FROM ENTERING STOMACH. THE INFLATABLE FACE MASK PROVIDES A TIGHT SEAL OVER PT'S MOUTH AND NOSE.

DO NOT USE EOA WHEN PT:

- IS CONSCIOUS AND/OR BREATHING
- HAS A GAG REFLEX
- IS UNDER 16 YRS OLD OR UNDER 5 FT. TALL
- HAS FACIAL INJURY PREVENTING TIGHT SEAL
- HAS KNOWN ESOPHAGEAL DISEASE
- HAS INGESTED KNOWN CAUSTIC

(1) IS EOA KIT COMPLETE? NEEDS WATER-BASE SURGICAL LUBRICANT.

(2) DRAW 35 CC OF AIR INTO SYRINGE. INSERT IT INTO ONE-WAY VALVE OF FACE MASK. INFLATE CUSHION.
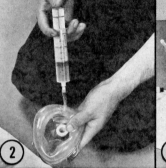

(3) TEST TUBE CUFF BY INJECTING 35 CC OF AIR THROUGH VALVE. IF CUFF IS USABLE, WITHDRAW AIR AND ATTACH TUBE TO MASK. LUBRICATE TIP OF TUBE.
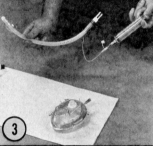

---

(4) LIFT JAW & TONGUE STRAIGHT UPWARD WITHOUT HYPEREXTENDING NECK.

(5) ADVANCE AIRWAY CAREFULLY BEHIND TONGUE & INTO PHARYNX & ESOPHAGUS.

(6) HOLD MASK IN PLACE WITH BOTH HANDS.

(7) TEST AIRWAY BY BLOWING INTO MOUTH PIECE. WATCH PT'S CHEST RISE. REMOVE & RE-INSERT IF CHEST DOES NOT RISE.

---

(8) INFLATE CUFF WITH 35 CC OF AIR FROM SYRINGE. REMOVE SYRINGE.
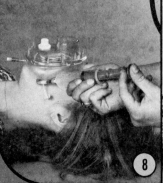

(9) VENTILATE PT BY MOUTH-TO-BAG, BAG-VALVE-MASK, OR POSITIVE PRESSURE OXYGEN DEVICE
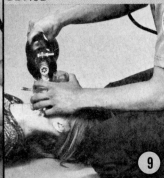

REMOVING AN EOA: BE ALERT FOR VOMITING. DO NOT DEFLATE CUFF OR REMOVE EOA UNTIL:
- PATIENT HAS RESUMED BREATHING
- ENDOTRACHEAL TUBE IS INSERTED & ITS CUFF IS INFLATED IN TRACHEA

WHEN THE TUBE IS REMOVED:
1. HAVE SUCTION EQUIPMENT READY FOR IMMEDIATE USE
2. TURN THE PATIENT ON HIS SIDE
3. INSERT SYRINGE INTO ONE-WAY VALVE & WITHDRAW AIR SLOWLY FROM THE CUFF
4. CAREFULLY REMOVE THE TUBE

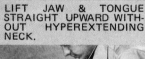
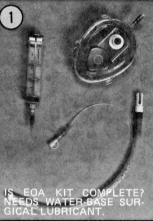
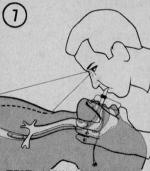
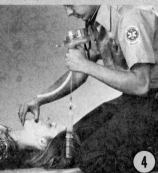

APPENDIX 4C
IV Therapy

INTRAVENOUS FLUID THERAPY

Two terms should be considered before we discuss the procedure associated with intravenous fluid therapy, *transfusion* and *infusion*.

Transfusion refers to the introduction of whole blood or whole blood components into the cardiovascular system. It is still a procedure that is seldom done outside a medical facility because of a number of complications that can arise. Thus, emergency medical personnel seldom participate in a blood transfusion effort.

Infusion is a technique that has been used for years and is a procedure that can be accomplished outside a medical facility by specially trained personnel. Infusion means the introduction into the cardiovascular system of a fluid other than blood—a fluid that will fill the system sufficiently to allow the heart to operate efficiently while new blood is manufactured by the life processes—in other words, a blood-volume expander.

There are several fluids available for intravenous therapy, including normal saline, Plasmalyte, D_5W (a 5% solution of dextrose in water), Dextran, and lactated Ringer's solution (a solution of salt, other electrolytes, and glucose in water). Lactated Ringer's solution does not have the red blood cells that carry life-sustaining oxygen to all parts of the body, but it can be used to replace up to two-thirds of the blood supply of a healthy individual before body functions start to fail.

Intravenous infusion is not a technique to be considered lightly. The procedure seems easy enough when reading about it. In the field, however, infusion may be made difficult by injuries, the lack of a suitable place to work, the possibility of contamination, and emotional and physical pressures.

Training must be undertaken in the proper setting (as in a hospital), and under the direction of a competent medical professional. Detailed lectures must be followed by carefully supervised practice sessions, during which trainees can practice on special training aids and each other. Examinations must be conducted to measure student progress, and proficiency must be maintained by means of supervised postgraduate practice sessions and update seminars. And, throughout a training program, emphasis must be given to the complications that can arise from IV therapy—complications that can be dangerous!

Supplies and Equipment
for IV Fluid Therapy

There is a variety of sterile infusion sets available today. The sets most commonly used by ambulance and rescue personnel are disposable. However, some medical facilities provide local ambulance services with replaceable sterile infusion sets. A sterile infusion set usually has the following items:

- A connector (that joins the set to the fluid container) with a protective cap
- A drip chamber
- A flow adjustment valve
- A port (where medication can be injected)
- A needle adapter that joins the set to the cannula

In addition to the containers of various fluids, other supplies are associated with IV therapy.

- An arm board to immobilize the insertion site when necessary.
- A tourniquet to restrict venous flow while an insertion site is selected.
- Tape to secure tubing to the patient's arm and to secure his arm to an arm board.
- An antiseptic solution to cleanse the insertion site.
- Gauze pads (2 × 2 in.) to cover the insertion site.
- Paper towels for clean-up.
- A pen and labels to identify containers.
- A prepared form or record book for recording information about the procedure.

Depending on local policy, some ambulance and rescue units carry a 20-ml syringe in which blood can be collected once the cannula is in place, containers for the blood samples, and an antibiotic ointment that can be spread over the insertion site.

The IV Fluid Infusion Procedure

The infusion of an IV fluid is accomplished in several steps.

Preparation of the Patient As in any emergency care procedure, preparation of the patient is an important step. Take a minute to explain the procedure to your patient and why it is important to him (that fluid must be replaced). Be calm, confident, and convincing in your presentation. A conscious, competent patient has a legal right to refuse your efforts to help him. And don't lie to your patient! IV's hurt, so don't tell him otherwise.

Selection of the Fluid It is vitally important that you select only the fluid that has been **ordered.** A good practice is for you to repeat your instructions over the radio so that the physician knows you understand.

If you are using a fluid that is packed in a plastic bag, follow the steps shown in Figures A4c-1 through A4c-3.

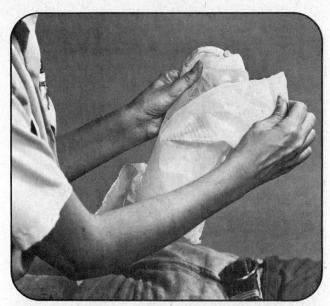

Figure A4c-1: Remove bag from protective envelope.

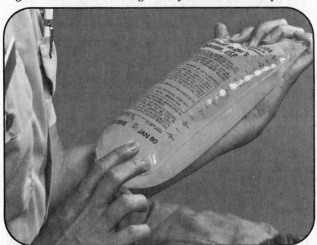

Figure A4c-2: Check that the fluid is the one ordered and note its expiration date.

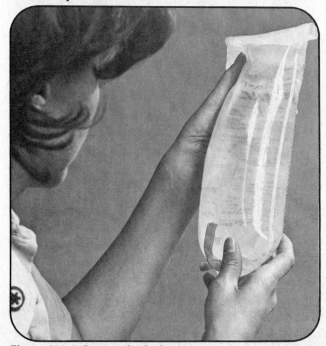

Figure A4c-3: Inspect for leaks.

If you are using fluid that is in a glass bottle, check the container for cracks and the fluid for clarity.

Preparation of the Infusion Set Remember that a macro-drip (standard) infusion set is needed for fluid replacement, and a micro-drip set is used for maintenance of a life-line and for use with children.

Open the infusion set and connect the extension tubing as shown in Figures A4c-4 through A4c-14.

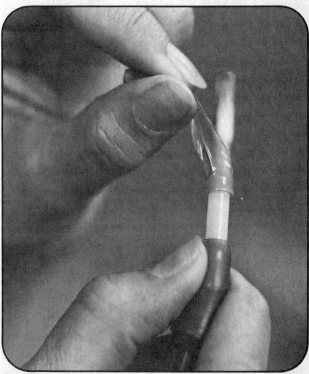

Figure A4c-4: Remove the protective covering from the adapter.

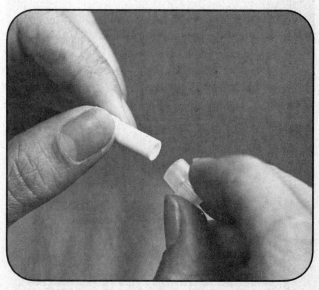

Figure A4c-5: Remove the protective cap from the extension tubing connector.

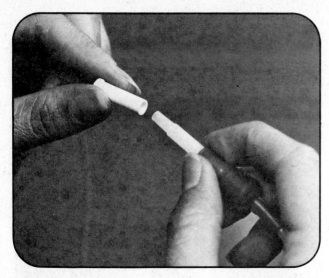

Figure A4c-6: Join the extension tubing to the infusion set.

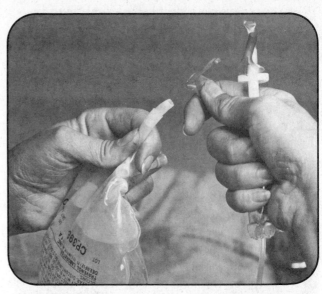

Figure A4c-8: Remove the protective covering from the port of the fluid bag.

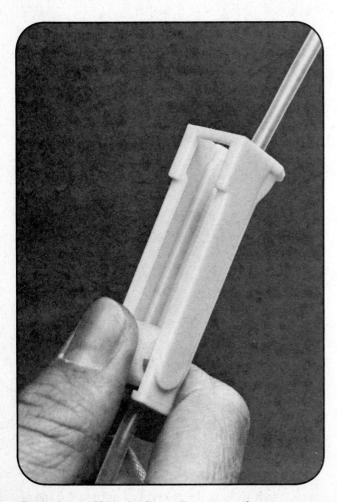

Figure A4c-7: Close the flow adjustment valve.

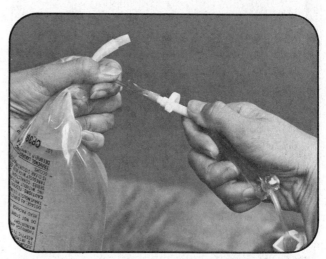

Figure A4c-9: Remove the protective covering from the spiked end of the infusion tubing.

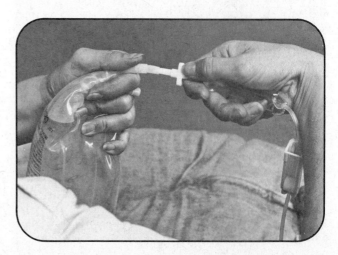

Figure A4c-10: Insert the spiked end of the infusion set into the fluid bag.

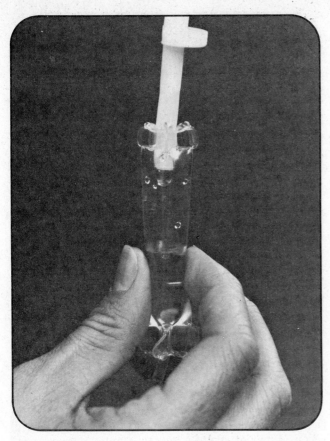

Figure A4c-11: Fill the drip chamber by squeezing and releasing it.

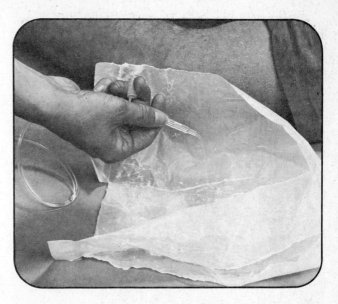

Figure A4c-13: Open the flow adjustment valve to flush air from the tubing.

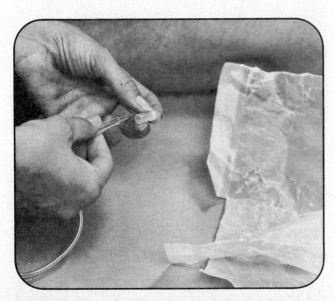

Figure A4c-12: Remove the protective cap from the needle adapter.

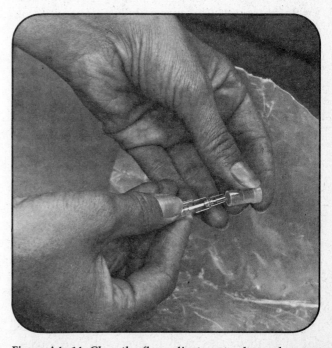

Figure A4c-14: Close the flow adjustment valve and recap the needle adapter.

Preparing the Tape That Will Secure the Cannula and Tubing   Cut or tear strips of tape to proper size *before* inserting the IV. Once you start the insertion, you should not stop until the fluid is running.

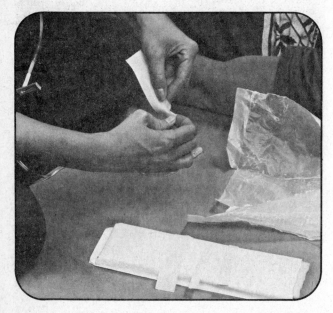

Figure A4c-15: Tear strips of tape to the appropriate length and place them on the arm board or the infusion set box.

Selection of the Cannula   An IV fluid can be infused in a number of ways: through a hollow needle inserted directly into a vein (as, for example, a "butterfly" needle); through a plastic catheter slipped over a hollow needle that has been inserted into a vein; or through a plastic catheter inserted into a vein through a hollow needle. A 14-16 gauge over-the-needle catheter is generally recommended for trauma victims. It can handle large quantities of fluid and is more readily stabilized in place than a hollow needle. Smaller needles are recommended for patients with medical problems when large quantities of fluids are neither indicated nor desired. Select the proper cannula and keep it close at hand.

Selection of the Insertion Site   Any accessible vein in the body can be selected to receive an IV. However, usually a vein in the forearm (below the crease of the elbow) is selected for IV insertion since vessels there are large, straight and easily punctured. If possible, a vein in the left forearm should be selected; that area is most easily accessible when the patient is on the ambulance stretcher.

Once you have the tourniquet in place, have the patient clench and unclench his fist several times. This will improve venous distention even more.

Preparing the Insertion Site   Disinfecting the site directly over the vein that is to be punctured is important. First scrub the area directly over the vein, and then move the swab in ever-widening circles away from the puncture site. If you use iodine

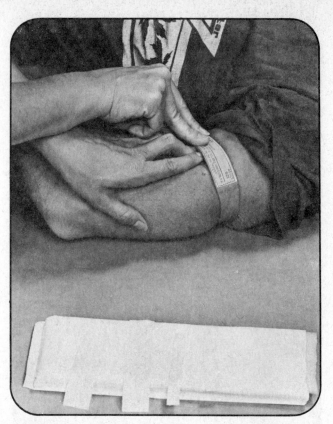

Figure A4c-16: Apply a tourniquet to the arm to cause venous distention. Palpate the radial pulse to be certain you have not stopped arterial flow.

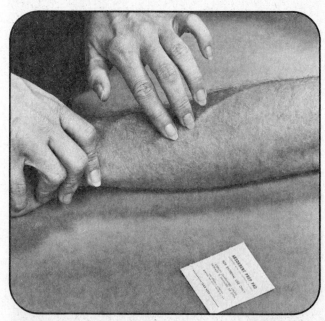

Figure A4c-17: Choose a vein that is well distended, fairly straight, well fixed (as opposed to one that rolls under your finger pressure) and springy when palpated.

swabs to disinfect, follow the scrubbing with a wipe-down with an alcohol sponge. This will reduce the possibility of an iodine reaction.

Preparation of the Cannula   Hollow needle and plastic catheters are packaged in different ways. Sterility is assured as long as the packages are un-

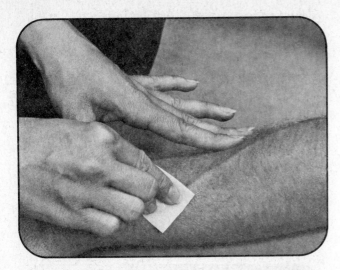

Figure A4c-18: Scrub the area with an antiseptic swab.

opened. Do NOT touch the needle with your fingers.

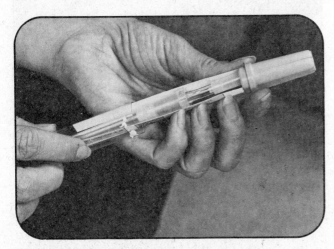

Figure A4c-19: Open the cannula package.

Insertion of the Cannula

1. Stabilize the vein by applying pressure on it with your thumb distal to the point where the needle will enter.

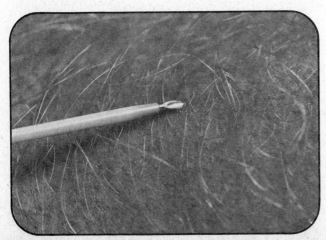

Figure A4c-20

2. Properly align the needle at an angle of 10-20°. The bevel must be up. (Fig. A4c-20)

3. Pierce the skin and insert the needle. (Fig. A4c-21). There will be little resistance as the needle passes through the skin, some resistance when the needle contacts the vein, and a loss of resistance when the needle passes through the wall of the vessel. The fact that the needle has entered the vein will be confirmed by a return of blood through the needle.

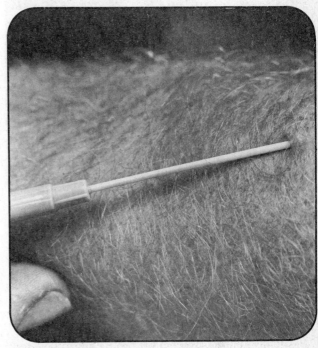

Figure A4c-21

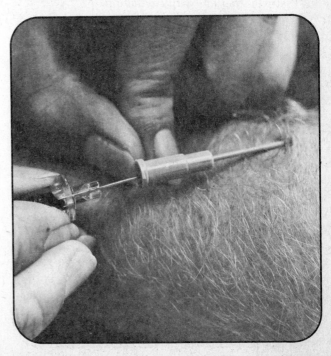

Figure A4c-22

NOTE: If you are using an over-the-needle or through-the-needle catheter, continue to insert the needle for just a few mm. more to make a sufficient opening for the catheter to pass through.

4. Slide the catheter into the vein. (Fig. A4c-22)

5. Remove the tourniquet. (Fig. A4c-23)

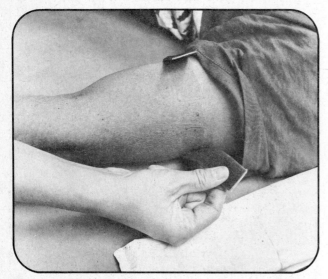

Figure A4c-23

6. Withdraw the needle (Fig. A4c-24)

NOTE: Compressing the vein with your thumb near the tip of the catheter as you support the patient's arm prevents blood loss through the catheter.

WARNING: Once you advance a plastic catheter over or through a needle, *never* pull it back. A piece of catheter may be sheared off by the sharp beveled edge of the needle point and become a plastic embolus that will interfere with circulation.

The procedure for inserting a hollow needle is essentially the same. The needle is inserted into the

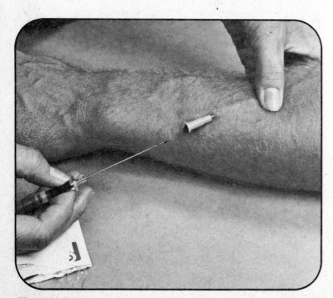

Figure A4c-24

vein. It is then leveled until it is virtually parallel to the vessel and pushed forward until at least $1/2$ in., but less than $3/4$ in. of the needle is in the vein.

Blood Sampling   In some areas, it is the policy for emergency medical personnel to draw blood samples at the time of an IV insertion.

If it is part of your standard operating procedures, collect blood samples. Stabilize the catheter with one hand, attach a 20 ml syringe, and distribute blood among the required number of collection tubes.

Starting the Infusion   After making a quick visual check to see that the system is ready.

1. Attach the needle adapter. (Fig. A4c-25)

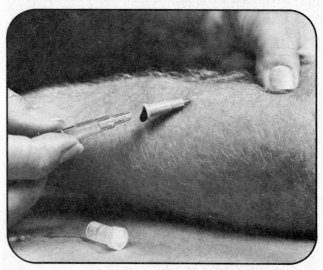

Figure A4c-25

2. Open the flow adjustment valve. If there is no flow, adjust the catheter slightly. (Fig. A4c-26)

Securing the Catheter

1. Cover the insertion site according to local policy. (Fig. A4c-27)

2. Tape the cannula and tubing in place. (Fig. A4c-28) Do NOT cover the junction of the tubing with the cannula.

3. Write on the tape the type of cannula used, the gauge, and time and date of the insertion. Do not write on the plastic fluid container, especially with a felt pen. Ink from a felt pen can permeate the bag and contaminate the fluid.

If necessary, immobilize the patient's arm on an arm board, a flattened magazine, or the box that the infusion set came in.

Regulation of the Flow Rate   The fluid flow rate must be adjusted according to the instructions of the physician. To do this, you must know 1) the volume of fluid that is to be infused; 2) the time over

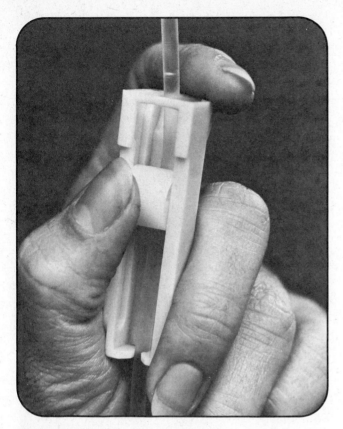

Figure A4c-26

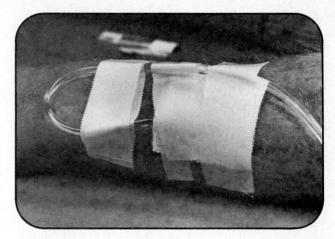

Figure A4c-28

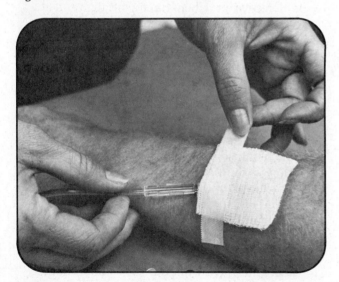

Figure A4c-27

which the volume is to be infused; and 3) the rate at which fluid is delivered by the particular infusion set being used.

Calculate the rate with the following formula:

$$\text{flow rate in drops/minute} = \frac{\text{Volume to be infused} \times \text{drops/minute that the set delivers}}{\text{Time of infusion in minutes}}$$

Thus, if the physician wants the patient to receive 1 liter (1000 ml) of a fluid in 2 hours and you have an infusion set that is capable of delivering 10 drops per

ml, you can calculate the flow rate in drops per minute like this:

$$\frac{1000 \text{ (ml)} \times 10 \text{ (drops per ml)}}{120 \text{ (minutes)}} = 83 \text{ drops per minute}$$

Troubleshooting an IV

If it appears that the IV fluid is not running properly (and there are no obvious kinks in the tubing), take the following corrective measures, starting with the patient's arm and working back to the fluid container.

- Assure that the tourniquet has been removed. Sometimes a sleeve slips down over a tourniquet and obscures it while the cannula is being inserted.
- Assure that the patient's arm is not bent in such a fashion that circulation is impeded.
- Inspect the IV site for swelling. *Infiltration* (the loss of blood into surrounding tissues) is not uncommon and occurs when a needle or catheter slips from a vein. If you suspect infiltration, lower the fluid container momentarily and watch for blood to appear in the tubing. If blood does appear, the cannula is in the vein. If there is no sign of blood, the cannula has slipped from the vessel. In either case, you must stop the infusion and remove the cannula.
- If there is no indication of infiltration, check to see that tape around the insertion site has not compressed any of the tubing. If this is not the problem. . .
- Check to see that the flow adjustment valve has not been accidentally closed. If it has not. . .
- Raise the fluid container. An increase in the height of a container is sometimes all that is

necessary to cause a sluggish IV to run properly.

- If these efforts do not result in a properly running fluid, discontinue the IV and start one in another site using a new infusion set, a new cannula and a new container of fluid.

NOTE: If infusion has occurred, a new site should be selected above, but never below, the original.

Complications of IV Therapy

Other than infiltration and plastic embolism there are other local and systemic complications that may arise during or after IV therapy.

Local Complications

- Pain is common because of the skin puncture and should be expected. Intense and continuing pain should be regarded as an indication of infiltration.

- Infection often results from the use of contaminated equipment or failure to use aseptic procedures. Local infection is not usually evident until a few days after the infusion.

- Accidental arterial puncture sometimes occurs when an artery lies close to the vein selected for puncture. Bright red blood spurting from the cannula indicates accidental arterial puncture. If you see this, quickly withdraw the cannula and apply pressure to the bleeding vessel until the flow stops (within a few minutes).

- Nerve damage and tissue sloughing are rare local complications.

Systemic Complications

- Simple fainting is usually nothing more than an emotional reaction to the insertion of the needle.

- Reactions occur when foreign proteins capable of producing fever are introduced into the cardiovascular system. If your patient experiences a sudden rise in temperature (perhaps up to 106°F), headache, backache, chills, nausea, and vomiting within a half hour or so after the start of IV therapy, discontinue the IV fluid immediately; the fluid may be contaminated. Start another IV in the other arm, using a new cannula, a new infusion set, and a new container of fluid. You can reduce the likelihood of fever-producing reaction by carefully inspecting IV fluid containers for leaks (through which contaminants can enter) and for contamination (evidenced by clouding).

- Thrombophlebitis is inflammation of a vein and often occurs when IV therapy is prolonged. The problem may be caused by the solution itself (some IV solutions are more irritating than others) or by excessive movement of the cannula in the vein. If you suspect thrombophlebitis because of pain along the vein and redness and swelling at the insertion site, stop the infusion and remove the cannula.

- Air embolism, although more likely to occur when blood is being transfused under pressure, may occur during an IV fluid infusion. Air can enter the cardiovascular system in a number of ways, as for example when tubing is defective or when tubing fittings are not tight, when the fluid container is allowed to run dry, or when negative pressure is created in the tubing. When a bubble of air forms and is carried to a swollen vessel, it forms an obstruction to circulation. Suspect air embolism when circulatory collapse occurs while an IV is running properly.

- Circulatory overload occurs when an excess of fluid is infused, perhaps because of miscalculation of the patient's needs. The symptoms of circulatory overload appear as those of congestive heart failure: dyspnea, rales, and distention of the jugular veins.

- Anaphylactic reaction may occur in some patients. The reaction is generally due to a medication included with the IV solution rather than the IV solution itself.

glossary

A-post—first roof pillar from the windshield of a vehicle.

Abandonment—to leave an injured or sick patient before care is assumed by an equally or more highly trained person. Leaving the scene without giving patient information may be viewed as a form of abandonment.

ABC Method—sequence of operations required in cardiopulmonary resuscitation. 'A' stands for airway, 'B' for breathe, and 'C' for circulate.

Abdomen (AB-do-men)—area of the body between the diaphragm and the pelvis.

Abdominopelvic (AB-dom-i-no-PEL-vik)—anterior body cavity inferior to the diaphragm.

Abduction—movement *away* from the midline of the body.

Abortion (ah-BOR-shun)—spontaneous (miscarriage) or induced delivery of the fetus and placenta before the 28th week of pregnancy.

Abrasion (ab-RAY-zhun)—*see* Scratch.

Acetone Breath—sweet breath with a fruit-like odor. A sign associated with diabetic coma.

Accident Zone—*see* Danger Zone.

Acidosis (AS-i-DO-sis)—condition of increased acidity.

Actual Consent—consent by the adult patient, usually in oral form, accepting emergency care. This must be informed consent.

Acute—to have a rapid onset. Sometimes used to mean severe.

Acute Abdomen—inflammation in the abdominal cavity producing intense pain.

Acute Myocardial Infarction (AMI) (my-o-KARD-e-al in-FARK-shun)—heart attack. The sudden death of heart muscle due to oxygen starvation. Usually caused by a narrowing or blockage of a coronary artery supplying the myocardium.

Adduction—movement *toward* the midline of the body.

Airway—the passageway for air from the nose and mouth to the exchange levels of the lungs. Can also mean artificial airways, such as S-tubes.

Alkalosis (AL-ke-LO-sis)—condition of an increase in base (alkaline).

Allergen (AL-er-jin)—any substance capable of inducing an allergic reaction.

Alveoli (Al-VE-o-li)—microscopic air sacs of the lungs where gas exchange takes place with the circulatory system.

Ambulance—vehicle for emergency care with a driver compartment and a patient compartment, carrying all equipment and supplies needed to provide basic EMT-level emergency care at the scene and en route to the emergency department.

Amniotic Sac—fluid-filled sac that surrounds the fetus.

Analgesic—pain reliever.

Anaphylactic (an-ah-fi-LAK-tik) Shock—allergy shock. The most severe type of allergic reaction in which a person goes into shock when he comes into contact with a substance to which he is allergic.

Anatomical Position—standard reference position for the body in the study of anatomy. The body is erect, facing the observer. The arms are down at the sides and the palms of the hands face forward.

Aneurysm (AN-u-riz'm)—blood-filled sac caused by the localized dilation of an artery or vein. The dilated or weakened section of an arterial wall.

Angina Pectoris (an-JI-nah PEK-to-ris)—chest pains often caused by an insufficient blood supply to the heart muscle.

Angulation—angle formed above and below a break in a bone. The fracture changes the straight line of a bone into an angle.

Anoxia—absence of oxygen. *See* Hypoxia.

Anterior—front surface of the body or body part.

Antiseptic—substance that will stop the growth of, or prevent the activities of germs (microorganisms).

Anus (A-nus)—outlet of the large intestine.

Aorta (a-OR-ta)—major artery of systemic circulation that carries blood from the heart out to the body.

Apical Pulse—heartbeat felt over the lower portion of the heart.

Apnea (ap-NE-ah)—suspension of breathing.

Apoplexy (AP-o-plek-see)—loss of consciousness, movement, and sensation that is caused by a stroke.

Appendicular (AP-pen-dik-u-ler) Skeleton—clavicles, scapulae, bones of the upper limbs, pelvis, and the bones of the lower limbs.

Arm—body part from shoulder to elbow.

Arrhythmia (ah-RITH-me-ah)—disturbance of heart rate and rhythm.

Arteriosclerosis (ar-TE-re-o-skle-RO-sis)—"hardening of the arteries" caused by calcium deposits.

Artery—any blood vessel carrying blood away from the heart.

Articulate—to unite to form a joint.

Ascites (a-SI-tez)—noticeable distention of the abdomen caused by accumulation of excessive fluids.

Aseptic—clean, free of particles of dirt and debris, but not necessarily sterile.

Asphyxia (as-FIK-si-ah)—loss of consciousness caused by too little oxygen reaching the brain. The functions of the brain, heart, and lungs will cease.

Aspiration—to inhale materials into the lungs. Often used to describe the breathing in of vomitus.

Asthma (AS-mah)—condition that constricts the bronchioles, causing a reduction of air flow and congestion. Air usually enters to the level of the alveoli, but it cannot be expired easily.

Atherosclerosis (ATH-er-o-skle-RO-sis)—build-up of fatty deposits and other particles on the inner wall of an artery.

This build-up is called "plaque." Calcium may deposit in the plaque, causing the wall to become hard and stiff.

Atrium (A-tree-um)—superior chamber of the heart. (plural—atria).

Avulsion (ah-VUL-shun)—piece of tissue or skin that is torn loose or pulled off by injury.

Axial (AK-si-al) **Skeleton**—skull, spine, sternum, and ribs.

B-post—second roof pillar from a vehicle's windshield

Bag-Valve-Mask Ventilator—aid for artificial ventilation. It has a face mask, a self-inflating bag, and a valve that allows the bag to refill while the patient exhales. It can be attached to an oxygen line.

Bandage—material such as gauze or tape used to hold a dressing in place.

Bile—fluid produced by the liver and sent to the small intestine. It may be stored in the gallbladder. Bile has many functions, including changing intestinal motility and helping to digest fatty foods.

Biological Death—when lung and heart activity stops and brain cells die. Changes in the brain cells and blood vessels usually begin within 4 to 6 minutes after breathing stops. Brain cell death typically begins within 10 minutes after respiratory arrest.

Bladder—usually referring to the urinary bladder located in the pelvic cavity.

Blanch—become pale.

Blood Pressure—pressure caused by blood exerting force on the walls of blood vessels. Usually, arterial blood pressure is measured.

Bolus—mass of chewed or partially chewed food that is ready to be swallowed.

Bowel—intestine.

Brachial (BRAY-key-al) **Pulse**—pulse produced by compressing the major artery of the upper arm. Used to detect heart action and circulation in infants.

Bradycardia (bray-de-KAR-de-ah)—abnormal condition where the heart rate is very slow. The pulse rate will be below 50 beats per minute.

Breech Birth—delivery where the buttocks of the baby are born first.

Bronchiole (BRONG-key-ol)—small branches of the airway that carry air to and from the alveoli.

Bronchus (BRONC-kus)—the portion of the airway connecting the trachea to the lungs (plural—bronchi).

Bruise—contusion

C-post—third roof pillar from a vehicle's windshield
Cannula—hollow tube that can be inserted into a cavity to allow for fluid drainage.
Capillary—microscopic blood vessel where exchange takes place between bloodstream and body tissues.

Cardiac (KAR-de-ak)—refers to the heart.

Cardiac Arrest—when the heart stops beating.

Cardiogenic (KAR-de-o-JEN-ik) **Shock**—failure of the cardiovascular system brought about when the heart can no longer develop the pressure needed to circulate blood to all parts of the body.

Cardiopulmonary Resuscitation (KAR-de-o-PUL-mo-ner-e re-SUS-ci-TA-shun) **(CPR)**—heart-lung resuscitation where there is a combined effort to restore or maintain respiration and circulation.

Carotid (kah-ROT-id) **Artery**—large neck artery. One is found on each side of the neck. Its pulse is of prime importance in the primary survey and CPR.

Carpals (KAR-pals)—wrist bones.

Catheter—flexible tube passed through body channels to allow for the drainage or withdrawal of fluids.

Cephalic (ce-FAL-ik)—refers to the head.

Cerebrospinal (ser-e-bro-SPI-nal) **Fluid**—clear watery fluid that helps to protect the brain and spinal cord.

Cervebrovascular Accident (CVA)—a stroke. The rupturing or blockage of a major blood vessel supplying or draining the brain.

Cervical (SER-ve-kal)—relating to the neck or to the inferior end of the uterus.

Cervix (SER-vicks)—inferior portion of the uterus, where it enters the vagina.

Chronic—opposite of acute. It can be used to mean long and drawn out or recurring.

Chronic Heart Failure—*see* Congestive Heart Failure.

Chronic Obstructive Pulmonary Disease (COPD)—group of diseases and conditions in which the lungs decline in their ability to exchange gases. COPD includes emphysema, chronic bronchitis, and miner's black lung.

Clavicle (KLAV-i-kul)—collarbone.

Clinical Death—state when breathing and heart action cease.

Clonic Phase—second phase of a convulsive seizure, with the patient exhibiting violent body jerks, drooling, and possibly cyanosis. Most convulsions last 1 to 2 minutes.

Closed Fracture—simple fracture where the skin is not broken by the fractured bones.

Closed Wound—injury where the skin is not broken, as in the case of a contusion.

Clot—formation of fibrin and entangled blood cells that act to stop bleeding from a wound.

Coccyx (KOK-siks)—lowermost bones of the vertebral column. They are fused into one bone in the adult.

Collarbone—clavicle.

Coma—state of complete unconsciousness.

Comminuted (KOM-i-nu-ted) **Fracture**—fracture where the bone is fragmented or turned to powder.

Concussion—mild state of stupor or temporary unconsciousness caused by a blow to the head. There is no laceration or bleeding in the brain.

Congestive Heart Failure—associated with lung conditions and diseases (e.g.: COPD), or heart disease. Excessive fluid build-up occurs in the lungs and/or body organs. The heart fails in its efforts to properly circulate blood and the lungs fail in their effort to properly exchange gases.

Constricting Band—used to restrict the flow of venom.

Contraindicated—condition, sign, or symptom that makes a particular course of treatment or procedure inadvisable.

Contusion (kun-TU-zhun)—bruise. The simplest form of closed wound where blood flows between tissues causing a discoloration.

Convulsion—uncontrolled muscle spasm, often violent.

COPD—chronic obstructive pulmonary disease.

Core Temperature—body temperature measured at a central point, such as within the rectum.

Cornea (KOR-ne-ah)—transparent covering over the iris and pupil of the eye.

Coronary (KOR-o-nar-e)—refers to the blood vessels that supply blood to the heart muscle. Many people use this term to mean heart attack.

CPR—cardiopulmonary resuscitation.

CPR Compression Site—mid-sternal point approximately two finger-widths superior to the xiphoid process. During CPR of adults, compressions are delivered to this site. In infants and children, this site is along the midline of the breastbone, between the nipples.

Cranial (KRAY-ne-al)—pertaining to the braincase of the skull.

Cranium (KRAY-ne-um)—braincase of the skull. Many people use the term skull when they mean cranium.

Crepitus (KREP-i-tus)—grating noise or the sensation felt caused by the movement of broken bone ends rubbing together.

Crowing—atypical sound made when a patient breathes. It usually indicates airway obstruction.

Crowning—when the presenting part of the baby first bulges out of the vagina opening. It is usually in reference to a normal head first delivery.

Cryotherapy—to treat with cold.

Cut—an open wound with smooth edges (incision) or jagged edges (laceration).

Cyanosis (sigh-ah-NO-sis)—when the skin color changes to blue or gray because of too little oxygen in the blood.

Danger Zone—at the scene of an accident, a circle with a 50-foot radius with the wreckage at the center of the circle. Special danger zones must be formed if the accident involves downed electrical wires, gas leaks, hazardous materials, fire, possible explosions, or radiation.

Debridement—surgical removal of dead, injured, or infected tissue from around a wound or a burn.

Deep Frostbite—*see* Freezing.

Diabetes (di-ah-BE-teez)—disease caused by the inadequate production of insulin.

Diabetic Coma—result of an inadequate insulin supply that leads to unconsciousness, coma, and eventually death unless treated.

Diaphoresis (DI-ah-fo-RE-sis)—profuse perspiration. The patient is said to be diaphoretic (DI-ah-fo-RET-ik).

Diaphragm (DI-ah-fram)—dome-shaped muscle that separates the thoracic cavity from the abdominopelvic cavity. It is the major muscle of respiration.

Diaphramatic Breathing—weak and rapid respirations with little movement of the chest wall and slight movement of the abdomen. An attempt to breathe with the diaphragm alone.

Diastolic (di-as-TOL-ik) **Pressure**—pressure exerted on the internal walls of the arteries when the heart is relaxing.

Dilation—to enlarge, expanding in diameter.

Disinfect—to destroy harmful microorganisms, but not necessarily their resistant spores.

Dislocation—displacement (pulling out) of a bone end that forms part of a joint.

Distal—away from a point of reference, such as the shoulder or the hip joint. More distant to.

Distended—inflated, swollen, or stretched.

Dressing—protective covering for a wound that will aid in the stoppage of bleeding and help to prevent contamination.

Duodenum (du-o-DE-num or du-OD-e-num)—first portion of the small intestine, connected to the stomach. More rigid than the other portions, causing it to receive greater injury in accidents.

Dyspnea (disp-NE-ah)—difficult or labored breathing.

Ecchymosis (EK-i-MO-sis)—discoloration of the skin because of internal bleeding. A "black and blue" mark.

Eclampsia (e-KLAM-se-ah)—convulsive state during pregnancy due to toxemia.

-ectomy (EK-toe-me)—word ending meaning surgical removal.

Edema (e-DE-mah)—swelling due to the accumulation of fluids in the tissues.

Embolism (EM-bo-liz-m)—movement and the lodgement of a blood clot or foreign body (fat or air bubble) inside a blood vessel. The foreign body is called an embolus (EM-bo-lus).

Emergency Medical Services System—EMS System. A chain of services linked together to provide care for the patient at the scene, during transport to the hospital, and upon entry at the hospital.

Emergency Medical Technician (EMT)—professional-level provider of emergency care. This individual has received formal training and is state certified.

Emesis—vomiting.

Emphysema (EM-fi-SEE-mah)—chronic disease where the lungs progressively lose their elasticity. *See* Chronic Obstructive Pulmonary Disease.

Epiglottis (EP-i-GLOT-is)—flap of cartilage and other tissues that is the superior structure of the larynx. It closes off the airway and diverts solids and liquids down the esophagus.

Epilepsy (EP-i-lep-see)—medical disorder characterized by attacks of unconsciousness, with or without convulsions.

Epistaxis (ep-e-STAK-sis)—nosebleed.

Esophageal Obturator Airway (EOA)—breathing tube inserted into the esophagus. The vents in the tube are positioned at the opening into the larynx.

Esophagus (e-SOF-ah-gus)—muscular tube leading from the pharynx to the stomach.

Eviscerate (e-VIS-er-ate)—usually applies to the intestine protruding through an incision or wound.

Expiration—breathing out. To exhale.

Extension—act of straightening.

Extrication—any actions that disentangle and free from entrapment.

Extruded—when an organ, bone, or vessel is pushed out of position.

Fainting—simple form of shock, occurring when the patient has a temporary, self-correcting, loss of consciousness caused by a reduced supply of blood to the brain. Also called psychogenic (SI-ko-JEN-ic) shock.

False Motion—movement of an extremity where there should be no motion, such as at the point of a fracture.

Febrile—feverish.

Femoral (FEM-o-ral) **Artery**—main artery of the thigh. A major pulse location and pressure point site.

Femur (FE-mer)—thigh bone.

Fetus (FE-tus)—developing unborn. It is an embryo until the third month, when it becomes a fetus until birth.

Fibrillation—uncoordinated contractions of the myocardium resulting from independent individual muscle fiber activity.

Fibrin (FI-brin)—fibrous protein material formed and utilized to produce a blood clot.

Fibula (FIB-yo-lah)—lateral leg bone.

First Degree Burn—mild partial thickness burn, only involving the outer layer of skin.

First Responder—individual who has received training in emergency care in order to provide for the patient before EMTs arrive.

Flail Chest—condition where the ribs and/or the sternum are fractured in such a way as to produce a loose section of the chest wall that will not move with the rest of the wall during breathing.

Flexion—bending. To lessen the angle of a joint.

Fracture—break, crack, split, or crumbling of a bone.

Freezing—deep frostbite. An injury due to cold involving the skin and subcutaneous layers. Deep structures such as bone and muscle can be involved.

Frostbite—*see* superficial frostbite.

Frostnip—incipient frostbite. Minor injury to the epidermis caused by exposure to cold.

Gallbladder—organ that attaches to the lower back of the liver. It stores bile.

Gastro- (GAS-tro)—used as a beginning of words in reference to the stomach.

Genitalia (jen-i-TA-le-ah)—external reproductive organs.

Good Samaritan Laws—series of laws written to protect emergency care personnel. These laws require a standard of care to be provided in good faith, to the level of training, and to the best of ability.

Grand Mal—severe epileptic seizure.

Greenstick Fracture—split along the length of a bone, giving the appearance of a green stick bent to its breaking point.

Gurgling—atypical sound of breathing made by patients having airway obstruction, lung disease, or lung injury due to heat.

Handoff—orderly transfer of the patient, patient information, and patient valuables to more highly trained personnel.

Hare Traction Splint—lower extremity splint that will apply a set amount of tension along the long axis of a lower extremity. This tension is limited by the windlass mechanism.

Heart Attack—usually the sudden blockage of a coronary vessel that can cause death to the heart muscle.

Heat Cramps—condition brought about by loss of body salts. Usually occurs in people working in hot environments. Muscle cramps occur in the lower extremities and abdomen.

Heat Exhaustion—condition where blood pools in the vessels of the skin. This is an attempt by the body to give off excessive heat. It causes an inadequate return of blood to the heart that can lead to collapse.

Heatstroke—true emergency caused by a failure of the body's heat-regulating mechanisms. The patient cannot cool his overheated body.

Heimlich Maneuver—*see* Manual Thrusts.

Hematemesis (HEM-ah-TEM-e-sis)—vomiting bright red blood.

Hematoma (hem-ah-TO-mah)—collection of blood under the skin or in the tissues as a result of an injured or broken blood vessel. Sometimes referred to as a "blood tumor."

Hematuria (HEM-ah-TU-ri-ah)—passing blood in the urine.

Hemorrhage (HEM-o-rej)—internal or external bleeding.

Hemorrhagic (HEM-o-RIJ-ic) **Shock**—*see* Hypovolemic Shock.

Hemothorax (he-mo-THO-raks)—condition of blood and bloody fluids in the area between the lungs and the walls of the chest cavity.

Hip—joint made between the pelvis and the femur.

Hives—slightly elevated red or pale areas of skin that often itch. Hives are transient, and often a reaction to certain foods, drugs, infection, or stress.

Humerus (HU-mer-us)—arm bone.

Hydroplaning—when a film of water develops between a vehicle's tires and the road surface so that the vehicle is riding in an uncontrolled fashion upon the water.

Hyperextension—overextension of a limb or body part.

Hyperglycemia (hi-per-gli-SEE-me-ah)—excess of sugar in the blood.

Hyperthermia—greatly increased body temperature.

Hyperventilation—increased rate and depth of breathing.

Hypoglycemia (hi-po-gli-SEE-me-ah)—too little sugar in the blood.

Hypothermia—general cooling of the body.

Hypovolemic Shock—state of shock brought about by an excessive loss of whole blood or plasma.

Hypoxia (hi-POK-se-ah)—inadequate supply of oxygen to the body tissues.

Implied Consent legal position that assumes an unconscious patient, or one so badly injured or ill that he cannot respond, would consent to receiving emergency care. Implied consent applies to children when parents or guardians are not at the scene.

Incipient Frostbite—*see* Frostnip.

Incision—*see* Cut.

Infarction—localized death of tissue resulting from the discontinuation of its blood supply.

Inferior—away from the top of the body. Usually compared with another structure which is closer to the top (superior).

Inflammation—pain, heat, redness, and swelling of tissues as they react to infection, irritation, or injury.

Informed Consent—actual consent given after the patient knows your level of training and what you are going to do.

Inspiration—breathe in, inhale.

Insulin (IN-su-lin)—hormone produced in the pancreas that is needed to move sugar from the blood into cells.

Insulin Shock—state of shock from too much insulin in the blood causing low sugar levels for the brain and nervous system. The high level of insulin can be due to overdose or from too low of a sugar intake (hypoglycemia).

Interposed Ventilation—artificial ventilations provided during CPR.

Intravenous (IV)—into a vein.

-itis (I-tis)—word ending used to mean inflammation.

Jaundice—yellowing of the skin, usually associated with liver or bile apparatus injury or disease.

Jaw-Thrust—method of opening the airway without lifting the neck or tilting the head.

Jugular Veins—large veins in the neck that drain blood from the head.

Ketoacidosis (KE-to-as-i-DO-sis)—when a diabetic's body breaks down too many fats trying to obtain energy, ketone bodies build in the blood and the blood becomes acid.

Kidneys—excretory organs located high in the back of the abdominal region. They are behind the abdominal cavity.

Labor—three stages of childbirth, including the beginning of contractions, delivery of the child, and delivery of the afterbirth (placenta, umbilical cord and some tissues of the lining of the uterus).

Laceration—jagged-edged open wound. *See* Cut.

Lacrimal (LAK-ri-mal) **Gland**—tear gland.

Laryngeal Edema—fluids invading the tissues of the larynx causing swelling.

Laryngectomy (lar-in-JEK-toe-me)—total or partial removal of the larynx. The patient is called a neck breather or a laryngectomee.

Larynx (LAR-inks)—airway situated between the pharynx and the trachea. The voice box.

Lateral—to the side, away from the midline of the body.

Ligament—fibrous tissue that connects bone to bone.

Liver—largest gland in the body, having many functions. Located in the upper right abdominal region, extending over to the central abdominal region.

Lumbar Spine—vertebrae of the lower back, consisting of 5 bones.

Manual Thrusts—abdominal or chest thrusts provided to expel an object causing an airway obstruction.

MAST—medical anti-shock trousers (garment).

Mechanical Pump Failure—inability of the heart to function properly due to damaged myocardial tissue.

Medial—toward the vertical midline of the body.

Mediastinum (me-de-as-TI-num or me-de-ah-STI-num)—central portion of the chest cavity (thoracic cavity) containing the heart, its greater vessels, part of the esophagus, and part of the trachea.

Medical Practices Act—laws requiring an individual to be licensed or certified in order to practice medicine or to provide certain levels of care.

Meninges (me-NIN-jez)—three membranes surrounding the brain and spinal cord.

Metabolic Shock—state of shock due to a loss of body fluids (dehydration) and a change in body chemistry.

Metacarpals (meta-KAR-pals)—hand bones.

Metatarsals (meta-TAR-sals)—foot bones.

Myocardium (mi-o-KAR-de-um)—heart muscle.

Neurogenic Shock—caused when the nervous system fails to control the diameter of the blood vessels. The vessels remain widely dilated, providing too great a volume to be filled by available blood.

Occlusion—blockage of an artery.

Occlusive Dressing—covering a wound and forming an airtight seal.

Open Fracture—when a bone is broken and bone ends or fragments cut through the skin. Listed in older references as a compound fracture.

Open Wound—when the skin is broken.

Oropharyngeal (or-o-fah-RIN-jee-al) **Airway**—curved breathing tube inserted into the patient's mouth. It will hold the base of the tongue forward.

Packaging—part of the procedure of preparation for removal in an accident. It can involve applying splints, dressings, and stabilizing impaled objects.

Pancreas (PAN-cre-as)—gland in the back of the upper portion of the abdominal cavity, behind the stomach. It produces insulin and digestive juices.

Paradoxical Respiration—associated with flail chest, where a loose segment of chest wall moves in the opposite direction to the rest of the chest during respiratory movements.

Paralysis—complete or partial loss of the ability to move a body part. Sensation in the area may also be lost.

Patella (pah-TEL-lah)—kneecap.

Pedal Pulse—foot pulse.

Penetrating Wound—puncture wound with only an entrance wound.

Perforating Wound—puncture wound with an entrance and an exit wound.

Pericardium (per-e-KAR-de-um)—sac that surrounds the heart.

Perineum (per-i-NE-um)—region of the body located between the genitalia and the anus.

Peritoneum (per-i-toe-NE-um)—membrane that lines the abdominal cavity.

Petit Mal—minor epileptic attack noted by a momentary loss of awareness.

Phalanges (fah-LAN-jez)—bones of the toes and fingers.

Pharynx (FAR-inks)—throat.

Placenta (plah-SEN-tah)—organ made of both maternal and fetal tissues to allow for exchange between the circulatory systems of the mother and fetus without having a mixing of blood.

Plasma (PLAZ-mah)—fluid portion of the blood. It is blood minus blood cells and other structures (formed elements).

Platelet (PLATE-let)—formed elements of the blood that release factors needed to form blood clots.

Pleura (PLOOR-ah)—double-membrane sac. The outer layer lines the chest wall and the inner layer covers the outside of the lungs.

Pneumothorax (NU-mo-THO-raks)—collection of air in the chest cavity to the outside of the lungs, caused by punctures to the chest wall or the lungs.

Posterior—back.

Postictal (post-IK-tal)—third phase of a convulsive seizure. Convulsions stop and the patient may be drowsy or remain unconscious for hours.

Priapism (PRE-ah-pizm)—persistent erection of the penis associated with spinal damage.

Primary Survey—first examination of a patient to detect life-threatening problems dealing with breathing, heartbeat, and profuse bleeding.

Prolapsed Cord—abnormal delivery where the umbilical cord is presented first.

Prone—lying face down.

Proximal—close to a point of reference such as the shoulder or hip joint. Used with distal, meaning away from.

Psychogenic Shock (SI-ko-JEN-ic)—*see* Fainting.

Pulmonary (PUL-mo-ner-e)—refers to the lungs.

Pulmonary Circulation—circuit of blood traveling from the right ventricle of the heart to the lungs and returning to the left atrium.

Pulse—alternate expansion and contraction of arterial walls as the heart pumps blood.

Puncture Wound—open wound tearing through the skin and destroying tissue in a straight line. *See* Penetrating Wound and Perforating Wound.

Radial Pulse—wrist pulse.

Radius—lateral forearm bone.

Rales (rahlz)—abnormal sound produced in the lungs as air moves through fluids in the bronchiole tree. The sound is like that made when you rub the hair near your ears.

Rectum (REK-tum)—lower portion of the large intestine ending with the anus.

Referred Pain—pain felt in a part of the body other than where the source or cause of the pain is located. For example, an inflammed gallbladder may have referred pain over the right scapula.

Respiratory Shock—state of shock caused by too little oxygen in the blood. Usually due to lung failure, where the patient is unable to adequately fill the lungs.

Resuscitation (re-SUS-ci-TA-shun)—any effort to restore or provide normal heart and/or lung function.

Rhonchi (RONG-ki)—coarse loud rales resulting from a partial obstruction of the bronchi or bronchioles.

Sacrum—fused vertebrae of the lower back, inferior to the lumbar spine.

Sanitize—rigid standard of cleaning, often to the point of practical sterilization.

Scapula (SKAP-u-lah)—shoulder blade.

Scratch—abrasion (ab-RAY-shun). An open wound that damages the surface of skin without breaking all the skin layers.

Secondary Survey—patient interview and the physical examination performed after the primary survey.

Second Degree Burn—partial thickness burn where the epidermis is burned through and the dermis is damaged.

Septic Shock—form of shock caused by severe infection. Toxins from the infection cause the blood vessels to dilate and plasma to be lost through vessel walls.

Shock—failure of the circulatory system to provide an adequate blood supply to all parts of the body.

Shoulder Dystocia (dis-TO-she-ah)—when a delivering baby with large shoulders wedges between its mother's sacrum and pubic bones.

Sign—any observed evidence of injury or illness.

Spleen—organ located to the left of the upper abdominal cavity, behind the stomach. It stores blood and destroys old blood cells.

Sphygmomanometer (SFIG-mo-mah-NOM-e-ter)—instrument used to measure blood pressure.

Splint—any device that will immobilize a fracture.

Sprain—injury in which ligaments are partially torn.

Sterile—free of all life forms.

Sternum (STER-num)—breastbone.

Stethoscope—instrument used to amplify body sounds.

Stoma (STO-mah)—opening in the neck of a neck breather.

Strain—injury to muscles caused by overexertion.

Subcutaneous (SUB-ku-TA-ne-us)—beneath the skin. Usually refers to the fatty and connective tissue layer found beneath the dermis.

Superficial Frostbite—injury due to cold involving the skin and the subcutaneous layers. The upper layers are frozen, but some elasticity remains in the tissues below the skin.

Superior—toward the top of the body. Often used in reference with inferior, meaning away from the top of the body.

Supine—lying flat on the back.

Symptom—evidence of injury or illness told to you by the patient.

Systemic (sis-TEM-ik)—refers to the entire body.

Systemic Hypothermia—generalized cooling of the body.

Systolic (sis-TOL-ik) **Blood Pressure**—force exerted by the blood on the artery walls when the heart is contracting.

Tachycardia (tak-e-KAR-de-ah)—rapid heartbeat, usually 120 or more beats per minute.

Tarsals (TAR-sals)—ankle bones.

Tendon—fibrous tissue that connects muscle to bone.

Thigh Bone—femur (FE-mur).

Third Degree Burn—full thickness burn, where all layers of the skin are damaged. Deep structures may also be burned.

Thoracic (tho-RAS-ik) **Cavity**—anterior body cavity above the diaphragm. It protects the heart and lungs.

Thorax (THO-raks)—chest.

Thrombosis (throm-BO-sis)—formation of a blood clot in a blood vessel or within a chamber of the heart.

Tibia (TIB-e-ah)—medial lower leg bone.

Tonic Phase—first stage of a convulsive seizure where the patient's body can become rigid for up to 30 seconds per episode.

Tourniquet—last resort used to control bleeding. A band or belt is used to constrict blood vessels to stop the flow of blood.

Trachea (TRA-ke-ah)—windpipe.

—part of the action taken to stabilize a broken bone to prevent any additional injury.

Trauma—injury caused by violence, shock, or pressure.

Traumatic Asphyxia—condition that arises from a broken sternum and ribs forcing blood out of the right side of the heart into the veins of the neck.

Triage—method of sorting patients according to the severity of their injuries.

Ulna (UL-nah)—medial forearm bone.

Umbilical (um-BIL-i-kal) **Cord**—structure that connects the body of the fetus to the placenta.

Umbilicus (um-BIL-i-kus)—navel.

Uterus (U-ter-us)—muscular structure in which the fetus develops. The womb.

Vagina (vah-JI-nah)—canal leading from the vulva to the cervix. The birth canal.

Vein—any blood vessel that returns blood to the heart.

Ventilation—supplying air to the lungs.

Ventral—front of the body or body part. *See* Anterior.

Ventricle—inferior chamber of the heart. Ventricles pump blood from the heart.

Vertebra (VER-te-brah)—bone of the spinal column.

Viscera (VIS-er-ah)—internal organs. Usually refers to the abdominal organs.

Vital Signs—in basic EMT-level care, pulse rate and character, breathing rate and character, blood pressure, and relative skin temperature.

Vitreous Fluid—transparent jelly-like substance filling the posterior cavity of the eye.

Vulva (VUL-vah)—external female genitalia.

Wheal—localized accumulation of fluid under the skin that may be accompanied by itching. A hive.

Wheeze—whistling respiratory sound. It can be caused in asthma when air is trapped in the alveoli and cannot be expired easily.

Womb—*See* Uterus.

Xiphoid (ZI-foyd)—inferior process of the sternum.

Zygomatic (zi-go-MAT-ik) **Bone**—cheek bone. Also called the malar (MA-lar).

bibliography

READINGS

The EMT-A Training Course

American Academy of Orthopaedic Surgeons, Committee on Allied Health: **Emergency Care and Transportation of the Sick and Injured.** 3rd ed. American Academy of Orthopaedic Surgeons, Chicago, 1981

Bergeron JD: **Self-Instructional Workbook for Emergency Care.** 3rd ed. Robert J. Brady Co., Bowie, MD, 1982

U.S. Department of Transportation: Emergency Medical Technician-A: Basic Training Program. Pamphlet no. HS 802 628. National Highway Traffic Safety Administration, Washington, DC, 1977

——: **Emergency Medical Technician-A: Basic Training Program: Course Guide,** 2nd ed. (050-003-00276-3), **Instructor Lesson Plans,** 2nd ed. (050-003-00277-1), **Student Study Guide,** 2nd ed. (050-003-00278-0). Government Printing Office, Washington, DC, 1977

The EMT and the EMS System

American Medical Association: Developing Emergency Medical Services: Guideline for Community Councils. Pub. no. OP-386. American Medical Association, Chicago

Bergeron JD: **First Responder.** Robert J. Brady Co., Bowie, MD, 1982

Farrington JD: Ambulance service. The EMT Journal Vol 1, No 1, p 37–39, March, 1977

Hampton OP: Categorization of hospital emergency capabilities. The EMT Journal Vol 1, No 1, p 47–49, March, 1977

Hanlon J: Emergency Medical Care as a Comprehensive System. Reprinted by the U.S. Department of Health and Human Services. Pub. no. HSA-742026. Government Printing Office, Washington, DC 1973

U.S. Department of Transportation: **Coordination in Developing an Effective Rural Emergency Medical Services Program.** National Highway Traffic Safety Administration, Washington, DC, 1977

——: **Emergency Medical Services: First Responder Training Course. Course Guide** (050-003-00360-3), **Instructor's Lesson Plans** (050-003-00361-1), **Student Study Guide** (050-003-00362-1). Government Printing Office, Washington, DC, 1979

——: **Emergency Medical Services: Instructor Training Course. Course Guide** (050-003-00351-4). Government Printing Office, Washington, DC, 1977

——: **Emergency Medical Technician: Refresher Training Program. Course Guide** (050-003-00363-8). Government Printing Office, Washington, DC, 1979

——: **Emergency Medical Technician-P: National Training Course. Course Guide** (050-003-00279-8). Government Printing Office, Washington, DC

Wiegenstein JG: Relationship of EMTs with Emergency Departments. The EMT Journal Vol 1, No 1, p 52, March, 1977

Anatomy, Physiology, and Medical Terminology

American Medical Association: **The Wonderful Human Machine.** American Medical Association, Chicago, 1967

Anthony CP, Kolthoff NJ: **Textbook of Anatomy and Physiology.** 9th ed. The C.V. Mosby Co., Saint Louis, Mo., 1975

The Robert J. Brady Company: **Brady's Programmed Orientation to Medical Terminology.** 2nd ed. Robert J. Brady Co., Bowie, MD, 1983

The Charles Press: **The Charles Press Handbook of Current Medical Abbreviations.** The Charles Press Publishers, Inc., Bowie, MD, 1976

Patient Assessment

Julihn: Patient Assessment. Journal of Emergency Medical Services, pp 44–46, March, 1980

Walraven G, et al: **Manual of Advanced Prehospital Care.** Robert J. Brady Co., Bowie, MD, 1978

Basic Life Support

American Heart Association: Standards and Guidelines for Cardiopulmonary Resuscitation (CPR) and Emergency Cardiac Care (ECC). Journal of the American Medical Association, Vol 244, No 5, pp 453–509, August, 1980 (Available as a supplement from the AHA.)

Geelhoed GW: Shock and its management. Emergency Medical Services, pp 42–49, November–December, 1976

Goldberg AH: Adjuncts for Airway and Breathing

(Ventilation). The EMT Journal, Vol 1, No 2, pp 31–36, June, 1977

International Association of Laryngectomees: **Neck Breathers' First Aid.** American Cancer Society, New York, 1971

National Academy of Sciences, Committee on EMS: Emergency management of the obstructed Airway. Journal of the American Medical Association, Vol 243, pp 1141–1142, March, 1980

National Research Council: Emergency airway management: respiratory assistance in upper airway Emergencies. The EMT Journal, Vol 1, No 2, pp 37–39, June, 1977

Phillips C: **Basic Life Support Manual.** 2nd ed. Robert J. Brady Co., Bowie, MD, 1982

Wilson RF: Management of shock. The EMT Journal, Vol 1, No 1, pp 52–53, March, 1977

Injuries

American College of Surgeons: A guide to the initial therapy of soft tissue wounds. Bulletin of the American College of Surgeons, September, 1977

Anast GT: Fractures and injuries of the cervical spine. The EMT Journal, Vol 2, No 3, pp 36–39, September, 1978

Barber JM: EMT Checkpoint: Spinal Cord Injury and Neurogenic Shock. The EMT Journal, Vol 2, No 3, pp 69–73, September, 1978

Browner BD, et al: The emergency treatment of musculoskeletal injuries, part I: the axial system. Emergency Medical Services, pp. 26–38, November–December, 1981

——: The emergency treatment of musculoskeletal injuries, part II: the appendicular system. Emergency Medical Services, pp. 10–28, March–April, 1982

Darin JC: The diagnosis and treatment of chest injuries. The EMT Journal, Vol 2, No 2, pp 52–56, June, 1978

Martina K: Management of joint fractures. The EMT Journal, Vol 3, No 4, pp 46–48, December, 1979

Rimel R, et al: Prehospital treatment of patient with spinal cord injuries. The EMT Journal, Vol 3, No 4, pp 49–54, December, 1979

Soll DB: A guide to emergency care of eye injuries. Bulletin of the American College of Surgeons, November, 1976

Medical Emergencies

Barber JM: EMT checkpoint: seizures. The EMT Journal, Vol 2, No 1, pp 75–79, March, 1978

Waldhour H: Management of the epileptic patient. The EMT Journal, Vol 2, No 1, pp 71–72, March, 1978

Werner C, Peace JS: The vial of life. The EMT Journal, Vol 2, No 3, pp 66–68, September, 1978

White RD: Part I: heart attack and emergency cardiac care. The EMT Journal, Vol 1, No 4, pp 42–45, December, 1977

White RD: Part II: components of basic and advanced cardiac life support. The EMT Journal, Vol 1, No 4, pp 46–50, December, 1977

Childbirth and Pediatrics

American Academy of Pediatrics, Committee on Disaster and Emergency Care: **Disaster and Emergency Medical Services for Infants and Children.** 2nd ed. American Academy of Pediatrics, Evanston, IL, 1975

Barber JM: EMT checkpoint: tips on assessment and management of pediatric trauma. The EMT Journal, Vol 4, No 1, pp 66–71, March, 1980

Barber JM: EMT checkpoint: Pediatric emergencies. The EMT Journal, Vol 4, No 4, pp 70–74, June, 1980

Hervada AR: Charting a pediatric head injury. Emergency Medicine, p. 143, September, 1976

National Institutes of Health: **Facts About Sudden Infant Death Syndrome.** Pub. no. 72-225. U.S. Department of Health and Human Services, Washington, DC

Wojslawowicz, JM: Emergency childbirth for emergency medical technicians. The EMT Journal, Vol 1, No 4, pp 66–67, December, 1977

Environmental Emergencies

American College of Surgeons: Assessment and initial care of burn patients. Bulletin of the American College of Surgeons, October, 1979

Edlich RF et al: Prehospital treatment of the burn patient. The EMT Journal, Vol 2, No 3, pp 42–48, September, 1978

Elliot DH et al: Acute decompression sickness. Lancet Vol 2, p 1193, 1974

Gray J: Prevention of heat injuries during distance running: a position statement from the american college of sports medicine. Journal of Sports Medicine, Vol 3, p 194, 1975

Myers E: **Chemistry of Hazardous Materials.** Prentice-Hall, Inc., Englewood Cliffs, NJ, 1977

U.S. Department of Transportation: **Hazardous Materials, The Emergency Response Handbook.** Pub.

no. DOT P 5800.2. Materials Transportation Bureau, Washington, DC, 1980

—: **Hypothermia and Cold Water Survival.** U.S. Coast Guard, Washington, DC

Whitcraft III DD, Karas S: Air embolism and decompression sickness in scuba divers. Journal of the American College of Emergency Physicians, Vol 5, p 355, 1976

Young RS et al: Neurological outcome in cold water drowning. Journal of the American Medical Association, Vol 244, pp 1233–1235, September, 1980

Special Patients and Situations

Burgess AW, Holmstrom LL: **Rape: Crisis and Recovery.** Robert J. Brady Co., Bowie, MD, 1979

Cryer L, Mattox K: Crisis management: The EMT and the sexual assault victim. The EMT Journal, Vol 3, No 4, pp 42–45, December, 1979

Hom MA: Disaster preparedness for medical emergencies. The EMT Journal, Vol 3, No 3, pp 53–58, September, 1979

Mitchell J, Resnik HL: **Emergency Response to Crisis.** Robert J. Brady Co., Bowie, MD, 1981

Motley RE: Disaster plans: the EMT as the vital link. The EMT Journal, Vol 1, No 1, pp 58–59, March, 1977

Warner C: **Conflict Intervention in Social/Domestic Violence.** Robert J. Brady Co., Bowie, MD, 1981

Preparation and Response

Clark JK Jr: **Emergency and High Speed Driving Techniques.** Gulf Publishing Co., Houston, 1976

General Services Administration–Federal Supply Service: **Federal Specifications (Revised) for the "Start of Life Ambulance."** Pub. no. KKK-A-1822-A. General services Administration, Washington, DC, April, 1982

Missouri Safety Center: **Instructors' Manual: Advanced Driver Education for Emergency Vehicle Operators.** Missouri Safety Center, Missouri State University, 1978

National Safety Council: **Driver Improvement Defensive Driving Course.** National Safety Council, Chicago, 1975

U.S. Department of Transportation: **Operation of Emergency Vehicles: Training Program. Course Guide** (050-003-00330-1), **Instructors Guide** (050-003-00332-8), **Study Guide** (050-003-00331-0). Government Printing Office, Washington, DC, 1979

Extrication and Rescue

Bruley ME: Guidelines for the selection and use of orthopedic (scoop) litters. The EMT Journal, Vol 2, No 2, pp 76–80, June, 1978

Conrad MB: Principles of extrication. The EMT Journal, Vol 3, No 4, pp 48–51, December, 1978

Folsom F: **Extrication and Casuality Handling Techniques.** J.B. Lippincott Co., Philadelphia, 1975

Grant HD: **Vehicle Rescue.** 2nd ed. Robert J. Brady Co., Bowie, MD, 1981

Gargan JB: **Trench Rescue.** Robert J. Brady Company, Bowie, MD, 1982

Hatfield L: Fundamentals of extrication. The EMT Journal, Vol 3, No 3, pp 42–44, September, 1979

MEDI-KED: How to Immobilize and Extricate with KED. MEDI-KED, Inc., El Cajon, CA, 1982

National Transportation Safety Board: Anatomy of an accident. The EMT Journal, Vol 3, No 3, pp 26–35, September, 1979

U.S. Department of Transportation: **Emergency Medical Technician: Crash Victim Extrication Training Course. Instructors Manual** (050-003-00343-3), **Student Manual** (050-003-00344-1). Government Printing Office, Washington, DC, 1979

—: **Emergency Medical Technician: Patient Handling Manual.** Pub. no. 050-003-00051-5. Government Printing Office, Washington, DC, 1979

Communications and Records

Boyd DR: Recordkeeping. The EMT Journal, Vol 1, No 1, pp 54–56, March, 1977

Gerold KB: Guidelines for reporting medical information to the resource hospital (a basic life support approach). The EMT Journal, Vol 3, No 3, pp 50–52, September, 1979

Kimball KF: Communications. The EMT Journal, Vol 1, No 1, pp 50–51, March, 1977

U.S. Department of Transportation: **Emergency Medical Technician: Dispatcher Training Course. Course Guide** (050-003-00239-9), **Instructors' Lesson Plans** (050-003-00237-2), **Student Study Guide** (050-003-00238-1). Government Printing Office, Washington, DC, 1977

Intermediate and Advanced Life Support

American College of Surgeons: Pneumatic counterpressure devices. Bulletin of the American College of Surgeons, February, 1980

American Heart Association: Standards and guidelines for cardiopulmonary resuscitation (CPR) and emergency cardiac care (ECC). Journal of the American Medical Association, Vol 244, No 5, pp 479–504, August, 1980 (Available as a supplement from the AHA.)

Huszar RJ: **Emergency Cardiac Care.** 2nd ed. Robert J. Brady Company, Bowie, MD, 1982

Philips C: **Paramedic Skills Manual.** Robert J. Brady Co., Bowie, MD, 1980

Walraven G: **Basic Arrhythmias.** Robert J. Brady Company, Bowie, MD, 1980

AUDIOVISUAL AIDS

Emergency Care, A Multimedia Approach. 3d ed. The Robert J. Brady Company, Bowie, MD, 1982

Emergency Childbirth. U.S. Department of Transportation, National Audiovisual Center, Washington, DC

New Pulse of Life/Revised. Pyramid Films. Available from the AHA.

index

Page numbers followed by the letter f indicate illustrations, those followed by the letter t indicate tables.